The Foot in Diabetes

Fourth Edition

Other titles in the Wiley Diabetes in Practice Series

The Foot in Diabetes

Fourth Edition

Edited by

Andrew J.M. Boulton
Manchester Royal Infirmary, Manchester, UK
Diabetes Research Unit
University of Miami, Florida, USA

Peter R. Cavanagh
The Cleveland Clinic Foundation
Cleveland, Ohio, USA

Gerry Rayman
Ipswich Hospital, Suffolk, UK

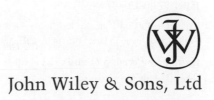

John Wiley & Sons, Ltd

Copyright © 2006 John Wiley & Sons Ltd,

        The Atrium, Southern Gate, Chichester,

        West Sussex PO19 8SQ, England

        Telephone   (+44) 1243 779777

Email (for orders and customer service enquiries): cs-books@wiley.co.uk

Visit our Home Page on www.wileyeurope.com or www.wiley.com

Reprinted April 2007, March and August 2008

All Rights Reserved. No part of this publication may be reproduced, stored in a retrieval system or transmitted in any form or by any means, electronic, mechanical, photocopying, recording, scanning or otherwise, except under the terms of the Copyright, Designs and Patents Act 1988 or under the terms of a licence issued by the Copyright Licensing Agency Ltd, 90 Tottenham Court Road, London W1T 4LP, UK, without the permission in writing of the Publisher. Requests to the Publisher should be addressed to the Permissions Department, John Wiley & Sons Ltd, The Atrium, Southern Gate, Chichester, West Sussex PO19 8SQ, England, or emailed to permreq@wiley.co.uk, or faxed to (+44) 1243 770620.

Designations used by companies to distinguish their products are often claimed as trademarks. All brand names and product names used in this book are trade names, service marks, trademarks or registered trademarks of their respective owners. The Publisher is not associated with any product or vendor mentioned in this book.

This publication is designed to provide accurate and authoritative information in regard to the subject matter covered. It is sold on the understanding that the Publisher is not engaged in rendering professional services. If professional advice or other expert assistance is required, the services of a competent professional should be sought.

Other Wiley Editorial Offices

John Wiley & Sons Inc., 111 River Street, Hoboken, NJ 07030, USA

Jossey-Bass, 989 Market Street, San Francisco, CA 94103-1741, USA

Wiley-VCH Verlag GmbH, Boschstr. 12, D-69469 Weinheim, Germany

John Wiley & Sons Australia Ltd, 33 Park Road, Milton, Queensland 4064, Australia

John Wiley & Sons (Asia) Pte Ltd, 2 Clementi Loop #02-01, Jin Xing Distripark, Singapore 129809

John Wiley & Sons Canada Ltd, 22 Worcester Road, Etobicoke, Ontario, Canada M9W 1L1

Wiley also publishes its books in a variety of electronic formats. Some content that appears in print may not be available in electronic books.

Library of Congress Cataloging-in-Publication Data

British Library Cataloguing in Publication Data

A catalogue record for this book is available from the British Library

ISBN 978-0-470-01504-9 (H/B)

Typeset in 10/12pt Times by TechBooks, New Delhi, India

Printed and bound in Great Britain by CPI Antony Rowe, Chippenham, Wiltshire

Cover images courtesy of the Cleveland Clinic Diabetic Foot Care Program

Contents

Foreword

FOR(E)WARD – NOT BACK

The editors in *The Foot in Diabetes* are taking a risk in inviting a retired elder statesman to contribute an introductory comment to the fourth edition of this hugely successful publication, which has been intimately linked to the Malvern Foot Conference. Having been out of clinical practice for nearly 5 years and having made little attempt to follow the literature, what can I say other than thank you for the compliment implied in your invitation! However, you do not need to be an avid reader of current literature to know that there has been continuing and highly effective progress in coping with the scourge of foot problems as they affect so many people with diabetes. The scientific and clinical understanding of the causes of foot ulceration and ischaemia in diabetes continues, thus allowing more logical approaches to prevention and treatment, and these are well reviewed in this publication. It is indeed rewarding for me to read the first copy of the book and see how much more is known and how sophisticated has treatment become. It was exciting in the 'old days' to gain satisfaction from realising that we were performing a simple but effective task in highlighting the extent of the disease and suffering associated with diabetic foot problems, which then brought more and more workers of many disciplines to become involved in that necessary understanding of pathology.

Any reader who has travelled to less fortunate countries will know that there is still a massive global task of producing awareness of the diabetic foot where quite unbelievable foot destruction exists. Somehow, dramatic medical needs relating to infection, the heart, cancer, AIDS and malnutrition always seem to demand priority over the foul infected foot and, in many ways, with some of these diseases this is understandable. The Malvern Conference and this publication have been a major source of encouragement to look at this more global problem and must continue to stimulate Western workers to think how they can do their bit in taking education, knowledge and understanding to the less fortunate and teach those in other countries to do it themselves.

What clearly has not changed in this challenging field is strong motivation and enthusiasm, which has always been the hallmark of the old and young working in this area. More than simply studying clinical science, these workers now and in the past exhibited a great empathy towards those people who suffered from the disease, and this made them try even harder to organise systems to prevent or at least minimise the progress to serious disease. It must still be the case that the focused use of educated eyes and hands, followed by effective education of those with the problem, will stop so much of the diabetic foot pathology. This approach is so simple and potentially effective, although it does and will require considerable organisation investment if a truly global attack is to continue. I have no doubt knowing the quality of those working in the field that more progress will be made towards a final resolution.

By far the most impressive feature of this area of medicine is the wonderful collaboration of so many disciplines of medicine and science. This is simply shown by reading the front index of the chapters and by those involved in their production. All those working in the field and writing in this book have a shared objective. I know of no other branch of medicine where this is so positively and highly developed and leaves no doubt in my mind that there will be continuing movement forward not back.

John D. Ward

Preface

While writing this introduction in late 2005, designated by the International Diabetes Federation as the 'Year of the Diabetic Foot', it was clear that much progress has been made in the 20 years since the first edition of this book was in preparation. At that time, the number of publications on the diabetic foot listed in *Index Medicus*, when expressed as a percentage of all papers on diabetes was less than 1%: this has increased fourfold in the last two decades. Moreover, the number of meetings focusing on the diabetic foot has increased dramatically. It is also apparent when reading this edition that the number of new treatments for foot lesions has increased rapidly in the last decade.

As in the previous edition, we have attempted to provide the reader with a concise clinical text, which it is anticipated will not only help in day-to-day clinical practice, but also provide a foundation for understanding the mechanisms that result in foot complications. The first few chapters cover the epidemiology, causation and classification of foot lesions. Practical issues surrounding the formation of a foot service both in the United Kingdom and in the United States are covered next. The closely related and pivotal topics of psychosocial issues and education are then presented. The following chapters discuss a range of investigational issues and treatment areas. Finally, after a report on the international developments from three continents, the ongoing International Consensus on the Diabetic Foot is reviewed.

We trust that having read this text the reader will be fully prepared to be an active member of the diabetic foot team.

Andrew J.M. Boulton
Peter R. Cavanagh
Gerry Rayman

Contributors

Zulfiqarali G. Abbas, Muhimbili University College of Health Science; and Abbas Medical Centre, Dar es Salaam, Tanzania

Lennox K. Archibald, University of Florida, Gainesville, Florida, USA

David G. Armstrong, Scholl's Centre for Lower Extremity Ambulatory Research (CLEAR), Rosalind Franklin University of Medicine and Science, Chicago, Illinois, USA

Gillian S. Ashcroft, Faculty of Life Sciences, University of Manchester, Manchester UK

Neil Baker, Ipswich Hospital, Heath Road, Suffolk IP5 4PD, UK

Karel Bakker, The IDF Consultative Section and International Working Group on the Diabetic Foot, KN Heemstede, the Netherlands

Anthony R. Berendt, Bone Infection Unit, Nuffield Orthopaedic Centre NHS Trust, Oxford, UK

Amman Bolia, Department of Radiology, Leicester Royal Infirmary NHS Trust, Leicester, UK

Andrew J.M. Boulton, University of Manchester, Manchester Royal Infirmary, Manchester, UK; and Division of Endocrinology, Metabolism and Diabetes, University of Miami, Miami, Florida, USA

James W. Brodsky, Baylor University Medical Centre (BUMC); and University of Texas Southwestern Medical School (UTSWMC), Dallas, Texas

Toby Carlsson, PACE Rehabilitation Ltd, Manchester UK

Peter R. Cavanagh, Diabetic Foot Care Program, Departments of Biomedical Engineering and Orthopaedic Surgery, and the Orthopaedic Research Centre, The Cleveland Clinic Foundation; and The Cleveland Clinic Lerner College of Medicine of Case Western Reserve University, Cleveland, Ohio, USA

Nish Chaturvedi, International Centre for Circulatory Health, National Heart and Lung Institute, Imperial College, London

Susan Chipchase, Foot Ulcer Trials Unit, Department of Diabetes and Endocrinology, City Hospital, Nottingham, UK

Michael Clark, Wound Healing Research Unit, Cardiff Medicentre, Cardiff, UK

Ryan C. Crews, Scholl's Centre for Lower Extremity Ambulatory Research (CLEAR), Rosalind Franklin University of Medicine and Science, Chicago, Illinois, USA

Jeffrey M. Davidson, Vanderbilt University School of Medicine; and VA Tennessee Valley Healthcare System, Nashville Campus, Nashville, Tennessee, USA

Maria Stela Oliveira Dias, Programme of Education and Control of Diabetes, Secretary of Health, Setor de Indístria e Abastecimento - Brasilia - Distrito Federal, Brasil

Mollie Donohoe, Royal Devon and Exeter Hospital, Exeter, Devon, UK

Michael Edmonds, Diabetic Foot Clinic, Kings College Hospital, London, UK

Alethea V.M. Foster, Diabetic Foot Clinic, Kings College Hospital, London, UK

Roger Gadsby, Warwick University, Coventry, UK

Fran L. Game, Foot Ulcer Trials Unit, Department of Diabetes and Endocrinology, City Hospital, Nottingham, UK

Matthew J. Hardman, Faculty of Life Sciences, University of Manchester, Manchester UK

Eva-Lisa Heinrichs, Wound Healing Research Unit, Cardiff Medicentre, Cardiff, UK

William J. Jeffcoate, Foot Ulcer Trials Unit, Department of Diabetes and Endocrinology, City Hospital, Nottingham, UK

Edward B. Jude, Diabetes Centre, Tameside General Hospital, Ashton-under-Lyne, Lancashire, UK

Ann Knowles, Manchester Diabetes Centre, Manchester, UK

Singhan T.M. Krishnan, Diabetes Centre, Ipswich Hospital, Suffolk, UK

Lawrence A. Lavery, Department of Surgery, Texas A&M University Health Science Centre College of Medicine, Scott and White Memorial Hospital, Temple, Texas, USA

Joseph W. LeMaster, Department of Family and Community Medicine, University of Missouri, Columbia, Missouri, USA

Benjamin A. Lipsky, University of Washington; and General Internal Medicine Clinic, Antibiotic Research, VA Puget Sound Health Care System (S-111-GIMC), Seattle, Washington, USA

Douglas P. Murdoch, Department of Surgery, Texas A&M University Health Science Centre College of Medicine, Scott and White Memorial Hospital, Temple, Texas, USA

Hermelinda Pedrosa, Programa de Diabetes, Setor de Endocrinologia e Diabetes – Hospital Regional de Taguatinga, Área Especial C Norte No 24 – CEP 72.119-900, Distrito Federal

Michael S. Pinzur, Loyola University Medical School, Maywood, Illinois, USA

Roy Powell, Peninsula Research and Development Support Unit, Exeter, UK

Kate Radford, Foot Ulcer Trials Unit, Department of Diabetes and Endocrinology, City Hospital, Nottingham, UK

Gerry Rayman, Diabetes Centre, Ipswich Hospital, Suffolk, UK

Gayle E. Reiber, VA Puget Sound Health Care System; and University of Washington, Seattle, Washington, USA

Jeffrey M. Robbins, Louis Stokes Cleveland VAMC, Cleveland, Ohio, USA

Michael L. Salamon, Department of Orthopaedics, University of Iowa Hospitals and Clinics, Iowa City, USA

Charles L. Saltzman, Department of Orthopaedic Surgery and Biomedical Engineering, Iowa City, USA

Nicolaas C. Schaper, University Hospital Maastricht, Maastricht, the Netherlands

Malcolm H. Simms, University Hospital Birmingham NHS Foundation Trust, Selly Oak Hospital, Birmingham, UK

Solomon Tesfaye, Sheffield Teaching Hospitals NHS Foundation Trust, Royal Hallamshire Hospital, Sheffield, UK

Stephen Thomas, ZooBiotic Ltd; and Princess of Wales Hospital, Bridgend

John Tooke, Peninsula Medical School, Plymouth, UK

Jan S. Ulbrecht, Department of Biobehavioral Health, and The General Clinical Research Centre, Pennsylvania State University, University Park, Pennsylvania 16802, USA

Ernest R.E. Van Ross, Withington Hospital, Manchester, UK

Carine van Schie, Department of Rehabilitation, Academic Medical Centre, University of Amsterdam, Amsterdam, the Netherlands; and University of Manchester, Manchester Royal Infirmary, Manchester, UK

Loretta Vileikyte, University of Manchester, Manchester, UK; Division of Diabetes, Endocrinology and Metabolism, University of Miami, Miami, Florida, USA; and Institute for Health and Centre for Health Beliefs and Behaviour, Rutgers University, New Brunswick, New Jersey, USA

Vijay Viswanathan, Diabetes Research Centre, Royapuram, Tamil Nadu, Chennai, India

Richard W. Whitehouse, Manchester Royal Infirmary, Manchester, UK

Stephanie C. Wu, Scholl's Centre for Lower Extremity Ambulatory Research (CLEAR), Rosalind Franklin University of Medicine and Science, Chicago, Illinois, USA

Robert J. Young, Hope Hospital, Salford UK

1 Epidemiology and Economic Impact of Foot Ulcers

Joseph W. LeMaster and Gayle E. Reiber

In the year 2005, most of the estimated 150 million people worldwide afflicted by diabetes mellitus lived in developing countries.[1] Diabetic foot ulcers will complicate the disease in more than 15% of these people during their lifetimes.[2,3] In prospective cohort studies conducted among those with diabetes, history of a foot ulcer increased the risk of subsequent amputation by two- to over three-fold.[4,5] Foot ulcers precede more than 80% of non-traumatic lower limb amputations.[6] In this chapter, we will review the definition of a 'foot ulcer' and the studies that estimate the incidence and prevalence of foot ulcers, making note of issues that need to be considered in their computation. We will also review risk factors for foot ulcers from well-conducted epidemiological studies, foot ulcer outcomes and the economic impact of foot ulcers.

FOOT ULCER DEFINITION AND CLASSIFICATION

In order to estimate accurately the occurrence of diabetic foot ulcers and risk factors associated with this diabetic complication, a common definition is needed. The International Consensus on the Diabetic Foot currently defines a diabetic foot ulcer as a full-thickness wound below the ankle in a patient with diabetes, irrespective of duration.[7] The International Working Group on the Diabetic Foot (IWGDF) also recommends that studies describing the occurrence of diabetic foot ulcers use a standard classification system to facilitate communication between health care providers, provide information about the healing potential of an ulcer and help guide management decisions. Use of such a system allows a patient to be followed up over time, allowing repeated classification of the foot ulcer. Classification systems should be sufficiently robust that intra- and inter-observer variability is low (i.e. the classification is reproducible) and should be applicable worldwide. This allows research results from one study to be compared to those of others, which is important in interpretability of results.[8] For foot ulcers, one challenge in this regard has been the numerous classification systems in existence. The most commonly used system internationally is Wagner's.[9] This system specifies ulcer depth and the presence of osteomyelitis or gangrene as a five-grade continuum:

Grade 0   Pre-ulcerative lesion

Grade 1   Partial-thickness wound up to but not through the dermis

The Foot in Diabetes, 4th Edition. Editors Andrew J.M. Boulton, Peter R. Cavanagh and Gerry Rayman.
© 2006 John Wiley & Sons, Ltd.

Grade 2   Full-thickness wound extending to tendons or deeper subcutaneous tissue but
           without bony involvement or osteomyelitis

Grade 3   Full-thickness wound extending to and involving bone

Grade 4   Localised gangrene

Grade 5   Gangrene of the whole foot

The University of Texas system adds to this assessment four stages that specify tissue perfusion and infection: clean wounds (stage A), non-ischaemic, infected wounds (stage B),
ischaemic, non-infected wounds (stage C) and ischaemic, infected wounds (stage D).[10] As
discussed in Chapter 7, Dr Jeffcoate and colleagues from Nottingham developed the S(AD)
SAD system, which adds to the Texas system cross-sectional area and the presence or absence
of neuropathy.[11] Most recently, the IWGDF has itself developed a classification system that
grades foot perfusion, wound size, depth, the presence of infection and sensation.[8] None of
these systems considers the duration of the foot ulcer,[12] which may be a factor in foot ulcer
treatment and time to healing.[13]

INCIDENCE AND PREVALENCE STUDIES

Reports of the incidence (new onset) and prevalence (history) of diabetic foot ulcers from
many countries have begun to appear in the medical literature. To identify these studies,
we conducted a literature review using the Ovid Information service, which includes Med-
line, the Cumulative Index to Nursing and Allied Health Literature, the Cochrane Controlled
Trials register and Current Contents. We searched for articles published between January
1964 and April 2005 that used the following phrases: diabetes or diabetic, incidence, prevalence, foot ulcer, foot and feet. We also searched the bibliography of each identified article. The published studies we reviewed include population-based cohort studies, large randomised controlled trials (from which we report foot ulcer incidence among the comparison
group) as well as clinic-based studies. We excluded studies that reported only lower limb
ulceration (without specifying foot ulcers),[14,15] those that did not specify a foot ulcer definition of any sort[13,16,17] and studies that described a series of foot ulcer patients without
clearly specifying a population base that would make it possible to estimate prevalence or
incidence.[18–21]

The lifetime risk for foot ulcers in people with diabetes has been estimated to be 15%.[2]
Table 1.1 shows that the annual, population-based incidence of foot ulcers among people with
diabetes ranges from less than 1% to 3.6% among people with type 1 or type 2 diabetes.[16,22–30]
Several methodological issues deserve consideration by those reviewing data or estimating
foot ulcer incidence and prevalence in a population:

1. A number of clinic-based studies have attempted to estimate the population prevalence
   (and in some cases the incidence) of diabetic foot ulcers for a geographic area.[17,30,31–44]
   Many of these studies were well conducted and required substantial coordination across
   health care systems. For example, in France, a cross-sectional survey was conducted on
   one day in May 2001 of all patients attending outpatient clinics or admitted by 16 hospital
   departments that were actively involved in managing such patients.[42] Clinic-based studies
   make use of accessible patients. When used to measure prevalence or incidence of foot
   ulcers for a geographical area in community-dwelling people with diabetes, however, this

Table 1.1 Selected population-based studies estimating incidence and prevalence of diabetic foot ulcers

Study (country)	Population base	N	Prevalence (%)	Annual incidence[a] (%)	Ulcer definition	Ulcer ascertainment method
Rith-Najarian et al.[22] (United States)	Chippewa Indian residents with diabetes	266	—	0.6 (Non-neuropathic subjects)	Full thickness plantar foot lesion	Retrospective review of medical records/clinical examinations
Walters et al.[23] (United Kingdom)	Registered patients with diabetes from 10 UK general practices	1077	2.9 (Current) 7.4 (History of ulcer)	—	Wagner grade ≥ 1 foot lesion	Direct examination and structured interview
Moss et al.[16] (United States)	Population-based sample of persons with diabetes	1834	10.6 (History of ulcers at baseline)	2.2	???	Medical history questionnaire administered at baseline and 4 years later
Kumar et al.[24] (United Kingdom)	Type 2 diabetes patients registered in three UK cities	811	1.4 (Current) 5.3 (History of ulcer)	—	Wagner grade ≥ 1 foot lesion	Direct exam by trained observers (current), and structured interview (history of ulcer)
Abbott et al.[25] (United Kingdom)	Randomised controlled trial cohort	1035	—	3.6	Full-thickness lesion requiring hospital treatment	Direct examination at least every 13 weeks
Ramsey et al.[26] (United States)	Registered adult type 1 or 2 diabetes patients in a large HMO (1992–1995)	8905	—	1.9	ICD-codes: 707.1 (ulcer of lower leg)	Medical billing record audit
Abbott et al.[27] (United Kingdom)	Registered type 1 and type 2 diabetes patients in six UK districts	9710	1.7 (Current)	2.2	Wagner grade ≥ 1 foot lesion	Clinical examination (plus chart review)
Muller et al.[28] (Netherlands)	1993–1998 registered type 2 diabetes patients	3827 person-years	—	2.1	Full-thickness skin loss on the foot	Abstracted medical records
Centers for Disease Control and Prevention[29] (United States)	US BRFSS respondents with diabetes, 2000–2002[b]	NS	11.8 (History of ulcer)	—	Foot sore that did not heal for >4 weeks	Random-digit-dialled telephone interview

???, not specified.
[a] Incidence is annualised unless otherwise noted.
[b] BRFSS, Behavioral Risk Factor Surveillance Survey.

information may be biased because not all those with diabetes attend clinics, and those who do attend are more likely to have complications when they attend, such as diabetic foot problems. Moreover, cross-sectional surveys of clinic attendees that select a random or consecutive sample of clinic attendees are more likely to sample patients with more severe disease, because these patients attend the clinic more frequently. The preferable strategy is to sample patients from a diabetes registry that enrolls all patients in a region or a large health system.

2. Foot ulcer prevalence will also be underestimated if care is not taken to sample only patients with previously diagnosed diabetes, because a substantial proportion of patients are diagnosed with diabetes only at the time they present to clinics with a foot ulcer. In the Congolese survey cited, Monabeka and colleagues found that diabetes was first diagnosed in 2.8% of patients admitted for diabetic foot problems,[36] while in the United Kingdom, 15% of patients admitted for amputation were first diagnosed with diabetes on admission to hospital.[45] Investigators should be sure to include the foot ulcer cases for which diabetes is diagnosed at the time of foot ulcer detection in the population denominator, when calculating incidence or prevalence.

3. Wherever possible, reported foot ulcers (either by patients in surveys or by providers in clinics) should be corroborated by direct examination by investigators to avoid possible misclassification. Routine administrative or clinical billing data are subject to reporting bias, because health professionals may fail to enter the correct diagnostic code, or assign codes to maximise reimbursement. Reimbursement and administrative systems are not well suited to tracking clinical information such as ulcer episodes. Foot ulcer occurrence will be underestimated if more severe presentations (such as cellulitis or gangrene) are not counted as foot ulcers when disease in such patients started as foot ulcers. In one survey of 1654 diabetes patients hospitalised with foot problems in the Congo, only 1.2% of the cases were classified as foot ulcers, while 70.4% had either local abscess or wet gangrene.[36]

4. Prospective studies that seek to estimate ulcer incidence in a population should define a cohort of individuals who are known to be free of foot ulcers at the onset of the study, and evaluate those individuals at a later time to determine the subsequent foot ulcer presence or absence, using a clear foot ulcer definition.

5. While randomised controlled trial cohorts allow for careful ascertainment of foot ulcer incidence, they may be unsuitable to estimate incidence in the overall population of people with diabetes in the region where the study was conducted (even in controls, or in a study where the intervention was not successful and the investigators attempt to draw conclusions from the total cohort) because the sample is often highly selected, i.e. very unlike the population from which the sampled participants are drawn. In one recent clinical trial sample that was used to estimate incidence of foot ulcers, participants must have been 18–70 years old, men or non-pregnant women, had a vibration perception threshold (VPT) of ≥ 25 V on at least one foot and have had no prior foot ulceration or lower limb amputation, only diabetic causes of neuropathy, and no history of alcohol abuse, previous treatment with radiotherapy or cytotoxic agents, uncontrolled hypertension or any renal disease.[25] While these criteria are suitable to enrolls participants into a controlled trial, they make it impossible to generalise results from such a study to estimate foot ulcer incidence in the general population of people with diabetes.

Table 1.2 Anatomic site and outcome of diabetic foot lesions in two prospective studies

	All lesions[a] (%) N = 314	Most severe lesion[b] (%) N = 302
Lesion site (%)		
Toes (dorsal and plantar surface)	51	52
Metatarsal heads, midfoot and heel	28	37
Dorsum of the foot	14	11
Multiple ulcers	7	NA
Total	100	100

[a] Ref. 46 (Apelqvist *et al.*); study included consecutive patients whose lesions were characterised according to Wagner criteria from superficial non-necrotic to major gangrene.
[b] Ref. 47 (Reiber *et al.*); study patients were enrolled with a lesion through the dermis that could extend to deeper tissue.

ANATOMIC LOCATION OF FOOT ULCERS

The anatomic site of foot ulcers varies according to the population from which the patients are drawn. Table 1.2 presents data from two prospective studies that reported foot ulcer site. Those studies using patients from general diabetes clinics found that the most common ulcer sites were the toes (dorsal and plantar surface), followed by the metatarsal heads.[46,47]

US COUNTRYWIDE ESTIMATES OF FOOT-ULCER-RELATED CONDITIONS

The ability to identify foot ulcers in individuals in clinics, offices and outpatient settings is difficult, due to limited surveillance systems. However, information on patients hospitalised with foot-ulcer-related conditions is available in many countries. In the United States, for example, the Healthcare Cost and Utilization Project Nationwide Inpatient Sample (NIS) reports a 20% stratified sample of US community hospitals discharges (excluding discharges from Department of Veterans Affairs and military hospitals). In Table 1.3 the data for 2001 and 2002 by International Classification of Diseases (ICD-9) codes, weighted to reflect the US civilian population, show that the leading reasons for hospitalisation among diabetic patients with foot-ulcer-related conditions are cellulitis and abscess, lower limb ulcers and osteomyelitis.[48]

RISK FACTORS FOR DIABETIC FOOT ULCERS

Independent risk factors for diabetic foot ulcers were identified from analytic and experimental studies that used multivariable modelling techniques and included a defined foot ulcer outcome. Results shown in Table 1.4 demonstrate that the most consistent independent foot ulcer risk factors were long diabetes duration, measures of peripheral neuropathy and peripheral vascular disease, prior foot ulcer and prior amputation. Long duration of diabetes, even after controlling for age, was a statistically significant finding in three studies.[16,23,24] The independent role of plantar foot pressure remains unclear.

Table 1.3 Frequency of foot-ulcer-related conditions in hospitalised individuals with diabetes, 2001–2002

Type of ulcer	ICD-CM code	Estimated US frequency, 2001	Estimated US frequency, 2002
Cellulitis, abscess or infected ulcer	681.1	26 685	29 347
Other cellulitis and abscess, foot, except toes	682.7	81 367	83 954
Ulcer of lower limbs, except decubitus	707.1	209 088	216 785
Osteomyelitis	730.07	60 989	66 591
	730.17		
	730.27		
	730.37		
	730.87		
	730.97		
Chronic non-healing ulcers	707.0	129 466	134 274
	707.9		
Atherosclerosis of lower limb with ulcer or gangrene	440.23	83 546	78 983
	440.24		

Source: Nationwide Inpatient Sample, 2001, 2002.[48]

Assessment of diabetic peripheral neuropathy is performed using several semi-quantitative and quantitative measures and neurological summary scores. Associations between peripheral neuropathy and foot ulcers are uniform across the studies reported in Table 1.4. Boyko and colleagues found an increased risk of ulcers in patients who were insensate to the 5.07 (10-g) monofilament, a semi-quantitative measure of light touch.[30,50] Kastenbauer and associates found that elevated VPT ≥ 25 V prospectively predicted foot ulcers in a cohort of type 2 patients followed up on average for more than 3 years.[37] In a randomised clinical trial that used VPT ≥ 25 V as an entry criteria, Abbott and colleagues found that VPT deficits and a combined neuropathy deficit score (NDS) that include both reflexes and muscle strength measures were significant predictors of incident ulcers.[25] Several years later, the same investigators, in a cohort study of 6613 diabetes patients from six UK health care districts, found similarly that NDS score, increasingly abnormal ankle reflexes and 10-g monofilament insensitivity all independently predicted new foot ulcers.[27] Carrington and associates found that peroneal motor nerve conduction velocity was strongly associated with foot ulcer risk even after controlling for sensory neuropathy.[39] Together these studies suggest that aberrations in the various sensory modalities and the presence of motor neuropathy independently predict increased foot ulcer risk.

Peripheral vascular function can be measured as absent pulses, transcutaneous oxygen tension ($TcpO_2$) decrements and low ankle–arm index (AAI). These variables predicted foot ulcers in several of the studies in Table 1.4. Low $TcpO_2$, indicating diminished skin oxygenation, and low AAI, indicating abnormal large vessel perfusion, were independent predictors of foot ulcers in the study by Boyko *et al.*[30] In Boyko and colleagues' study, laser Doppler flowmetry did not predict foot ulcer. Kumar *et al.* defined peripheral vascular involvement as the absence of two or more foot pulses or a history of previous peripheral revascularisation.[24] They reported that this variable was a significant predictor of foot ulcers. Walters *et al.* found that an absent dorsalis pedis pulse was associated with a 6.3-fold increased risk of foot ulcer (95% CI 5.57–7.0).[23] Abbott and colleagues found that having two or less palpable pedal pulses on

Table 1.4 Risk factors for foot ulcers in patients with diabetes mellitus from the final analysis models of selected studies

Study (type of analysis)	Study design, diabetes type	Long DM duration	Neuropathy (monofilament, reflex, vibration or neurological deficit score)	Low AAI, TcpO$_2$ or absent pulses	High HbA$_{1c}$	Deformity	Smoking	History of ulcer	Amputation
Moss et al.[16] (Logistic regression)	Cohort, patients with early- and late-onset diabetes = 2990	Borderline older			+		Borderline younger		
Walters et al.[23] (Logistic regression)	Cohort, 10 UK general practices type 1 and 2 patients = 1077	+	+ Absent light touch + Impaired pain Perception 0 VPT	+ Absent pulses 0 Doppler			0		
Litzelman et al.[49] (GEE)	RCT Type 2 patients = 352	0	+ Monofilament		0	0		+	Exclusion criteria
Kumar et al.[24] (Logistic regression)	Cross-sectional UK general practices type 2 patients = 811	+	+ NDS	+			0	0	+
Carrington et al.[39] (Cox regression analysis)	Cohort, single UK diabetes clinic attendees Non-diabetes = 22 Type 1 = 83 Type 2 = 86	0	+ Motor neuropathy 0 VPT 0 Pressure sensation 0 Thermal (All were in the model simultaneously)	Exclusion criteria	0			0	Exclusion criteria

(Continued)

Table 1.4 (*Continued*)

Study (type of analysis)	Study design, diabetes type	Long DM duration	Neuropathy (monofilament, reflex, vibration or neurological summary score)	Low AAI, TcpO$_2$ or absent pulses	High HbA$_{1c}$	Deformity	Smoking	History of ulcer	Amputation
Abbott et al.[25] (Cox regression analysis)	RCT, patients with VPT ≥ 25 V (United States, United Kingdom, Canada) Type 1 = 255 Type 2 = 780	0	0 Monofilament + VPT + Reflex	Exclusion criteria				Exclusion criteria	Exclusion criteria
Boyko et al.[30] (Cox regression analysis)	Cohort, veterans Type 1 = 48 Type 2 = 701	0	+ Monofilament	+ AAI +TcpO$_2$	0	+ Charcot	0	+	+
Kastenbauer et al.[37] (Logistic regression)	Cohort Type 2 = 187	0	0 Monofilament + VPT	Exclusion criteria	0	0	0	Exclusion criteria	Exclusion criteria
Abbott et al.[27] (Cox regression analysis)	Cohort, United Kingdom registered diabetes patients from six UK health districts Type 1 or 2 = 6613	0	0 VPT + Monofilament + NDS + Reflex	+	0	+	0	+	

Blank, not studied; +, statistically significant; 0, no statistically significant finding; AAI, ankle–arm index; DM, diabetes mellitus; HbA$_{1c}$, haemoglobin A$_{1c}$; RCT, randomised controlled trial; TcpO$_2$, transcutaneous oxygen tension; VPT, vibration perception threshold; NDS, neuropathy disability score.

both feet (at the dorsalis pedis or posterior tibial arteries) predicted increased foot ulcer risk, after controlling for neuropathy measures, history of prior foot ulcer and foot deformity.[27]

The proportion of foot ulcers with both neuropathy and ischaemia is fairly consistent internationally. In the United Kingdom, Kumar et al. found neuropathy alone in 46% of those with a history of foot ulcer, ischaemia alone in 12%, neuropathy and ischaemia (neuroischaemia) in 30% and neither in 12%.[24] Similarly, Walters et al., also working in the United Kingdom, and Nyamu et al. in a carefully conducted clinic-based study in Kenya found that the greatest proportion of foot ulcers were neuropathic, followed by neuroischaemic and lastly by ischaemic ulcers, and that ischaemia was present in about half the ulcers overall.[23,40] On the other hand, the proportion of foot ulcers that are ischaemic is less in some lesser developed countries, compared to more developed countries. Morbach et al., in a study comparing foot ulcers classified by the Wagner system across several countries, found that peripheral vascular disease was present in 48% of foot ulcers in Germany, but in only 11% of ulcers in Tanzania and 10% in India.[51]

The risk associated with a prior history of ulcers was assessed in five studies. Boyko et al., Litzelman et al. and Abbott et al. reported that a prior history of foot ulcers significantly increased the likelihood of a subsequent ulcer.[27,30,49] Kumar et al. reported a relationship between prior amputation and subsequent ulcer.[24] Rith-Najarian and colleagues (though they did not use a multivariate approach and hence their study is not shown in Table 1.4) found an incidence rate of foot ulcers of 6/1000 person-years at risk among people with diabetes who had no history of prior foot ulcer, intact foot sensation and no foot deformity, whereas the rate was 330/1000 person-years at risk if all three of these criteria were present.[22]

Health care access and availability of diabetes education have been reported to influence development of foot ulcers. In a randomised trial conducted by Litzelman et al. in a county hospital population, diabetes patients were randomised to education, behavioural contracts and reminders, while concurrently their providers received special education and chart prompts. The control population in this study received usual care and education. After 1 year, patients in the intervention group reported more appropriate foot self-care behaviours, including inspection of feet and shoes, washing of feet and drying between toes. Not all desirable behaviours were adopted. There was no significant difference between patient groups in testing of bath water temperature and reporting of foot problems. Patients in the intervention group developed fewer serious foot lesions including ulcers than did those in the control group.[49] Among the five studies reported in Table 1.4 that included glycosylated haemoglobin (HbA$_{1c}$, indicating medium-term glycaemic control) in their analyses,[16,30,37,39,49] only HbA$_{1c}$ or blood glucose levels was positively associated and foot ulcers: Moss et al. found a statistically significant association between increasingly poor HbA$_{1c}$ and subsequent foot ulcers in their cohort study, with an odds ratio of 1.6 (95% CI 1.3–2.0) for every 2% deterioration in this measure.[16]

The relationship between smoking and foot ulcers was assessed in six studies reported in Table 1.4;[23,24,27,30,37,39] however, it was only of borderline significance in the younger population in the Wisconsin study.[16] Moss and colleagues found that current smokers younger than 30 years were more likely to ulcerate, with odds ratio 2.3 (95% CI 1.0–5.6).[16] Kastenbauer and colleagues found that daily intake of alcohol also increased ulcer risk.[37] The cohort study by Boyko et al. also identified higher body weight, insulin use and history of poor vision as three additional independent predictors of foot ulcer.[30]

Four of the studies reported in Table 1.4 address the relationship between deformity and subsequent foot ulcer.[27,30,37,49] The study by Boyko et al. found an independent association between Charcot deformity and foot ulcer, but other foot deformities were not independent ulcer predictors.[30] Foot deformity did not enter the final analytic model in the studies by Litzelman et al.[49] or Kastenbauer et al.[37] A number of other studies not presented in Table 1.4 have assessed the role of elevated foot pressure in foot ulcer development, using case–control comparisons. As long ago as 1963, Bauman and Brand found elevated plantar pressures under the feet of people with neuropathic insensitivity, foot deformities and foot ulcers.[52] Mueller and colleagues found that patients with diabetes and a history of foot ulcers had significantly reduced ankle dorsiflexion and subtalar joint range of motion, compared to those without diabetes.[53] In a similar study, Zimny et al. found that those with diabetic neuropathy but no history of foot ulcers also had reduced dorsiflexion and subtalar motion, compared to non-diabetic controls.[54] Recently, Robertson et al. found, using spiral computerised tomography, that plantar tissue muscle density was decreased and that metatarso-phalangeal arthropathy (especially hammer toe deformity) was more likely to be present in those with diabetic peripheral neuropathy and a history of plantar ulcer than in normal controls ($P < 0.001$).[55] In another study by the same group, Mueller et al. found that peak plantar pressure during walking was significantly greater in those who had both diabetic peripheral neuropathy and hammer toes than in normal controls.[56] Van Schie et al. found a greater frequency of both foot deformities (hammer toes, claw toes, prominent metatarsal heads and high medial arch) and foot muscle weakness (in both intrinsic and extrinsic muscles) ($P < 0.001$, Kruskal–Wallis test for trend in both types of comparisons) in those with a history of diabetic foot ulcers than in diabetic, non-neuropathic and non-diabetic controls.[57]

In reports from prospective cohort studies, progressively higher plantar pressure predicts increasing foot ulcer risk.[35,58] Despite these associations, prospective studies have been unable to demonstrate an optimal cut-point for increasing plantar pressure, above which the probability of foot ulceration is substantially increased.[43,59] This may be the case because other factors, such as weight-bearing activity, act together with plantar pressure to increase foot ulcer risk. Maluf and Mueller in a case–control study found that cumulative plantar tissue stress (which they defined as the combination of plantar pressure and total daily weight-bearing activity) was *reduced* in those with a history of diabetic neuropathic ulcers compared to either those with neuropathy alone or non-diabetic controls ($P = 0.03$).[60] The authors speculated that plantar tissues in those who ulcerated may have been more vulnerable to ulceration due to disuse atrophy. That study measured plantar pressure once at study onset, and measured weight-bearing activity over the ensuing week. Ledoux et al. investigated the relationship between ulcer location and peak plantar pressure at one Veterans Affairs (VA) medical centre in 549 individuals with diabetes, each of whom had in-shoe plantar pressure measured using the F-scan plantar pressure measurement device. After an average of 2.5 years of follow-up, there were 42 patients who developed plantar ulcers. In an analysis that considered whether plantar pressure differed within each foot site by foot ulcer occurrence, no significant difference was seen for peak pressure. Sites at which ulcers developed had higher mean pressure than other sites, but the site of highest pressure was unrelated to the foot ulcer site.[61] Together, these studies represent a substantial shift over time in our understanding of the role of plantar pressure and foot ulceration. It is becoming clear that while foot deformities and associated plantar pressure are important risk factors for diabetic foot ulcer, other as yet unidentified factors probably play an important synergistic role with plantar pressure in the development of foot ulcers. Further prospective studies are needed to investigate the joint role of plantar pressure and weight-bearing activity using technology that measures cumulative plantar tissue stress continuously, via an in-shoe system. Such systems are being developed[62] and will greatly improve investigation in this area.

ULCER OUTCOMES

Table 1.5 shows the outcomes of incident ulcers reported from three prospective studies of foot ulcers. The proportion of patients with diabetic foot ulcer who progress to at least partial amputation ranges from 11 to 24%, depending on ulcer severity and length of follow-up.[26,28,46,47,63] Factors associated with amputation once foot ulcer occurs will be reviewed in the next chapter. Later chapters will review therapeutic strategies for treatment of diabetic foot ulcer; however, a number of studies have found that, given similar care, ulcer surface area and ulcer duration prior to the start of treatment delay ulcer healing.[13,63–66] In a study of 194 ulcers that were re-examined weekly for 6–18 months, Oyibo and colleagues found that ulcer surface area differed strongly and significantly between ulcers that healed, did not heal or proceeded to amputation (larger ulcers having worse outcomes and taking longer to heal). Patient gender, age and duration of diabetes at presentation, and site of the ulcer on the foot did not affect time to healing. Neuroischaemic ulcers took longer to heal (20 vs 9 weeks) and were three times more likely to lead to amputation.[63] Margolis and colleagues found, after pooling data from the control arms of five related randomised studies investigating new ulcer-healing therapies, that neuropathic wounds were more likely to heal within 20 weeks if they were smaller (<2 cm^2), had existed for a shorter period before they were treated (<6 months) or if the patients were of non-White ethnicity.[13] Gender, age and glycosylated haemoglobin level had no effect in their multivariable regression model. In an analysis that utilised medical records from 150 wound care facilities in 38 US states, these same investigators confirmed that among 72 525 diabetic foot wounds in 31 106 patients, wounds that were older, larger and deeper in grade (especially Wagner grade ≥ 3) were more likely to take more than 20 weeks to heal, after adjustment for gender and age.[64] Pecoraro and colleagues described the importance of a 4-week reduction in ulcer volume and reported that low levels of periwound TcpO$_2$ and CO$_2$ were significantly associated with initial rate of healing, while an average periwound TcpO$_2$ <20 mm Hg was associated with a 39-fold increased risk of early healing failure.[66] Sheehan and colleagues similarly found, among 276 patients with Wagner grade ≥ 1 diabetic foot ulcers of 30 days duration, that change in ulcer area within 4 weeks of treatment onset strongly predicted complete wound healing by 12 weeks.[65] All patients in each of these studies received similar ulcer care, which included offloading, wound debridement and moist wound dressings.[13,63–65]

Foot ulcer recurrences were addressed in a UK study by Mantey and colleagues.[67] Diabetic patients with an initial foot ulcer and two ulcer recurrences were compared with diabetic patients who had only one ulcer and no recurrences over a 2-year interval. The authors reported greater peripheral sensory neuropathy and poor diabetes control in the ulcer recurrence group. Members of the ulcer recurrence group had higher glycosylated haemoglobin levels, waited longer after observing a serious foot problem until seeking care and consumed more alcohol than did the group without ulcer recurrences. Several years later, Connor and Mahdi reported on their cohort analysis of 83 patients followed up for 2–10 years after their initial foot ulcer.[68] They found that the 37% of patients with a higher rate of recurrence (≥3.5 ulcers per foot per 10 years) accounted for 68% of all inpatient days and 75% of all amputations. These patients fell into two distinct groups: those with neuroarthropathy, who were more likely to wear non-orthotic footwear and had problems with footwear or orthoses, and those without neuroarthropathy, who attended clinic irregularly. Both groups had poorer glycaemic control than those with less ulcer recurrence.

Table 1.5 Frequency of lesion outcomes for diabetic foot ulcers in three prospective studies

	All lesions followed until final outcome[a]	All lesions followed for 6–18 months[b]	Most severe lesion followed until final outcome[c]
Number of ulcers	314	194	302
Re-epithelialisation/primary healing (%)	63	65	81
Amputation at any level (%)	24	15	14
Remained unhealed (%)	0	16	0
Death (%)	13	3.5	5
Total (%)	100	100	100

[a] Ref. 46 (Apelqvist *et al.*); lesions were characterised according to Wagner criteria from superficial non-necrotic to major gangrene.
[b] Ref. 63 (Oyibo *et al.*); lesions were grade 1 or deeper in the S(AD) SAD foot ulcer classification system.
[c] Ref. 47 (Reiber *et al.*); study patients were enrolled with a lesion through the dermis that could extend to deeper tissue.

ECONOMIC CONSIDERATIONS FOR FOOT ULCERS

Studies on foot-ulcer-related conditions usually report only direct patient costs or charges such as outpatient visits, procedures, pharmaceuticals and hospitalisations, since indirect costs (value of lost income from work, pain, suffering and family burden) are difficult to measure. Two studies assessed the economic impact of ulcers and amputations, and followed the lesion from the onset of the ulcer episode to each lesion's final resolution. Ramsey conducted a nested case–control study in a large health maintenance organisation (HMO) that involved 8905 patients with diabetes. Of this group, 514 individuals developed one or more foot ulcers, and 11% of these patients required amputation. Costs were computed for the year prior to the ulcer and the two years following the ulcer, for both cases and controls. The excess cost attributed to foot ulcers and their sequelae averaged $27 987 per patient for the 2-year period following ulcer presentation.[26] Apelqvist followed 314 patients across their ulcer episode, and reported healing was achieved in ≤2 months in 54% of patients, in 3–4 months in 19% of patients and in ≥5 months in 27% of patients. There were 63% of patients who healed without surgery at an average cost of $6664. Lower limb amputation was required for 24% of patients at an average cost of $44 790. The 13% of patients who died prior to final ulcer resolution were excluded from this analysis. The proportion of all costs that were related to hospitalisation was 39% among ulcer patients and 82% among amputees.[69]

Direct costs for US patients with private insurance are available from the Medstat group, who manages a large US integrated administrative claims system affiliated with private health insurance plans. Table 1.6 shows reimbursement to hospitals for patients with selected foot conditions by Diagnostic Related Group (DRG). For example, for DRG 271, i.e. skin ulcers, patients with private insurance averaged 11-day hospitalisation at a cost of $11 638, while those whose coverage was Medicare had an average 7.3-day length of stay and an average

Table 1.6 Reimbursement to hospitals for patients with and without diabetes, 2002

| DRG | Condition | Medstat (private) | | Medicare | |
		LOS	Average reimbursement (in $)	LOS	Average reimbursement (in $)
277	Cellulitis, age >17 with complications	4.8	6 823	5.7	4 000
278	Cellulitis, age >17 without complications	3.4	4, 426	4.2	2 192
271	Skin ulcers	11.0	11 638	7.3	5 227
238	Osteomyelitis	5.9	9 913	8.7	7 376

Source: Medstat group, Thompson Corporation, 2005[70]; Centers for Medicare and Medicaid Services, 2005[71]. DRG, Diagnostic Related Group; LOS, length of stay.

hospital reimbursement of $5227 according to the Centers for Medicare and Medicaid Services. Payment for the health care providers is not included in these figures.[70,71]

In summary, foot ulcer prevalence and incidence is increasing globally and is challenging to measure, due to a lack of outpatient- and clinic-based surveillance systems. Peripheral neuropathy and its sequelae, a long duration of diabetes and peripheral vascular disease are the most consistent risk factors for predicting a foot ulcer. Re-ulceration occurs in about 60% of persons with prior ulcers and is more common among those with more severe peripheral neuropathy, increased alcohol consumption, poorer blood glucose control and delays in seeking ulcer care. Costs are high to the patient and the health care system.

REFERENCES

1. King H, Aubert RE, Herman WH. Global burden of diabetes, 1995–2025: prevalence, numerical estimates, and projections. *Diabetes Care* 1998;21:1414–1431.
2. Palumbo PJ, Melton LJ III. Peripheral vascular disease and diabetes. In: National Diabetes Data Group (US), National Institute of Diabetes and Digestive and Kidney Diseases (United States), eds. *Diabetes in America.* Bethesda, MD: National Institutes of Health, National Institute of Diabetes and Digestive and Kidney Diseases; 1995:401–408.
3. Singh N, Armstrong DG, Lipsky BA. Preventing foot ulcers in patients with diabetes. *JAMA* 2005;293:217–228.
4. Adler AI, Boyko EJ, Ahroni JH, *et al.* Lower-extremity amputation in diabetes. The independent effects of peripheral vascular disease, sensory neuropathy, and foot ulcers. *Diabetes Care* 1999;22:1029–1035.
5. Moss SE, Klein R, Klein BE. The 14-year incidence of lower-extremity amputations in a diabetic population. The Wisconsin Epidemiologic Study of Diabetic Retinopathy. *Diabetes Care* 1999;22:951–959.
6. Pecoraro RE, Reiber GE, Burgess EM. Pathways to diabetic limb amputation. Basis for prevention. *Diabetes Care* 1990;13:513–521.
7. Apelqvist J, Bakker K, van Houtum WH, *et al. International Consensus on the Diabetic Foot.* Maastricht, the Netherlands: International Working Group on the Diabetic Foot; 1999.
8. Schaper NC. Diabetic foot ulcer classification system for research purposes: a progress report on criteria for including patients in research studies. *Diabetes Metab Res Rev* 2004;20:S90–S95.

9. Wagner FW Jr. The dysvascular foot: a system for diagnosis and treatment. *Foot Ankle* 1981;2:64–122.

10. Lavery LA, Armstrong DG, Harkless LB. Classification of diabetic foot wounds. *J Foot Ankle Surg* 1996;35:528–531.

11. Treece K, Macfarlane R, Pound N, *et al.* Validation of a new system of foot ulcer classification in diabetes mellitus. Nottingham, UK: Department of Diabetes and Endocrinology, City Hospital; 2005.

12. Macfarlane RM, Jeffcoate WJ. Factors contributing to the presentation of diabetic foot ulcers. *Diabet Med* 1997;14:867–870.

13. Margolis DJ, Kantor J, Santanna J, *et al.* Risk factors for delayed healing of neuropathic diabetic foot ulcers: a pooled analysis. *Arch Dermatol* 2000;136:1531–1535.

14. Wong I. Measuring the incidence of lower limb ulceration in the Chinese population in Hong Kong. *J Wound Care* 2002;11:377–379.

15. Andersson E, Hansson C, Swanbeck G. Leg and foot ulcer prevalence and investigation of the peripheral arterial and venous circulation in a randomised elderly population. An epidemiological survey and clinical investigation. *Acta Derm Venereol* 1993;73:57–61.

16. Moss SE, Klein R, Klein BE. The prevalence and incidence of lower extremity amputation in a diabetic population. *Arch Intern Med* 1992;152:610–616.

17. Tseng CH. Prevalence and risk factors of diabetic foot problems in Taiwan: a cross-sectional survey of non-type 1 diabetic patients from a nationally representative sample. *Diabetes Care* 2003;26:3351.

18. Gulam-Abbas Z, Lutale JK, Morbach S, *et al.* Clinical outcome of diabetes patients hospitalized with foot ulcers, Dar es Salaam, Tanzania. *Diabet Med* 2002;19:575–579.

19. Yalamanchi H, Yalamanchi S. Profile of diabetic foot infections in a semiurban area of a developing country. *Diabetologia* 1997;40:A468.

20. Akanji AO, Adetuyidi A. The pattern of presentation of foot lesions in Nigerian diabetic patients. *West Afr J Med* 1990;9:1–5.

21. Benotmane A, Mohammedi F, Ayad F, *et al.* Diabetic foot lesions: etiologic and prognostic factors. *Diabetes Metab* 2000;26:113–117.

22. Rith-Najarian SJ, Stolusky T, Gohdes DM. Identifying diabetic patients at high risk for lower-extremity amputation in a primary health care setting. A prospective evaluation of simple screening criteria. *Diabetes Care* 1992;15:1386–1389.

23. Walters DP, Gatling W, Mullee MA, *et al.* The distribution and severity of diabetic foot disease: a community study with comparison to a non-diabetic group. *Diabet Med* 1992;9:354–358.

24. Kumar S, Ashe HA, Parnell LN, *et al.* The prevalence of foot ulceration and its correlates in type 2 diabetic patients: a population-based study. *Diabet Med* 1994;11:480–484.

25. Abbott CA, Vileikyte L, Williamson S, *et al.* Multicenter study of the incidence of and predictive risk factors for diabetic neuropathic foot ulceration. *Diabetes Care* 1998;21:1071–1075.

26. Ramsey SD, Newton K, Blough D, *et al.* Incidence, outcomes, and cost of foot ulcers in patients with diabetes. *Diabetes Care* 1999;22:382–387.

27. Abbott CA, Carrington AL, Ashe H, *et al.* The North-West Diabetes Foot Care Study: incidence of, and risk factors for, new diabetic foot ulceration in a community-based patient cohort. *Diabet Med* 2002;19:377–384.

28. Muller IS, de Grauw WJ, van Gerwen WH, *et al.* Foot ulceration and lower limb amputation in type 2 diabetic patients in Dutch primary health care. *Diabetes Care* 2002;25:570–574.

29. Centers for Disease Control and Prevention. History of foot ulcer among persons with diabetes – United States, 2000–2002. *MMWR Morb Mortal Wkly Rep* 2003;52:1098–1102.

30. Boyko EJ, Ahroni JH, Stensel V, *et al.* A prospective study of risk factors for diabetic foot ulcer. The Seattle Diabetic Foot Study. *Diabetes Care* 1999;22:1036–1042.

31. Holewski JJ, Moss KM, Stess RM, *et al.* Prevalence of foot pathology and lower extremity complications in a diabetic outpatient clinic. *J Rehabil Res Dev* 1989;26:35–44.

32. Wikblad K, Smide B, Bergstrom A, *et al*. Outcome of clinical foot examination in relation to self-perceived health and glycaemic control in a group of urban Tanzanian diabetic patients. *Diabetes Res Clin Pract* 1997;37:185–192.
33. Nielsen JV. Peripheral neuropathy, hypertension, foot ulcers and amputations among Saudi Arabian patients with type 2 diabetes. *Diabetes Res Clin Pract* 1998;41:63–69.
34. Vijay V, Narasimham DV, Seena R, *et al*. Clinical profile of diabetic foot infections in south India – a retrospective study. *Diabet Med* 2000;17:215–218.
35. Pham H, Armstrong DG, Harvey C, *et al*. Screening techniques to identify people at high risk for diabetic foot ulceration: a prospective multicenter trial. *Diabetes Care* 2000;23:606–611.
36. Monabeka HG, Nsakala-Kibangou N. Epidemiological and clinical aspects of the diabetic foot at the Central University Hospital of Brazzaville. *Bull Soc Pathol Exot* 2001;94:246–248.
37. Kastenbauer T, Sauseng S, Sokol G, *et al*. A prospective study of predictors for foot ulceration in type 2 diabetes. *J Am Podiatr Med Assoc* 2001;91:343–350.
38. Gulliford MC, Mahabir D. Diabetic foot disease and foot care in a Caribbean community. *Diabetes Res Clin Pract* 2002;56:35–40.
39. Carrington AL, Shaw JE, van Schie CH, *et al*. Can motor nerve conduction velocity predict foot problems in diabetic subjects over a 6-year outcome period? *Diabetes Care* 2002;25:2010–2015.
40. Nyamu PN, Otieno CF, Amayo EO, *et al*. Risk factors and prevalence of diabetic foot ulcers at Kenyatta National Hospital, Nairobi. *East Afr Med J* 2003;80:36–43.
41. Stein H, Yaacobi E, Steinberg R. The diabetic foot: update on a common clinical syndrome. *Orthopedics* 2003;26:1127–1130.
42. Malgrange D, Richard JL, Leymarie F, *et al*. Screening diabetic patients at risk for foot ulceration. A multi-centre hospital-based study in France. *Diabetes Metab* 2003;29:261–268.
43. Lavery LA, Armstrong DG, Wunderlich RP, *et al*. Predictive value of foot pressure assessment as part of a population-based diabetes disease management program. *Diabetes Care* 2003;26:1069–1073.
44. Lavery LA, Armstrong DG, Wunderlich RP, *et al*. Diabetic foot syndrome: evaluating the prevalence and incidence of foot pathology in Mexican Americans and non-Hispanic whites from a diabetes disease management cohort. *Diabetes Care* 2003;26:1435–1438.
45. Deerochanawong C, Home PD, Alberti KG. A survey of lower limb amputation in diabetic patients. *Diabet Med* 1992;9:942–946.
46. Apelqvist J, Larsson J, Agardh CD. Long-term prognosis for diabetic patients with foot ulcers. *J Intern Med* 1993;233:485–491.
47. Reiber GE, Lipsky BA, Gibbons GW. The burden of diabetic foot ulcers. *Am J Surg* 1998;176:5S–10S.
48. HCUP Databases. *Healthcare Cost and Utilization Project (HCUP). Nationwide Inpatient Sample.* Rockville, MD: Agency for Healthcare Research and Quality; June 2005. Available from: www.hcup-us.ahrq.gov/nisoverview.jsp. (updated 2005 Jun 20; cited 2005 Aug 14).
49. Litzelman DK, Slemenda CW, Langefeld CD, *et al*. Reduction of lower extremity clinical abnormalities in patients with non-insulin-dependent diabetes mellitus. A randomized, controlled trial. *Ann Intern Med* 1993;119:36–41.
50. McNeely MJ, Boyko EJ, Ahroni JH, *et al*. The independent contributions of diabetic neuropathy and vasculopathy in foot ulceration. How great are the risks? *Diabetes Care* 1995;18:216–219.
51. Morbach S, Lutale JK, Viswanathan V, *et al*. Regional differences in risk factors and clinical presentation of diabetic foot lesions. *Diabet Med* 2004;21:91–95.
52. Bauman JH, Girling JP, Brand PW. Plantar pressures and trophic ulceration: an evaluation of footwear. *J Bone Joint Surg Br* 1963;45B:652–673.
53. Mueller MJ, Diamond JE, Delitto A, *et al*. Insensitivity, limited joint mobility, and plantar ulcers in patients with diabetes mellitus. *Phys Ther* 1989;69:453–459.
54. Zimny S, Schatz H, Pfohl M. The role of limited joint mobility in diabetic patients with an at-risk foot. *Diabetes Care* 2004;27:942–946.

55. Robertson DD, Mueller MJ, Smith KE, *et al.* Structural changes in the forefoot of individuals with diabetes and a prior plantar ulcer. *J Bone Joint Surg Am* 2002;84A:1395–1404.
56. Mueller MJ, Hastings M, Commean PK, *et al.* Forefoot structural predictors of plantar pressures during walking in people with diabetes and peripheral neuropathy. *J Biomech* 2003;36:1009–1017.
57. van Schie CH, Vermigli C, Carrington AL, *et al.* Muscle weakness and foot deformities in diabetes: relationship to neuropathy and foot ulceration in Caucasian diabetic men. *Diabetes Care* 2004;27:1668–1673.
58. Veves A, Murray HJ, Young MJ, *et al.* The risk of foot ulceration in diabetic patients with high foot pressure: a prospective study. *Diabetologia* 1992;35:660–663.
59. Armstrong DG, Peters EJ, Athanasiou KA, *et al.* Is there a critical level of plantar foot pressure to identify patients at risk for neuropathic foot ulceration? *J Foot Ankle Surg* 1998;37:303–307.
60. Maluf KS, Mueller MJ. Novel Award 2002. Comparison of physical activity and cumulative plantar tissue stress among subjects with and without diabetes mellitus and a history of recurrent plantar ulcers. *Clin Biomech (Bristol, Avon)* 2003;18:567–575.
61. Ledoux WR, Cowley MS, Ahroni JH, *et al.* No relationship between plantar pressure and diabetic foot ulcer incidence after adjustment for ulcer location. *Diabetes* 2005;54:A17.
62. Maluf KS, Morley RE Jr, Richter EJ, *et al.* Monitoring in-shoe plantar pressures, temperature, and humidity: reliability and validity of measures from a portable device. *Arch Phys Med Rehabil* 2001;82:1119–1127.
63. Oyibo SO, Jude EB, Tarawneh I, *et al.* The effects of ulcer size and site, patient's age, sex and type and duration of diabetes on the outcome of diabetic foot ulcers. *Diabet Med* 2001;18:133–138.
64. Margolis DJ, Allen-Taylor L, Hoffstad O, *et al.* Diabetic neuropathic foot ulcers: the association of wound size, wound duration, and wound grade on healing. *Diabetes Care* 2002;25:1835–1839.
65. Sheehan P, Jones P, Caselli A, *et al.* Percent change in wound area of diabetic foot ulcers over a 4-week period is a robust predictor of complete healing in a 12-week prospective trial. *Diabetes Care* 2003;26:1879–1882.
66. Pecoraro RE, Ahroni JH, Boyko EJ, *et al.* Chronology and determinants of tissue repair in diabetic lower-extremity ulcers. *Diabetes* 1991;40:1305–1313.
67. Mantey I, Foster AV, Spencer S, *et al.* Why do foot ulcers recur in diabetic patients? *Diabet Med* 1999;16:245–249.
68. Connor H, Mahdi OZ. Repetitive ulceration in neuropathic patients. *Diabetes Metab Res Rev* 2004;20:S23–S28.
69. Apelqvist J, Ragnarson-Tennvall G, Persson U, *et al.* Diabetic foot ulcers in a multidisciplinary setting. An economic analysis of primary healing and healing with amputation. *J Intern Med* 1994;235:463–471.
70. Center for Medicare Services. *Diagnostic Related Groups Inpatient Billing Data*; 2005. Available from: www.cms.hhs.gov/statistics/medpar/DRG500_02_i.pdf. (updated 2003 Jun; cited 2005 Aug 14).
71. Medstat. *Diagnostic Related Groups Billing Data 2002.* Ann Arbor, MI: Medstat; 2005.

2 The Epidemiology of Amputations and the Influence of Ethnicity

Nish Chaturvedi

INTRODUCTION

Despite encouraging trends,[1,2] rates of non-traumatic amputation in people with diabetes remain some 10–20-fold higher than in those without diabetes.[3,4] Costs associated with diabetes-related amputation are high,[5] due to prolonged inpatient stays and co-morbidity, and risks of further limb surgery are greater than in non-diabetic individuals with amputation (37% vs 20%).[4] Post-amputation mortality risks rival those of cancer, the median survival duration being 2–5 years.[6–9]

WHY STUDY THE EPIDEMIOLOGY OF AMPUTATION?

Examination of the epidemiology of amputation is valuable for a number of reasons. Firstly, it facilitates dissection of key risk factors, and allows us to understand their relative importance, thus providing evidence for the likely benefit of interventions. Secondly, geographical differences in rates and time trend data demonstrate potential and actual impacts of changes in risk factors, and effect of interventions.[3] Such analysis is particularly important in the study of complex conditions, of which amputation is a good example. There is no one single risk factor for non-traumatic diabetes-related amputation; rather, it is the end point of a series of complex inter-relationships between diabetes-specific factors, including general environmental risk factors, such as smoking, quality of health care services, and personal commitment to disease prevention. These will be discussed in more detail later in the chapter.

INTERPRETING EPIDEMIOLOGICAL STUDIES OF AMPUTATION

Estimating Amputation Rates

Before demonstrating what epidemiological studies have told us about the risks and aetiology of amputation, it is first worth considering the strengths and limitations of study design. Estimation

The Foot in Diabetes, 4th Edition. Editors Andrew J.M. Boulton, Peter R. Cavanagh and Gerry Rayman.
© 2006 John Wiley & Sons, Ltd.

of amputation rates for comparative purposes, either at the same time point across different locations, or in a single location over time, would at first glance appear simple. The end point is easy to identify, and the sources of information that need to be consulted are limited by the fact that some type of surgical intervention is required. However, even here there is evidence that limiting the search to operating lists, hospital discharge systems or referrals to limb-fitting centres will miss a number of cases.[10,11] For a given location, searches must be made on neighbouring hospital databases, to ensure that all cross-boundary outcomes are captured. In addition, some locations will release only anonymised data, and so repeat amputations and incident (i.e. first-time) amputations are difficult to identify unless detailed case note review is performed on all cases. Correct classification of diabetes status, even perhaps surprisingly in amputees, is complicated by inappropriate or missing notification of diabetes on computerised databases or in clinical records and even in some instances where diabetes has not been formally tested for.[11] Prospective data collection is preferred to retrospective, as this is thought to improve the quality of the data and overcome some of the limitations described above.

There are several different opinions as to how to classify amputations, from quite detailed anatomical location to a dichotomisation between major and minor. One of the valuable tasks performed by the Lower Extremity Amputation (LEA) Study Group is to agree to a set of definitions for amputation level.[12]

Probably the most difficult problem is access to high-quality, age- and gender-specific data on diabetes prevalence in these locations, which provide the denominator for calculation of incidence rates. Unless a high-quality population-based register exists, as it does, for example, for The Diabetes Audit and Research in Tayside Scotland – Medicines Monitoring Unit (DARTS–MEMO) group,[4] the investigator is forced to rely on extrapolations from specific prevalence studies or national health surveys, where they exist.[10] Estimation of incidence of amputation using routine census data may result in data that are difficult to interpret, as variations could be due to either differences in underlying prevalence of diabetes, or a true difference in amputation risk.

Exploring Risk Factors for Amputation

The approach employed to understand risk factors for amputation, rather than incidence rates, is somewhat different. Here, the need is not so much of a comprehensive collection of all cases within a given location, but of proper attention to high-quality data on risk factors in a sample of cases with amputation. Many studies have utilised a case–control approach to identify risk factors for amputation. To qualify as a risk factor, a potential aetiological agent would have to be more prevalent in cases (people with diabetes who had had an amputation), compared to controls (people with diabetes and no history of amputation). This is a logical epidemiological approach to the study of rare diseases, but has major potential for bias. Selecting a source population for controls is problematic, as choosing individuals in hospital for reasons other than amputation, on the face of it an easily accessible source of controls, may restrict selection to individuals with quite severe diabetes complications, making it difficult to tease out any differences between cases and controls. Assessment of risk factors is often dependent on previously collected data, with varying quality control. Assigning a temporal relationship between risk factor and disease may prove difficult if, for example, all that is available is a glucose level at the time of amputation, and incidence, i.e. rates of new disease, cannot be estimated.

A better study design is a cohort study, where risk factors of interest are measured to a standardised protocol in a large number of individuals, who are then followed up to determine development of amputation. Risk factor profiles are then compared between those who did and did not develop amputations, and their impact on the incidence of amputation can be established. The major drawback of this study design is that a large number of people with diabetes, probably in their thousands, need to be included, and follow-up would need to continue for a number of years in order to yield sufficient cases. Ideally, changes in risk factors, such as repeated estimates of glycaemic control, and incidence and progression of neuropathy and peripheral arterial disease (PAD), need to be measured.

From previous studies, it is clear that the duration of follow-up in part determines the relative statistical importance of risk factors. For example, a 4-year follow-up of the Wisconsin Epidemiologic Study of Diabetic Retinopathy (WESDR) cohort indicated that blood pressure and glycated haemoglobin were related to amputation risk, but microvascular complications were not.[13] In contrast, in the longer term follow-up in the World Health Organisation Multinational Study of Vascular Disease in Diabetes (WHO MSVDD) study (around 9 years), microvascular complications dominated.[14] It is likely that microvascular complications, representing a long-term measure of vascular damage, which change modestly over time, will act as better predictors over long periods of time than factors such as glycated haemoglobin and blood pressure, which vary substantially over quite short periods of time, and given the historical context of these earlier cohort studies, were more likely to be altered due to treatment than the microvascular complications. Older studies have the difficulty that assessment of the two key risk factors, peripheral neuropathy and PAD, was somewhat crude, leaving scope for residual confounding, i.e. inability to wholly account for the effects of a risk factor, due to inadequate measurement. Newer studies, where assessment of such complications is more accurate, are beset by the fact that as amputation rates have declined, the numbers of individuals required for well-powered cohort studies have increased. A potential solution is to study a high-risk population, where prevalence of diabetes is high so that recruitment is facilitated. This explains why a large part of our understanding of the aetiology of amputation comes from study of special groups, such as native American populations.

But even when the gold standard cohort approach is employed, comparisons of findings between each individual study are limited due to differences in definition of both the outcome (amputation) and the risk factors, in particular neuropathy. Time trend comparisons of risk factors are complex, as methods to detect risk factors, such as neuropathy and PAD, have changed, largely to increased sensitivity and improved objectivity. Not all risk factors can be easily measured, and the complex interactions between factors mean that a whole host of factors need to be assembled, some associated with health care access and delivery and some related to preventive self-foot care. These factors are difficult to assess objectively.[11]

Risk Factors For Amputation

Major environmental risk factors for amputation

From these previous epidemiological studies, it is clear that the key clinical risk factors for amputation in diabetes are the complications of peripheral neuropathy and PAD (Figure 2.1).[15] The exact mechanism by which these complications occur and interact to reach the stage of amputation is again complex and not fully understood. Clearly, abnormal glucose levels and

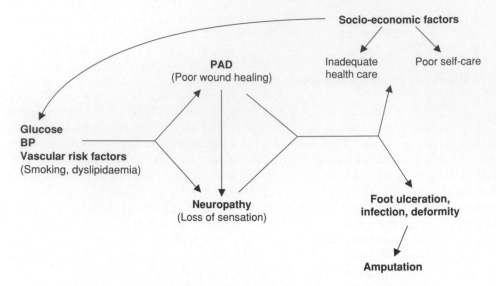

Figure 2.1   Inter-relationships between risk factors for diabetic limb amputation

toxic products associated with elevations of glucose, such as advanced glycation end products, play a role,[16] an assertion supported by the observation that strict glycaemic control can improve peripheral neuropathy.[17] In addition to glucose, as expected, cardiovascular disease (CVD) risk factors, in particular smoking, are the key risk factors for PAD.[18–21] It is often difficult to tease out which factors are specific to neuropathy, and which to PAD, as there is a tight within-individual correlation between presence of PAD and peripheral neuropathy,[22] which may simply reflect coexistence of complications due to upstream risk factors, such as abnormal blood glucose, rather than a causative relationship. But there is an increasing evidence that the microcirculation plays a direct role in the aetiology of neuropathy, with abnormalities of the vasa vasorum, the microcirculation surrounding peripheral nerve fibres responsible for the diffusion of nutrients and clearance of waste products, resulting in nerve damage.[23] Strong evidence for a vascular contribution to diabetic neuropathy comes from an intervention study with an angiotensin-converting enzyme inhibitor, which had a beneficial effect on neuropathy compared to placebo.[24]

The impact of peripheral neuropathy on amputation risk is in large part due to loss of peripheral sensation.[25] This has a number of adverse consequences. Repeated trauma to pressure points results in foot deformities, and loss of sensation means that such abnormalities and any wounds are not sensed. These unnoted injuries progress to chronic ulceration. PAD compounds these problems. Wound healing is poor due to poor circulation, and osteomyelitis and gangrene are common sequelae of infection. Advanced infection and ulceration, therefore, threaten the viability of the limb, and amputation has to be considered.[26]

Unalterable risk factors for amputation

Unavoidable risk factors for amputation are age and male gender.[4,27–30] Men with diabetes consistently have rates of amputation that are twice those of women.[31] The reasons for this are largely differences in the key risk factors, peripheral neuropathy[32] and PAD, the latter in large part due to gender differences in smoking rates.

Role of socio-economic status and care provision

Non-clinical factors also make a contribution to amputation risk. There are marked geographical and socio-economic variations in amputation rates, which cannot be accounted for by clinical risk factors alone.[3] The impact of patient and health care factors is apparent at all points of the amputation pathway. Good-quality health care and patient concordance with medical advice can normalise blood glucose levels and reduce vascular risk by proper management of blood pressure, dyslipidaemia and cessation of smoking.[33] Further along the disease pathway, attention to regular foot inspections, foot hygiene and appropriate footwear reduces the progression of early diabetic foot disease, including development of foot deformities, and highlights the presence of infection or injury at an early stage, where treatment is more likely to be successful.[34] Early presentation also means that conservative surgery, or vascular reconstructive surgery, can be undertaken, in order to save the foot.

There are clear indications that poor socio-economic status, measured by education, income or occupation, is a strong predictor of amputation.[31,35] It is not surprising that people of low socio-economic status are at a disadvantage at all points of the care process. A lack of education means that it is less likely that these individuals will be aware of the importance of preventive measures.[36] Attendance at primary and secondary care facilities is likely to be infrequent, as physical barriers to getting to such sources of care are greater for these individuals, and getting time off work to attend clinics is likely to be harder. In addition, the quality of care provided to these high-risk groups is likely to be poorer, the so-called inverse care law.[37] This is true in countries where access to high-quality health care depends on the ability to pay, as in the United States, but also in countries where in theory, care is freely available to all, regardless of financial status.

Further, even when there are few barriers to care, variations in practice, capacity, and availability of surgical services may also influence amputation rate.[3,38]

TIME TRENDS IN AMPUTATION RATES

Apart from establishing aetiological risk factors, epidemiological investigation can also help to determine the impact of intervention. Examinations of recent time trend data[1,2] show marked reductions in rates of amputation. An absolute reduction in all amputations (i.e. in those with and without diabetes) of 41% between 1984 and 2000 has been reported.[2] Over the same time period, infrainguinal reconstructions rose by 372%. It was postulated by the authors that the latter largely explained the former, a suggestion supported by others.[39,40] However, in this particular study in Finland, the decline in amputation was also preceded by the establishment of a diabetic foot care team, and one cannot be certain that the decline in amputation was due to surgery alone. Indeed, there is clear evidence that the decline in amputation rates is rather largely due to better-quality foot care.[41] This question was examined in the Netherlands, where the analysis could be restricted just to people with diabetes. Here, there was an almost doubling in provision of podiatrists and multidisciplinary foot teams occurring from 1995 to 2000, which coincided with a nearly 40% reduction in amputation risk.[1] The number of surgical interventions for PAD did not increase during this period, leading the authors to conclude that it was the provision of more foot care teams that resulted in the marked decline in amputation rates.

WHY STUDY ETHNIC DIFFERENCES IN DIABETES-RELATED AMPUTATION?

The study of ethnic differences in amputation can contribute substantially to our understanding of this condition. Given the close correlation and interdependence of the risk factors for amputation, determining which factors are causally independent, which are downstream on the causal pathway, and which are simple confounders is therefore challenging. Observational studies of interethnic differences in disease are therefore extremely valuable in this regard. Risks and correlates of disease may differ by ethnicity, breaking the natural confounding between disease and risk factors found in majority populations. For example, people of Black African descent in Africa, the Caribbean, and the United Kingdom have relatively high risks of stroke, but relatively low risks of coronary disease, compared with White European populations.[42] Study of this natural breakdown of concordance of cardiovascular disease helps to establish which risk factors are particularly important for stroke, and which for coronary disease. Such questions could not be addressed by simple examination of a White European population, where concordance between stroke and heart disease is high. Further, confirming that a particular risk factor plays a key role in determining amputation likelihood in a number of different populations provides reassurance that that factor is an important causal agent.

ETHNIC DIFFERENCES IN DIABETES-RELATED AMPUTATION RISK

American Indians

American Indians have one of the highest rates of diabetes-related amputation in the world.[6,14,43–46] Risks of amputation are eightfold higher in type 1 diabetes and threefold higher in type 2 diabetes, compared with European populations.[14] Risk factors appear to be similar however *within* each of these ethnic groups. In type 2 diabetes, these were disease duration, glucose, male gender, the presence of other microvascular complications, in particular retinopathy and nephropathy, and dyslipidaemia, in particular raised triglyceride, which increased amputation risk.[6,14,31,44] There were indications that interactions may exist, i.e. the presence of one risk factor, such as poor glycaemic control, may substantially compound the effect of another, such as renal disease, on amputation.[31] None of these factors singly or in combination could account for differences *between* American Indians and Europeans. Residual ethnic differences in amputation risk after statistical adjustment for risk factors may be due to incomplete measurement of, and thus incomplete adjustment for, key risk factors.

Hispanic Americans

Amputation risk in Hispanic Americans has been variously reported to be equivalent to,[47] lower than,[48] or 1.2–2-fold higher than that of the non-Hispanic White population in the United

States.[49–52] This disparity may be due to variable differences between Hispanic and non-Hispanic populations in self-care and access to high-quality medical care.[53] But this may not be the whole explanation. While key risk factors, such as prevalence of peripheral neuropathy and PAD, did not differ between these ethnic groups, intervention types did. Mexican Americans were less likely to undergo lower extremity bypass surgery, more likely to be categorised as unsuitable for a bypass, and more likely to have a failed bypass.[50] So, although differential access to high-quality health care, and poor self-foot care, in Mexican Americans is clearly a problem, and has been shown in other studies to account for ethnic differences,[54] the authors also hypothesised that higher amputation rates in Mexican Americans reflected a greater prevalence of non-reconstructable distal vessels.[50,55]

Populations of Black African Descent

Study of people of Black African descent worldwide has provided useful insights into the balance of diabetes-related risk factors, cardiovascular risk factors, and the importance of high-quality health care. Comparative interethnic data first emerged from the United States, where diabetes-related amputation rates in African Americans were found to be two- to threefold greater than the rates in US Whites.[27,35,48,56] Interestingly, non-diabetes-related amputation rates were not different. Conventional risk factors could not wholly account for the interethnic difference in amputation rates. It is well known that people of Black African descent have poorer access to good-quality health insurance, are less likely to be offered preventive screening and are less likely to undergo lower extremity revascularisation.[57–59] When insurance status or indeed educational status (both proxies for access to health care) is taken into account, several, but not all, studies suggested that the ethnic difference in amputation risk disappeared.[35,53,54,60] These striking findings indicate that poor-quality care increases risk of amputation twofold, and highlights the scope that health care interventions can have to reduce the risk.

In contrast, studies in the United Kingdom tell quite a different story. The United Kingdom is a setting where access to health care should be equitable, being free at the point of delivery. Thus, we would anticipate that people of Black African descent in the United Kingdom (African Caribbeans) would have equivalent diabetes-related amputation rates to Europeans. In fact, rates of amputation in African Caribbean men were around a third that of European men.[61] In women though, risks did not differ by ethnicity. The marked ethnic difference in men but not women provides a clue as to why amputation rates are so low in people of Black African descent in the United Kingdom. As stated above, African Caribbeans have particularly low rates of ischaemic heart disease (IHD).[14,42] This is more pronounced in men than in women. This protection from IHD is related to low rates of PAD in African Caribbeans, with again the ethnic difference being more pronounced in men. Indeed, ethnic differences in PAD could account for much of the protection from amputation observed in African Caribbeans, with low smoking and neuropathy rates further contributing to the low risk, such that the risk of amputation in African Caribbeans compared to Europeans was 0.97 when these protective factors were taken into account. This confirms findings from the United Kingdom Prospective Diabetes Study (UKPDS), where African Caribbeans with newly diagnosed diabetes had less PAD, and less neuropathy, at least as assessed by biothesiometry, than Europeans.[62] Why is this not the case in the United States? In the early part of the twentieth century, African Americans were protected from heart disease to a similar extent to that observed in current

African Caribbeans in the United Kingdom. However, the ethnic difference in IHD risk in the United States has attenuated over time, such that rates are either equivalent to or even higher than the rates in US Whites. Rates of PAD are similarly high.[63] In addition, neuropathy rates do not differ between African Americans and US Whites.[64] The reasons for this are not known, but acculturation and miscegenation, given the longer duration of residence of people of Black African descent in the United States compared to the United Kingdom, could play a role. Notably, smoking rates do not differ by ethnicity to the same extent in the United States as they do in the United Kingdom.

Strikingly, rates of amputation in the Caribbean are high, with around 75% of all amputations being performed in people with diabetes. Rates were around 950 per 100 000 population,[65] equivalent to those found in the United States,[48] but at least threefold higher compared to UK rates.[61] This is puzzling, given that much of the UK African Caribbean populations in the at-risk age group are first-generation migrants largely from the Caribbean. Investigation of risk factors suggested that the most important was the use of ill-fitting footwear (both soft or no shoes worn daily, coupled with tight shoes worn once weekly to church), which increased the risk of amputation threefold. In addition, inadequate self-foot inspection increased risk, emphasising the importance of this simple activity in reducing risk. Clinical predictive factors included glycated haemoglobin, PAD, and neuropathy. From the study, it was clear that around a quarter of all amputees had been admitted to hospital the previous year, and thus should have been well known to the health care system; yet delays of around a week occurred before the individual sought help after noting an injury or ulcer, and the median time to admission post-injury was 3 weeks. Again, studies like these provide clear evidence of the need for and benefits of intervention targeted at both the patient and the health care professional.

Amputation associated with diabetes was until recently a rare event in Africa itself, but there are now indications, with increasing development, that the contribution of diabetes to amputation has now increased; current estimates stand at 30% of all amputations being due to diabetes.[66] Of note is the young mean age at amputation in these populations, which at around 59 years[67] is substantially younger than that for comparator United Kingdom (63 years) and Caribbean (70 years) populations.[61,65]

Such striking disparities within a given ethnic group but between different locations do not support a genetic explanation for variations in risk. As described above, many of the differences observed between populations of Black African descent in different locations are due to access to health care, socio-economic status or, in the case of the Caribbean, greater exposure to infection and minor trauma. Of course the lower PAD rates observed in the UK African Caribbean population, consonant with the lower IHD rates compared to Europeans, may have a genetic component. But again, an argument against this statement is that in the last century, IHD rates were also lower in African Americans compared to US Whites, and that is not consistently the case now.[68] A genetic explanation for low IHD rates could not conceivably have altered in such a short space of time, and it is likely that environmental factors have played a major role in this IHD risk reversal.

Indian Asians

Studies of the UK South Asian population provide a very different contrast to the story for UK African Caribbeans. South Asian people worldwide share an elevated risk of stroke, diabetes and insulin resistance,[69,70] and thus resemble the disease profile of African Caribbeans in many regards. However, unlike the African Caribbeans, South Asians have markedly elevated risks of IHD compared to White Europeans.[42] At first glance, this would lead us to believe that South Asians would also have elevated risks of amputation. But studies in the United Kingdom consistently show a much lower risk of diabetes-related amputation, being about a quarter that of the host population.[7,71,72] Key risk factors that account for this ethnic difference are the lower rates of PAD, peripheral neuropathy, and smoking in South Asians, attenuating the risk ratio from 0.26 in favour of South Asians to just 0.84.[72] Low rates of PAD in South Asians have been reported both from the United Kingdom[62,73] and from India.[74,75] The reasons for these ethnic differences in neuropathy and PAD are unclear, and the latter particularly surprising given the high rates of both IHD and stroke. However, it is clear that CVD risk factors have different impacts on atherosclerosis, depending upon site. Smoking is a strong risk factor for PAD,[18] and its impact may be greater here than on IHD. In contrast, abnormal lipids are weaker predictors of PAD than they are of IHD. This has implications for understanding the paradoxical low risk of PAD, but high risk of IHD in South Asian populations. South Asian groups in general smoke either a lot less or just as much as European-origin populations, but dyslipidaemia, in particular elevated triglyceride levels, is more pronounced.[70]

At first glance, data from the United States would support UK findings of lower risks of amputation in Asian populations,[52,54] in part at least explained by lower rates of peripheral neuropathy in one of these studies[54] PAD was not assessed in either study. However, on closer inspection, these data refer to individuals of Far East Asian descent, largely Filipino, and cannot be compared with the Indo-Asian populations discussed above. The former are known to have lower rates of myocardial infarction in particular, which may account for a degree of protection from amputation, but this situation is not comparable to the situation in Indo-Asians, who have a greater risk of IHD.

CONCLUSIONS

Although absolute risk is declining, given the large numbers of people surviving to older age and increasing incidence of diabetes particularly in the young, resulting in greater duration of exposure to diabetes, it is likely that absolute numbers of people requiring amputation will increase rather than decrease.

REFERENCES

1. van Houtum WH, Rauwerda JA, Ruwaard D, Schaper NC, Bakker K. Reduction in diabetes-related lower-extremity amputations in The Netherlands: 1991–2000. *Diabetes Care* 2004;27:1042–1046.
2. Eskelinen E, Lepantalo M, Hietala EM, *et al.* Lower limb amputations in Southern Finland in 2000 and trends up to 2001. *Eur J Vasc Endovasc Surg* 2004;27:193–200.
3. Wrobel JS, Mayfield JA, Reiber GE. Geographic variation of lower-extremity major amputation in individuals with and without diabetes in the Medicare population. *Diabetes Care* 2001;24:860–864.
4. Morris AD, McAlpine R, Steinke D, *et al.* Diabetes and lower-limb amputations in the community. A retrospective cohort study. DARTS/MEMO Collaboration. Diabetes Audit and Research in Tayside Scotland/Medicines Monitoring Unit. *Diabetes Care* 1998;21:738–743.
5. Waugh NR. Amputations in diabetic patients – a review of rates, relative risks and resource use. *Community Med* 1988;10:279–288.

6. Lee JS, Lu M, Lee VS, Russell D, Bahr C, Lee ET. Lower-extremity amputation. Incidence, risk factors, and mortality in the Oklahoma Indian Diabetes Study. *Diabetes* 1993;42:876–882.

7. Deerochanawong C, Home PD, Alberti KGMM. A survey of lower limb amputation in diabetic patients. *Diabet Med* 1992;9:942–946.

8. Aulivola B, Hile CN, Hamdan AD, *et al.* Major lower extremity amputation: outcome of a modern series. *Arch Surg* 2004;139:395–399.

9. Lindegard P, Jonsson B, Lithner F. Amputations in diabetic patients in Gotland and Umea counties 1971–1980. *Acta Med Scand Suppl* 1984;687:89–93.

10. Rayman G, Krishnan ST, Baker NR, Wareham AM, Rayman A. Are we underestimating diabetes-related lower-extremity amputation rates? Results and benefits of the first prospective study. *Diabetes Care* 2004;27:1892–1896.

11. van Houtum WH, Lavery LA. Methodological issues affect variability in reported incidence of lower extremity amputations due to diabetes. *Diabetes Res Clin Pract* 1997;38:177–183.

12. The LEA Study Group. Comparing the incidence of lower extremity amputations across the world: the Global Lower Extremity Amputation Study. *Diabet Med* 1995;12:14–18.

13. Moss SE, Klein R, Klein BEK. The prevalence and incidence of lower extremity amputation in a diabetic population. *Arch Intern Med* 1992;152:610–616.

14. Chaturvedi N, Stevens LK, Fuller JH, Lee ET, Lu M. Risk factors, ethnic differences and mortality associated with lower-extremity gangrene and amputation in diabetes. The WHO Multinational Study of Vascular Disease in Diabetes. *Diabetologia* 2001;44:S65–S71.

15. Reiber GE, Pecorraro RE, Koepsell TD. Risk factors for amputation in patients with diabetes mellitus: a case–control study. *Ann Intern Med* 1992;117:97–105.

16. Carrington AL, Litchfield JE. The aldose reductase pathway and nonenzymatic glycation in the pathogenesis of diabetic neuropathy: a critical review for the end of the 20th century. *Diabetes Rev* 1999;7:275–299.

17. Amthor K-F, Dahl-Jorgensen K, Berg TJ, *et al.* The effect of 8 years strict glycaemic control on peripheral nerve function in IDDM patients: the Oslo Study. *Diabetologia* 1994;37:579–584.

18. Fowkes FG, Housley E, Riemersma RA, *et al.* Smoking, lipids, glucose intolerance, and blood pressure as risk factors for peripheral atherosclerosis compared with ischaemic heart disease in the Edinburgh Artery Study. *Am J Epidemiol* 1992;135:331–340.

19. Wattanakit K, Folsom AR, Selvin E, *et al.* Risk factors for peripheral arterial disease incidence in persons with diabetes: the Atherosclerosis Risk in Communities (ARIC) Study. *Atherosclerosis* 2005;180:389–397.

20. Hamalainen H, Ronnemaa T, Halonen JP, Toikka T. Factors predicting lower extremity amputations in patients with type 1 or type 2 diabetes mellitus: a population-based 7-year follow-up study. *J Intern Med* 1999;246:97–103.

21. Moss SE, Klein R, Klein BE. The 14-year incidence of lower-extremity amputations in a diabetic population. The Wisconsin Epidemiologic Study of Diabetic Retinopathy. *Diabetes Care* 1999;22:951–959.

22. Carrington AL, Abbott CA, Griffiths J, *et al.* Peripheral vascular and nerve function associated with lower limb amputation in people with and without diabetes. *Clin Sci* 2001;101:261–266.

23. Tesfaye S, Malik R, Ward JD. Vascular factors in diabetic neuropathy. *Diabetologia* 1994;37:847–854.

24. Malik RA, Williamson S, Abbott C, *et al.* Effect of angiotensin-converting-enzyme (ACE) inhibitor trandolapril on human diabetic neuropathy: randomised double-blind controlled trial. *Lancet* 1998;352:1978–1981.

25. Adler AI, Ahroni JH, Boyko EJ, Smith DG. Lower extremity amputation in diabetes: the independent effects of peripheral vascular disease, sensory neuropathy, and foot ulcers. *Diabetes Care* 1999;22:1029–1035.

26. Pecoraro RE, Reiber GE, Burgess EM. Pathways to diabetic limb amputation. Basis for prevention. *Diabetes Care* 1990;13:513–521.

27. Most RS, Sinnock P. The epidemiology of lower extremity amputations in diabetic individuals. *Diabetes Care* 1983;6:87–91.
28. Siitonen OI, Niskanen LK, Laakso M, Siitonen JT, Pyorala K. Lower-extremity amputations in diabetic and non diabetic patients. A population based study in Eastern Finland. *Diabetes Care* 1993;16:16–20.
29. Armstrong DG, Lavery LA, van Houtum WH, Harkless LB. The impact of gender on amputation. *J Foot Ankle Surg* 1997;36:66–69.
30. Group TG. Epidemiology of lower extremity amputation in centres in Europe, North America and East Asia. The global lower extremity amputation study group. *Br J Surg* 2000;87:328–337.
31. Resnick HE, Carter EA, Lindsay R, *et al.* Relation of lower-extremity amputation to all-cause and cardiovascular disease mortality in American Indians: the Strong Heart Study. *Diabetes Care* 2004;27:1286–1293.
32. Sorensen L, Molyneaux L, Yue DK. Insensate versus painful diabetic neuropathy: the effects of height, gender, ethnicity and glycaemic control. *Diabetes Res Clin Pract* 2002;57:45–51.
33. Loveman E, Cave C, Green C, Royle P, Dunn N, Waugh N. The clinical and cost-effectiveness of patient education models for diabetes: a systematic review and economic evaluation. *Health Technol Assess* 2003;7:iii, 1–190.
34. Mayfield JA, Reiber GE, Sanders LJ, Janisse D, Pogach LM. Preventive foot care in people with diabetes. *Diabetes Care* 1998;21:2161–2177.
35. Resnick HE, Valsania P, Phillips CL. Diabetes mellitus and nontraumatic lower extremity amputation in black and white Americans: the National Health and Nutrition Examination Survey Epidemiologic Follow-up. *Arch Intern Med* 1999;159:2470–2475.
36. Adams AS, Mah C, Soumerai SB, Zhang F, Barton MB, Ross-Degnan D. Barriers to self-monitoring of blood glucose among adults with diabetes in an HMO: a cross sectional study. *BMC Health Serv Res* 2003;3:6.
37. Hart JT. The inverse care law. *Lancet* 1971;i:405–412.
38. Wennberg JE. Understanding geographic variations in health care delivery. *N Engl J Med* 1999;340:52–53.
39. Lindholt JS, Bovling S, Fasting H, Henneberg EW. Vascular surgery reduces the frequency of lower limb major amputations. *Eur J Vasc Surg* 1994; 8:31–35.
40. Pedersen AE, Bornefeldt OB, Krasnik M, *et al.* Halving the number of leg amputations: the influence of infrapopliteal bypass. *Eur J Vasc Surg* 1994;8:26–30.
41. Larsson J, Apelqvist J, Agardh CD, Stenstrom A. Decreasing incidence of major amputation in diabetic patients: a consequence of a multidisciplinary foot care team approach? *Diabet Med* 1995;12:770–776.
42. Wild S, McKeigue P. Cross sectional analysis of mortality by country of birth in England and Wales, 1970–92. *BMJ* 1997;314:705–710.
43. Freeman WL, Hosey GM. Diabetic complications among American Indians of Washington, Oregon, and Idaho. Prevalence of retinopathy, end-stage renal disease, and amputations. *Diabetes Care* 1993;16:357–360.
44. Nelson RG, Gohdes DM, Everhart JE, *et al.* Lower-extremity amputations in NIDDM. 12-yr follow-up study in Pima Indians. *Diabetes Care* 1988;11:8–16.
45. Valway SE, Linkins RW, Gohdes DM. Epidemiology of lower extremity amputations in the Indian Health Service, 1982–1987. *Diabetes Care* 1993;16:354–356.
46. Rith-Najarian SJ, Valway SE, Gohdes DM. Diabetes in a northern Minnesota Chippewa Tribe. Prevalence and incidence of diabetes and incidence of major complications, 1986–1988. *Diabetes Care* 1993;16:266–270.
47. Krapfl H, Gohdes D. Lower extremity amputation episodes among persons with diabetes – New Mexico, 2000. *JAMA* 2003;289:1502.
48. Lavery LA, Ashry HR, van Houtum W, Pugh JA, Harkless LB, Basu S. Variation in the incidence and proportion of diabetes-related amputations in minorities. *Diabetes Care* 1996;19:48–52.

49. Lavery LA, van Houtum WH, Ashry HR, Armstrong DG, Pugh JA. Diabetes-related lower-extremity amputations disproportionately affect Blacks and Mexican Americans. *South Med J* 1999;92:593–599.

50. Lavery LA, Armstrong DG, Wunderlich RP, Tredwell J, Boulton AJ. Diabetic foot syndrome: evaluating the prevalence and incidence of foot pathology in Mexican Americans and non-Hispanic whites from a diabetes disease management cohort. *Diabetes Care* 2003;26:1435–1438.

51. Collins TC, Johnson M, Henderson W, Khuri SF, Daley J. Lower extremity nontraumatic amputation among veterans with peripheral arterial disease: is race an independent factor? *Med Care* 2002; 40:I106–I116.

52. Young BA, Maynard C, Boyko EJ. Racial differences in diabetic nephropathy, cardiovascular disease, and mortality in a national population of veterans. *Diabetes Care* 2003;26:2392–2399.

53. Wachtel MS. Family poverty accounts for differences in lower-extremity amputation rates of minorities 50 years old or more with diabetes. *J Natl Med Assoc* 2005;97:334–338.

54. Karter AJ, Ferrara A, Liu JY, Moffet HH, Ackerson LM, Selby JV. Ethnic disparities in diabetic complications in an insured population. *JAMA* 2002;287:2519–2527.

55. Toursarkissian B, Jones WT, D'Ayala MD, *et al.* Does the efficacy of dorsalis pedis artery bypasses vary among diabetic patients of different ethnic backgrounds? *Vasc Endovasc Surg* 2002;36:207–212.

56. Miller AD, Van BA, Verhoek-Oftedahl W, Miller ER. Diabetes-related lower extremity amputations in New Jersey, 1979 to 1981. *J Med Soc N J* 1985;82:723–726.

57. Kahn KL, Pearson ML, Harrison ER, *et al.* Health care for black and poor hospitalized Medicare patients. *JAMA* 1994;271:1169–1174.

58. Schneider EC, Zaslavsky AM, Epstein AM. Racial disparities in the quality of care for enrollees in medicare managed care. *JAMA* 2002;287:1288–1294.

59. Guadagnoli E, Ayanian JZ, Gibbons G, McNeil BJ, Logerfo FW. The influence of race on the use of surgical procedures for treatment of peripheral vascular disease of the lower extremities. *Arch Surg* Apr 1995;130:381–386.

60. Selby JV, Zhang D. Risk factors for lower extremity amputations in persons with diabetes. *Diabetes Care* 1995;18:509–516.

61. Leggetter S, Chaturvedi N, Fuller JH, Edmonds ME. Ethnicity and risk of diabetes-related lower extremity amputation: a population-based, case control study of African Caribbeans and Europeans in the United Kingdom. *Arch Intern Med* 2002;162:73–78.

62. UK Prospective Diabetes Study Group. UK Prospective Diabetes Study Paper XII: Differences between Asian, Afro-Caribbean and White Caucasian Type 2 diabetic patients at diagnosis of diabetes. *Diabet Med* 1994;11:670–677.

63. Newman AB, Siscovick DS, Manolio TA, *et al.* Ankle–arm index as a marker of atherosclerosis in the Cardiovascular Health Study. Cardiovascular Health Study (CHS) Collaborative Research Group. *Circulation* 1993;88:837–845.

64. Veves A, Sarnow MR, Giurini JM, *et al.* Differences in joint mobility and foot pressures between black and white diabetic patients. *Diabet Med* 1995;12:585–589.

65. Hennis AJ, Fraser HS, Jonnalagadda R, Fuller J, Chaturvedi N. Explanations for the high risk of diabetes-related amputation in a Caribbean population of black african descent and potential for prevention. *Diabetes Care* 2004;27:2636–2641.

66. Solagberu BA. The scope of amputations in a Nigerian teaching hospital. *Afr J Med Med Sci* 2001;30:225–227.

67. Lester FT. Amputations in patients attending a diabetic clinic in Addis Abeba, Ethiopia. *Ethiop Med J* 1995;33:15–20.

68. Gillum RF. Coronary heart disease in black populations, I: mortality and morbidity. *Am Heart J* 1982;104:839–851.

69. McKeigue PM, Miller GJ, Marmot MG. Coronary heart disease in south Asians overseas: a review. *J Clin Epidemiol* 1989;42:597–609.

70. McKeigue PM, Shah B, Marmot MG. Relation of central obesity and insulin resistance with high diabetes prevalence and cardiovascular risk in South Asians. *Lancet* 1991;337:382–386.
71. Gujral JS, McNally PG, O'Malley BP, Burden AC. Ethnic differences in the incidence of lower extremity amputation secondary to diabetes mellitus. *Diabet Med* 1993;10:271–274.
72. Chaturvedi N, Abbott CA, Whalley A, Widdows P, Leggetter SY, Boulton AJ. Risk of diabetes-related amputation in South Asians vs Europeans in the UK. *Diabet Med* 2002;19:99–104.
73. Nicholl CG, Levy JC, Mohan V, Rao PV, Mather HM. Asian diabetes in Britain: a clinical profile. *Diabet Med* 1986;3:257–260.
74. Mohan V, Premalatha G, Sastry NG. Peripheral vascular disease in non-insulin-dependent diabetes mellitus in south India. *Diabetes Res Clin Pract* 1995;27:235–240.
75. Premalatha G, Shanthirani S, Deepa R, Markovitz J, Mohan V. Prevalence and risk factors of peripheral vascular disease in a selected South Indian population: the Chennai Urban Population Study. *Diabetes Care* 2000;23:1295–1300.

3 Diabetic Neuropathy

Solomon Tesfaye

INTRODUCTION

Polyneuropathy is one of the commonest complications of the diabetes and the commonest form of neuropathy in the developed world. Diabetic neuropathy encompasses several neuropathic syndromes the commonest of which is chronic distal sensorimotor symmetrical neuropathy (abbreviated to 'distal symmetrical neuropathy'), the main initiating factor for foot ulceration. The epidemiology of distal symmetrical neuropathy has recently been reviewed.[1] The European Diabetes (EURODIAB) Prospective Complications Study, which involved the examination of 3250 type 1 patients, from 16 European countries, found a prevalence rate of 28% for distal symmetrical neuropathy.[2] Indeed, several clinic-[2,3] and population-based studies[4,5] show surprisingly similar prevalence rates for distal symmetrical neuropathy, affecting about 30% of all diabetic people at any time and 50% after 15 years of diabetes.

There is now little doubt that glycaemic control is a key determinant of the development of the microvascular complications of diabetes, including distal symmetrical neuropathy.[2,6–8] Age[2,4] and duration[2,4,5] of diabetes are well-established correlates of distal symmetrical neuropathy. Cigarette smoking,[2,4] both background and proliferative retinopathy[2,4,5] and microalbuminuria[2] have also been reported to be associated with distal symmetrical neuropathy.

However, most of the studies with regard to the epidemiology of distal symmetrical neuropathy have been cross-sectional and thus the observed associations with the various risk factors can be misleading, as true causality can be demonstrated only in a prospective fashion. To date, few studies have assessed risk factors for neuropathy prospectively, and findings have been conflicting. Hypertension was observed to be a strong risk factor for distal symmetrical neuropathy in 463 young, type 1 subjects in the Epidemiology of Diabetes Complications (EDC) follow-up study.[9] In contrast, in type 2 patients, hypoinsulinaemia was identified as a key risk factor for neuropathy incidence,[10] while a mixed population follow-up suggested that the type of diabetes and microvascular disease were associated with the severity of distal symmetrical neuropathy.[11]

Recently the results of the EURODIAB Prospective Study, which included a large cohort of type 1 patients, were published: After excluding those with neuropathy at baseline, the study showed that over a 7-year period, about one quarter of type 1 diabetic patients developed distal symmetrical neuropathy, with age, duration of diabetes and poor glycaemic control being the major determinants.[12] The development of neuropathy was also associated with potentially

The Foot in Diabetes, 4th Edition. Editors Andrew J.M. Boulton, Peter R. Cavanagh and Gerry Rayman.
© 2006 John Wiley & Sons, Ltd.

modifiable cardiovascular risk factors such as serum lipids, hypertension, body mass index and cigarette smoking.[12] Furthermore, cardiovascular disease at baseline carried a twofold risk of neuropathy, independent of cardiovascular risk factors.

In summary, based on recent epidemiological studies, correlates of diabetic neuropathy include increasing age, increasing duration of diabetes, poor glycaemic control, retinopathy, albuminuria and vascular risk factors (hypertension, obesity, smoking and hyperlipidaemia).[1,2,4,12]

DISTAL SYMMETRICAL NEUROPATHY

This is the commonest neuropathic syndrome affecting over 90% of diabetic patients with neuropathy and this is what is meant in clinical practice by the phrase 'diabetic neuropathy'. Sensory loss starts in the toes and then extends to involve the feet and legs in a 'stocking' distribution. When sensory loss is well established in the legs, the upper limbs may be involved in a 'glove' distribution, starting with the fingers. Diabetes can affect the autonomic nervous system, and in patients with distal symmetrical neuropathy subclinical autonomic neuropathy is common, although clinical autonomic neuropathy is rare. With disease progression, motor manifestations such as wasting of the small muscles of the hands and limb weakness become apparent.

The main clinical presentation of distal symmetrical neuropathy is sensory loss, which the patient may not be aware of, or may be described as 'numbness' or 'dead feeling'. However, some may experience a progressive build-up of unpleasant sensory symptoms including tingling (paraesthesiae); burning pain; shooting pains down the legs (like 'electric shock'); lancinating (knife-like) pains; contact pain or hypersensitivity often with daytime clothes and bedclothes (allodynia); pain on walking often described as 'walking barefoot on marbles', or 'walking barefoot on hot sand'; sensations of heat or cold in the feet; persistent achy feeling in the feet and cramp-like sensations in the legs. Within a 24-h period the same patient with painful diabetic neuropathy may perceive a variety of painful symptoms including seemingly contradictory sensations of intense heat and cold in the feet. To the external observer these may seem inherently contradictory but as Huskisson remarked 'pain is a purely subjective experience and the external observer cannot play any part in its assessment'[13] and so we have no choice but to take the patient's word for it. In addition, a patient may experience dull aching pain and 'numbness' or 'dead feeling' of the lower limbs (a 'negative' symptom as opposed to 'positive' symptoms of burning, shooting and lancinating pains). Occasionally, pain can extend above the feet and may involve the whole of the legs, and when this is the case there is usually upper limb involvement also. It is also important to appreciate that there is a large spectrum of severity of these symptoms, ranging from minor complaints such as tingling in a toe or two, to severe painful neuropathy involving both legs. This has implications on management strategy for the patient.

Painful diabetic neuropathy is characteristically more severe at night, and often prevents sleep.[14,15] Some patients may be in a constant state of tiredness because of sleep deprivation.[14,15] Others are unable to maintain full employment.[14–17] Severe painful neuropathy can occasionally cause marked reduction in exercise threshold, which interferes with daily activities. This is particularly the case when there is an associated disabling, severe postural hypotension due to autonomic involvement. Not surprisingly therefore, depressive symptoms are not uncommon.[17]

As discussed in Chapter 6, it is important to appreciate that many subjects with distal symmetrical neuropathy may not have any of the above symptoms, and their first presentation may be with a foot ulcer.[18] This underpins the need for carefully examining and screening the feet of all diabetic people, in order to identify those at risk of developing foot ulceration. The insensate foot is at risk of developing mechanical and thermal injuries, and patients must therefore be warned about these and given appropriate advice with regard to foot care.[18,19] In those with advanced neuropathy, there may be sensory ataxia. The unfortunate sufferer is affected by unsteadiness on walking, and even falls, particularly if there is associated visual impairment due to retinopathy.

A curious feature of the neuropathic foot is that both numbness and pain may occur, the so-called 'painful, painless' leg.[19] This may be perceived as a paradox, as the patient with a large foot ulcer may also have severe neuropathic pain. However, it is now clear that one does not need to have sensation intact to experience pain. Many patients with severe numb legs and a vibration perception threshold (VPT) of over 40 V or complete absence of the 10-g monofilament test may have severe painful symptoms. Damage to the large A-beta nerve fibres leads to loss of sensation, but it is the C-fibre (small-fibre) damage and the consequent ectopic generation of impulses, peripheral and central sensitisation that lead to neuropathic pain.[20] Thus, this apparent paradox of pain and insensitivity is not in fact a paradox.

Neuropathy is usually easily detected by simple clinical examination.[21-23] Shoes and socks should be removed and the feet examined at least annually and more often if neuropathy is present. The most common presenting abnormality is a reduction or absence of vibration sense in the toes. As the disease progresses, there is sensory loss in a stocking and sometimes in a glove distribution, involving all modalities. When there is severe sensory loss, proprioception may also be impaired, leading to a positive Romberg's sign. Ankle tendon reflexes are lost and with more advanced neuropathy, knee reflexes are often reduced or absent. Scored clinical examination and bedside tests to detect (diagnose) neuropathy, such as the 10-g monofilament test and biothesiometry, are described in Chapter 6.[22,23]

Muscle strength is usually normal early during the course of the disease, although mild weakness may be found in toe extensors. However, with progressive disease, there is significant generalised muscular wasting, particularly in the small muscles of the hand and feet. The fine movements of fingers would then be affected, and there is difficulty in handling small objects. Wasting of dorsal interossei may also be due to entrapment of the ulnar nerve at the elbow. The clawing of the toes is believed to be due to unopposed (because of wasting of the small muscles of the foot) pulling of the long extensor and flexor tendons. This scenario results in elevated plantar pressure points at the metatarsal heads that are prone to callus formation and foot ulceration.[18] Deformities such as bunions can form the focus of ulceration and with more extreme deformities, such as those associated with Charcot arthropathy, the risk is further increased.[24] As one of the most common precipitants to foot ulceration is inappropriate footwear, a thorough assessment should also include examination of shoes for poor fit, abnormal wear and internal pressure areas or foreign bodies.

Autonomic neuropathy affecting the feet can cause a reduction in sweating and consequently dry skin that is likely to crack easily, predisposing the patient to the risk of infection.[18] The 'purely' neuropathic foot is also warm due to arterio-venous shunting, first described by Ward.[19] This results in the distension of foot veins that fail to collapse even when the foot is elevated.[25] It is not unusual to observe a gangrenous toe in a foot that has bounding arterial pulses, as there is impairment of the nutritive capillary circulation due to arterio-venous shunting. The oxygen tension of the blood in these veins is typically raised.[26] The increasing blood flow brought about by autonomic neuropathy can sometimes result in neuropathic oedema, which is often resistant to treatment with diuretics.

Natural History of Distal Symmetrical Neuropathy

The natural history of chronic distal symmetrical neuropathy remains poorly defined, as there are only a limited number of small prospective studies. The lack of simple, accurate and readily reproducible methods of measuring neuropathy, unlike in diabetic retinopathy and nephropathy, may be a contributory factor.[12] A study by Boulton et al.[27] reported that neuropathic symptoms remain or get worse over a 5-year period in patients with chronic distal symmetrical neuropathy. A major drawback of this study was that it involved highly selected patients from a hospital base. A more recent study reported improvements in painful symptoms over 3.5 years.[28] Neuropathic pain was assessed using a visual analogue scale, and small-fibre function by thermal limen, heat pain threshold and weighted pinprick threshold. At follow-up 3.5 years later, one third of the 50 patients at baseline had died or were lost to follow-up. Clearly this is a major drawback. There was symptomatic improvement in painful neuropathy in majority of the remaining patients. Despite this symptomatic improvement, however, small-fibre function as measured by the above tests deteriorated significantly, suggesting a dichotomy in the evolution of neuropathic symptoms and neurophysiological measures.

Differential Diagnosis of Distal Symmetrical Neuropathy

Diabetic peripheral neuropathy presents in a similar way to neuropathies of other causes, and thus the physician needs to carefully exclude other common causes before attributing the neuropathy to diabetes. Absence of other complications of diabetes, rapid weight loss, excessive alcohol intake and other atypical features in either the history or clinical examination should alert the physician to search for other causes of neuropathy. Table 3.1 shows differential diagnoses for distal symmetrical neuropathy.

ACUTE PAINFUL NEUROPATHIES

These are transient neuropathic syndromes characterised by an acute onset of pain in the lower limbs. Acute neuropathies present in a symmetrical fashion and are relatively uncommon. Pain is invariably present and is usually distressing to the patient, and can sometimes be incapacitating. There are two distinct syndromes, the first of which occurs within the context of poor glycaemic control, and the second with rapid improvements in metabolic control.[29] Thankfully, these resolve within 12 months,[21] unlike the more common chronic painful diabetic neuropathy.[27]

ASYMMETRICAL (FOCAL) DIABETIC NEUROPATHIES

Asymmetrical or focal neuropathies are well-recognised complications of diabetes, and include proximal motor, cranial, thoraco-abdominal and entrapment neuropathies.[30] They have a relatively rapid onset, and complete recovery is usual except in entrapment neuropathies such as carpal tunnel syndrome where surgical release may be required. This contrasts with chronic distal symmetrical neuropathy, where there is usually no improvement in symptoms 4 years

Table 3.1   Differential diagnosis of distal
symmetrical neuropathy

Metabolic
Diabetes
Amyloidosis
Uraemia
Myxoedema
Porphyria
Vitamin deficiency (thiamin, B_{12}, B_6, pyridoxine)

Drugs and chemicals
Alcohol
Cytotoxic drugs
Anti-tuberculous drugs

Neoplastic disorders
Bronchial or gastric carcinoma
Lymphoma

Infective or inflammatory
Leprosy
Guillain–Barre syndrome
Chronic inflammatory demyelinating polyneuropathy
Polyarteritis nodosa

Genetic
Charcot–Marie–Tooth disease
Hereditary sensory neuropathies

after onset.[27] Unlike chronic distal symmetrical neuropathy they are often unrelated to the presence of other diabetic complications.[31] Asymmetrical neuropathies are more common in men and tend to predominantly affect older patients.[32] A careful history is mandatory in order to identify any associated symptoms that might point to another cause for the neuropathy.

Proximal Motor Neuropathy (Amyotrophy)

This affects both type 1 and type 2 patients older than 50 years.[33,34] The syndrome of progressive asymmetrical proximal leg weakness and atrophy was first described by Garland,[33] who coined the term 'diabetic amyotrophy'. This condition has also been named as 'proximal motor neuropathy', 'femoral neuropathy' or 'plexopathy'. The patient presents with severe pain, which is felt deep in the thigh, but can sometimes be of burning quality and extends below the knee. The pain is usually continuous and often causes insomnia and depression.[34] There is an associated weight loss, which can sometimes be very severe and can raise the possibility of an occult malignancy.

On examination there is profound wasting of the quadriceps with marked weakness in these muscle groups, although hip flexors and hip abductors can also be affected.[35] Thigh adductors, glutei and hamstring muscles may also be involved. The knee jerk is usually reduced or absent.

The profound weakness can lead to difficulty in getting out of a low chair or climbing stairs. Sensory loss is unusual, and if present indicates a coexistent distal sensory neuropathy.

Careful exclusion of other causes of quadriceps wasting, such as nerve root and cauda equina lesions, and an occult malignancy is mandatory. An erythrocyte sedimentation rate, an X-ray of the lumbar–sacral spine, a chest X-ray and an ultrasound of the abdomen may be required. Electrophysiological studies may demonstrate increased femoral nerve latency and active denervation of affected muscles. Magnetic resonance imaging (MRI) of the lumbo-sacral spine is now recommended to exclude focal nerve root entrapment.

Management is largely symptomatic and supportive. Patients should be encouraged and reassured that this condition is likely to resolve. There is still controversy as to whether the use of insulin therapy influences the natural history of this syndrome.[34] Some patients benefit from physiotherapy that involves extension exercises aimed at strengthening the quadriceps. The management of pain in proximal motor neuropathy is similar to that of chronic or acute distal symmetrical neuropathies (see below).

PATHOGENESIS OF DISTAL SYMMETRICAL NEUROPATHY

The pathogenesis of diabetic neuropathy remains undetermined.[36] Historically, there have been two distinct views with regard to the pathogenesis of distal symmetrical neuropathy. The first view regards metabolic factors to be primarily important in the pathogenesis of distal symmetrical neuropathy; the second contends vascular factors to be the determining aetiological factors for neuropathy.[37–39] However, most authorities now agree that the truth is probably in the middle and that both metabolic and vascular factors are important (Table 3.2).

MANAGEMENT OF PAINFUL DIABETIC NEUROPATHY

Managing the diabetic patient with lower limb pain can pose a considerable challenge. A careful history and peripheral neurological/vascular examination of the patient is essential in order to exclude other possible causes of leg pain such as peripheral vascular disease, prolapsed intervertebral discs, spinal canal stenosis and cauda equina lesions. Unilateral leg pain should arouse a suspicion that the pain may be due to lumbar–sacral nerve root compression. These patients may well need to be investigated with a lumbar–sacral MRI. The quality and severity should be assessed preferably using a suitable scale, so that response to treatment may be evaluated. An empathic approach with a multidisciplinary support is crucial, as psychological

Table 3.2 Proposed hypotheses of diabetic peripheral nerve damage

Chronic hyperglycaemia
Nerve microvascular dysfunction
Protein kinase C hyperactivity
Increased free-radical formation
Polyol pathway hyperactivity
Non-enzymatic glycation
Abnormalities of nerve growth

dysfunction in diabetic patients is an important factor in increasing the suffering associated with all aspects of the disease.

Glycaemic Control and Management of Cardiovascular Risk Factors

There is now little doubt that good blood sugar control prevents/delays the onset of diabetic neuropathy.[6–8,12] In addition, painful neuropathic symptoms are also improved by improving metabolic control, if necessary with the use of insulin in type 2 diabetes.[40] Thus, the first step in the management of painful neuropathy is a concerted effort aimed at improving glycaemic control, although there are no controlled studies to confirm this view.[40] Traditional markers of large vessel disease including hypertension, obesity, hyperlipidaemia and smoking also appear to be independent risk factors for neuropathy and therefore need to be effectively managed.[14]

Tricyclic Compounds and Serotonin Norepinephrine Reuptake Inhibitors

Tricyclic compounds continue to be regarded as the first-line treatment for painful diabetic neuropathy.[15,41] A number of double-blind clinical trials have confirmed their effectiveness beyond any doubt. As these drugs do have unwanted side effects such as drowsiness, anticholinergic side effects such as dry mouth, and dizziness due to postural hypotension in those who have autonomic neuropathy, patients should be started on imipramine or amitriptyline at a low dose (25–50 mg taken before bed), the dose gradually titrated, if necessary, up to 150 mg/day. The mechanism of action of tricyclic compounds in improving neuropathic pain is not known, but their effect does not appear through their antidepressant property, as they appear to be effective even in those with a depressed mood.[41] Recently, the seretonin and norepinephrine re-uptake inhibitor (SNRI), Duioxetine (60 mg–120 mg/d) was found effective with reasonable side effect profile.[41a]

Anticonvulsants

Anticonvulsants, including carbamazepine, phenytoin, gabapentin,[42] and more recently pregabalin,[43] have also been found effective in the relief of more severe neuropathic pain. Unfortunately, treatment with anticonvulsants is often complicated with troublesome side effects such as sedation, dizziness and ataxia, and therefore treatment should be started at a relatively low dose and gradually increased to maintenance dose of these drugs, while carefully looking for side effects. However, pregabalin and gabapentin appear to have less unwanted side effects and are hence better tolerated.[42,43]

Opiates

The opiate derivative tramadol has been found effective in relieving neuropathic pain.[44] Another opiod, oxycodone, has also been shown to be effective in the management of neuropathic pain.[45]

Recently, the combination of morphine and gabapentin was found to be more effective than either, in the management of neuropathic pain.[46]

Topical Capsaicin

Topical capsaicin (0.075%) applied sparingly three to four times per day to the affected area has also been found to relieve neuropathic pain. Topical capsaicin works by depleting substance 'P' from nerve terminals, and there may be worsening of neuropathic symptoms for the first 2–4 weeks of application.[47]

Intravenous Lignocaine and Oral Mexiletine

Intravenous lignocaine at a dose of 5 mg/kg body weight, with another 30 min with a cardiac monitor *in situ*, has also been found to be effective in relieving neuropathic pain for up to 2 weeks.[48] This form of treatment is useful in subjects who are having severe pain that is not responding to the above agents, although it does necessitate bringing the patient into hospital for a few hours. Oral mexiletine, which has similar structure to lignocaine, may have a beneficial effect at reducing neuropathic pain, although in the author's experience treatment is disappointing.

α-Lipoic Acid

Infusion of the antioxidant α-lipoic acid at a dose of 600 mg intravenously per day over a 3-week period has also been found to be useful in reducing neuropathic pain.[49]

Isosorbide Dinitrate Spray and Glyceryl Trinitrate Patch

Two studies have shown that nitrate spray[50] and patch[51] applications in the lower limbs lead to a significant improvement of neuropathic pain in diabetic patients. These results are promising and hopefully will be confirmed by larger, multicentre randomised controlled trials (RCTs).

Non-pharmacological Treatments

Lack of response and unwanted side effects of conventional drug treatments force many sufferers to try alternative therapies such as acupuncture,[52] near-infrared phototherapy,[53] low-intensity laser therapy,[54] magnetic field therapies[55] and transcutaneous electrical stimulation[52] and, as a last resort, implantation of electrical spinal cord stimulator.[16] Recently, Bosi *et al.* recommended the use of frequency-modulated electromagnetic neural stimulation therapy and reported a significant improvement in pain scores and some measures of nerve function.[56] Another recent study by Reichstein *et al.* also demonstrated the effectiveness of high-frequency external muscle stimulation in relieving neuropathic pain.[57] However, most of these studies need to be confirmed by multicentre RCTs.

Management of Disabling Painful Neuropathy not Responding to Pharmacological Treatment

Neuropathic pain can sometimes be extremely severe, interfering significantly with patients' sleep and daily activities. Unfortunately, some patients are not helped by conventional pharmacological treatment. Such patients pose a major challenge, for they are severely distressed and sometimes wheelchair bound. A recent study has demonstrated that such patients may respond to electrical spinal cord stimulation, which relieves both background and peak neuropathic pain.[16] This form of treatment is particularly advantageous, as the patient does not have to take any other pain-relieving medications, with all their side effects. A recent follow-up of patients fitted with electrical spinal cord stimulators found that stimulators continued to be effective 10 years after implantation.[58]

REFERENCES

1. Shaw JE, Zimmet PZ. The epidemiology of diabetic neuropathy. *Diabetes Rev* 1999;7:245–252.
2. Tesfaye S, Stephens L, Stephenson J, Fuller J, Platter ME, Ionescu-Tirgoviste C, Ward JD. The prevalence of diabetic neuropathy and its relation to glycaemic control and potential risk factors: the EURODIAB IDDM Complications Study. *Diabetologia* 1996;39:1377–1384.
3. Young MJ, Boulton AJM, Macleod AF, Williams DRR, Sonksen PH. A multicentre study of the prevalence of diabetic peripheral neuropathy in the United Kingdom hospital clinic population. *Diabetologia* 1993;36:150–154.
4. Maser RE, Steenkiste AR, Dorman JS, *et al.* Epidemiological correlates of diabetic neuropathy. Report from Pittsburgh Epidemiology of Diabetes Complications Study. *Diabetes* 1989;38:1456–1461.
5. Ziegler D. Diagnosis, staging and epidemiology of diabetic peripheral neuropathy. *Diabetes Nutr Metab* 1994;7:342–348.
6. The Diabetes Control and Complications Trial Research Group. The effect of intensive treatment of diabetes on the development and progression of long-term complications in insulin-dependent diabetes mellitus. *N Engl J Med* 1993;329:977–986.
7. Diabetes Control and Complications Trial Research Group. The effect of intensive diabetes therapy on the development and progression of neuropathy. *Ann Intern Med* 1995;122:561–568.
8. United Kingdom Prospective Diabetes Study Group. Intensive blood glucose control with sulphonylureas or insulin compared with conventional treatment and risk of complications in patients with type 2 diabetes. *Lancet* 1998;352:837–853.
9. Forrest KY, Maser RE, Pambianco G, Becker DJ, Orchard TJ. Hypertension as a risk factor for diabetic neuropathy: a prospective study. *Diabetes* 1997;46:665–670.
10. Partanen J, Niskanen L, Lehtinen J, Mervaala E, Siitonen O, Uusitupa M. Natural history of peripheral neuropathy in patients with non-insulin-dependent diabetes mellitus. *N Engl J Med* 1995;333:89–94.
11. Dyck PJ, Davies JL, Wilson DM, Service FJ, Melton LJ, O'Brien PC. Risk factors for severity of diabetic polyneuropathy: intensive longitudinal assessment of the Rochester Diabetic Neuropathy Study cohort. *Diabetes Care* 1999;22:1479–1486.
12. Tesfaye S, Chaturvedi N, Eaton SEM, Witte D, Ward JD, Fuller J. Vascular risk factors and diabetic neuropathy. *N Engl J Med* 2005;352:341–350.
13. Huskisson EC. Measurement of pain. *Lancet* 1974;2:1127–1131.
14. Watkins PJ. Pain and diabetic neuropathy. *Br Med J* 1984;288:168–169.
15. Tesfaye S, Price D. Therapeutic approaches in diabetic neuropathy and neuropathic pain. In: Boulton AJM, ed. *Diabetic Neuropathy.* Lancaster: Marius Press; 1997:159–181.

16. Tesfaye S, Watt J, Benbow SJ, Pang KA, Miles J, MacFarlane IA. Electrical spinal cord stimulation for painful diabetic peripheral neuropathy. *Lancet* 1996;348:1696–1701.
17. Quattrini C, Tesfaye S. Understanding the impact of painful diabetic neuropathy. *Diabetes Metab Res Rev* 2003;19:S1–S8.
18. Boulton AJM, Kirsner RS, Viliekyte L. Neuropathic diabetic foot ulcers. *N Engl J Med* 2004;351: 48–55.
19. Ward JD. The diabetic leg. *Diabetologia* 1982;22:141–147.
20. Tesfaye S, Kempler P. Painful diabetic neuropathy. *Diabetologia* 2005;48:805–807.
21. Tesfaye S. Diabetic neuropathy: achieving best practice. *Br J Vasc Dis* 2003;3:112–117.
22. Eaton SEM, Tesfaye S. Clinical manifestations and measurement of somatic neuropathy. *Diabetes Rev* 1999;7:312–325.
23. Scott LA, Tesfaye S. Measurement of somatic neuropathy for clinical practice and clinical trials. *Curr Diabetes Rep* 2001;1:208–215.
24. Rajbhandari SM, Jenkins R, Davies C, Tesfaye S. Charcot neuroarthropathy in diabetes mellitus. *Diabetologia* 2002;45:1085–1096.
25. Ward JD, Simms JM, Knight G, Boulton AJM, Sandler DA. Venous distension in the diabetic neuropathic foot (physical sign of arterio-venous shunting). *J R Soc Med* 1983;76:1011–1014.
26. Boulton AJM, Scarpello JHB, Ward JD. Venous oxygenation in the diabetic neuropathic foot: evidence of arterial venous shunting? *Diabetologia* 1982;22:6–8.
27. Boulton AJM, Armstrong WD, Scarpello JHB, Ward JD. The natural history of painful diabetic neuropathy – a 4 year study. *Postgrad Med J* 1983;59:556–559.
28. Benbow SJ, Chan AW, Bowsher D, McFarlane IA, Williams G. A prospective study of painful symptoms, small fibre function and peripheral vascular disease in chronic painful diabetic neuropathy. *Diabet Med* 1994;11:17–21.
29. Tesfaye S, Malik R, Harris N, Jakubowski J, Mody C, Rennie IG, Ward JD. Arteriovenous shunting and proliferating new vessels in acute painful neuropathy of rapid glycaemic control (insulin neuritis). *Diabetologia* 1996;39:329–335.
30. Ward JD, Tesfaye S. Pathogenesis of diabetic neuropathy. In: Pickup J, Williams G, eds. *Textbook of Diabetes*. Vol. 2. Blackwell Science; 1997:49.1–49.19.
31. Watkins PJ, Edmonds ME. Clinical features of diabetic neuropathy. In: Pickup J, Williams G, eds. *Textbook of Diabetes*. Vol. 2. Blackwell Science; 1997:50.1–50.20.
32. Matikainen E, Juntunen J. Diabetic neuropathy: epidemiological, pathogenetic, and clinical aspects with special emphasis on type 2 diabetes mellitus. *Acta Endocrinol Suppl (Copenh)* 1984;262:89–94.
33. Garland H. Diabetic amyotrophy. *Br Med J* 1955;2:1287–1290.
34. Coppack SW, Watkins PJ. The natural history of femoral neuropathy. *Q J Med* 1991;79:307–313.
35. Subramony SH, Willbourn AJ. Diabetic proximal neuropathy. Clinical and electromyographic studies. *J Neurol Sci* 1982;53:293–304.
36. Cameron NE, Eaton SE, Cotter MA, Tesfaye S. Vascular factors and metabolic interactions in the pathogenesis of diabetic neuropathy. *Diabetologia* 2001;44:1973–1988.
37. Tesfaye S, Malik R, Ward JD. Vascular factors in diabetic neuropathy. *Diabetologia* 1994;37:847–854.
38. Tesfaye S, Harris N, Jakubowski J, *et al.* Impaired blood flow and arterio-venous shunting in human diabetic neuropathy: a novel technique of nerve photography and fluorescein angiography. *Diabetologia* 1993;36:1266–1274.
39. Tesfaye S, Harris N, Wilson RM, Ward JD. Exercise induced conduction velocity increment: a marker of impaired nerve blood flow in diabetic neuropathy. *Diabetologia* 1992;35:155–159.
40. Boulton AJM, Drury J, Clarke B, Ward JD. Continuous subcutaneous insulin infusion in the management of painful diabetic neuropathy. *Diabetes Care* 1982;5:386–390.
41. Max MB, Culnane M, Schafer SC, *et al.* Amitriptyline relieves diabetic neuropathy pain in patients with normal or depressed mood. *Neurology* 1987;37:598–596.

41a. Goldstein DJ, Lu Y, Detke MJ, *et al.* Duloxetine vs. placebo in patients with painful diabetic neuropathy. *Pain* 2005;116:109–118.

42. Backonja M, Beydoun A, Edwards KR, *et al.* Gabapentin for the symptomatic treatment of painful neuropathy in patients with diabetes mellitus: a randomized controlled trial. *JAMA* 1998;280:1831–1836.

43. Lesser H, Sharma U, LaMoreaux L, Poole RM. Pregabalin relieves symptoms of painful diabetic neuropathy: a randomized controlled trial. *Neurology* Dec 2004;63:2104–2110.

44. Harati Y, Gooch C, Swenson M, Edelman S, Greene D, Raskin P, Donofrio P, Cornblath D, Sachdeo R, Siu CO, Kamin M. Double-blind randomized trial of tramadol for the treatment of the pain of diabetic neuropathy. *Neurology* Jun 1998;50:1842–1846.

45. Watson CP, Moulin D, Watt-Watson J, Gordon A, Eisenhoffer J. Controlled-release oxycodone relieves neuropathic pain: a randomized controlled trial in painful diabetic neuropathy. *Pain* Sep 2003;105:71–78.

46. Gilron I, Bailey JM, Tu D, Holden RR, Weaver DF, Houlden RL. Morphine, gabapentin, or their combination for neuropathic pain. *N Engl J Med* Mar 2005;352:1324–1334.

47. Capsaicin Study Group. The effect of treatment with capsaicin on daily activities of patients with painful diabetic neuropathy. *Diabetes Care* 1992;15:159–165.

48. Kastrup J, Angelo H, Petersen P, Dejgard A, Hilsted J. Treatment of chronic painful neuropathy with intravenous lidocaine infusion. *Br Med J* 1986;292:173.

49. Zeigler D, Hanefeld M, Ruhnau KJ, *et al.* Treatment of symptomatic diabetic peripheral neuropathy with anti-oxidant alpha-lipoic acid: a 3-week multicentre randomised controlled trial (ALADIN Study). *Diabetologia* 1995;38:1425–1433.

50. Yuen KC, Baker NR, Rayman G. Treatment of chronic painful diabetic neuropathy with isosorbide dinitrate spray: a double-blind placebo-controlled cross-over study. *Diabetes Care* Oct 2002;25:1699–1703.

51. Rayman G, Baker NR, Krishnan ST. Glyceryl trinitrate patches as an alternative to isosorbide dinitrate spray in the treatment of chronic painful diabetic neuropathy. *Diabetes Care* Sep 2003;26:2697–2698.

52. Abuaisha BB, Costanzi JB, Boulton AJ. Acupuncture for the treatment of chronic painful peripheral diabetic neuropathy: a long-term study. *Diabetes Res Clin Pract* Feb 1998;39:115–121.

53. Leonard DR, Farooqi MH, Myers S. Restoration of sensation, reduced pain, and improved balance in subjects with diabetic peripheral neuropathy. A double-blind, randomized, placebo-controlled study with monochromatic near-infrared treatment. *Diabetes Care* 2004;27:168–172.

54. Zinman L, Ngo M, Ng ET, Nwe KT, Gogov S, Bril V. Low-intensity laser therapy for painful symptoms of diabetic sensorimotor polyneuropathy. A controlled trial. *Diabetes Care* 2004;27:921–924.

55. Weintraub MI, Wolfe GI, Barohn RA, *et al.* Static magnetic field therapy for symptomatic diabetic neuropathy: a randomized, double-blind, placebo-controlled trial. *Arch Phys Med Rehabil* 2003;84:736–746.

56. Bosi E, Conti M, Vermigli C, *et al.* Effectiveness of frequency-modulated electromagnetic neural stimulation in the treatment of painful diabetic neuropathy. *Diabetologia* 2005;48:817–823.

57. Reichstein L, Labrenz S, Ziegler D, Martin S. Effective treatment of symptomatic diabetic polyneuropathy by high-frequency external muscle stimulation. *Diabetologia* 2005;48:824–828.

58. Daousi C, Benbow SJ, MacFarlane IA. Electrical spinal cord stimulation in the long-term treatment of chronic painful diabetic neuropathy. *Diabet Med* 2005;22:393–398.

FURTHER READING

Boulton AJM, Malik RA, Arezzo JC, Sosenko JM. Diabetic somatic neuropathies. *Diabetes Care* 2004;27:1458–1486.

4 Microcirculation and Diabetic Foot

Singhan T.M. Krishnan and Gerry Rayman

INTRODUCTION

The importance of microvascular disease in the development of foot ulceration and in wound healing has long been debated.[1] In this chapter we explore this relationship from a historical perspective and review recent studies of microvascular function in the diabetic foot.

SMALL VESSEL DISEASE

In 1959, Goldenberg concluded from studies of amputated legs that endothelial cell proliferation is a feature of the diabetic vasculature and that this could lead to small vessel occlusion. He suggested that these occlusions could have an important role in the development of foot ulceration.[2] This led to the concept of 'small vessel disease', which was purported as the cause of foot ulceration and gangrene in the presence of normal pedal pulses. As a result, a nihilistic approach towards the management of diabetic foot problems prevailed for several decades until challenged by LoGerfo and Coffman in 1984. They demonstrated that when careful and appropriate revascularisation techniques are used, good, long-term outcomes similar to those of non-diabetic subjects could be achieved.[3] Subsequently, Goldenberg's studies have received much criticism and indeed other investigators have failed to confirm his findings. However, although capillary occlusions were not observed, other structural small vessel abnormalities were found. Furthermore, studies using physiological methods demonstrated functional microvascular abnormalities supporting the involvement of microvascular disease in foot ulceration. From these observations and observations in other tissues, Parving put forward the 'haemodynamic hypothesis' to explain the development of microangiopathy in diabetes (Figure 4.1).[4]

According to this hypothesis, in the early stages of diabetes there is blood flow dysregulation leading to increased microvascular flow and capillary pressure. This results in an injury response within the endothelial cells of the microvasculature, consequently causing microvascular sclerosis.[5,6] In addition to arteriolar hyalinosis and sclerosis, subsequent studies using electron microscopy demonstrated thickening of the basement membrane now recognised as the hallmark of diabetic microangiopathy.[7,8] These abnormalities have been shown to relate to

The Foot in Diabetes, 4th Edition. Editors Andrew J.M. Boulton, Peter R. Cavanagh and Gerry Rayman.
© 2006 John Wiley & Sons, Ltd.

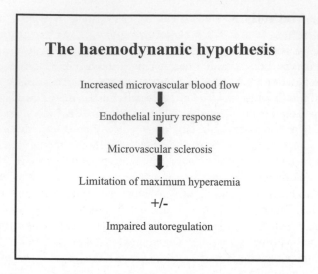

Figure 4.1   The haemodynamic hypothesis. (Adapted from Parving *et al.*[4])

capillary pressure, and are thus more marked in the lower limb, due to hydrostatic influences of the upright posture.[9,10] It has been suggested that microvascular sclerosis leads to a 'structural locking' of capillary wall, impairing vasodilatation and disrupting other vascular responses particularly in the lower limbs.

RECENTLY DESCRIBED FUNCTIONAL MICROVASCULAR DEFECTS IN THE FOOT

Technological advances in the last few decades have enabled more detailed evaluation of the microcirculation to further explore the above hypothesis and to gain a better understanding of the aetiopathogenesis of foot complications. These methods include laser Doppler flowmetry, video capillaroscopy, transcutaneous oxygen tension (TcpO$_2$) measurements and more recently laser Doppler imaging. The abnormalities described include impairment in vasodilatory responses to skin heating and other forms of injury, reduced post-occlusive hyperaemia, defective responses to iontophoresis of vasoactive substances and impaired vasoconstrictor responses to a variety of stimuli including postural changes.[11–13] The more important of these abnormalities are described in the following sections.

IMPAIRED MICROVASCULAR RESPONSE TO TISSUE INJURY IN DIABETES

Local skin heating to >42 °C has been shown to overcome the influence of central vasoconstrictor reflexes on the microcirculation in the heated area and to produce maximal microvascular vasodilation.[14] This maximum hyperaemia response has received considerable attention and has been extensively investigated using various techniques including laser Doppler flowmetry and TcpO$_2$, as described below.

Laser Doppler Methods

Rayman *et al.* in 1986 were the first to describe the maximum hyperaemic response and to show that it is impaired in type 1 diabetes. Furthermore, they showed that the degree of abnormality was related to the duration of diabetes and the severity of complications.[15] The same group also demonstrated a relationship between the severity of the impairment and the degree of basement membrane thickening, suggesting that the abnormality could in part be related to a structural limitation in vasodilatory capacity, in keeping with the haemodynamic hypothesis.[16] Since then, numerous investigators using a variety of different stimuli have confirmed that the microvascular hyperaemic response is impaired in type 1 diabetes.[17,18] Thus, Shore *et al.* demonstrated reduced hyperaemia in children, and Khan *et al.* showed that the hyperaemia to heating is reduced in the adolescents and young adults with type 1 diabetes.[19,20]

In type 2 diabetes, Sandemann *et al.* demonstrated that the maximum hyperaemic response is impaired even at the time of diagnosis.[21] Although considered to be surprising at that time, this is in accordance with more recent observations that people with type 2 diabetes have a pre-diabetic stage of impaired glucose tolerance for at least 10 years prior to diagnosis, and that microvascular abnormalities may be present during this stage.[22]

Transcutaneous Oxygen Tension

Early studies with this technique demonstrated reduced $TcpO_2$ in the skin of people with diabetes and were thought to indicate abnormalities of oxygen diffusion. However, it is now recognised that in the absence of large vessel disease the measurement reflects the maximum microvascular responses. This is because the estimation of blood oxygen tension with this technique involves heating the skin to 44°C to maximise oxygen delivery to the skin. Railton *et al.* described reduced $TcpO_2$ in foot skin of young, type 1 diabetic patients without peripheral arterial disease or neuropathy,[23] and in type 2 diabetic subjects, reduced $TcpO_2$ has been demonstrated in those with and without autonomic neuropathy.[24] These findings mirror those with the laser Doppler methods previously described.

In summary, numerous studies using $TcpO_2$ and laser Doppler methods in both type 1 and type 2 diabetes at various stages have universally demonstrated impairment of the maximal hyperaemic response. This injury response has long been considered to be an important event in normal wound healing, and its impairment in diabetes has thus been suggested to explain the propensity to foot ulceration in the absence of large vessel disease.

INCREASED RESTING BLOOD FLOW AND 'THE CAPILLARY STEAL' IN DIABETES

Studies using various techniques including plethysmography, Doppler ultrasound and laser Doppler have shown that lower limb blood flow is increased in those with diabetic neuropathy. Increased resting blood flow has been suggested to be secondary to sympathetic denervation with loss of vasoconstriction. Sympathetic denervation also leads to loss of regulation of blood flow through arterio-venous anastomotic blood vessels. This has been suggested to lead to a 'capillary steal', whereby blood is shunted away from the capillaries through these vessels, resulting in reduced skin nutrition. This hypothesis was thought to explain the paradox of neuropathic ulceration despite increased skin blood flow. Although attractive, the 'capillary steal' theory was not supported by direct measurement of nail-fold capillary blood flow using capillary microscopy. Investigators have reported either no difference or increased blood flow at rest in patients with peripheral neuropathy.[25]

In contrast, later studies using both capillaroscopy and laser Doppler methods have shown important differences in nutritional and non-nutritional blood flow in the toes, following is-chaemia. Although, as with the study previously described, there was no difference in the capillary or total blood flow at rest, after release of occlusion, peak capillary blood velocity was markedly reduced in those with diabetes whereas the total blood flow was unaffected.[26] This suggests that after an ischaemic insult there may be a 'capillary steal' with shunting of blood through subpapillary vessels.

Thus, impaired post-ischaemic hyperaemia has been suggested but not proven to contribute to the development of neuropathic ulceration.

REFLEX VASOCONSTRICTION IN THE MICROCIRCULATION

A variety of sympathetic vasoconstrictive reflexes have been shown to be impaired in subjects with diabetes, including postural reflex vasoconstriction, response to deep inspiration, cold temperature challenge and mental and emotional stress.[27,28]

The postural vasoconstriction reflex (veno-arteriolar reflex) is of particular significance. On standing, venous and arteriolar pressures increase due to the height of the column of blood between the heart and foot, resulting in an increase in the capillary pressure in the foot. This should rapidly result in interstitial oedema. Oedema is prevented by a local vasoconstrictor reflex mediated by a local sympathetic axon reflex and a myogenic response.[29] Using laser Doppler flowmetry, several investigators have shown that this veno-arteriolar reflex is reduced in subjects with diabetic autonomic neuropathy, causing oedema and orthostatic hypotension.

Thus, loss of postural regulation of blood flow and raised capillary pressure may have important consequences in the diabetic foot due to increased fluid filtration and oedema formation. In addition and more importantly in accordance to the 'haemodynamic hypothesis' these abnormalities may initiate microvascular damage and contribute to the development of foot complications.[30]

AXON REFLEX AND ENDOTHELIUM-DEPENDENT AND -INDEPENDENT VASODILATATION

In 1927, Sir Thomas Lewis described the axon-reflex-mediated flare, the response that follows a firm stroke applied to the skin. First, the skin blanches, and is then briefly followed by the appearance of a red line due to capillary dilatation. Twenty to forty seconds later, a red flare surrounds this line due to arteriolar dilatation. This flare is mediated through a local axon reflex, whereby stimulation of C-nociceptive fibres causes antidromic impulses to stimulate adjacent C-fibres to release vasodilatatory neuropeptides such as histamine, calcitonin gene-related peptide (CGRP), substance P and bradykinin (Figure 4.2).[31,32] This injury response has been

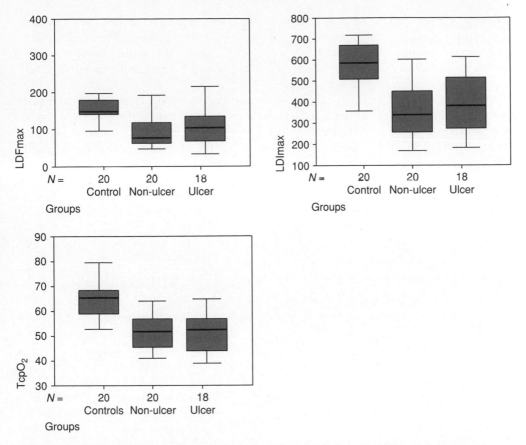

Figure 4.2 Microvascular hyperaemia in diabetic subjects with and without foot ulceration. All the microvascular measurements were significantly lower ($p < 0.0001$) in both the diabetic groups (non-ulcer and ulcer) compared to controls. There was no significant difference in any of the measurements between the diabetic groups. LDFmax, mean maximum hyperaemia using laser Doppler flowmeter in perfusion units; LDImax, mean maximum hyperaemia using laser Doppler imager in perfusion units; TcpO₂, transcutaneous partial pressure of oxygen in millimetres of mercury. (Adapted from Krishnan *et al.*)

shown to be diminished in people with diabetes and has been suggested to have implications on wound healing and ulceration.[33]

The axon reflex has been studied using a variety of stimuli and a number of techniques. The initial studies were crude, relying on visual assessment of vasodilatation. More recent studies have used the laser Doppler method to assess microvascular dilation and have employed iontophoresis of vasoactive substances to deliver the stimulus.[32,34]

Iontophoresis of acetylcholine causes vasodilatation by two mechanisms. It stimulates C-fibres to elicit axon-reflex-mediated vasodilatation within and beyond the skin to which the acetylcholine has been iontophoresed (the indirect response). It also causes vasodilatation directly in the area of iontophoresis by release of endothelium-derived hyperpolarising factor, production of prostaglandin and nitric oxide (NO) (endothelium dependent or direct response).[35]

In contrast, sodium nitroprusside acts as a donor of NO and acts directly on the smooth muscle cells.[36] Iontophoresis of this substance is used to assess endothelium-independent vasodilatation.

A variety of investigators have studied these vasodilatory responses in different stages of the diabetic process. Investigators have demonstrated both impaired endothelium-dependent and -independent vasodilatation in patients with peripheral neuropathy and have suggested that these abnormalities may be important in the development of foot ulceration.[20] In contrast, and not supporting this suggestion, other studies have shown abnormal responses in children and young adults with type 1 diabetes, who at this stage are not at risk of foot ulceration.[37] Furthermore, studies in type 2 diabetes demonstrated these same abnormalities before the development of complications.[38] Of importance, Caballero *et al.* showed that impaired responses are present in people at risk of developing type 2 diabetes, before they develop hyperglycaemia.[39]

Most of the above-mentioned studies were performed using a single-point laser Doppler and so were able to measure only change in blood flow rather than the extent of the axon-reflex-mediated flare in terms of the area over which it spreads. Recently, Krishnan *et al.* described a novel method (the LDIflare to assess the extent of the axon reflex flare (the indirect response) in response to skin heating, using laser Doppler imaging. In contrast to iontophoresis, this method is more physiological and has been shown to be more reproducible. This group has shown that the LDIflare area is markedly reduced in type 2 diabetic subjects with neuropathy. Furthermore, they have shown that patients without clinical neuropathy have significantly reduced flare responses compared to healthy controls, albeit not as markedly reduced as those with neuropathy (Figure 4.3, Plate 1). This study again confirms that the C-fibre dysfunction occurs relatively early in type 2 diabetes.[40]

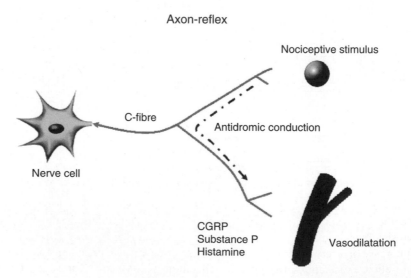

Figure 4.3   Stimulation of the C-nociceptive nerve fibres leads to antidromic conduction to the adjacent C-fibres, which secrete substance P, calcitonin gene-related peptide (CGRP) and histamine that cause vasodilatation and increased blood flow in the adjacent blood vessels

MICROVASCULAR DEFECTS AND FOOT ULCERATION

Thus, as previously described, abnormalities of the skin microcirculation are a feature of diabetes. Because of the importance of the microcirculation to skin nutrition, it is not surprising that this has been linked to the development of diabetic foot ulceration. However, until recently only a few studies have specifically examined the microcirculation in patients with foot ulceration to explore this relationship; furthermore, there have been no studies to determine whether these tests are of value in identifying those at risk. Krishnan *et al.* evaluated the relative roles of neuropathy and microvascular dysfunction in foot ulceration in type 2 diabetes, by examining patients with and without ulceration (Figure 4.4). Maximum blood flow to skin heating was assessed by laser Doppler scanning, the single-point laser Doppler probe and indirectly by TcpO$_2$ measurement. Both the diabetic groups were found to have impaired microvascular hyperaemic responses as assessed by the laser Doppler methods described and by TcpO$_2$ measurements. Of importance, those without foot ulceration had responses that were as severe as the responses in those with a history of foot ulceration. Furthermore, neither TcpO$_2$ nor the more sophisticated measurements of microvascular hyperaemic responses to skin heating were able to identify those with or without ulceration and thus could not be use to screen for those at risk. In contrast, both large- and small-fibre dysfunctions were predictive of foot ulceration. It was thus concluded that microvascular dysfunction by itself may not play an aetiological role in the development of foot ulceration. However, this does not exclude a role for microcirculatory abnormalities in the delayed wound healing in diabetes.

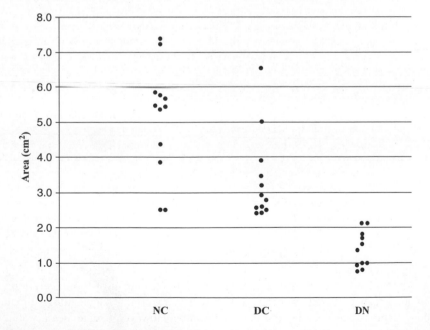

Figure 4.4 LDIflare areas (cm^2) in the three groups of subjects. LDIflare was reduced in both diabetic groups compared to NC (DN − $p < 0.0001$, DC − $p = 0.01$, respectively) and was also significantly reduced in DN compared to DC ($p < 0.0001$). NC, normal controls; DC, diabetic controls; DN, diabetic with neuropathy. (Adapted from Krishnan *et al.*[38])

WOUND HEALING IN DIABETES

Wound healing has been extensively studied in a variety of animal models. Most studies have focused on the cellular and growth factors involved in wound healing and have demonstrated reduced production of a variety of these factors including insulin-like growth factor I (IGF-I), IGF-II, keratinocyte growth factor and platelet-derived growth factor (PDGF). Other studies have shown that application of growth factors to wounds in diabetic animals had a beneficial effect. More recent work has concentrated on the enzymatic processes involved in wound healing, demonstrating increased levels of matrix metalloproteinases in the chronic ulcers in diabetic subjects and in animal models of diabetes. Surprisingly, the role of the microcirculation in wound healing has received little experimental attention in either animal models or human studies.

We have attempted to examine this by studying wound healing and microvascular responses in subjects with type 2 diabetes undergoing 3-mm foot skin biopsy for assessment of neuropathy.[41] In this study, wound closure was assessed by measuring wound area, using digital microscopy immediately after biopsy, and at day 3 and day 10 (Table 4.1).

In addition, the maximum hyperaemia to dorsal foot skin heating (44°C) was assessed using a laser Doppler imager. Against expectations and in contrast to findings in animal models, the rate of wound closure was identical in the two groups despite the subjects with diabetes having significantly impaired maximal hyperaemia responses and diabetic neuropathy. These observations do not support an influence of impaired hyperaemic responses on wound healing in diabetes.

Table 4.1 Maximum hyperaemia to heating and wound area in mm^2 in healthy controls and subjects with diabetic neuropathy

	Controls	Neuropaths	p value
LDImax (PU)	577.4 ± 125.3	310.33 ± 97.3	<0.0001
Area (mm^2)			
Day 0	6.28 ± 0.3	6.17 ± 0.5	0.78
Day 3	4.89 ± 0.8	4.63 ± 0.4	0.56
Day 10	3.01 ± 0.7	2.93 ± 0.5	0.95

CONCLUSION

A variety of microvascular abnormalities are present in people with diabetes, including structural changes and impaired vasodilatation and vasoconstriction to a variety of stimuli including trauma. Although considered to be important in the development of foot ulceration and impaired wound healing, there have been no studies that support this suggestion. Animal models of diabetes demonstrate clear defects in wound healing. However, to date the only study to examine the relationship between wound closure and the microcirculation in human diabetes has confirmed neither delayed closure nor any relationship between closure rate and hyperaemic responses. Further studies are required to confirm or refute these important observations and to explore the relationship between microvascular function and other aspects of wound healing.

REFERENCES

1. Flynn MD, Tooke JE. Diabetic neuropathy and the microcirculation. *Diabet Med* 1995;12:298–301.
2. Goldenberg S, Alex M, Joshi RA, Blumenthal HT. Nonatheromatous peripheral vascular disease of the lower extremity in diabetes mellitus. *Diabetes* Jul 1959;8:261–273.
3. LoGerfo FW, Coffman JD. Current concepts. Vascular and microvascular disease of the foot in diabetes. Implications for foot care. *N Engl J Med* 1984;311:1615–1619.
4. Parving HH, Viberti GC, Keen H, Christiansen JS, Lassen NA. Hemodynamic factors in the genesis of diabetic microangiopathy. *Metabolism* Sep 1983;32:943–949.
5. Rayman G, Malik RA, Sharma AK, Day JL. Microvascular response to tissue injury and capillary ultrastructure in the foot skin of type I diabetic patients. *Clin Sci (Colch)* 1995;89:467–474.
6. Silhi N. Diabetes and wound healing. *J Wound Care* Jan 1998;7:47–51.
7. Braverman IM. Ultrastructure and organization of the cutaneous microvasculature in normal and pathologic states. *J Invest Dermatol* 1989;93:2S–9S.
8. Malik RA, Newrick PG, Sharma AK, *et al.* Microangiopathy in human diabetic neuropathy: relationship between capillary abnormalities and the severity of neuropathy. *Diabetologia* 1989;32:92–102.
9. Sandeman DD, Shore AC, Tooke JE. Relation of skin capillary pressure in patients with insulin-dependent diabetes mellitus to complications and metabolic control. *N Engl J Med* Sep 1992;10:760–764.
10. Jorneskog G, Brismar K, Fagrell B. Pronounced skin capillary ischemia in the feet of diabetic patients with bad metabolic control. *Diabetologia* 1998;41:410–415.
11. Hamdy O, Abou-Elenin K, LoGerfo FW, Horton ES, Veves A. Contribution of nerve-axon reflex-related vasodilation to the total skin vasodilation in diabetic patients with and without neuropathy. *Diabetes Care* 2001;24:344–349.
12. Vinik AI, Erbas T, Park TS, Pierce KK, Stansberry KB. Methods for evaluation of peripheral neurovascular dysfunction. *Diabetes Technol Ther* 2001;3:29–50.
13. Shore AC, Price KJ, Sandeman DD, Tripp JH, Tooke JE. Posturally induced vasoconstriction in diabetes mellitus. *Arch Dis Child* Jan 1994;70:22–26.
14. Johnson JM, O'Leary DS, Taylor WF, Kosiba W. Effect of local warming on forearm reactive hyperaemia. *Clin Physiol* Aug 1986;6:337–346.
15. Rayman G, Williams SA, Spencer PD, Smaje LH, Wise PH, Tooke JE. Impaired microvascular hyperaemic response to minor skin trauma in type I diabetes. *Br Med J (Clin Res Ed)* 1986;292:1295–1298.
16. Rayman G, Malik RA, Sharma AK, Day JL. Microvascular response to tissue injury and capillary ultrastructure in the foot skin of type I diabetic patients. *Clin Sci (Colch)* 1995;89:467–474.
17. Rendell MS, Finnegan MF, Healy JC, *et al.* The relationship of laser-Doppler skin blood flow measurements to the cutaneous microvascular anatomy. *Microvasc Res* Jan 1998;55:3–13.
18. Morris SJ, Shore AC. Skin blood flow responses to the iontophoresis of acetylcholine and sodium nitroprusside in man: possible mechanisms. *J Physiol (Lond)* 1996;496:531–542.
19. Shore AC, Price KJ, Sandeman DD, Green EM, Tripp JH, Tooke JE. Impaired microvascular hyperaemic response in children with diabetes mellitus. *Diabet Med* 1991;8:619–623.
20. Khan F, Elhadd TA, Greene SA, Belch JJ. Impaired skin microvascular function in children, adolescents, and young adults with type 1 diabetes. *Diabetes Care* 2000;23:215–220.
21. Sandeman DD, Pym CA, Green EM, Seamark C, Shore AC, Tooke JE. Microvascular vasodilatation in feet of newly diagnosed non-insulin dependent diabetic patients. *BMJ* 1991;302:1122–1123.
22. Jaap AJ, Shore AC, Tooke JE. Relationship of insulin resistance to microvascular dysfunction in subjects with fasting hyperglycaemia. *Diabetologia* Feb 1997;40:238–243.
23. Railton R, Newman P, Hislop J, Harrower AD. Reduced transcutaneous oxygen tension and impaired vascular response in Type 1 (insulin-dependent) diabetes. *Diabetologia* 1983;25:340–342.
24. Uccioli L, Monticone G, Russo F, *et al.* Autonomic neuropathy and transcutaneous oxymetry in diabetic lower extremities. *Diabetologia* 1994;37:1051–1055.

25. Flynn MD, Edmonds ME, Tooke JE, Watkins PJ. Direct measurement of capillary blood flow in the diabetic neuropathic foot. *Diabetologia* 1988;31:652–656.
26. Jorneskog G, Brismar K, Fagrell B. Skin capillary circulation severely impaired in toes of patients with IDDM, with and without late diabetic complications. *Diabetologia* Apr 1995;38:474–480.
27. Aso Y, Inukai T, Takemura Y. Evaluation of skin vasomotor reflexes in response to deep inspiration in diabetic patients by laser Doppler flowmetry. A new approach to the diagnosis of diabetic peripheral autonomic neuropathy. *Diabetes Care* 1997;20:1324–1328.
28. Stansberry KB, Hill MA, Shapiro SA, McNitt PM, Bhatt BA, Vinik AI. Impairment of peripheral blood flow responses in diabetes resembles an enhanced aging effect. *Diabetes Care* 1997;20:1711–1716.
29. Ubbink DT, Jacobs MJ, Tangelder GJ, Slaaf DW, Reneman RS. Posturally induced microvascular constriction in patients with different stages of leg ischaemia: effect of local skin heating. *Clin Sci (Colch)* 1991;81:43–49.
30. Jorneskog G, Brismar K, Fagrell B. Skin capillary circulation is more impaired in the toes of diabetic than non-diabetic patients with peripheral vascular disease. *Diabet Med* 1995;12:36–41.
31. Schmelz M, Michael K, Weidner C, Schmidt R, Torebjork HE, Handwerker HO. Which nerve fibers mediate the axon reflex flare in human skin? *Neuroreport* Feb 28, 2000;11:645-648.
32. Caselli A, Rich J, Hanane T, Uccioli L, Veves A. Role of C-nociceptive fibers in the nerve axon reflex-related vasodilation in diabetes. *Neurology* Jan 28, 2003;60:297–300.
33. Walmsley D, Wales JK, Wiles PG. Reduced hyperaemia following skin trauma: evidence for an impaired microvascular response to injury in the diabetic foot. *Diabetologia* 1989;32:736–739.
34. Morris SJ, Shore AC. Skin blood flow responses to the iontophoresis of acetylcholine and sodium nitroprusside in man: possible mechanisms. *J Physiol* Oct 15, 1996;496:531–542.
35. Vallance P, Collier J, Moncada S. Effects of endothelium-derived nitric oxide on peripheral arteriolar tone in man. *Lancet* 1989;2:997–1000.
36. Veves A, Akbari CM, Primavera J, *et al*. Endothelial dysfunction and the expression of endothelial nitric oxide synthetase in diabetic neuropathy, vascular disease, and foot ulceration. *Diabetes* 1998;47:457–463.
37. Lim SC, Caballero AE, Smakowski P, LoGerfo FW, Horton ES, Veves A. Soluble intercellular adhesion molecule, vascular cell adhesion molecule, and impaired microvascular reactivity are early markers of vasculopathy in type 2 diabetic individuals without microalbuminuria. *Diabetes Care* 1999;1:1865–1870.
38. Krishnan ST, Rayman G. The LDIflare: a novel test of C-fiber function demonstrates early neuropathy in type 2 diabetes. *Diabetes Care* 2004;27:2930–2935.
39. Caballero AE, Arora S, Saouaf R, *et al*. Microvascular and macrovascular reactivity is reduced in subjects at risk for type 2 diabetes. *Diabetes* 1999;48:1856–1862.
40. Krishnan ST, Baker NR, Carrington AL, Rayman G. Comparative roles of microvascular and nerve function in foot ulceration in type 2 diabetes. *Diabetes Care* 2004;27:1343–1348.
41. Rayman G, Baker NR, Krishnan STM. Wound healing and microvascular responses in the foot skin of type 2 diabetic subjects with neuropathy. Diabetic Foot Study Group, 5th Scientific Meeting; 2005; Chalkidiki, Greece.

5 The Pathway to Ulceration: Aetiopathogenesis

Andrew J.M. Boulton

> *Coming events cast their shadows before*
> — Thomas Campbell

INTRODUCTION

As the lifetime incidence of foot ulceration in diabetic patients was recently estimated to be as high as 25%,[1] understanding the pathways that result in the development of an ulcer is increasingly important. Although not referring to diabetic foot ulcers when writing the above lines, the Scottish poet Thomas Campbell's words can usefully be applied to the breakdown of the diabetic foot. Ulceration does not occur spontaneously; rather, it is the combination of causative factors that result in the development of a lesion. There are many warning signs or 'shadows' that can identify those at risk. The famous Boston diabetes physician Elliot Joslin realised this over 70 years ago when, after observing many clinical cases of diabetic foot disease, he remarked 'diabetic gangrene is not heaven-sent, but earth-born'.[2] Thus, it is not an inevitable consequence of having diabetes that foot ulceration will eventually occur: ulcers invariably occur as a consequence of an interaction between specific pathologies in the lower limb and environmental hazards.

Those various pathologies that affect the feet and ultimately interact to increase vulnerability to ulceration will be considered in this chapter. A clear understating of the aetiopathogenesis of ulceration is essential if we are to succeed in reducing the incidence of foot ulceration, and ultimately amputations. Although some countries such as the Netherlands have achieved a reduction in diabetes-related lower limb amputations in recent years,[3] this has not been a universal finding. In Germany, for example, no change in the incidence of amputations could be observed in the 9 years until 2000.[4] As the vast majority of amputations are preceded by foot ulcers,[5] a thorough understanding of the causative pathways to ulceration is essential if we are to reduce the depressingly high incidences of ulceration and amputation. Moreover, as lower limb complications are the commonest precipitants of hospitalisation of diabetic patients in most countries, there are potential economic benefits to be gained from preventative strategies, as noted in the previous chapters. Potential economic savings of a successful amputation

The Foot in Diabetes, 4th Edition. Editors Andrew J.M. Boulton, Peter R. Cavanagh and Gerry Rayman.
© 2006 John Wiley & Sons, Ltd.

prevention programme were estimated to be between $2 million and $3 million over 3 years in a hypothetical cohort of 10 000 diabetic individuals.[6] Finally, a successful screening programme based upon early identification of those at risk should impact on the appreciable morbidity, and even mortality, of diabetic foot disease, as emphasised by Krentz et al.[7]

The breakdown of the diabetic foot traditionally has been considered to result from an interaction of peripheral vascular disease (PVD), peripheral neuropathy and some form of trauma. More recently, other contributory causes, such as psychosocial factors (Chapter 11) and abnormalities of pressures and loads under the foot,[5] have been implicated. The interaction between neuropathy and foot pressure abnormalities will be considered and, although covered in great detail in Chapter 21, the importance of vascular disease will be discussed briefly. There is no compelling evidence that infection is a direct cause of ulceration: it is likely that infection becomes established once skin breaks occur, and so this topic will not be considered here. Detailed discussion of infection can be found in Chapters 13 and 14.

PERIPHERAL VASCULAR DISEASE

A number of large epidemiological studies have confirmed the frequency of all forms of ischaemic vascular disease in diabetes.[8,9] The Diabetes Audit and Research in Tayside Scotland (DARTS) study from Scotland, for example, reported the annual incidence for the development of PVD in diabetic patients to be 5.5/1000 patients in those with type 1 diabetes, and 13.6/1000 in type 2 diabetes.[9] In the US National Health and Nutrition Examinations Survey, 1999–2000, the prevalence of PVD in the general population was 4.3%, but having diabetes was positively associated with prevalent PVD (odds ratio 2.83).[10] PVD tends to occur at a younger age in diabetic patients and is more likely to involve distal vessels. Reports from the United States and Finland have confirmed that PVD is a major contributory factor in the pathogenesis of foot ulceration and subsequent major amputations.[11,12] In the assessment of PVD, simple clinical assessment of the distal circulation and non-invasive tests of the circulation by a hand-held Doppler ultrasound stethoscope can be useful in the assessment of outcome.[8]

In the pathogenesis of ulceration, PVD itself, in isolation, rarely causes ulceration: as will be discussed for neuropathy, it is the combination of risk factors with minor trauma that inevitably leads to ulceration (Figure 5.1). Thus, minor injury and subsequent infection increase the demand for blood supply beyond the circulatory capacity, and ischaemic ulceration and the risk of amputation ensue. Early identification of those at risk and education in good foot care habits are therefore potentially protective. In recent years, neuroischaemic ulcers in which combination of neuropathy and PVD exists in the same patient, together with some form of trauma, are becoming increasingly common in diabetic foot clinics. Whereas at the time of publication of the first edition of this volume (1987), neuropathic ulcers were most frequently seen in diabetic foot clinics, this has changed in the twenty-first century, with neuroischaemic ulcers now being the commonest in most clinics.

Although the United Kingdom Prospective Diabetes Study (UKPDS) suggested that tight control of blood glucose and blood pressure might influence the development of certain cardiovascular end points such as stroke and sudden death, statistical evidence that these influence the progression of PVD was not forthcoming.[13,14] However, educational strategies aimed at the cessation of smoking and control of dyslipidaemia therefore remain of paramount importance. Moreover, in view of the trends observed in the UKPDS, optimal glycaemic and blood pressure control should be aimed for.

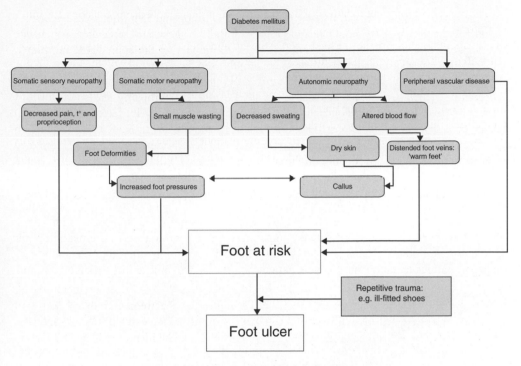

Figure 5.1 Pathways to diabetic foot ulceration

DIABETIC NEUROPATHY

As discussed in Chapter 3, the diabetic neuropathies represent the commonest of the long-term complications of diabetes, affect different parts of the nervous system and may present with diverse clinical manifestations.[15] Most common among the neuropathies are chronic sensorimotor distal symmetric polyneuropathy and the autonomic neuropathies. It is the common chronic sensorimotor neuropathy and peripheral autonomic sympathetic neuropathy that together play an important part in the pathogenesis of ulceration, and these will be discussed in some detail. The association between peripheral neuropathy and foot ulceration has been recognised for many years: Pryce, a surgeon working in Nottingham over 120 years ago, remarked that 'it is abundantly clear to me that the actual cause of the perforating ulcer was a peripheral nerve degeneration', and 'diabetes itself may play an active part in the causation of the perforating ulcers'.

Sensorimotor Neuropathy

Chronic sensorimotor neuropathy, which commonly occurs in both major types of diabetes, may be defined as 'the presence of symptoms and/or signs of peripheral nerve dysfunction in people with diabetes after exclusion of other causes'. The diagnosis cannot be made without a careful clinical examination of the lower limbs, as absence of symptoms can never be equated with absence of signs.[16]

The onset of chronic neuropathy is gradual and insidious, and indeed, on occasions, the initial symptoms may go unnoticed by patients. Typical symptoms, which may be present in up to half of all patients, include paraesthesia, hyperaesthesia, and sharp stabbing, shooting and burning pain, all of which are prone to nocturnal exacerbation. Whereas in some patients these uncomfortable symptoms predominate, others may never experience any symptoms. Clinical examination usually reveals a sensory deficit in a stocking distribution, and signs of motor dysfunction, including small muscle wasting and absent ankle reflexes, are usually present.[15] A particularly dangerous situation, originally described by J.D. Ward, is the 'painful–painless leg' in which the patient experiences painful or paraesthetic symptoms, but on examination has severe sensory loss to pain and proprioception; such patients are at great risk of painless injury to their feet.

The threshold of sensation that protects normal feet holds a very delicate balance. The purpose of pain sensation as described by Brand[17] is not to cause pain but to enable the body to use its strength to the maximum short of damage. Thus, a person who has lost some pain sensation has not totally lost the ability to feel pain – he simply feels pain at a higher level of stress. Thus it takes more pressure or temperature or more prolonged ischaemia before the residual nerve fibres are activated and warn higher centres. It must therefore be emphasised that neuropathic ulceration may occur in patients who still have some ability to perceive stimuli to various modalities. It is extremely difficult in practice to define exactly what a 'significant' loss of sensation is, or at what level of sensory loss a patient's foot becomes 'at risk'.

There is a spectrum of symptomatic severity in sensorimotor neuropathy: at one extreme, patients experience severe symptoms whereas others experience mild symptoms or even none at all. Thus, whereas a history of typical symptoms is strongly suggestive of a diagnosis of neuropathy, *absence of symptoms cannot exclude neuropathy and must never be equated with a lack of foot ulcer risk*. Therefore, *assessment of foot ulcer risk must always include a careful foot examination whatever the history*.[15–17]

Peripheral Sympathetic Autonomic Neuropathy

Sympathetic autonomic neuropathy affecting the lower limbs leads to reduced sweating and results in both dry skin that is prone to crack and stroke or fissure, and also to increased blood flow (in the absence of large vessel PVD) with arterio-venous shunting leading to the warm foot. The complex interactions of sympathetic neuropathy and other contributory factors in the causation of foot ulcers are summarised in Figure 5.1.

The warm, insensitive and dry foot that results from a combination of somatic and autonomic dysfunction often provides the patient with a false sense of security, as most patients still perceive vascular disease as the main cause of ulcers. It is such patients who may present with insensitive ulceration, as they have truly painless feet. Perhaps, the highest risk foot is the pulseless insensitive foot, because it indicates somatic and autonomic neuropathy together with PVD.

NEUROPATHY: THE MAJOR CONTRIBUTORY FACTOR IN ULCERATION

Cross-sectional data from established UK foot clinics in London and Manchester presented in the second edition of this volume suggested that neuropathy was present in up to 90% of foot ulcers in patients attending physician – or podiatrist – led services. Thus, most foot ulcers were considered to be of neuropathic or neuroischaemic aetiology. Confirmation of these facts in recent years has come from several European and North American studies. Patients with sensory loss appear to show an increase in risk of developing ulcers of up to sevenfold, compared with non-neuropathic, diabetic individuals.[18–20] In the large North-West Diabetes Foot Care Study, for example, a cohort of 10 000 patients was followed for 2 years in the community.[20] Whereas the overall incidence of new foot ulceration in the cohort was 2.2%, when divided into those with and without neuropathy at baseline, the annual incidence of ulceration was 1.1% in those without neuropathy compared with greater than 6% in those with neuropathy. Other prospective trials have confirmed the pivotal role of both large-fibre (e.g. proprioceptive deficits) and small-fibre (e.g. loss of pain and temperature sensation) neurological deficits in the pathogenesis of ulceration.[18–21] Poor balance and instability are also increasingly being recognised as troublesome symptoms of peripheral neuropathy, presumably secondary to proprioceptive loss. The relationship between sway, postural instability and foot ulceration has also been confirmed.[22]

Considering the above data, there can be little doubt that neuropathy causes foot ulcers with or without ischaemia, but it must be remembered that the neuropathic foot does not spontaneously ulcerate; it is the combination of neuropathy and either extrinsic factors (such as ill-fitting footwear) or intrinsic factors (such as high foot pressures, Chapter 6) that results in ulceration. The other risk factors that are associated with ulceration will now be considered.

OTHER RISK FACTORS FOR FOOT ULCERATION

Age and Duration of Diabetes

The risk of ulcers and amputation increases two- to fourfold with both age and duration of diabetes.[23] The relationship of diabetes duration to prevalence of ulceration and amputation appears to be similar for people with both type 1 and type 2 diabetes.

Sex

The male sex has been associated with a 1.6-fold increased risk of ulcers[20,23] and an even higher risk of amputation[23] in most studies of people with type 2 diabetes. The mechanism by which men are at greater risk of these complications is yet to be explained.

Previous Foot Ulceration

Several studies have confirmed that foot ulceration is most common in those patients with a past history of similar lesions or amputation, and also in patients from a poor social background.[23] Indeed, in many diabetic foot clinics, more than 50% of patients with new foot ulcers have a past history of similar problems. In one randomised controlled trial, Litzelman found that a history of an ulcer increased the risk of new ulceration 13-fold.[21] In another prospective study, the risk of ulceration was highly associated with a history of previous ulcers (odds ratio 56.8).[24] Similarly, a history of prior ulceration is associated with a two- to tenfold higher risk of amputation.[23]

Other Diabetic Microvascular Complications

It has been recognised for many years that patients with retinopathy and/or renal impairment are at increased risk of foot ulceration. However, it is now confirmed that patients at all stages of diabetic nephropathy, even microalbuminuria, have an increased risk of foot ulceration.[25] Indeed, diabetes was recently shown to be the strongest risk factor for lower extremity amputation in new dialysis patients.[26]

Race

Data from cross-sectional studies in Europe suggest that foot ulceration is commoner in Europid subjects when compared to groups of other racial origins. Recent data from the North-West Diabetes Foot Care Study showed that the age-adjusted prevalence of diabetic foot ulcers (past or present) for Europeans, South Asians and African Caribbeans was 5.5, 1.8 and 2.7%, respectively.[27] The reasons for these ethnic differences certainly warrant further investigation. In contrast, in the southern United States, ulceration was much more common in Hispanic Americans and native Americans than in non-Hispanic Whites.[28] However, there is no suggestion that within Europe the risk is related to any geographical differences: Veves *et al.*, for example, showed no differences in risk factors for ulceration according to location, for different European centres.[29]

Motor Neuropathy

Although the commonest neuropathy of diabetes is 'chronic sensorimotor neuropathy', most reviews focus exclusively on the sensory components. Thus, special mention is made here of the motor component: small muscle wasting in the feet is common in neuropathy, and atrophy of foot muscles is closely related to the severity of neuropathy.[30] Moreover, small muscle dysfunction secondary to neuropathy may contribute to ulcer risk through altered gait and foot pressure changes.

Oedema

The presence of peripheral oedema impairs local blood supply and has been associated with increased risk of ulceration.[31]

Callus

The presence of plantar callus, especially in the neuropathic foot, is associated with an increased risk of ulceration: in one study, the risk was 77-fold in the cross-sectional part, whereas in the prospective follow-up, ulceration occurred only at sites of callus, representing an infinite increase in risk.[32]

Deformity

Any deformity occurring in a diabetic foot with other risk factors, such as prominence of the metatarsal heads, clawing of the toes, Charcot prominences or hallux valgus, increases ulcer risk. Evidence to support this statement comes from the prospective North-West Diabetes Foot Care Study in which foot deformities were independently related to the risk of new foot ulcers.[20]

ASSESSMENT OF FOOT ULCER RISK

For one mistake made for not knowing, ten mistakes are made for not looking
                                                                                    – J.A. Lindsay

The above aphorism could have been written specifically for diabetic foot problems, as many foot lesions are missed because the clinician fails to examine the feet. Paul Brand (1914–2003) emphasised this when he was asked, at a US Department of Health Conference, to recommend how amputations could be reduced in diabetic patients. Expecting an answer promoting vascular surgery or modern medications, the questioner was surprised at the answer, 'remove the shoes and socks and examine the feet every time you see a patient with diabetes'.[17]

The traditional model of disease is that a patient goes to the doctor with symptoms, treatment is then prescribed and the patient recovers. As this cannot apply to insensate feet, health care professionals have difficulty comprehending the diabetic foot syndrome: they find it difficult to take the initiative and look for early lesions or warning signs of imminent breakdown. Many doctors regard these patients as stupid – how can a sensible individual walk on a swollen red foot with an active ulcer? What we must realise is that an insensitive foot not only is painless, but also does not feel as if it belongs to the individual.[17] In screening for 'at-risk' feet, it is our job to identify patients at risk of ulceration and help them understand and cope with this health state and thus avoid exposure to environmental hazards that may result in injury (often unperceived) and eventual breakdown.

As with other microvascular complications, there may be no symptoms to suggest to the patient that they have foot problems. The concept of the 'annual review' for diabetic patients is now well established.[33] Thus, all patients should be screened for retinopathy, hypertension, nephropathy and risk of foot lesions, annually. For the foot, the following are recommended according to the level of care (Table 5.1).

1. History – important in the annual review
   (a) Neuropathic symptoms?
   (b) Past history of ulcer?
   (c) Other diabetic problems, especially retinopathy/impaired vision?
   (d) History of claudication/rest pain/vascular surgery?
   (e) Home circumstances – e.g. living alone?

2. Examination – essential in the annual review
   (a) Inspection: shoes and socks must be removed
       (i) Skin status: colour, thickness, dryness, cracking?
       (ii) Sweating?

Table 5.1 Screening techniques for identifying the 'at-risk' foot

	Primary care	Secondary care	Clinical research
History			
(symptoms of neuropathy/PVD)	+++	+++	+
Clinical exam	+++	+++	+++
Monofilament	+++	++	++
Vibration perception	++	++	+++
Quantitative sensory tests	−	+	++
Electrophysiology	−	−	++
Pressuremat			
(e.g. PressureStat)	++	+++	++
Quantitative foot pressure	−	+	++

+++, recommended; ++, useful if available; +, occasionally required; −, not recommended.

    (iii) Infection: check between the toes as well.
    (iv) Ulceration?
    (v) Deformity, e.g. Charcot changes or clawing of the toes?
    (vi) Foot shape.
    (vii) Small muscle wasting?
    (viii) Skin temperature: compare the feet. A unilateral, warm swollen foot with intact skin would suggest the possibility of acute Charcot neuroarthropathy. Moreover, prior to neuropathic ulceration there would be a local increase in temperature.[34]
    (ix) The patient's footwear and gait should also be assessed. Walking without a limp with a plantar ulcer is diagnostic of neuropathy.
(b) Neurological assessment
    (i) Neuropathy can easily be documented by a simple clinical exam of large-fibre function (e.g. 128-Hz tuning fork for vibration), small-fibre function (e.g. pinprick, hot/cold rods) and ankle reflexes. A simple composite score comprising these measures (Table 5.2) has been shown to be useful in the prediction of those at risk of future ulceration.[20]
    (ii) 10-g monofilament: This tests pressure perception and is frequently used to assess foot ulcer risk status.[35] Although simple to perform, general agreement is lacking as to which site should be tested and not all filaments accurately assess pressure at 10 g.[36] Moreover, the number of sites that should be tested is unknown: for example, the 128-Hz tuning fork vibration assessment tested at two sites was recently shown to be as sensitive as the monofilament tested at eight sites.[37]
(c) Vascular assessment
    (i) Posterior tibial and dorsalis pedis pulses should be palpated.
    (ii) Bedside assessment of the circulation using a Doppler ultrasound probe can be useful. However, the presence of diabetes and neuropathy make the usual tests such as the ankle pressure index less efficacious: wave form analysis and pressures are more effective.[38]

3. Other assessments
  (a) Quantitative sensory testing (QST)

Table 5.2 The Modified Neuropathy Disability Score

Neuropathy Disability Score (NDS)		
	Right	Left
Vibration perception threshold 128-Hz tuning fork; apex of big toe; normal = can distinguish vibrating/not vibrating		
Temperature perception on dorsum of the foot Use tuning fork with beaker of ice/warm water; normal = can distinguish hot from cold	Normal = 0 Abnormal = 1	
Pinprick Apply pin proximal to big toenail just enough to deform the skin; trial pair = sharp, blunt; normal = can distinguish sharp/not sharp		
Achilles reflex		
	Present = 0 Present with reinforcement = 1 Absent = 2 NDS total out of 10	

   (i) Vibration assessment: The biothesiometer, neurothesiometer and vibration perception threshold meters are simple, hand-held tests of vibration perception that can easily be used in the outpatient setting: loss of vibration as assessed with these instruments is strongly predictive of subsequent ulceration.[19]

   (ii) Temperature perception: A new hand-held instrument, the NeuroQuick,[39] that tests cold sensation is now available. This may in future be useful in screening for early neuropathy.

  (iii) Other QST instruments: Other more elaborate equipment to assess distal sensory function are available.[16] However, most of these are expensive and time consuming and are restricted to clinical research usage.

  (iv) Electrophysiology: Although nerve conduction studies strongly predict future ulcers,[40] their use is generally restricted to clinical research studies.

(b) Foot pressure studies

   (i) Simple semi-quantitative mat systems: PressureStat is a simple, inexpensive, semi-quantitative foot print mat that takes a minute or two to measure plantar pressures. Images can be identified immediately (Figure 5.2) and as higher pressure areas are darker, this provides a powerful educational tool to help patients understand which areas of their feet are at particular risk.[41]

  (ii) Detailed foot pressure analysis: A number of complex mats and in-shoe systems are available for foot pressure analysis. These are covered in Chapter 7.

4. Guidelines – a number of guidelines on foot assessment are available as published reviews.[16,23,33,42]

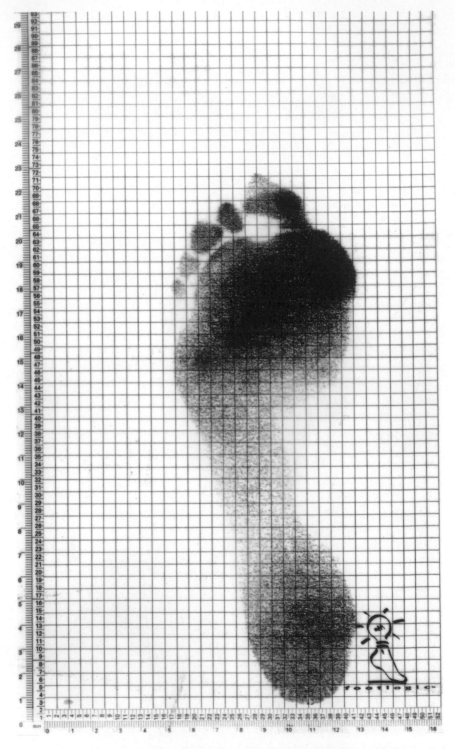

Figure 5.2   An example of a PressureStat Foot Print. The darker areas represent higher foot pressures

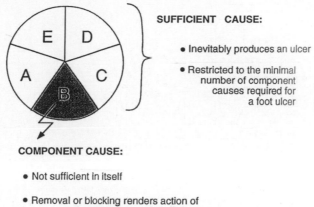

SUFFICIENT CAUSE:

- Inevitably produces an ulcer

- Restricted to the minimal
  number of component
  causes required for
  a foot ulcer

COMPONENT CAUSE:

- Not sufficient in itself

- Removal or blocking renders action of
  other components insufficient

Figure 5.3 Diagram of sufficient and component causes of diabetic foot ulcers. A–E represent causes that are not sufficient in themselves but that are the required components of a sufficient cause that will inevitably produce the affect. (Copyright © 1999 American Diabetes Association. From Diabetes Care, Vol, 22, 1999; 157–162. Reprinted with permission from The American Diabetes Association.)

THE PATHWAY TO ULCERATION

It is the combination of two or more risk factors that ultimately results in diabetic foot ulceration. Both Pecoraro *et al.*[11] and later Reiber *et al.*[31] have taken the Rothman model for causation and applied this to amputation and foot ulceration in diabetes. The model is based upon the concept that a component cause (e.g. neuropathy) is not sufficient in itself to lead to ulceration, but when the component causes act together, they result in a sufficient cause, which will inevitably result in ulceration (Figure 5.3). In their study of amputations, Pecoraro *et al.*[11] described five component causes that lead to amputation: neuropathy, minor trauma, ulceration, faulty healing and gangrene.

Reiber *et al.* subsequently applied this model to foot ulceration, and a number of causal pathways were identified: the commonest triad of component causes, present in 63% of incident cases, was neuropathy, deformity and trauma (Figure 5.4). Oedema and ischaemia were also common component causes.

Other simple examples of two-component pathways to ulceration are neuropathy and mechanical trauma, e.g. standing on a nail (Figure 5.5), ill-fitting footwear (Figure 5.6); neuropathy and thermal trauma; and neuropathy and chemical trauma, e.g. the inappropriate use of chemical 'corn cures'. Similarly, the Rothman model can be applied to neuroischaemic ulceration, where the three component parts comprising ischaemia, trauma and neuropathy are often seen.[11,31]

MECHANICAL FACTORS AND NEUROPATHIC FOOT ULCERATION

The insensitive neuropathic foot does not ulcerate spontaneously: traumatic or extrinsic ulcers result as a consequence of trauma to the insensitive foot, as shown in Figure 5.6. In contrast,

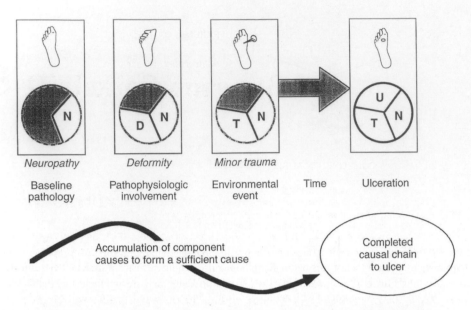

Figure 5.4   The commonest causal pathway to incident diabetic foot ulcers. (Copyright © 1999 American Diabetes Association. From Diabetes Care, Vol, 22, 1999; 157–162. Reprinted with permission from The American Diabetes Association.)

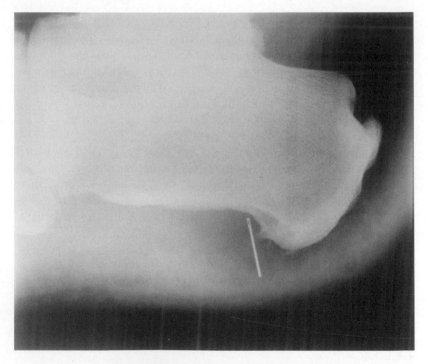

Figure 5.5   Radiograph of patient presenting with a recurrent discharging heel lesion. On enquiry, the patient remembered some trauma to the heel but did not realise that he had part of a needle in the subcutaneous tissue under the calcaneum – an example of a traumatic ulcer in the insensitive foot, which could have been prevented by wearing appropriate footwear

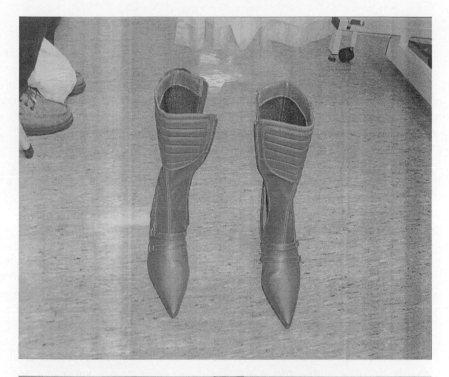

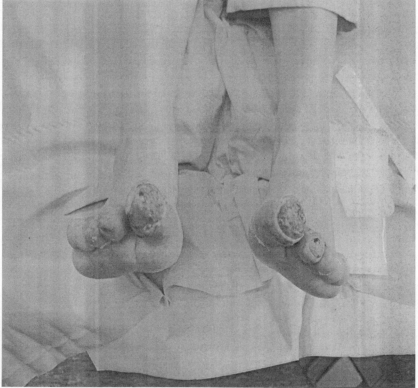

Figure 5.6 Inappropriate footwear for a female patient with insensitive feet (left) that resulted in toe lesions (right)

intrinsic or pressure ulcers occur as a result of pressure that would not normally cause ulceration, but which, because of intrinsic abnormalities in the neuropathic foot, leads to plantar ulceration when repetitively applied. As stated in the next chapter, abnormalities of pressures and loads under the diabetic foot are very common. Both prospective and cross-sectional studies have confirmed that high plantar pressures are a major aetiological factor in neuropathic foot ulceration.[5,43] Pressure ulcers tend to occur under areas such as the metatarsal heads, as a result of repetitive pressure application during walking. Callus tissue that forms under the dry foot (as a consequence of autonomic neuropathy) may itself further aggravate the problem. An example of a foot at high risk of intrinsic neuropathic foot ulceration, with insensitivity, prominent metatarsal heads, clawed toes and resultant high foot pressure, is provided in Figure 5.7. Recent evidence suggests that high foot pressures occur early in the natural history of diabetes, often before clinical neuropathy is apparent.[44]

Two additional component causes for intrinsic foot ulcers are callus and limitation of joint mobility. This latter abnormality, originally described in the hand, also occurs in the feet and contributes to abnormalities of foot pressure.

The five component causes leading to intrinsic foot ulcers are therefore somatic peripheral neuropathy, sympathetic peripheral neuropathy, limited joint mobility, callus and high foot pressure. There is therefore potential for preventing such ulcers: callus can be removed by the podiatrist; high foot pressures can be reduced by callus removal, protective insoles and hosiery; and the incidence of neuropathy can be reduced by near-normoglycaemia from the time of diagnosis of diabetes. Thus, many if not most neuropathic and neuroischaemic ulcers are potentially preventable.

THE PATIENT WITH SENSORY LOSS

It should now be possible to achieve a significant reduction of foot ulcer and amputation in diabetes. Guidelines now exist for the diagnosis and management of neuropathy[15,16] and foot problems.[16,42] However, much work is still required in the assessment and management of psychosocial factors (Chapter 11) and, as is well known, guidelines will be of use only if properly implemented.

However, a reduction in neuropathic foot problems will be achieved only if we remember that patients with insensitive feet have lost their warning signal – pain – that ordinarily brings the patients to their doctors. Thus, as stated earlier, the care of a patient with no pain sensation is a new challenge for which we have no training. It is difficult for us to understand, for example, that an intelligent patient would buy and wear a pair of shoes three sizes too small and come to our clinic with an extensive shoe-induced ulcer (Figure 5.6). The explanation however is simple: with reduced sensation, a very tight fit stimulates the remaining pressure nerve endings and this is interpreted as a normal fit – hence the common complain when we provide patients with custom-designed shoes is 'these shoes are too loose'. We can learn much about the management from the treatment of patients with leprosy[17]; if we are to succeed, we must realise that with loss of pain there is also diminished motivation in the healing of, and prevention of, injury.

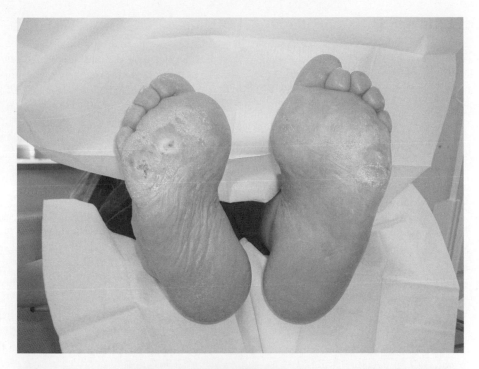

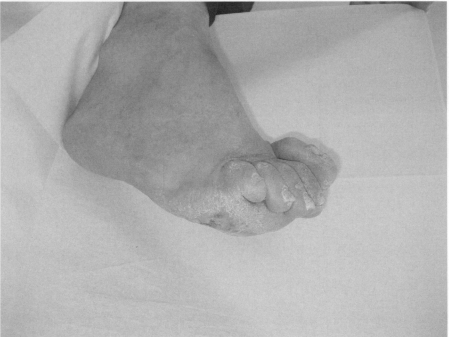

Figure 5.7 The high-risk neuropathic foot (plantar and lateral views). This foot displays a marked prominence of the metatarsal head with clawing of the toes and is at high risk of pressure-induced ulceration

REFERENCES

1. Singh N, Armstrong DG, Lipsky BA. Preventing foot ulcers in patients with diabetes. *JAMA* 2005;293:217–228.
2. Joslin EP. The menace of diabetic gangrene. *N Engl J Med* 1934;211:16–20.
3. van Houtum WH, Rawerda JA, Ruwaard D, *et al.* Reduction in diabetes-related lower-extremity amputations in the Netherlands: 1991–2000. *Diabetes Care* 2004;27:1042–1046.
4. Trautner C, Haastert B, Spraul M, *et al.* Unchanged incidence of lower-limb amputations in a German city 1990–1998. *Diabetes Care* 2001;24:855–859.
5. Boulton AJM, Kirsner RS, Vileikyte L. Neuropathic diabetic foot ulcers. *N Engl J Med* 2004;351:48–55.
6. Ollendorf DA, Kotsanos JG, Wishner WJ, *et al.* Potential economic benefits of lower-extremity amputation prevention strategies in diabetes. *Diabetes Care* 1998;21:1240–1245.
7. Krentz AJ, Acheson P, Basu A, *et al.* Morbidity and mortality associated with diabetic foot disease: a 12 month prospective study of hospital admission in a single UK centre. *Foot* 1997;7:144–177.
8. Young MJ, Boulton AJM. Peripheral vascular disease. In: Dyck PJ, Thomas PK, Ashbury AK, Winegrad AI, Porte D, eds. *Diabetic Neuropathy*. Philadelphia: WB Saunders; 1999:105–122.
9. McAlpine RR, Morris AD, Emslie-Smith A, *et al.* The annual incidence of diabetic complications in a population of patients with type 1 and type 2 diabetes. *Diabet Med* 2005;22:348–352.
10. Selvin E, Erlinger TP. Prevalence of and risk factors for peripheral arterial disease in the United States: results from the National Health and Nutrition Examination Survey, 1999–2000. *Circulation* 2004;110:738–743.
11. Pecoraro RE, Reiber RE, Burgess EM. Pathways to diabetic limb amputation: basis for prevention. *Diabetes Care* 1990;13:510–521.
12. Siitonen OI, Niskanen LK, Laakso M, *et al.* Lower extremity amputation in diabetic and non-diabetic patients: a population-based study in Eastern Finland. *Diabetes Care* 1993;16:16–20.
13. UKPDS. Intensive blood glucose control with sulphonylurea or insulin compared with conventional treatment and risk of complications in type 2 diabetes. UKPDS 33. *Lancet* 1998;352:837–853.
14. UKPDS. Tight blood pressure control and risk of macrovascular and microvascular complications in type 2 diabetes. UKPDS 38. *BMJ* 1998;317:703–713.
15. Boulton AJM, Malik RA, Arezzo JC, Sosenko JM. Diabetic somatic neuropathies. *Diabetes Care* 2004;27:1458–1486.
16. Boulton AJM, Vinik AI, Arezzo JC, *et al.* Diabetic neuropathies: a statement by the American Diabetes Association. *Diabetes Care* 2005;28:956–964.
17. Brand PW. Diabetic foot. In: Ellenberg M, Rifkin H, eds. *Diabetes Mellitus: Theory and Practice.* 3rd edn. New York: Medical Examination Publishing; 1983:829–849.
18. Young MJ, Veves A, Breddy JL, Boulton AJM. The prediction of diabetic neuropathic foot ulceration using vibration perception threshold: a prospective study. *Diabetes Care* 1994;17:557–560.
19. Abbott CA, Vileikyte L, Williamson S, *et al.* Multicentre study of the incidence of and predictive factors for diabetic foot ulceration. *Diabetes Care* 1998;21:1071–1078.
20. Abbott CA, Carrington AL, Ashe H, *et al.* The North-West Diabetes Footcare Study: incidence of, and risk factors for, new diabetic foot ulcers in a community-based cohort. *Diabet Med* 2002;20:377–384.
21. Litzelman DK, Marriott DJ, Vinicor F. Independent physiological predictors of foot lesions in patients with NIDDM. *Diabetes Care* 1997;14:296–300.
22. Katoulis EC, Ebdon-Parry M, Hollis S, *et al.* Postural instability in diabetic patients at risk of foot ulceration. *Diabet Med* 1997;14:296–300.
23. Mayfield JA, Reiber GE, Sanders LJ, *et al.* Preventative foot care in people with diabetes. *Diabetes Care* 1998;12:2161–2178.
24. McNeely MJ, Boyko EJ, Ahroni JH, *et al.* The independent contributions of diabetic neuropathy and vasculopathy in foot ulceration. *Diabetes Care* 1995;18:216–219.

25. Fernando DJS, Hutchinson A, Veves A, *et al.* Risk factors for non-ischaemic foot ulceration in diabetic nephropathy. *Diabet Med* 1991;8:223–225.

26. Speckman RA, Frankenfield DL, *et al.* Diabetes is the strongest risk factor for lower-extremity amputation in new hemodialysis patients. *Diabetes Care* 2004;27:2198–2203.

27. Abbott CA, Garrow AP, Carrington AL, *et al.* Foot ulcer risk is lower in South Asian and African-Caribbean compared to European diabetic patients in the UK: the North-West Diabetes Footcare Study. *Diabetes Care* 2005;28:1869–1875.

28. Lavery LA, Armstrong DG, Wunderlich RP, *et al.* Diabetic foot syndrome: evaluating the prevalence and incidence of foot pathology in Mexican-Americans and non-Hispanic whites from a diabetes management cohort. *Diabetes Care* 2003;26:1435–1438.

29. Veves A, Uccioli L, Manes C, *et al.* Comparison of risk factors for foot ulceration in diabetic patients attending teaching hospital out-patient clinics in four different European states. *Diabet Med* 1996;11:709–711.

30. Anderson H, Gjerstad MD, Jakobsen J. Atrophy of foot muscles: a measure of diabetic neuropathy. *Diabetes Care* 2004;27:2382–2385.

31. Reiber GE, Vileikyte L, Boyko EJ, *et al.* Causal pathways for incident lower extremity ulcers in patients with diabetes from two settings. *Diabetes Care* 1999;22:157–162.

32. Murray HJ, Young MJ, Boulton AJM. The relationship between callus formation, high foot pressures and neuropathy in diabetic foot ulceration. *Diabet Med* 1996;16:979–982.

33. Boulton AJM. The annual review – here to stay. *Diabet Med* 1992;9:887.

34. Lavery LA, Higgins KR, Lanctot DR, *et al.* Home monitoring of foot skin temperatures to prevent ulceration. *Diabetes Care* 2004;27:2642–2647.

35. Mayfield JE, Sugarman JR. The use of the Semmes–Weinstein monofilament and other threshold tests for preventing foot ulceration and amputation in people with diabetes. *J Fam Pract* 2000;49:S17–S29.

36. Booth J, Young MJ. Differences in the performance of commercially available monofilaments. *Diabetes Care* 2000;23:984–988.

37. Miranda-Palma B, Sosenko JM, Bowker JH, *et al.* A comparison of the monofilament with other testing modalities for foot ulcer susceptibility. *Diabetes Res Clin Pract* 2005;70:8–12.

38. Williams DT, Harding KG, Price P. An evaluation of methods used in screening for lower limb arterial disease in diabetes. *Diabetes Care* 2005;28:2206–2210.

39. Ziegler D, Siekierka EK, Meyer B, *et al.* Validation of a novel screening device (NeuroQuick) for quantitative assessment of small fiber dysfunction as an early feature of diabetic neuropathy. *Diabetes Care* 2005;28:1169–1174.

40. Carrington AL, Shaw JE, van Schie CH, *et al.* Can motor conduction velocity predict foot problems in diabetic subjects over a 6 year period? *Diabetes Care* 2002;25:2010–2105.

41. van Schie CH, Abbott CA, Vileikyte L, *et al.* A comparative study of the Podotrack and the optical pedobarograph in the assessment of pressures under the diabetic foot. *Diabet Med* 1999;16:154–159.

42. Pinzur MS, Slovenkai MP, Trepman E, *et al.* Guidelines for diabetic footcare. *Foot Ankle Int* 2005;26:113–119.

43. Veves A, Murray HJ, Young MJ, Boulton AJM. The risk of foot ulceration in diabetic patients with high foot pressure: a prospective study. *Diabetologia* 1992;35:660–663.

44. Pataky Z, Assal JP, Conne P, *et al.* Plantar pressure distribution in type 2 diabetic patients without peripheral neuropathy and peripheral vascular disease. *Diabet Med* 2005;22:762–767.

6 What the Practising Clinician Should Know About Foot Biomechanics

Peter R. Cavanagh and Jan S. Ulbrecht

INTRODUCTION

Biomechanics is a branch of the life sciences concerned with the consequences of forces applied to living tissues. This field is clearly relevant to diabetic foot disease, since the majority of foot ulcers result from mechanical stress, which, because of loss of protective sensation (LOPS) to pain,[1] is not perceived by the patient. The relevance of biomechanics to the practising clinician who treats diabetic foot problems can be stated very clearly: many of the recalcitrant diabetic foot ulcers that fail to heal in a typical practice fail not because of medical issues, in which the clinician is well versed (infection, impaired immunity, vascular disease, etc.), but because of simple biomechanical issues, which were often not discussed during medical training. Thus, a few minutes spent becoming familiar with those biomechanical issues will pay considerable dividends in improved patient care. Biomechanical considerations are important in all three phases of care of the diabetic foot: primary prevention, healing foot ulcers and secondary prevention (prevention of ulcer recurrence).

  This chapter discusses several very practical concepts that can be applied to diabetic feet; it does not address the more quantitative areas of biomechanics (such as tissue property characterisation and modelling). It should also be pointed out that there is an entire field of foot biomechanics, which is concerned with 'balancing' structural abnormalities in non-neuropathic feet. The types of interventions typically used by practitioners of that field (such as rigid 'corrective' orthoses) are not relevant to our present discussion. Most of this chapter will concern itself with the most common diabetic foot ulcer, the neuropathic plantar ulcer. Skin breakdown due to penetrating injuries, burns and dorsal surface injuries due to ill-fitting footwear are all also common, but will be addressed only briefly (see Chapter 28 for a more complete discussion of footwear).

STRESS AND STRESS CONCENTRATION

Because force and stress (force divided by the arrea over which it is applied – which we shall call *pressure*) cannot be seen without the aid of specialised instruments, it is easy to overlook

The Foot in Diabetes, 4th Edition. Editors Andrew J.M. Boulton, Peter R. Cavanagh and Gerry Rayman.
© 2006 John Wiley & Sons, Ltd.

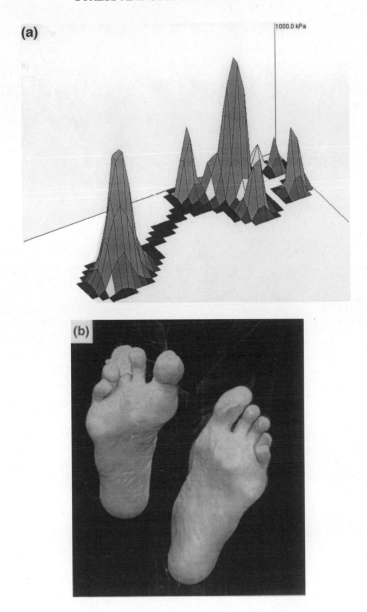

Figure 6.1 Postero-medial view of a peak pressure distribution (a) measured during barefoot walking, under the foot, and (b) of a patient with a prior ulcer at a prominent second MTH (MTH2).

the dramatic concentrations of load that can occur at bony prominences on the plantar aspect of the foot. In the single-limb support phase of gait, the total force under the foot will always be approximately 110% of body weight (the extra 10% comes from the 'inertial' component as the body decelerates and accelerates throughout the gait cycle). Since a typical man's size-10 foot has a total area of approximately 130 cm^2, the average pressure under the foot of a 100-kg person would be 0.77 kg/cm^2 (force/area) or, stated in the more usual units, approximately 75 kPa (kilopascals). Figure 6.1 shows an actual pressure distribution measured during barefoot walking under the foot of a patient who had a prior ulcer at a prominent metatarsal head (MTH). The actual peak pressure is almost 15 times greater than if calculated as above, using the simple force/area argument. In units that might be easier to comprehend, this peak pressure under this patient's foot is approximately 160 pounds per square inch or 11.2 kg/cm^2. Pressures under the foot during running and turning while walking can be 40% greater than those encountered during walking.[2]

Another important mechanical quantity that has the potential to damage tissue is shear stress, which results from the forces exerted parallel to the skin and tends to cause a tear.[3] Because only a few rudimentary measurements of shear stress have been made,[4] we have no clear idea of the role of shear stress in foot injury, although most authorities believe that it is a significant factor.

NEUROPATHY AND HIGH PRESSURE – THE KEY COMBINATION

As discussed elsewhere in this volume (Chapters 3 and 5), peripheral neuropathy results in what has been called a 'loss of protective sensation' (LOPS). The loss of sensation to touch, temperature, pain and deep pressure can be so dense that patients, without being aware of it, can allow objects to penetrate completely through the foot from plantar surface to the dorsum, or they can burn their feet with hot water, etc.

However, most injuries or ulcers in patients with diabetes and LOPS occur at sites of high plantar pressure. High pressures, such as those shown in Figure 6.1, are not usually seen in healthy feet and would result in pain during ambulation for an individual with adequate sensation. For example, patients with bony deformities from rheumatoid arthritis can experience such pressures[5] without ulceration because they either adjust their gait to avoid bearing load on a prominent and painful area and/or choose footwear that will reduce the pressure (see below).

However, the repetitive application of high pressures to the same soft tissue overlying a bony prominence in the setting of LOPS is believed to cause tissue damage that begins deep (close to the bone).[6] Callus frequently forms on the skin surface. When a patient presents with callus exhibiting a shadowy dark base to visual examination, this is usually an indication that there is a deep ulcer causing haemorrhage into the callus.[7] This 'pre-ulcer' will then usually develop into an ulcer, with further walking. Thus, high pressure alone is not sufficient for plantar ulceration, and neither is neuropathy – it is the combination of the two that provides the necessary and sufficient conditions for ulceration.

Since most clinicians will encounter neuropathic diabetic patients who are hospitalised for non-foot-related complaints, it is important to mention here that low pressure applied for long periods of time to feet with LOPS can also cause devastating lesions. The most common manifestation is deep bilateral pressure ulcers, often penetrating to tendon and bone, on the heels of patients who have been bedridden for a period of time. A similar result can occur in just a few hours in patients who have been lying supine during a surgical procedure. In both situations, the ulcers are entirely iatrogenic, caused by failure of the clinician to insist on load relief for neuropathic patients, and the failure of the nursing staff to either recognise or act on the knowledge that the patient was neuropathic.

MECHANISMS FOR ELEVATED PRESSURE

Over time, people with diabetes can develop areas of abnormally high pressure under the foot during weight-bearing activities, and this can result from a number of intrinsic, extrinsic and

Table 6.1 Biomechanical factors that can lead to elevated plantar pressure under the foot during walking

Intrinsic	Extrinsic	Behavioural
Foot architecture	Poor footwear	Walking without shoes
Long second toe	Tight or loose shoes	
High arch	Shoes with hard soles	
Soft tissue alterations	Accidents and incidents	Poor choice of shoes
Callus		
Glycosylation (presumed)		
Migration of tissue		
Thin tissue		
Limited joint mobility	Prior surgery	Inadequate callus care
Foot deformity		Walking patterns
Claw toes		
Hallux valgus		
Charcot fracture		

behavioural factors (Table 6.1). According to Edmonds et al.,[8] most neuropathic ulcers occur on the toes (39%), the hallux (30%) and the MTHs (24%); these areas, therefore, are of principal concern in both understanding the causes of elevated pressure and how intervention might be accomplished successfully. There is some debate about the critical magnitude of plantar pressure that is required for tissue damage. Veves et al.[9] believe that a value of over 1000 kPa during barefoot walking is required, but other studies report ulceration at values below 500 kPa. Armstrong et al.[10] have suggested that a threshold of 700 kPa is the best compromise between sensitivity and specificity. It is, however, likely that each patient's threshold is different and that the more active a patient is, the less pressure is needed at each step to cause ulceration. Also, since most studies have measured barefoot pressure, the footwear chosen by an individual patient can clearly make the difference between ulceration and no ulceration. It is likely that the pressure between the foot and the shoe is the most important variable to minimise.[11]

Intrinsic Factors

Certain foot structures predispose an individual to elevated pressures. Some, like a long second metatarsal (Morton's toe) and a high arch,[12,13] are not diabetes related. Callus appears to concentrate pressure rather, as if it were a foreign body under the foot.[14] Studies have shown that the presence of callus increases the risk of ulceration by over 11 times.[7] Thus, callus should be regularly removed.

There are some indications that the properties of the plantar soft tissue may be adversely affected by glycosylation end products, although much remains to be explored in this area.

Palpation of the MTHs in a patient with claw toes often reveals an exquisitely thin layer of soft tissue overlying the bone, which is directly exposed to high pressures during walking and thus easily damaged unless countermeasures are undertaken (see below). In fact, the lack of adequate thickness of soft tissue under bony prominences has been shown to be an extremely important determinant of elevated pressure in normal subjects.[13] Clawing of the toes in diabetic patients appears to result in the plantar fat pads being displaced anteriorly, leaving the condyles

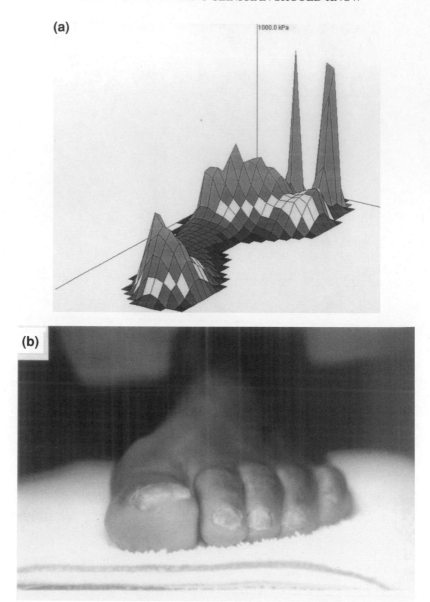

Figure 6.2 Postero-medial view of a peak pressure distribution (a) measured during barefoot walking showing elevated pressure at the tips of a clawed second toe. Note that the pressures under toe 2 and the hallux are approximately equal. The foot is shown in part (b).

of the MTHs 'exposed'. This has been shown to lead to higher than normal plantar pressures.[15] The tips of claw toes can themselves be locations of ulcers due to concentrated pressure (Figure 6.2). Toe deformities (claw toes, hammer toes, hallux valgus) also tend to result in higher pressures.

  The range of motion at many joints has been shown to be decreased in patients with diabetes.[16] This is not a neuropathic complication, but probably another effect of glycosylation whereby the collagen in joint capsules is stiffened by the glycosylation process. The consequence of reduced range of motion at the major joints of the foot and ankle (such as the first metatarso-phalangeal (MTP), sub-talar and talo-crural joints) is likely to be increased plantar pressures under the forefoot.[6] The most frequently problematic joint in this regard is the first MTP.[17] Invariably, a patient with a neuropathic ulcer under the pad of the hallux will be found to have reduced capacity for dorsiflexion at this joint[18] (Figure 6.3).

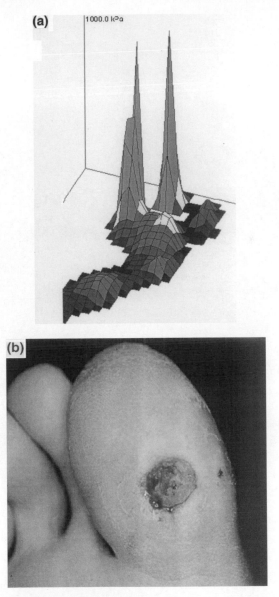

Figure 6.3 Postero-lateral view of a peak pressure distribution (a) measured during barefoot walking, from a patient with a neuropathic ulcer under the pad of the hallux (b) secondary to a reduced capacity for dorsiflexion at the first MTP joint (Reprinted from Cavanagh PR, Ulbrecht JS, Caputo GM. Biomechanics of the foot in diabetes mellitus. In: Bowker JH, Pfiefer M, eds. *The Diabetic Foot* 6th edn, Copyright © (2000) Elsevier). Note that the MTH1 and hallux pressures are approximately equal, although this patient has never experienced an ulcer under MTH2.

Despite the above emphasis on the forefoot, a number of conditions can cause elevated pressure in other regions of the foot. Charcot fractures of the midfoot[20,21] typically result in a 'rocker bottom' foot, which bears load principally on the collapsed region of the midfoot (Figure 6.4). Certain surgical procedures that are intended to reduce loads at primary areas of ulceration can have a secondary effect of increasing pressure in other areas. For example,

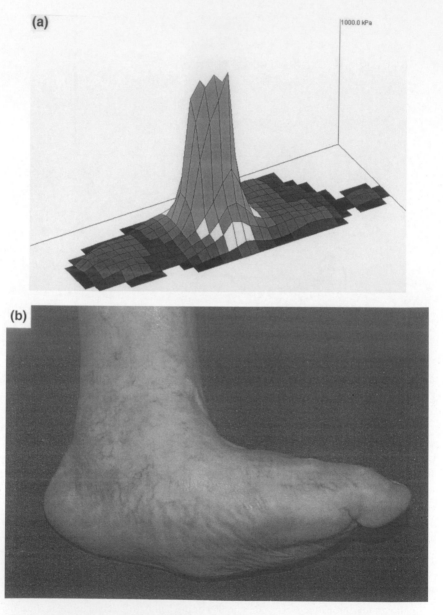

Figure 6.4   Postero-medial view of a peak pressure distribution (a) under a 'rocker bottom' foot and (b) during barefoot walking. Load is principally borne on the collapsed region of the midfoot. Other regions in the rearfoot and forefoot receive almost no load throughout the entire contact phase.

lengthening of the Achilles tendon, which is sometimes performed following forefoot surgery, can result in what is known as a 'calcaneus gait', in which elevated heel pressure occurs during much of the stance phase (Figure 6.5). Removing MTHs because of ulceration in that region can also lead to higher pressures under the remaining MTHs.

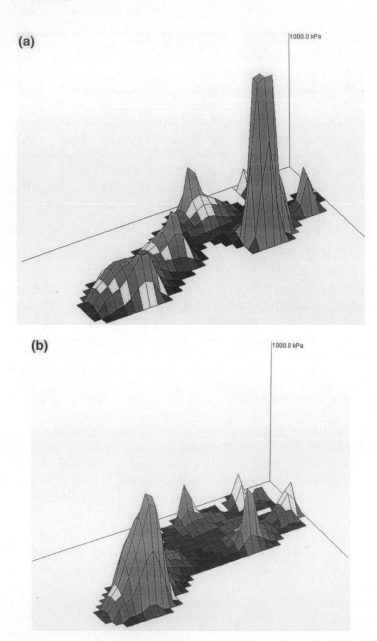

Figure 6.5 Postero-medial view of peak pressure distributions (a) before and (b) 3 months after surgery that included an osteotomy of the first metatarsal and a lengthening of the Achilles tendon. Note the reduction in forefoot pressures and the increase in the heel peak pressure post-surgically.

The effects of motor neuropathy are often underestimated, but a number of studies have shown dramatic atrophy of the intrinsic muscles of the feet (Figure 6.6).[22,23] This atrophy alters the biomechanics of the foot and may lead to instability during standing and walking. Postural stability is markedly degraded in neuropathic patients,[24] probably because of both sensory and motor neuropathy, and patients need to be warned that they may lose their balance under conditions such as poor lighting or uneven surfaces.[25,26]

Extrinsic Factors

In terms of the pressures that the soft tissues are exposed to, footwear is the single most important extrinsic determinant of elevated pressure. While appropriate footwear can be of great benefit in preventing ulcers (see below; Chapter 28), incorrect footwear can actually cause ulceration.[27] The two major deficiencies most frequently seen in shoes are incorrect sizing (too loose or too tight) and inadequate cushioning. Tight shoes can cause ulceration at a number of locations. Lesions commonly occur over dorsal deformities such as a bunion or a dorso-lateral prominence of the fifth MTH (MTH5). The tips of the interphalangeal joints on claw or hammer toes are prime at-risk sites, and ulcers in the spaces between the toes can be caused by the toes being crushed together in a shoe with incorrect contours. Loose shoes, which allow the foot to slip, can also result in ulcers.

The term 'cushioning' of the neuropathic foot is usually defined in static terms and can be equated with 'thickness' of 'soft' material under the foot. It has been shown that walking in shoes with leather soles is roughly equivalent to walking barefoot, whereas walking in simple sports shoes (trainers) can reduce Plantar pressure by up to 50%, compared to barefoot walking.[28] Thus, the wrong choice or prescription of shoes can be devastating for the integrity of the diabetic foot.

Activity Profiles

It is widely believed that barefoot walking is a principal cause of plantar ulceration that is amenable to behavioural intervention. As mentioned above, we do not know the number of steps and the magnitude of pressure that will exceed an individual's threshold for ulceration. However, experience suggests that there are some patients who protect their feet adequately in footwear throughout the day, and yet ulcerate because of just a few steps of barefoot walking, e.g. to urinate during the night. Thus, at least for some patients, even a few steps of barefoot walking are too many. Taking showers barefoot is another dangerous behaviour. Advising the patient to consistently use padded slippers, which can be donned easily, is a simple way to intervene in such cases.

In the last 5 years, technology has been applied to monitor patient activity profiles,[29] and this has led to a number of theories about the relationship between what might be called the 'dose' of activity[30] and the risk of ulceration[31–33] (Chapter 25). Surprisingly, a direct relationship between number of steps per day and risk of ulceration has not emerged from these early studies. It has been suggested that either a change in level of activity[32] or variability in activity[31] may be important risk factors for ulceration.

There are some indications that neuropathic patients have altered gait patterns,[34] but it is not yet clear whether this results in elevated plantar pressure. Brand[35] hypothesised that

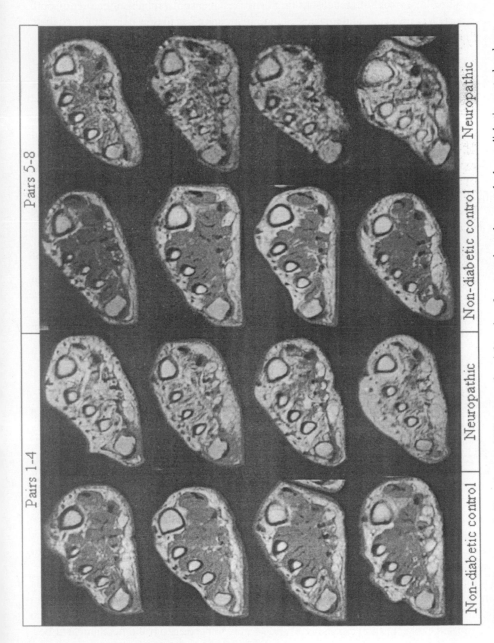

Figure 6.6 Anatomically referenced T2 images for eight pairs of age- and gender-matched non-diabetic control and neuropathic subjects. The remarkable loss of muscle tissue and the fatty infiltration in the neuropathic subject are apparent. (Reproduced with permission from Ref. 23)

neuropathic gait would be less variable and that this would result in continued application of stress to the same plantar location, but this has not been found to be the case.[36] Regardless, patients with LOPS will not consciously alter their gait because they feel no pain developing in high-pressure areas, from too much walking. There is also some evidence that neuropathic patients experience more falls and injuries due to falls than matched non-neuropathic diabetic patients.[37,38] Balance[34] and limb-position sense[39] are also impaired, and these two factors may lead to more frequent traumatic injuries to the feet of neuropathic patients.

PRIMARY PREVENTION: THE 30-SECOND FOOT EXAMINATION

We have established above that most foot ulcers that the practising clinician will see result from mechanical insult to tissue deprived of normal sensation. Although we have emphasised neuropathic injury, diminished lower extremity pulses identify another group of patients at risk because of ischaemia. Thus, the most important issues in prevention of foot pathology are to identify patients who have lost protective sensation and patients with significant ischaemia. These assessments are also recommended in the United Kingdom by the National Institute for Clinical Excellence guidelines (http://www.nice.org.uk/pdf/CG010NICEguideline.pdf; Chapters 10 and 36). Loss of such protective sensation is most simply assessed with a 10-g monofilament,[40] using the procedure described in the International Practical Guidelines in Chapter 35. We recommend that the examination described in Table 6.2 be performed annually. If the examination shows that the patient has protective sensation and foot pulses and therefore is judged not to be at risk, then 30 seconds is all the time that is needed. During this initial assessment, the presence of significant deformity should also be noted, as this may affect treatment decisions even in the absence of significant neuropathy.

PRIMARY PREVENTION: THE 2-MINUTE FOOT EXAMINATION

If the initial examination determines that protective sensation has been lost, the biomechanics of the foot and shoes become critical issues in the patient's future. The examination must now be extended to look for the factors discussed above, and for other non-biomechanical factors discussed elsewhere in this volume, which could contribute to ulceration. Surprisingly, this need not be a lengthy examination – it is remarkable how much can be achieved in a short time if the clinician has a well-defined set of goals in advance of the foot examination. In approximately 2 minutes, an examination can cover all of the components shown in Table 6.3 for a patient who is at risk of foot injury.

The surface examination of the foot is fairly straightforward. The clinician must identify ulcers, callus, haemorrhage into callus, breaks or cracks in the skin, skin infection, maceration between toes and elevated surface temperature. The latter may be an indication of infection or of an active Charcot process (Chapters 22 and 23), as can oedema or erythema. Toenail care should be assessed, and the presence of ingrown or long nails, nail fungal infections and injuries from self-nail care should be noted. While some of these are not biomechanical issues, their importance is self-evident; most of these topics are covered elsewhere in this volume.

One does not have to be a chiropodist or a foot orthopaedic surgeon to identify the major deformities that can lead to elevated pressure. Those shown in Figure 6.7, including prominent MTHs, claw or hammer toes, excessive callus, hallux valgus and prior amputation, can,

Table 6.2 The 30-second foot examination (assess on both feet)

Evaluation component	Details	Action
1. Ascertain if the patient has had any previous diabetes-related foot lesions	Ask about ulcers or blisters that *were not perceived as particularly painful*; ask about foot lesions that required vascular procedures to heal; look for toe or partial foot amputations.	If there is a history of previous foot problems, consider the patient as at risk.
2. Vascular status/pulses	Feel for Pulse in posterior tibial artery behind medial maleolus Pulse in dorsalis pedis artery on the dorsum of the foot	If both pulses are absent in either foot, consider further evaluation, particularly if other symptoms or signs of vascular disease are present (Chapter 4)
3. Loss of protective sensation: inability to feel the touch of a 10g monofilament	In a quiet room, test multiple forefoot plantar sites, in particular, toes and MTHs; avoid callused areas; ask the patient to tell you every time he/she can feel the touch (*do not ask for a response only when you are touching the patient*); with the patient's eyes closed, bend monofilament against the skin for 1 s; repeat questionable sites; apply monofilament with random cadence; the patient's relative/caregiver can observe to reinforce abnormal findings for the patient.	If the patient cannot feel the monofilament at even one site, label the patient as 'at risk'. If you are concerned about questionable or hesitant responses, repeat the test at each clinic visit till the result is clearer, or classify the patient as 'at risk'.
4. Look for significant foot deformity	See the examples shown in Figure 6.6.	Appropriate footwear or referral should be suggested, even in the absence of neuropathy.

Note: If the patient has no history of previous problems, can feel touch at all sites and has *one palpable pulse in each foot*, the 30-s examination can end here. Repeat in 1 year, or sooner, if findings were questionable. If the patient has a history of previous problems, has absent pulses or cannot feel touch at even one site, then he/she is at risk for foot injury. Proceed with the additional '2-min examination'.

in combination with neuropathy, lead to ulceration (see also rocker bottom deformity from Charcot neuroarthropathy in Chapters 22 and 23). The identification of these deformities will also be important in decisions related to prescription footwear (see below).

Looking at the patient's footwear is a key component of the examination. Shoes and socks should be removed. The socks should be examined for evidence of drainage from a wound, and the shoe insoles should be studied to see if they have 'bottomed out' and no longer

Table 6.3 The 2-minute foot examination (both feet examined)

Evaluation component	Details	Action

1. Examine all surfaces	Look for
	Ulcer
	Callus
	Haemorrhage into callus
	Blister
	Maceration between toes
	Other breaks in the skin
	Skin infection
	Oedema, erythema, elevated
	    temperature
		Prescribe offloading device to heal
		    ulcer (Figures 6.8 and 6.9).
		Remove callus (sharp debridement
		    and/or Dremmel or emery board).
		Treat skin infection or injury. Refer
		    if Charcot fracture suspected.

6. Examine the toenails	Look for Fungal infections Ingrown toenails Evidence of injury from self-nail care	Consider treating fungal infections. Advise against self-care of nails. Suggest chiropody/podiatry care.

7. Identify foot deformity	Look for
	Prominent metatarsal heads
	Claw or hammer toes
	Rocker bottom foot deformity
	Hallux valgus and bunions
	Prior amputation
		The presence of foot deformity will
		    dictate footwear specifications (see
		    text and Table 6.4).

8. Examine the shoes
Observe mobility of the
patient putting on his/her
shoes and socks as the
last component of the
examination. This will
show the patient's ability
to examine his/her own
feet.
	Look for
	Drainage into socks
	Worn-out (flattened) insoles
	Shoes that are leaning badly to
	    one side
	Poorly fitting shoes (too tight,
	    too loose, too short, not
	    enough room for the toes)
	Gait pattern
		Prescribe appropriate footwear if
		    necessary (see text and Table 6.4).
		Suggest replacement shoes if
		    necessary.

9. Establish need for
patient education
	Ask:
	Why do you think I am
	    concerned about your feet?
	Do you walk without shoes at
	    home?
	Who takes care of your toenails?
		Schedule patient for education visit
		    with diabetes educator/nurse if
		    understanding is lacking or if
		    behaviours are unacceptable.

Note: This follows on from the examination in Table 6.2 if the patient has had previous foot problems, has lost protective sensation or has significant vascular disease.

provide adequate cushioning. The size of the shoe should be compared to the size of the foot, particularly the height and curvature of the forefoot region. At the end of the examination, the patient should be asked to put shoes and socks on, so that the examiner can assess the patient's mobility during this process, as this factor will give an indication of the patient's ability to examine his or her own feet. At some point during the exam, the clinician should ask a few key questions that will elicit information regarding the patient's understanding of the disease process and indicate his or her educational needs. Questions such as 'Why do you think I am

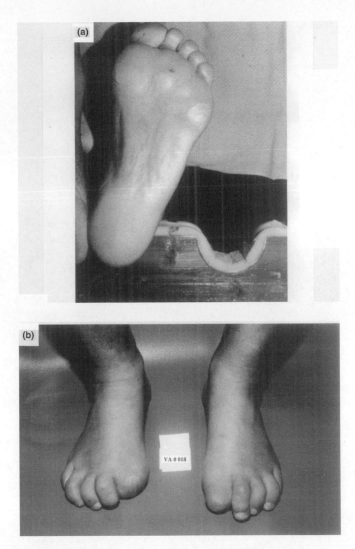

Figure 6.7 Common foot deformities that should be identified during a brief foot examination. In combination with neuropathy, these conditions can lead to ulceration. (a) Prominent MTHs; (b) clawed toes; (c) hallux valgus and excessive plantar callus; (d) partial amputation.

concerned about your feet?', 'Do you walk without shoes at home?' and 'Who takes care of your toenails?' can be helpful in this regard. A brief observation of the patient's gait, watching for obvious abnormalities, will complete the examination. A final determination of shoe fit during load bearing should also be performed at this time.

Action Based on the 'At-Risk' Examination

Appropriate actions based on the findings of the examination are listed in Table 6.2. These include referral for problems that require specialist care (e.g. symptomatic vascular

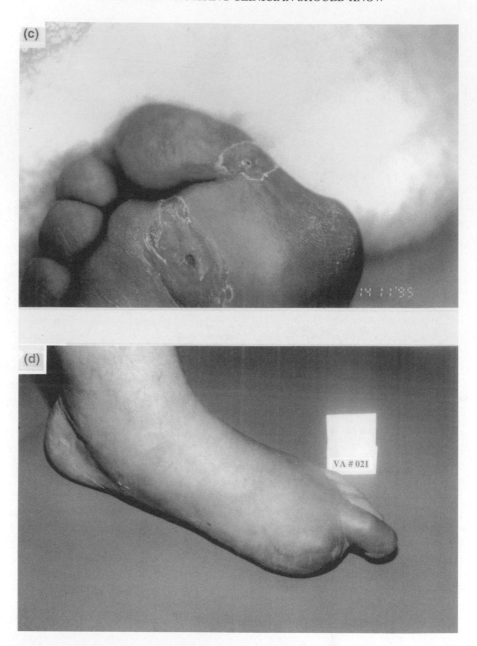

Figure 6.7 *Continued*

impairment, suspected Charcot fracture or periodic care by a chiropodist/podiatrist), immediate treatment for ulcers and infections (see below), the prescription of therapeutic footwear
(see below) and patient education (Chapters 11 and 12). Callus can be trimmed by a trained
health care provider in the clinician's office, using a number-15 scalpel and an emery
board.

BIOMECHANICAL ISSUES IN TREATING A PLANTAR ULCER

One of the most often heard complaints by specialists in diabetic foot clinics is that ulcers referred to as 'non-healing' are often simply badly treated ulcers that could have been healed many months previously. This finding can be verified in the literature where studies of, for example, the total contact cast (TCC; see below) show that ulcers that had existed often for more than a year were healed by casting in approximately 6 weeks.[41] This result can be compared to studies of 'standard care', where healing is typically remarkably poor.[42,43]

There is little doubt that the TCC (Figure 6.8), in combination with good wound care, is the 'gold standard' for healing neuropathic ulcers.[41,44,45] This combination accomplishes a number of goals that are important to wound healing: reduction in oedema, load relief at the ulcer site, enforced compliance with load relief and encouragement for the patient to keep a return appointment. However, some drawbacks of TCC use are that specially trained staff are required to apply and remove the cast, patients with infection should not generally be casted and casting can result in additional lesions, either on the other foot or on the casted foot if the cast becomes too loose.

Thus, in a typical clinical practice, the TCC is not a realistic method of healing ulcers. Therefore, if referral for casting is impossible, the goals of wound healing in such a setting should be to provide conditions that approximate those in a TCC, by using some other approach. Of the various requirements discussed above for healing neuropathic ulcers, the most critical is compliance with non-weight-bearing. Bedrest would be ideal, but this is rarely realistic.

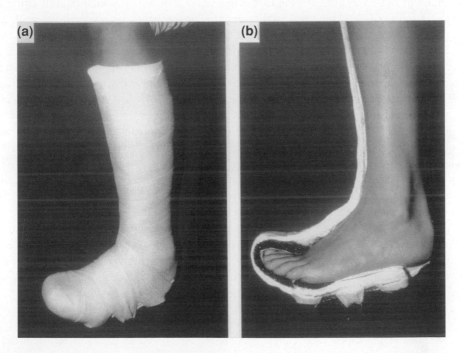

Figure 6.8 A total contact cast, also shown in cutaway view. This is the 'gold standard' for wound healing of diabetic foot ulcers. Note the soft foam wrapped around the forefoot and the way in which this mechanically isolates the forefoot from load bearing.

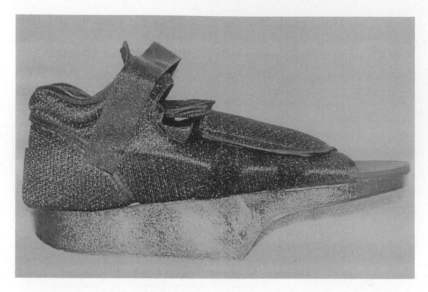

Figure 6.9   Shoe designed to provide offloading of a forefoot plantar ulcer.

The patient with an ulcer must not be allowed to walk away from an examination in the shoes that helped to cause the lesion in the first place. As obvious as this sounds, it is a rule that is frequently broken. A wound that receives continual mechanical stress will not heal, as is apparent from the duration of ulcers prior to entry in the studies mentioned above. Among the ways of achieving offloading of forefoot ulcers are shoes that have only a rear platform (Figure 6.9). Similar devices with heel cutouts are available for rearfoot ulcers. Leg braces or 'walkers' that both transfer some load from the foot to the leg and provide a cavity in the insole that mechanically isolates the lesion can also be useful (Figure 6.10). All of these devices need to be used with crutches or a wheelchair if adequate unloading of the ulcer is to be achieved. Patients need to understand that they have been provided with load-relieving devices to allow them to perform only the most basic activities of daily living. The foot must never touch the ground or wear a regular shoe until the ulcer is healed.

The way in which the footwear is used can also affect its efficacy. For example, if a patient rocks forward on the shoe shown in Figure 6.9, the forefoot can be loaded. It is likely that more offloading is needed to heal an ulcer than to prevent an ulcer. Thus, footwear in the usual sense of the word, and even 'specialised' footwear, as discussed below for prevention of ulcers, is unlikely to be adequate to achieve healing.

Compliance with a regimen of load relief is likely to be the primary determinant of healing. The patient needs to understand the rationale for unloading the foot, and caregivers need to be sensitised to the need to keep the foot completely clear of the ground. If a primarily neuropathic ulcer is not healing after a course of 6–8 weeks of debridement and unloading, it can be assumed that the patient is not being compliant to the load relief regimen or that the regimen is inadequately designed. Patients in general do not believe that a few steps per day on an ulcer to get coffee or to go to the bathroom can prevent healing. Unfortunately, recent studies have shown that patients' adherence with removable devices is very poor,[46] and this finding has led some to suggest that irremovable devices may always be necessary (Chapter 25).

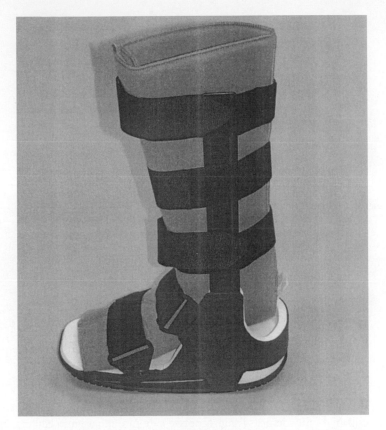

Figure 6.10   A brace designed to transfer some load to the leg and to provide space for a thick insole with mechanical relief in the ulcerated area. The outsole is of a 'roller design' (Figure 6.13).

Non-plantar ulcers are easier to heal, though the principles are the same: avoidance of ongoing mechanical injury, usually from footwear or from a support surface during rest, is key. Clinicians should be alert to the potential for ulceration in the patient with a lateral malleolus or a lateral MTH5 lesion, who sleeps on that same side.

PRIMARY AND SECONDARY PREVENTION – THE IMPORTANCE OF FOOTWEAR

Patients who have experienced a foot ulcer must pay special attention to footwear for the remainder of their lives. It is only after an ulcer has healed through one of the load-relieving methods discussed above that definitive therapeutic footwear can be provided. Specifying the details of prescription footwear is often considered to be a task that the clinician delegates to others – but there are many settings in which specialised footwear assistance is not available. It is important, therefore, for the clinician who is the primary provider of foot care to have a clear idea of the options available. Unfortunately, many clinicians regard footwear prescription as somewhat of a mystery. This should not be the case, because more than 80% of patients

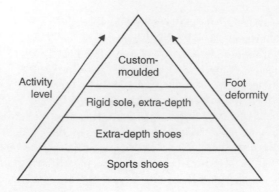

Figure 6.11 The 'footwear pyramid' showing a schematic distribution of all cases of prescription footwear. Many cases can be managed in sports shoes (trainers). The next category, extra-depth shoes, can be modified to provide additional pressure relief by making the outsoles rigid and rockered. Custom-moulded shoes will need to be made by an experienced orthopaedic shoe technician, but the treating clinician can provide all other categories. (Reprinted from Cavanagh PR, Ulbrecht JS, Caputo GM. Biomechanics of the foot in diabetes mellitus. In: Bowker JH, Pfiefer M, eds. *The Diabetic Foot.* 6th edn, Copyright © (2000) Elsevier.)

can be successfully managed in either 'over-the-counter' sport shoes (trainers) or extra-depth shoes with prescribed flat or customised insoles. Only patients with severe foot deformity or other special problems will require custom-moulded shoes (and perhaps braces), which only a specialist such as pedorthist, orthotist or orthopaedic shoemaker can provide. This is shown schematically in the 'footwear pyramid' in Figure 6.11. The approach to footwear prescription is shown in Table 6.4. Shoes are listed in order of increasing complexity and expense, and the clinician should aim to provide the simplest footwear solution that will keep the patient ulcer

Table 6.4   Footwear for the neuropathic patient (in order of complexity)

Footwear	Modification	Comment
Sports shoe (trainers)	Can replace supplied insole with flat foam insole.	Make sure that there is enough dorsal room for the tips of toes.
Extra-depth shoe with flat 0.25-in. insole	Often supplied with just a 'spacer' insole; this should be replaced with a prescribed flat foam insole.	Make sure that there is enough dorsal room for the tips of toes, particularly if thicker insole is used.
Extra-depth shoe with custom insole		Insole will need to be made by a specialist technician, but the mould can be made in the clinician's office.
Extra-depth shoe with custom insole and rigid roller or rocker outsole	Any experienced shoemaker can make the sole rigid and produce a rocker sole, as shown in Figure 6.11.	Make sure that the axis of the rocker is behind the MTH of interest.
Custom footwear		This will need to be measured and made by an experienced orthopaedic shoe technician.

free and active. A more detailed discussion of footwear can be found in Chapter 28, but a few general biomechanical principles[47] will be discussed here.

The clinical goals of footwear for a diabetic patient are either to prevent the development of an initial ulcer (in the case of primary prevention)[48] or to prevent a recurrence of ulceration at the same site or new ulceration at a different site (in secondary prevention). Footwear can also give patients the freedom to live an active life, but the more active the patient is, the more 'sophisticated' the footwear needs to be (see earlier discussion on the likely relationship between pressure, activity/number of steps and ulceration risk; specialised footwear can be made for golf, horse riding, etc.). The biomechanical goals are to provide load relief or 'cushioning' at sites of elevated pressure and sometimes to transfer load from one site to another. These goals can often be accomplished quite simply using 0.25-in.-thick (6.5-mm-thick) flat foam insoles of various densities to accommodate to plantar deformity. Probably the most important aspect of material selection is that it should be durable and should not 'bottom out' particularly. Since thicker insoles are required than what is available inside a typical shoe, extra-depth shoes (Figure 6.12) are the mainstay of prescribed footwear. These shoes are built with the same shape as regular shoes, with a roomy toe box if viewed from above, but when looked at from the side, it is apparent that they have a much higher toe box so that insoles can be worn without forcing the toes against the upper of the shoe. Thicker socks, which can also be accommodated in extra-depth shoes, have been shown to offer additional pressure relief.[49] As discussed earlier, even the cushioning available in simple off-the-shelf sports shoes (trainers) provides significant pressure relief compared to leather-soled shoes, and the use of such sports shoes has been shown to reduce the appearance of calluses.

Most authorities believe that moulded insoles provide a superior reduction of load compared to flat insoles. Our research has shown that modifications such as a build-up of the insole height behind the MTHs, a high-arch support or a depression to relieve specific high-pressure areas can be effective in removing load from at-risk areas and distributing it to other regions of the

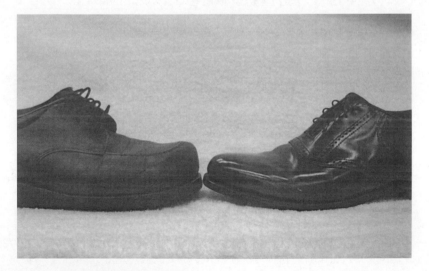

Figure 6.12 A comparison of the toe box region of an extra-depth shoe (left) with a typical leather Oxford shoe. Note that the extra-depth shoe has sufficient space to allow a thick insole to be placed in the shoe while still leaving space to ensure that the dorsal surfaces of the toes are not pushed against the shoe's upper.

foot.[11] On the other hand, simple moulding without attention to the anatomy of the particular foot may not be beneficial. While the fabrication of moulded insoles is beyond the scope of a typical office practice, several in-office methods for obtaining an impression of the shape of the foot are available. Such impressions can then be sent to an orthotic manufacturer, who will return custom-moulded insoles to fit directly into extra-depth shoes.

The next level of complexity is to provide the patient with extra-depth shoes and custom insoles where the outsole of the shoe has been made rigid and contoured. This produces a 'roller' or 'rocker' shoe (Figure 6.13). Both these shoes allow walking without flexion of the

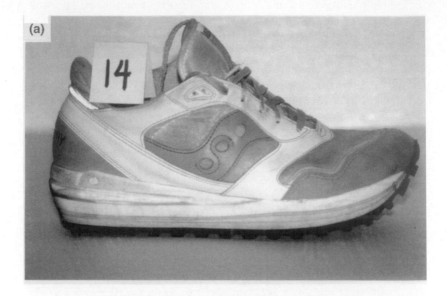

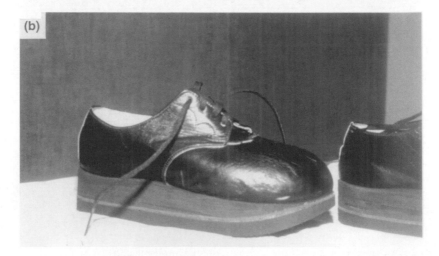

Figure 6.13   Shoes with rigid and contoured outsoles: (a) a roller shoe with a continuous curve; (b) a rocker shoe with a clear pivot point. Both these shoes allow walking without flexion of the MTP joints, thus reducing plantar pressure markedly.

MTP joints, thus reducing MTH plantar pressure markedly. This modification is a relatively simple one, which can be performed by a local shoemaker who is given the correct instructions. The axis of the rocker shoe is generally placed approximately 2 cm behind the MTH of interest. The patient must be taught how to walk correctly in the shoe, allowing the shoe to rock forward during late support but not dwelling on the wedge area in the forepart. The simplest way to encourage patients to do this is to ask them to take smaller than usual strides.

Methods are available for the measurement of plantar pressure inside footwear,[50] but the equipment needed is not widely available. As a result, footwear prescription is somewhat of a trial-and-error process for most clinicians, who must try to discern by eye whether or not a particular shoe reduces load at a critical area of pressure. Patients with new footwear must therefore be followed very closely during the first few weeks, and they should also be encouraged to increase the use of the shoes slowly and progressively during this time, starting with just 1 h/day. Frequent self-examinations of the feet should also be encouraged, to look for signs of tissue damage (redness, inflammation, warmth, blisters, callus, haemorrhage into callus and in the extreme, of course, ulceration). If none of the footwear interventions described above prove satisfactory, referral of the patient to a specialised centre is warranted.

SUMMARY

This brief review has presented a number of biomechanical issues that have direct relevance to treatment of the diabetic foot. An understanding of the role that mechanical stress plays in tissue damage can lead to better treatment and to more successful primary and secondary prevention of foot ulcers.

REFERENCES

1. Birke JA, Sims DS. Plantar sensory threshold in the ulcerative foot. *Lepr Rev* 1986;57:261–267.
2. Rozema A, Ulbrecht JS, Pammer SE, Cavanagh PR. In-shoe plantar pressures during activities of daily living: implications for therapeutic footwear design. *Foot Ankle Int* 1996;17:352–359.
3. Davis BL. Foot ulceration: hypotheses concerning shear and vertical forces acting on adjacent regions of skin. *Med Hypotheses* 1993;40:44–47.
4. Perry JE, Hall JO, Davis BL. Simultaneous measurement of plantar pressure and shear forces in diabetic individuals. *Gait Posture* 2002;15:101–107.
5. Masson EA, Hay EM, Stockley I, Veves A, Betts RP, Boulton AJ. Abnormal foot pressures alone may not cause ulceration. *Diabet Med* 1989;6:426–428.
6. Delbridge L, Ctercteko G, Fowler C, Reeve TS, Le Quesne LP. The aetiology of diabetic neuropathic ulceration of the foot. *Br J Surg* 1985;72:1–6.
7. Murray HJ, Young MJ, Hollis S, Boulton AJ. The association between callus formation, high pressures and neuropathy in diabetic foot ulceration. *Diabet Med* 1996;13:979–982.
8. Edmonds ME, Blundell MP, Morris ME, Thomas EM, Cotton LT, Watkins PJ. Improved survival of the diabetic foot: the role of a specialized foot clinic. *Q J Med* 1986;60:763–771.
9. Veves A, Murray HJ, Young MJ, Boulton AJ. The risk of foot ulceration in diabetic patients with high foot pressure: a prospective study. *Diabetologia* 1992;35:660–663.
10. Armstrong DG, Peters EJ, Athanasiou KA, Lavery LA. Is there a critical level of plantar foot pressure to identify patients at risk for neuropathic foot ulceration? *J Foot Ankle Surg* 1998;37:303–307.

11. Bus SA, Ulbrecht JS, Cavanagh PR. Pressure relief and load redistribution by custom-made insoles in diabetic patients with neuropathy and foot deformity. *Clin Biomech (Bristol, Avon)* 2004;19:629–638.

12. Ahroni JH, Boyko EJ, Forsberg RC. Clinical correlates of plantar pressure among diabetic veterans. *Diabetes Care* 1999;22:965–972.

13. Morag E, Cavanagh PR. Structural and functional predictors of regional peak pressures under the foot during walking. *J Biomech* 1999;32:359–370.

14. Young MJ, Cavanagh PR, Thomas G, Johnson MM, Murray H, Boulton AJ. The effect of callus removal on dynamic plantar foot pressures in diabetic patients. *Diabet Med* 1992;9:55–57.

15. Bus SA, Maas M, de Lange A, Michels RP, Levi M. Elevated plantar pressures in neuropathic diabetic patients with claw/hammer toe deformity. *J Biomech* 2005;38:1918–1925.

16. Andersen H, Mogensen PH. Disordered mobility of large joints in association with neuropathy in patients with long-standing insulin-dependent diabetes mellitus. *Diabet Med* 1997;14:221–227.

17. Birke JA, Cornwall MA, Jackson M. Relationship between hallux limitus and ulceration of the great toe. *J Orthop Sports Phys Ther* 1988;10:172–176.

18. Dinh TL, Veves A. A review of the mechanisms implicated in the pathogenesis of the diabetic foot. *Int J Low Extrem Wounds* 2005;4:154–159.

19. Cavanagh PR, Ulbrecht JS, Caputo GM. Biomechanics of the foot in diabetes mellitus. In: Bowker JH, Pfiefer M, eds. *The Diabetic Foot*. 6th edn. Philadelphia: WB Saunders; 2000.

20. Myerson MS, Henderson MR, Saxby T, Short KW. Management of midfoot diabetic neuroarthropathy. *Foot Ankle Int* 1994;15:233–241.

21. Pinzur MS, Sage R, Stuck R, Kaminsky S, Zmuda A. A treatment algorithm for neuropathic (Charcot) midfoot deformity. *Foot Ankle* 1993;14:189–197.

22. Andersen H, Gjerstad MD, Jakobsen J. Atrophy of foot muscles: a measure of diabetic neuropathy. *Diabetes Care* 2004;27:2382–2385.

23. Bus SA, Yang QX, Wang JH, Smith MB, Wunderlich R, Cavanagh PR. Intrinsic muscle atrophy and toe deformity in the diabetic neuropathic foot: a magnetic resonance imaging study. *Diabetes Care* 2002;25:1444–1450.

24. Simoneau GG, Ulbrecht JS, Derr JA, Becker MB, Cavanagh PR. Postural instability in patients with diabetic sensory neuropathy. *Diabetes Care* 1994;17:1411–1421.

25. Corriveau H, Hebert R, Raiche M, Dubois MF, Prince F. Postural stability in the elderly: empirical confirmation of a theoretical model. *Arch Gerontol Geriatr* 2004;39:163–177.

26. Maurer MS, Burcham J, Cheng H. Diabetes mellitus is associated with an increased risk of falls in elderly residents of a long-term care facility. *J Gerontol A Biol Sci Med Sci* 2005;60:1157–1162.

27. Apelqvist J, Larsson J, Agardh CD. The influence of external precipitating factors and peripheral neuropathy on the development and outcome of diabetic foot ulcers. *J Diabetes Complications* 1990;4:21–25.

28. Perry JE, Ulbrecht JS, Derr JA, Cavanagh PR. The use of running shoes to reduce plantar pressures in patients who have diabetes. *J Bone Joint Surg Am* 1995;77:1819–1828.

29. Armstrong DG, Gildenhuys A, Holtz-Neiderer K. Computerized activity monitoring preoperatively and postoperatively. *J Foot Ankle Surg* 2004;43:131–133.

30. Armstrong DG, Boulton AJ. Activity monitors: should we begin dosing activity as we dose a drug? *J Am Podiatr Med Assoc* 2001;91:152–153.

31. Armstrong DG, Lavery LA, Holtz-Neiderer K, *et al.* Variability in activity may precede diabetic foot ulceration. *Diabetes Care* 2004;27:1980–1984.

32. Lott DJ, Maluf KS, Sinacore DR, Mueller MJ. Relationship between changes in activity and plantar ulcer recurrence in a patient with diabetes mellitus. *Phys Ther* 2005;85:579–588.

33. Maluf KS, Mueller MJ. Novel Award 2002. Comparison of physical activity and cumulative plantar tissue stress among subjects with and without diabetes mellitus and a history of recurrent plantar ulcers. *Clin Biomech (Bristol, Avon)* 2003;18:567–575.

34. Petrofsky J, Lee S, Bweir S. Gait characteristics in people with type 2 diabetes mellitus. *Eur J Appl Physiol* 2005;93:640–647.

35. Brand PW. The insensitive foot (including Hansen's disease). In: Jahss MH, ed. *Disorders of the Foot and Ankle and Their Surgical Management*. 2nd edn. Vol. 3. Philadelphia: WB Saunders; 1991:2170–2186.

36. Cavanagh PR, Perry JE, Ulbrecht JS, Derr JA, Pammer SE. Neuropathic diabetic patients do not have reduced variability of plantar loading during gait. *Gait Posture* 1998;7:191–199.

37. Cavanagh PR, Derr JA, Ulbrecht JS, Maser RE, Orchard TJ. Problems with gait and posture in neuropathic patients with insulin-dependent diabetes mellitus. *Diabet Med* 1992;9:469–474.

38. Richardson JK, Ching C, Hurvitz EA. The relationship between electromyographically documented peripheral neuropathy and falls. *J Am Geriatr Soc* 1992;40:1008–1012.

39. Simoneau GG, Derr JA, Ulbrecht JS, Becker MB, Cavanagh PR. Diabetic sensory neuropathy effect on ankle joint movement perception. *Arch Phys Med Rehabil* 1996;77:453–460.

40. Rith-Najarian SJ, Stolusky T, Gohdes DM. Identifying diabetic patients at high risk for lower-extremity amputation in a primary health care setting. A prospective evaluation of simple screening criteria. *Diabetes Care* 1992;15:1386–1389.

41. Mueller MJ, Diamond JE, Sinacore DR, *et al.* Total contact casting in treatment of diabetic plantar ulcers: controlled clinical trial. *Diabetes Care* 1989;12:384–388.

42. Margolis DJ, Allen-Taylor L, Hoffstad O, Berlin JA. Healing diabetic neuropathic foot ulcers: are we getting better? *Diabet Med* 2005;22:172–176.

43. Margolis DJ, Kantor J, Berlin JA. Healing of diabetic neuropathic foot ulcers receiving standard treatment. A meta-analysis. *Diabetes Care* 1999;22:692–695.

44. Coleman WC, Brand PW, Birke JA. The total contact cast. A therapy for plantar ulceration on insensitive feet. *J Am Podiatry Assoc* 1984;74:548–552.

45. Petre M, Tokar P, Kostar D, Cavanagh PR. Revisiting the total contact cast: maximizing off-loading by wound isolation. *Diabetes Care* 2005;28:929–930.

46. Armstrong DG, Lavery LA, Kimbriel HR, Nixon BP, Boulton AJ. Activity patterns of patients with diabetic foot ulceration: patients with active ulceration may not adhere to a standard pressure off-loading regimen. *Diabetes Care* 2003;26:2595–2597.

47. Ulbrecht JS, Cavanagh PR. Shoes and insoles for at-risk people with diabetes. In: Armstrong DG, Lavery LA, eds. *Clinical Care of the Diabetic Foot*. Alexandria, VA: American Diabetes Association.

48. Chantelau E, Kushner T, Spraul M. How effective is cushioned therapeutic footwear in protecting diabetic feet? A clinical study. *Diabet Med* 1990;7:355–359.

49. Veves A, Masson EA, Fernando DJ, Boulton AJ. Use of experimental padded hosiery to reduce abnormal foot pressures in diabetic neuropathy. *Diabetes Care* 1989;12:653–655.

50. Cavanagh PR, Ulbrecht JS. Clinical plantar pressure measurement in diabetes: rationale and methodology. *Foot* 1994;4:123–135.

7 The Description and Classification of Diabetic Foot Lesions: Systems for Clinical Care, for Research and for Audit

William J. Jeffcoate and Fran L. Game

INTRODUCTION

The causes of diabetic foot lesions are multiple and their relative importance differs from case to case.[1–4] Since the balance of causative factors varies, so does the presentation – as well as the outcome. It is therefore important to have a simple but precise system for describing and classifying such lesions in clinical practice. Unfortunately, no such system is currently in widespread use. This problem has continued to tax those interested in the field,[5–9] and although there has been a slow move towards consensus,[10] no robust solution has yet been found. The structure of potential classifications will be reviewed in this chapter. The value and limitations of existing systems are assessed, and a possible new hybrid solution proposed.

AIMS AND SPECIFICATIONS OF CLASSIFICATION SYSTEMS

Systems for classification (or description) can be used in three broad ways: routine clinical care, research and audit. The first is concerned with an individual lesion, while the second and third are concerned with groups.

Clinical Care

In routine clinical care the aim is to facilitate note keeping and communication between professionals. The use of such a system would have the secondary benefit of increasing the precision with which lesions are assessed in clinical practice and hence the appropriate choice of treatments.

The Foot in Diabetes, 4th Edition. Editors Andrew J.M. Boulton, Peter R. Cavanagh and Gerry Rayman.
© 2006 John Wiley & Sons, Ltd.

Clinical Research

The purpose of a research classification is to identify groups of similar lesions for inclusion in prospective, controlled intervention trials. In this case, the system will identify appropriate cases from the whole, and is essentially selective. This contrasts with systems for audit – which are essentially all-inclusive.

Clinical Audit

The purpose of clinical audit may vary from simply counting events (e.g. referrals, number of cases of osteomyelitis, incidence of amputation) to seeking associations between different ulcer types and outcome. If the performance between different centres is to be compared, it is important to establish that the population managed by each is similar. Because the cohort studied in each case will be large, the items recorded must be simple, unambiguous and easily documented. Systems for audit are therefore by far the most challenging, since they require prospective accumulation of reliable data on a large number of people, and this information will need to be recorded during the course of busy clinical practice.

WHAT IS CLASSIFIED?

The 'At-Risk' foot

It is known that in diabetes the foot is predisposed to problems due to a combination of factors, including neuropathy, peripheral arterial disease, microvascular disease, deformity and co-morbidity.[1–4] Those at greatest risk are the ones who have been affected by earlier ulceration. While all of the classifications in current use include the option for defining lesions in which the skin is intact, this is not always the same as identifying the foot or person thought to be 'at risk' (from, for instance, any combination of neuropathy, ischaemia and deformity). The classification, or definition, of the 'at risk' foot has been addressed by others[11,12] and will not be considered further in this review.

Ulcers, Lesions and Wounds

The word 'ulcer' applies only to a condition in which the skin is broken (Latin *ulcus* – open sore). The term should not be used when the skin is intact as, for instance, in the acute Charcot foot, or in cases of cellulitis with no apparent portal of entry. In such cases it might be more precise to use the word 'lesion' (Latin *laesionem* – a hurt, damage or flaw). The word lesion could also be extended to include 'pre-ulcers' (areas at high risk of imminent ulceration – such as haemorrhage into an area of plantar callus). The term 'wound' (Old English *wund*) is sometimes used but, strictly, it should apply to penetrating injuries caused by a sharp object. It is worth noting that the words chosen may also occasionally have a disproportionate effect on some patients: some may be reasonably reassured by a chronic problem of the foot – provided it is not called 'an ulcer'.

The importance of deciding whether the system is for 'ulcers' or for 'lesions'

The distinction between these words is of more than just semantic importance. This is especially true when a classification system is used in attempting to audit all clinical activity in a certain specialist unit. Take, for example, the case where a patient may present with a single gangrenous toe, triggered by soft tissue infection, which itself was a complication of pre-existing tinea pedis. If the system employed was of 'lesions' rather than 'ulcers', the obvious dominant problem is either the infection or the gangrene. If the clinician was asked to define either area or depth, he/she would have to decide what was the area covered by the gangrene, for example, or the depth of tissue involved in the infection. On the other hand, if the system was primarily for classifying 'ulcers', then the area and depth should apply purely to the ulcer, or break in the skin, which led to the infection. In this case, the cellulitis and gangrene should properly be logged as complications, rather than episodes in their own right. This issue must be considered carefully at the outset by all who wish to use such systems for the purpose of audit. It should be noted, however, that difficulties will arise when gangrene occurs without a preceding ulcer, or when the ulcer that leads to infection is not apparent.

Multiple Ulcers or Lesions

Another issue to be addressed is that of multiple lesions. If the system of classification is used simply as an aid to clinical practice and to improve communication, then it can be applied to every lesion that exists. If, however, the intention is to use the system to link ulcer type with outcome (as in research or audit), then the issue is slightly more complex. If the chosen outcome relates to the lesion (such as healing, or incidence of secondary infection), then every ulcer could be considered. If, however, the outcome is person centred (such as well-being, or survival), then it will usually be invalid to classify all ulcers, and one (the largest or the most recent, for instance) must be selected as the index lesion. This is relevant to the question of timing of the classification when the exercise is undertaken for the purposes of audit (see below).

THE TIMING OF THE CLASSIFICATION

Clinical Care

When the classification system is to be used to define a strategy for managing a lesion in clinical practice, it can be applied and changed as often as necessary. Thus, an ulcer that is clean and uninfected could be categorised as such, and management principles defined accordingly. If, however, it becomes infected, then its classification (or description) should change to reflect the change in clinical priorities.

Clinical Research

The question of timing also presents little problem in the selection of lesions for prospective research – because the only concern is whether a lesion meets the criteria for selection at the time of recruitment to the study, and it matters little how much it has changed in the period prior to selection.

Clinical Audit

Timing presents a major problem, however, when a classification system is used as the basis of audit. The problem hinges, once again, on whether the system is being applied to 'ulcers' or to 'lesions'. If the aim of the exercise is to determine the outcome of all ulcers or lesions seen in a certain clinic or community (and possibly to compare the results with those from another centre), then – depending on the chosen outcome – each ulcer or lesion episode or person can be counted only once. The time when this is done is likely to be arbitrary – when, for instance, a person is first referred to the specialist unit.

This dependence of audit on timing poses a special problem when the character of a foot lesion changes. Thus, a lesion may present as a clean, uncomplicated ulcer and be classified as such. If, however, it becomes complicated by secondary osteomyelitis, the prognosis changes. Such osteomyelitis may be managed by amputation, and the patient could then be left with an amputation site that fails to heal and with a new ulcer – which is different from the first, even though it is the result of it. While all these stages can obviously be logged as complications or outcomes of the original index lesion, they themselves may also become the subjects of other studies – of, for example, the outcome of osteomyelitis, or of amputation.

The difficulties posed by the evolution of chronic foot lesions are peculiar to the needs of audit, but can be overcome by adopting what may be called the 'lesion narrative'. An example that describes a fictitious case is shown in Table 7.1. Using such a method, it is possible to flag

Table 7.1 An example of a lesion narrative

	Problem 1	Problem 2	Problem 3	Problem 4	Problem 5
01/02/05	**Ulcer under 1MT head (R)**	Ulcer tip third toe (R)			
01/03/05	Persists	Complicated by problem 3	**Osteomyelitis third toe (R)**		
01/04/05	Persists		**Toe amp**	Open wound (R)	
01/05/05	Persists		Complicated by problem 4	**Infected**	
01/06/05				Complicated by problem 5	**BKA (R)**
01/07/05					**Unhealed amp site**
01/08/05		Death of patient from myocardial infarction			

This illustration of the complications that occur in the management of a fictitious patient presenting with two neuropathic ulcers shows how the audit process can be used to document the complications, and outcome, of the initial dominant lesion. However, the documentation of other significant episodes (highlighted in **bold**) means that these too could be used as the basis of independent study. Key: 1MT, first metatarsal; R, right; BKA, below-knee amputation.

dominant or significant events electronically such that both individual lesions and individual conditions (e.g. osteomyelitis, amputation) can later be used as the basis of separate analysis.

COMPONENT DATASETS

Need for Multiple Criteria

The factor that renders classifications of foot lesions so complex is the need to include reference to multiple types of information: there is no single feature that allows clear distinction of lesions of different type or severity. Some of the information is either nominal or categorical (i.e. divided into mutually exclusive categories, such as 'Neuropathy present/absent'), while others form part of a continuum that may be either ordinal or continuous (e.g. measures of area or depth). Moreover, the actual choice of criteria will vary, depending on the purpose of the classification system: whether it is for clinical care, for research or for audit. But although the use of a combination of a larger number of different personal and clinical features confers greater specificity on the system, it is done at the expense of simplicity, and this will mean that it is less attractive to the less committed specialist. A classification will not be used unless it can be easily understood, remembered and applied.

The information that may be used is of three broad types: (a) demographic and personal details of a person's diabetes and co-morbidities, (b) specific features that have contributed to the onset of the lesion and that may delay healing and (c) details of the condition of an established lesion (Table 7.2). It is a matter of preference as to how much information is stored on an independent foot register.

Table 7.2   Datasets that may be variously used in classifying or recording patients, limbs and ulcers/lesions for the purposes of clinical practice, research and audit

1. Features of the person
     Demographic
     Social
     Diabetes related
2. Features that contribute to the onset of an ulcer/lesion, and that may delay healing
     Deformity
     Co-morbidity
     Unrelated disease or treatment
3. Features of the limb or the ulcer/lesion
     Limb
        Site, side
        Ischaemia
        Neuropathy
     Ulcer/lesion
        Bacterial infection
        Area
        Depth

Features of the Person

Aspects of an individual may determine the outcome of any established lesion. These may include demographic details, details of the diabetes, its management and its complications, other co-morbidities, and social factors such as social deprivation, occupational risk and use of tobacco and alcohol. Not all are relevant to every circumstance (or may not be captured on a routine basis), and the items can be selected to meet the needs of individual practice. Some of the detail may also vary with time: for example, new co-morbidities may arise, and the quality of glycaemic control may change. In general terms, it is better to record less than more.

Features that Contribute to the Onset of an Ulcer/Lesion, and that May Delay Healing

Three abnormalities of the limb can both contribute to the development of an ulcer or lesion and affect its rate of healing. These are deformity, co-morbidity and unrelated disease (Table 7.3).

Table 7.3 Features that may contribute to the onset of an ulcer/lesion, and that may delay healing

Deformities of the foot
(a) Changes in the nails
(b) Deformity leading to increased forces applied to the bones and joints of the foot (e.g. consequences of motor neuropathy, shortening of the Achilles tendon or of previous surgery)
(c) Other deformity
Co-morbidity (e.g. immobilisation from other illness, oedema, varicose veins)
Unrelated disease of the skin or treatment, e.g. eczema or psoriasis, systemic glucocorticoids

Features of the Limb and the Ulcer/Lesion

The limb

Site and side

It will be necessary to define the site and side for the purposes of both communication and record keeping. It may also be required for population definition, even though there is currently no evidence that outcome is affected by the site of the lesion.[13,14]

Arterial disease

The diagnosis of significant peripheral arterial disease is essentially clinical, and relies on recognised signs of ischaemia associated with loss of palpable pedal pulses. Although the use of pedal pulses is known to be poorly reproducible[15] and is of even less value in the presence of peripheral oedema, it is a method that is easily applied and may in practice be no less robust than quantitative measures that appear to be more precise. A good correlation with both ulcer incidence[16] and ulcer outcome[17-19] has been demonstrated when the extent of peripheral arterial disease has been assessed using pulse palpation alone. The value of documenting ankle–brachial pressure index (ABPI) is limited by false elevation of the apparent systolic pressure as a result of arteriosclerosis. Systolic pressure in the toe is a more reliable guide to reduced perfusion but can be difficult to determine. Transcutaneous oxygen tension (TcpO$_2$) predicts outcome in limbs that are known to be ischaemic,[20,21] and has been shown to be reproducible,[22] but it is time consuming and the equipment is not widely available. The result is that no single measure is sufficiently reliable for use on its own.

Subclassification (grading) of peripheral arterial disease. Given the imprecision of the clinical methods, and the limitations of investigational tools, it can be difficult to grade the severity of peripheral arterial disease. The options are to grade peripheral arterial disease (or tissue ischaemia) in one of the following ways:

  (i) Present/Absent;

 (ii) in some form of subjective ranking (such as None, Slight, Moderate, Severe); or

(iii) by some means of objective measure of microcirculatory function (e.g. ABPI, toe pressure, TcpO$_2$).

The aim is to use a system of grading that is as precise as possible, and also practicable. The problem with using objective measures of peripheral limb blood flow is that they can be time consuming and impractical during the course of routine clinical care. They are, therefore, really applicable only to research. But even when used in a research classification, their value can be limited by their unreliability (poor reproducibility) and lack of specificity, and any attempt to overcome these limitations may result in a formula that appears unduly complicated (see Table 7.4).

Table 7.4 Potential subclassification of peripheral arterial disease

Grade 1	No symptoms or signs of peripheral arterial disease *plus*
	Both pedal pulses palpable *or*
	ABPI >0.9 and <1.1
	Toe brachial pressure index >0.6 *or*
	TcpO$_2$ >60 mm Hg
Grade 2	Symptoms or signs of peripheral arterial disease, but without critical limb ischaemia:
	Intermittent claudication (confirmed by arterial imaging) *or*
	ABPI <0.9 *but* with ankle pressure >50 mm Hg *or*
	Toe–brachial pressure index <0.6 *but* systolic toe pressure >30 mm Hg *or*
	Other test results compatible with peripheral arterial disease but not critical limb ischaemia
Grade 3	Critical limb ischaemia:
	Systolic ankle pressure <50 mm Hg *or*
	Systolic toe pressure <30 mm Hg *or*
	TcpO$_2$ <30 mm Hg

Adapted from Schaper[10].
These criteria were designed to overcome the inherent imprecision of individual methods, as well as to be compliant with the TASC guidelines for critical limb ischaemia.

Neuropathy

In practice, the assessment of peripheral neuropathy for this purpose is largely based on documentation of loss of sensation. While the modified Neuropathy Disability Score (NDS) is the best validated in terms of correlation both with other measures of nerve damage and with outcome,[16,23] it is time consuming in practice because of its reliance on different measures (temperature sensation, vibration perception threshold (VPT), pinprick and ankle tendon reflexes). Measurement of temperature sensation (warm or cold) threshold is impractical in routine practice and this alone limits the use of the NDS to research. For the detection of VPT, some will have access to a quantitative measure (e.g. biothesiometer or neurosthesiometer), while the majority will rely on the use of a 128-Hz tuning fork. VPT correlates with ulcer incidence.[16,23,24] For assessment of fine touch (pinprick) sensation, the majority now use a 10-g monofilament, although products such as the Neurotip® and Neuropen® are also used. Remarkably, and despite considerable study, there is no consensus as to which, and to how many, sites these stimuli should be applied, and how the results are interpreted. Guidelines exist,[25] but these are based more on opinion and pragmatism than on scientific evidence. The evidence to date suggests that testing for fine touch can be limited to two sites – under the first and fifth metatarsal heads[26] – or even to one – at the base of the hallux nail.[27] At the moment, it has to be accepted that measures of loss of protective sensation from neuropathy are imperfect, but that VPT (biothesiometer), tuning fork, Neurotip and 10-g monofilament all have potentially equivalent and acceptable receiver-operating characteristics.[27]

Subclassification (grading) of neuropathy. As in the case of arterial disease, the option exists for grading sensation as simply Present/Absent, or to attempt some form of subjective grading into None, Mild, Moderate or Severe. It is acknowledged that significant nerve damage may be present, even when the results of clinical testing are normal.[28]

Features of the Limb and the Ulcer/Lesion

The ulcer/lesion

Bacterial infection

The definition, or exclusion, of bacterial infection can also be difficult. Microbiological studies cannot be used to diagnose infection – only to help identify (some or all of) the organisms that are present: the diagnosis is essentially clinical. The clinical signs are dependent on (i) local signs – pus, exudate and smell, (ii) evidence of soft tissue inflammation, and (iii) systemic reaction – fever, ill health. Systemic reaction is, however, rare. The signs of inflammation may also be misleading, because they may be attenuated in those with poor peripheral arterial flow. On the other hand, patients with neuropathy may have redness and swelling that persist for some weeks after the apparently successful elimination of an infective episode.

Subclassification of infection. Cases of bacterial infection can be subdivided in one of two ways: into the tissues affected or into grades of severity. The overlap between the two is only partial. If the first – subclassification according to tissues affected – is used, a distinction may be made between

(i) superficial colonisation (slough and debris on the wound surface without signs of clinical infection);

(ii) infection of soft tissue;

(iii) infection of bone and joints.

It is worth noting, however, that one detailed audit found no difference in overall outcome between ulcers covered with superficial slough and those that were clean.[19] This might suggest that it is unnecessary (for the purposes of audit) to specify the appearance of the wound surface, and that superficial colonisation is of little relevance in terms of healing. In the case of (ii) and (iii), thought should be given to including the option of specifying infection as either 'definite' or 'possible', and to changing the categorisation when further information is available.

On the other hand an infection may be graded in terms of severity, and in line with the guidelines published by the International Working Group on the Diabetic Foot.[29] This approach has been proposed as part of the attempt to reach international consensus on classification (Table 7.5).[10] Once again, the need for precise definition results in the whole appearing rather complex. Moreover, it should be noted that classification guidelines that are based on severity will not necessarily distinguish between infection of deep soft tissue and of bone, and this is a significant limitation. Systemic symptoms and signs probably occur less frequently in patients with osteomyelitis than in those with soft tissue infection, and yet the presence of osteomyelitis has major implications for limb salvage.

Table 7.5   Categorisation of infection according to severity, rather than tissues affected

Grade 1	No symptoms or signs of infection
Grade 2	Infection involving skin and subcutaneous tissue only, with *at least two* of *the following* (having excluded other possible causes): Local swelling or induration Erythema >0.5 and <2.0 cm around the ulcer Local tenderness and pain Local warmth Purulent discharge
Grade 3	Erythema >2.0 cm around the ulcer *plus* One or more of the items listed in grade 1, *or* Infection involving tissues deeper than skin and subcutaneous tissue
Grade 4	Any infection associated with systemic signs – i.e. *two or more of* Temperature >38 or <36°C Heart rate >90 beats/min Respiratory rate >20 breaths/min $PaCO_2$ <32 mm Hg White cell count >12 000 or <4000/mm^3 >10% immature neutrophils

Adapted from Schaper.[10]

Wound bed appearance

It is debatable whether it is necessary to include the appearance of the wound bed in any classification. However, this appearance is a crucial part of clinical assessment, and plays an important part in determining local management. The state of the wound bed may also correlate with outcome, although this has not yet been conclusively proved. It has been suggested that the appearance of the wound bed can be described under four separate headings: percent visible granulation tissue, percent covered by fibrin and debris, percent covered by hard eschar and the presence or otherwise of exudate.[30] Consideration of such features may well form a part of the selection of lesions for both clinical description and selection of ulcers/lesions for prospective research.

Cross-sectional area

Cross-sectional area may be determined with reasonable precision either by tracing the circumference of the ulcer or, in a more rough and ready way, by taking the two maximum widths of the wound at an angle of 90° to each other, and multiplying them as if the ulcer were rectangular in shape. It is, however, very easy to obtain more precise measures using digital imaging with appropriate software, such as 'Mouseyes'.[31]

Depth

Judging the depth of the wound can be very difficult, as many clinicians have only an approximate understanding of the divisions between the various soft tissue layers. It can thus be difficult to decide when an ulcer is confined to 'skin and subcutaneous tissue only' and when it becomes 'deep – but without involving bone and joint capsule'. Moreover, deep structures such as joint capsule and periosteum may be very close to the skin in some parts (as the medial aspect of the first metatarso-phalangeal joint) and relatively distant from it in others (the plantar aspect of the heel). In practice, all three of the recently published classifications use the same criteria to grade depth.[8,10,19] Two of them also include the option for lesions of zero depth – in which the epithelium is intact. Such lesions might include blisters, cellulitis with no obvious portal of entry and the acute Charcot foot.

There is no precise means of measuring (as opposed to describing) depth. Even if there were, it would be debatable whether a measure of depth in millimetres was necessarily meaningful, given the variation in thickness of different tissue layers at different sites on the foot.

FRAMEWORK FOR THE IDEAL SYSTEM

It is apparent that very similar measures are used when a classification is for the purpose of clinical care, research and audit, even though they may be used in different ways. For the purposes of clinical care, the aim is to ensure that any ulcer or lesion is described with clarity and simplicity – such that its status is immediately apparent to any clinician who has not seen it. The system should also convey to the clinician an impression of severity and of the urgency required for intervention. Site and side should be specified in order to eliminate confusion when multiple lesions are present. When a system is intended for research, the overriding concern is the need for precision, with clear definition of the clinical measures used. However, the greatest difficulty is encountered when choosing a classification system for the purpose of audit. The ideal system needs to be both simple and precise: simple enough to be remembered and applied on a routine basis in busy clinical practice, and yet precise enough to generate data that are meaningful.

PUBLISHED CLASSIFICATIONS

Previous published classifications have been well reviewed.[9] The Meggitt–Wagner system[32,33] suffers from lack of specificity. Meggitt–Wagner grades 1, 2 and 3 are essentially measures of increasing ulcer depth (with or without infection), while 4 and 5 refer to localised and extensive gangrene, respectively. Although the Meggitt–Wagner classification has been used for almost 30 years, it is insufficiently precise for modern purposes.

University of Texas

The University of Texas (UT) system for ulcer classification[8] is also primarily based on depth and, as a result, has been shown to correlate well with the Wagner system.[34] However, the inclusion of an additional option of scoring an ulcer by the presence of ischaemia or infection greatly enhances its usefulness (Table 7.6). Different grades of ulcers (from superficial and non-infected in a foot with good blood supply, to deep and infected in an ischaemic foot) have a close correlation with later amputation – which is, perhaps, not surprising. Being based on simple clinical criteria, the UT system is eminently easy to use in clinical practice, and is being increasingly adopted as a means of describing ulcers and for defining best management. However, the UT classification suffers from one main limitation: the omission of any reference to cross-sectional area, when it is known that there is a clear association between cross-sectional area and outcome at baseline.[14,19,35]

Another factor that limits the application of the UT classification for the purposes of either research or systematic audit is the omission of any reference to neuropathy.[9] Neuropathy is undoubtedly a major causative factor in the majority of cases – although it is more true to say that it is not so much neuropathy as a single entity that contributes, as the various features of peripheral nerve damage: motor, sensory and vasomotor. The reason for its exclusion is that

Table 7.6 The University of Texas (UT) classification of ulcers

		0	1	2	3
		Skin intact	Superficial	Deep but not involving bone or joint	Involving bone or joint
A	Not infected, not ischaemic				
B	Infected but not ischaemic				
C	Ischaemic but not infected				
D	Both infected and ischaemic				

the presence of neuropathy (either in isolation or in association with ischaemia) does not really dictate treatment – since offloading is part of the management of all ulcers, irrespective of aetiology. Despite this, the classical neuropathic or mal perforans ulcer is a discrete and well-recognised clinical entity, and it would therefore be odd to exclude it either from any system attempting comprehensive audit of clinical practice, or from a research classification. It follows that the omission of reference to neuropathy and cross-sectional area from the UT system means that its application is effectively limited to the description of ulcers in the process of clinical care.

S(AD) SAD System

The S(AD) SAD system evolved from the experience gained in trying to maintain a comprehensive register of all ulcers managed in a single centre over a protracted period. It was as a result of this process that it was progressively refined until just five features were identified: features that were thought to be key to distinguishing between groups of lesions. It was from these five elements that the (rather ugly) acronym derives: Size, (Area, Depth), infection (Sepsis), ischaemia (Arteriopathy) and neuropathy (Denervation) (Table 7.7). Like the UT system, this system has undergone some form of validation by seeking correlations without outcome.[19] Unlike the UT system, however, the S(AD) SAD system was validated against a variety of end points (healing, failure to heal, amputation and death), rather than just against amputation. The strength of the correlation between baseline measures and outcomes varied, with the strongest associations being found with ischaemia, area and depth. The absence of strong association with infection conflicted with the results of the validation of the UT system, and this was almost certainly the result of the use of different end points and, to a lesser extent, different patterns of care. In the United States, it has been usual to consider surgery early in the process of managing bone infection, whereas the unit in Nottingham has tended to favour a non-surgical approach.[36,37] The absence of a strong association with infection when other outcomes are used suggests that its undoubted importance may be obscured by the effectiveness of appropriate antibiotic prescription. Nevertheless, a weak correlation between infection and eventual outcome does not mean that infection is not a key factor distinguishing different types of lesions.

The main drawbacks of the S(AD) SAD classification (apart from its name) are the apparent complexity of a grid-based system and the irregularity (part ordinal, part nominal) with which

Table 7.7 The S(AD)SAD Classification

| Grade | Size | | Sepsis | Arteriopathy | Denervation |
	Area	Depth			
0	Skin Intact	Skin Intact.	None	Pedal pulses present	Pin pricks intact
1	<1 cm^2	Superficial (skin and subcutaneous tissue).	Surface	Pedal pulses reduced or one missing	Pin pricks reduced
2	1–3 cm^2	Tendon, periosteum, joint capsule.	Cellulitis	Absence of both Pedal pulses	Pin pricks absent
3	>3 cm^2	Bone or joint space	Osteomyelitis	Gangrene	Charcot

components (area, depth, infection, ischaemia and neuropathy) are subclassified, and the imprecision of the clinical methods used. The system also includes the Charcot foot (as a grade of neuropathy), even though others have argued (with good reason) that the Charcot foot is a separate and highly complex condition that does not need to be included in any classification of ulcers.[9]

The PEDIS System

The PEDIS system is the result of an attempt to reach international consensus, and has been published in preliminary form.[10] It includes the same five components as the S(AD) SAD system, although using different terms to create the acronym: Perfusion (ischaemia), Extent (area), Depth, Infection, Sensation (neuropathy). It differs from the UT and S(AD) SAD systems in being designed specifically for the purpose of population selection in prospective research. As such, it abandons the symmetry of both UT and S(AD) SAD and uses strict definitions for the proposed grades of peripheral arterial disease and infection (Tables 7.4 and 7.5). This gives the system the appearance of complexity, but that is not a major disadvantage if it is being used – as intended – only for the purposes of prospective research. Those using it in research will be interested specialists who are studying rather smaller populations. Having said that, those planning prospective research will inevitably consider their own criteria for inclusion and exclusion and would not necessarily feel the need to rely on the PEDIS framework. The main value of this consensus work, however, lies in the formulation of working definitions for each of the parameters that might be classified.

IS IT POSSIBLE TO HAVE A SINGLE SYSTEM THAT MIGHT BE USED FOR ALL THREE PURPOSES?

The omission of neuropathy from the UT system means that it cannot be used for audit, and its place is effectively restricted to clinical care. Even for this purpose, the UT system is limited by the lack of reference to ulcer area. On the other hand, the S(AD)SAD system incorporates both neuropathy and area, and has a proven track record in clinical audit – even though its structure is far from ideal. But as both UT and S(AD) SAD systems are based on much the same elements, it is not impossible that they could be combined, with the hybrid being based on the better points of each. The PEDIS system is based on the same clinical elements and is not in competition – being concerned mainly with the clear definition of subgrades of the component parts. Precise definitions, such as those explored in the PEDIS system, are desirable for implementation of any such new hybrid scheme.

Blueprint for a Hybrid

All three classifications variously use a combination of categorical (infection, ischaemia or both) and ordinal (area, depth) scales. In attempting to incorporate all of the features listed above, it will be apparent that – in addition to site and side – there are three that are categorical (binomial) and three that are semi-quantitative or ordinal. The three that are categorical (infection, ischaemia, neuropathy) are strictly all features of the limb or foot, whereas the three

Table 7.8 The SINBAD system for classifying foot lesions

Site and side			
Ischaemic ?	Yes/No	If Yes, is the ischaemia critical*?	Yes/No
Neuropathy ?	Yes/No	If Yes, has the patient got Charcot?	Yes/No
Bacterial infection	Yes/No	If Yes, is there osteomyelitis?	Yes/No
	0	1	2	3
Area	Skin intact	<1 cm^2	1–3 cm^2	>3 cm^2
Depth*	Skin intact	Superficial	Deep	Bone

*Categories as defined in UT, S(AD) SAD and PEDIS.

that are semi-quantitative are features of the ulcer (Table 7.8). The option exists for defining infection, ischaemia and neuropathy simply as binomial (Yes/No) options. Alternatively, it is possible to subclassify each, as shown in Table 7.8.

Note that the issue relating to whether or not the system is used for 'ulcer' or for 'lesions' is not considered at this stage – despite its importance in using these systems in practice.

SUMMARY

Clinical Care

A system is needed for the routine description of foot lesions – whether the purpose is description in routine in clinical practice, or more structured classification for audit and in population selection for prospective research. Each of these has differing requirements and these determine the structure of any classification used – even though many of the components are shared. Any system used in routine clinical practice must be simple enough to be remembered and easily applied, and the UT classification is suitable. Its specificity would be improved by including reference to area and to neuropathy, but this would inevitably compromise its appealing two-dimensional structure and make it rather more complex and less easy to use.

Clinical Research

The PEDIS system has refined the definitions that might be used when considering criteria for inclusion and exclusion for prospective research projects, and it emphasises the reliance of any working system on five specified criteria: area, depth, infection, neuropathy and ischaemia. It remains, however, in the development stage and has not yet been subjected to any form of validation.

Clinical Audit

There is a great need for an agreed system for clinical audit because this will allow comparisons to be made between different centres, and the results of these comparisons will generate the hypotheses which will ultimately lead to improved clinical management. The specification of a system of audit presents, however, the greatest difficulty – since it needs to be simple enough to be applied easily to a large number of lesions in routine practice, and yet, it also needs to be precise enough to be meaningful. The issues of timing and of clinical progression need to be addressed, as suggested by the introduction of the concept such as the 'lesion narrative'. The Nottingham (or S(AD) SAD) system has been shown to be both feasible and useful in routine practice, and the software is freely available (www.futu.co.uk).

Nevertheless, it is possible that the best features of both the UT and S(AD) SAD systems could be combined and used for both routine clinical care and comparing performance between different centres. A new hybrid of the two, called the SINBAD system, is suggested. The use of a single system for routine clinical description, for audit and – subject to the suggested definitions incorporated in the PEDIS system – for research, would have great advantages.

REFERENCES

1. Reiber GE, Vileikyte L, Boyko EJ, *et al.* Causal pathways for incident lower-extremity ulcers in patients with diabetes from two settings. *Diabetes Care* 1999;22:157–162.
2. Jeffcoate WJ, Harding KG. Diabetic foot ulcers. *Lancet* 2003;361:1545–1551.
3. Boulton AJ. The diabetic foot: from art to science. The 18th Camillo Golgi Lecture. *Diabetologia* 2004;47:1343–1353.
4. Singh N, Armstrong DG, Lipsky BA. Preventing foot ulcers in patients with diabetes. *JAMA* 2005;293:217–228.
5. Pecoraro RE, Reiber GE. Classification of wounds in diabetic amputees. *Wounds* 1990;2:65–73.
6. Jeffcoate WJ, Macfarlane RM, Fletcher EM. The description and classification of diabetic foot lesions. *Diabet Med* 1993;10:676–679.
7. Macfarlane RM, Jeffcoate WJ. Factors contributing to the presentation of foot ulcers. *Diabet Med* 1997;14:867–870.
8. Armstrong DG, Lavery LA, Harkless LB. Validation of a diabetic wound classification system: contribution of depth, infection, and vascular disease to the risk of amputation. *Diabetes Care* 1998;21:855–859.
9. Armstrong DG, Peters EJ. Classification of wounds of the diabetic foot. *Curr Diabetes Rep* 2001;1:233–238.
10. Schaper NC. Diabetic foot ulcer classification system for research purposes: a progress report on criteria for including patients in research studies. *Diabetes Metab Res Rev* 2004;20:S90–S95.
11. Peters EJ, Lavery LA. Effectiveness of the diabetic foot risk classification of the International Working Group on the Diabetic Foot. *Diabetes Care* 2001;24:1442–1447.
12. Malgrange D, Richard JL, Leymarie F, for the French Working Group on the Diabetic Foot. Screening diabetic patients at risk for foot ulceration. A multi-centre hospital-based study in France. *Diabet Metab* 2003;29:261–268.
13. Apelqvist J, Castenfors J, Larsson J, Stenstrom A, Agardh CD. Wound classification is more important than site of ulceration in the outcome of diabetic foot ulcers. *Diabet Med* 1989;6:526–530.
14. Oyibo SO, Jude EB, Tarawneh I, *et al.* The effects of ulcer size and site, patient's age, sex and type and duration of diabetes on the outcomes of diabetic foot ulcers. *Diabet Med* 2001;18:133–138.
15. de Heus-van Putten MA, Schaper NC, Bakker K. The clinical examination of the diabetic foot in daily practise. *Diabet Med* 1996;13:S55–S57.
16. Abbott CA, Carrington AL, Ashe H, *et al.* The North-West Diabetes Foot Care Study: incidence of, and risk factors for, new diabetic foot ulceration in a community-based patient cohort. *Diabet Med* 2002;19:377–384.

17. Apelqvist J, Larsson J, Agardh CD. The importance of peripheral pulses, peripheral oedema and local pain for the outcome of diabetic foot ulcers. *Diabet Med* 1990;7:590–594.

18. Edelman D, Hough DM, Glazebrook KN, Oddone EZ. Prognostic value of the clinical examination of the diabetic foot ulcer. *J Gen Intern Med* 1997;12:537–543.

19. Treece KA, Macfarlane RM, Pound P, Game FL, Jeffcoate WJ. Validation of a system of foot ulcer classification in diabetes mellitus. *Diabet Med* 2004;21:987–991.

20. Carrington AL, Shaw JE, Van Schie CH, Abbott CA, Vileikyte L, Boulton AJ. Can motor nerve conduction velocity predict foot problems in diabetic subjects over a 6-year outcome period? *Diabetes Care* 2002;25:2010–2015.

21. Ubbink DT, Spincemaille GH, Reneman RS, Jacobs MJ. Prediction of imminent amputation in patients with non-reconstructible leg ischemia by means of microcirculatory investigations. *J Vasc Surg* 1999;30:114–121.

22. Jorneskog G, Djavani K, Brismar K. Day-to-day variability of transcutaneous oxygen tension in patients with diabetes mellitus and peripheral arterial occlusive disease. *J Vasc Surg* 2001;34:277–282.

23. Pham H, Armstrong DG, Harvey C, Harkless LB, Giurini JM, Veves A. Screening techniques to identify people at high risk for diabetic foot ulceration: a prospective multicenter trial. *Diabetes Care* 2000;23:606–611.

24. Young MJ, Breddy JL, Veves A, Boulton AJ. The prediction of diabetic neuropathic foot ulceration using vibration perception thresholds. A prospective study. *Diabetes Care* 1994;17:557–560.

25. *International Consensus on the Diabetic Foot: Practical Guidelines* (book on CD-ROM). Noordwijkerhuit, the Netherlands: International Working Group on the Diabetic Foot; 1999.

26. McGill M, Molyneaux L, Spencer R, Heng LF, Yue DK. Possible sources of discrepancies in the use of the Semmes–Weinstein monofilament. Impact on prevalence of insensate foot and workload requirements. *Diabetes Care* 1999;22:598–602.

27. Perkins BA, Olaleye D, Zinman B, Bril V. Simple screening tests for peripheral neuropathy in the diabetes clinic. *Diabetes Care* 2001;24:250–256.

28. Arrezzo JC. New developments in the diagnosis of diabetic neuropathy. *Am J Med* 1999;107:9S–16S.

29. Lipsky BA. Diagnosing and treating diabetic foot infections. *Diabetes Metab Res Rev* 2004;20:S56–S64.

30. Schultz GS, Sibbald RG, Falanga V, *et al*. Wound bed preparation: a systematic approach to wound management. *Wound Repair Regen* 2003;11:1–28.

31. Taylor RJ. 'Mouseyes': an aid to wound measurement using a computer. *Wound Care* 1997;6:123–126.

32. Meggitt B. Surgical management of the diabetic foot. *Br J Hosp Med* 1976;16:227–232.

33. Wagner FW. The dysvascular foot: a system for diagnosis and treatment. *Foot and Ankle* 1981;2:64–122.

34. Oyibo SO, Jude EB, Tarawneh I, Nguyen HC, Harkless LB, Boulton AJ. A comparison of two diabetic foot ulcer classifcation systems: the Wagner and the University of Texas wound classification systems. *Diabetes Care* 2001;24:84–88.

35. Zimny S, Pfohl M. Healing times and prediction of wound healing in neuropathic diabetic foot ulcers: a prospective study. *Exp Clin Endocrinol Diabetes* 2005;113:90–93.

36. Venkatesan P, Lawn S, Macfarlane RM, Fletcher EM, Finch RG, Jeffcoate WJ. Conservative management of osteomyelitis in the feet of diabetic patients. *Diabet Med* 1997;14:487–490.

37. Jeffcoate WJ, Lipsky BA. Controversies in diagnosing and managing osteomyelitis in diabetes. *Clin Infect Dis* 2004;39:S115–S122.

8 Providing a Diabetes Foot Care Service: Lessons from the Veterans Health Affairs in the United States

Jeffrey M. Robbins

INTRODUCTION

The Veterans Health Administration (VHA) has a significant advantage over most other US-managed health care systems in that it is a closed system of care with a defined population that is not profit driven. It is, however, limited by the resource allocations it receives from the US Congress. This forces the system to be as cost-effective and time-efficient as possible, in order to provide the right care to its cohort of patients at the right time and at the right place. One of the biggest challenges is to provide care to its increasing population of patients with diabetes in general and foot-related complications in particular. Moulik *et al.* reported on 5-year mortality rates for new-onset diabetic ulcers. Of those that went on to an amputation, the mortality rate was 47%; however, of those patients whose ulcers healed, the mortality rate was 43%.[1] Tentolouris *et al.* reported slightly higher mortality rates in both diabetic (61%) and non-diabetic (54.3%) patients suffering amputation.[2] In both studies, peripheral vascular disease and neuropathy were found to be the main causes of amputation and cardiovascular disease as the main cause of mortality. These studies highlight the vital importance of a system of care that addresses the multidisciplinary management of diabetes from the initial diagnosis through the continuum of care.

DEVELOPMENT OF PRESERVATION, AMPUTATION CARE AND TREATMENT PROGRAMME

The VHA has long recognised the need to establish a system of care to deal with morbid limb-threatening foot problems in patients with diabetes. Since the late 1980s, VHA has evolved a process of care beginning with the Special Team Amputation Mobility Prosthetics (STAMP) programme that ultimately developed into the Preservation, Amputation Care and Treatment

The Foot in Diabetes, 4th Edition. Editors Andrew J.M. Boulton, Peter R. Cavanagh and Gerry Rayman.
© 2006 John Wiley & Sons, Ltd.

(PACT) programme. This programme was mandated in 1992 by the *Veterans Medical Programs Amendments of 1992* (Public Law 102-405).[3] It emphasised the importance of the highest quality amputee care as well as recognising the need to identify veterans with amputations as a special disability group. It also chartered an oversight committee to ensure compliance, known as the *Advisory Committee on Prosthetics and Special Disabilities*.

In the process of complying with this mandate, VHA recognised the changing needs of the ageing veteran population who were now suffering fewer traumatic amputations and more amputations secondary to diabetes and peripheral vascular diseases. To do this, the PACT programme was initiated in 1993 to establish a model of care to prevent or delay amputations while taking care of those who had already suffered an amputation. The need to be proactive and identify 'at-risk' patients early became a hallmark of the programme. 'At-risk' patients are defined as those patients at potential risk to develop limb-threatening complications such as foot infections and ulcers within the general patient populations. This would include patients with diabetes, peripheral vascular disease and end-stage renal disease, at a minimum. Patients with 'high-risk' feet are defined as those with significant neuropathy, ischaemia and/or deformity that would place them at more immediate risk of a limb-threatening event. Each medical centre determines if other cohorts should be included in the 'at-risk' population. Finally, a system to track patients who are 'at risk', 'high risk' or who have already suffered an amputation from the date of entry into the health care system, through the system of care and back to the community was also mandated.

The directive called for the establishment of this system of care in each medical centre and was to include a coordinator and multidisciplinary care for patients. In 1996, the directive was re-issued and was tied to performance measures, specifically visual inspection for foot deformities, palpation of pedal pulses and testing for protective sensation. The latest iteration of the directive was issued in 2001 and called for improved measures such as a high-risk foot registry.[4]

SYSTEMS OF CARE

Nelson *et al.* have studied the concept of the microsystem of care, which they define as a small functional, front-line unit of health care providers who work together to provide health care to patients. In our case, it is a subpopulation of patients who are at risk for limb loss. They studied 20 such microsystems in North America and discovered nine success characteristics related to high performance as measured by high-quality care in a positive work environment. These included *leadership, culture, macro-organisational support of the microsystem, patient focus, staff focus, interdependence of care team, information and information technology, process improvement and performance patterns.*[5]

Recognising the complex nature of the prevention of amputation, the VHA embarked on a quest to develop a resource-based system of care designed to not only prevent first amputation and subsequent amputation, but also maintain the highest functional capacity and quality of life. It was recognised that this process had to be multidisciplinary, patient centred and well coordinated in order to be effective. The PACT directive established national, regional and local leadership with specific oversight, programme review and quality improvement responsibilities. This includes regular review of the national directive, local directives, amputation rates and other patient care data. The informatics system of the VHAs is quite extensive and includes national, regional and local databases, as well as the computerised patient record system (CPRS). CPRS allows for a significant improvement over the paper medical record, in

PACT clinical foot risk score						
Risk score	Neuropathy As evidenced by loss of protection sensation via Semmes–Weinstein monofilament	PVD As evidenced by no palpable pedal pulses	Specified deformity As evidenced by visual inspection, i.e. bunion, hammer toe, claw toe, mallet toe, metatarsal head deformity, etc.	Ulcer or osteomyelitis or amputation	Intermittent claudication or rest pain, gangrene, peripheral bypass surgery or angiography	ESRD
0 Normal risk Diagnosis of qualifying at risk condition, i.e. diabetes						
1 Low risk (one of three)		X	X			
2 Moderate risk (two of three)	X	X	X			
3 Highest risk Prior ulcer, osteomyeleitis or amputation or severe PVD or all three risk factors (N, PVD, D)	X	X	X	X	X	X

A history of smoking, although not shown to be an independent risk factor for lower extremity amputation, clearly raises the risk level for other morbid vascular complications such as *peripheral vascular disease*, stroke and myocardial infarction and as such aggressive smoking cessation counselling is recommended.

Figure 8.1   PACT clinical foot risk score.

the ability to access all patient information including progress notes, consultation, laboratory studies, etc., at one time from the provider's computer terminal. In addition, clinical reminders appear automatically to facilitate mandatory screening of patients with diabetes and peripheral vascular disease for foot-related problems. The ability to use these databases to retrieve information allows national, regional and local PACT teams to measure their progress. This is accomplished by reviewing both process and outcome measures to evaluate effectiveness and make changes and adjustments to their system of care.

Numerous studies suggest that limb preservation consists of well-timed interventions. These include early screening, risk assessment, foot care education, timely and appropriate referral, revascularisation and limb salvage.[6–11] That said, in a closed managed care system like the VHA with inconsistent access to specialists such as surgical podiatry, vascular surgery, orthopaedics and specialised wound care clinics, a consistent design was not possible. To address this issue, the PACT directive was written in general terms and left to each medical centre to comply with each element. These elements included a model of care which was multidisciplinary and provided screening for those patients considered 'at risk', the assignment of a foot risk score (FRS) (Figure 8.1)[12–17] and timely and appropriate referral as defined by a decision tree, care map or algorithm (Tables 8.1 and 8.2).[18–24] Multidisciplinary care is coordinated by the directors of surgical, medical, podiatry, primary care, nursing and social work services.

COMPONENTS OF PREVENTION AND CARE

The foot screening process involves the palpation of pedal pulses, a sensory examination to determine protection sensation (i.e. Semmes–Weinstein 5.07 monofilament, vibratory exam,

Table 8.1   Risk assessment level

'At risk' is defined, at a minimum, as patients who have had an amputation for any reason, patients with diabetes, peripheral vascular disease and end-stage renal disease, who are considered susceptible to ulcer development.

(a) Level 0, low risk. These patients have no evidence of sensory loss, diminished circulation, foot deformity, ulceration or history of ulceration or amputation. Diabetic patients should receive foot care education and annual foot care. These patients do not need therapeutic footwear.

(b) Level 1, at risk. These individuals demonstrate *one* of the following:
   1. diminished circulation
   2. foot deformity or minor foot infection (and a diagnosis of diabetes).

   Patient education and preventative care are required. The patients in this category and the following two categories (level 2 and level 3) should not walk barefoot. Special attention is to be directed to shoe style and fit. These individuals do not need therapeutic footwear.

(c) Level 2, at risk. These individuals demonstrate sensory loss and one additional:
   1. evidence of sensory loss (inability to perceive the Semmes–Weinstein 5.07 monofilament) or
   2. diminished circulation
   3. foot deformity or minor foot infection (and a diagnosis of diabetes).

   These individuals require therapeutic footwear and orthosis to accommodate foot deformities, to compensate for soft tissue atrophy and to evenly distribute plantar foot pressures. Patient education, regular preventive foot care and annual foot screening are required.

(d) Level 3, at risk. These individuals demonstrate *all three* of the following:
   1. evidence of sensory loss (inability to perceive the Semmes–Weinstein 5.07 monofilament) or
   2. diminished circulation
   3. foot deformity or minor foot infection (and a diagnosis of diabetes).

   or any of the following by itself

   4. Prior ulcer, osteomyelitis or amputation
   5. Severe PVD (*intermittent claudication, rest pain, gangrene, peripheral bypass surgery* or *angiography*)
   6. End-stage renal disease

These individuals are at highest risk of lower extremity events. Individuals in this category require extra-depth footwear with soft moulded inserts. They may require custom-moulded shoes and braces (e.g. double upright brace, patella-tendon-bearing orthosis, etc.). More frequent clinic visits are required with careful observation, regular preventive foot care and footwear modifications.

  'In the case of the traumatic amputee, at least one follow-up visit annually to evaluate prosthetic fit and componentry, maintain optimal functional status and prevent secondary complications is required. The follow-up visit may be made through a direct consultation in the clinic or through a telephone consultation.'

---

sharp/dull) and inspection for foot deformities. The assignment of an FRS provides a guide for the most appropriate referral. A 3- or 4-point scale is used to assign normal risk, low risk, moderate risk or high risk that is coupled with a referral algorithm that provides guidance for follow-up care (Figure 8.1). In order to facilitate this screening process, some conditions and findings lead to an automatic assignment as a high-risk foot. These include a history of prior ulceration or amputation, gangrene, vascular surgery, intermittent claudication and end-stage renal disease. Once the assignment of a high-risk foot is made, yearly repeat screenings are unnecessary and some type of regularly scheduled foot care is established.

  Prevention and treatment interventions are based on the foot risk score and include, at a minimum, patient education and preventive care. Implicit in preventive care are such things

Table 8.2   Module F: PACT algorithms

Patients initially screened in general medicine (FIRM) clinics or other clinic that serves as the entry point to the health care system (geriatrics, woman's health, etc.):

(a) FRS = 0, normal risk
  • diabetes control
  • self-care patient education
  • determine patient's willingness and refer to smoking cessation if applicable
  • annual foot inspection (should include ABI)

(b) FRS = 1, low risk
  • diabetes control
  • self-care patient education
  • determine patient's willingness and refer to smoking cessation if applicable
  • refer to podiatry clinic for regularly scheduled preventive care as needed
  • annual foot inspection (should include ABI)

(c) FRS = 2, moderate risk
  • diabetes control
  • self-care patient education
  • determine patient's willingness and refer to smoking cessation if applicable
  • refer to podiatry clinic for regularly scheduled preventive care as needed
  • refer to prosthetics for proper footwear
  • annual foot inspection (should include ABI)

(d) FRS = 2, high risk
  • diabetes control
  • self-care patient education
  • determine patient's willingness and refer to smoking cessation if applicable
  • patients with claudication symptoms, rest pain or other signs of vascular disease should be referred to vascular surgery for revascularisation work-up
  • page podiatry resident for immediate care if ulceration and/or superficial infection are present
  • page vascular resident if significant tissue loss and/or infection are present in a patient with peripheral vascular disease
  • refer to podiatry clinic for regularly scheduled preventive care within 24–48 h, if non-emergent and no history of ulceration
  • refer to prosthetics for proper footwear

From Ref. 24.

as glycaemic control, self-foot care education, smoking cessation counselling and nutrition counselling. Risk-score-specific interventions (Table 8.1) include the following:

• Risk score 0, normal risk – should receive patient education and annual foot screenings;

• Risk score 1, low risk – should receive patient education and annual foot screenings, specific advise about not walking barefoot and proper shoe fit;

• Risk score 2, moderate risk – should receive patient education and annual foot screenings, and these patient should receive therapeutic footwear;

• Risk score 3, high risk – should receive patient education and annual foot screenings, and these patient should receive therapeutic footwear and possibly custom-moulded shoes. More intensive foot care may also be required.

The timing for referral to foot care specialist as a result of the risk assessment is based on the foot risk score and the presence or absence of specific foot problems. For example, an FRS of 1 or 2 in the absence of any active pathology may be scheduled within a pre-determined time frame (i.e. 2–8 weeks from the time of the initial care, i.e. for subsequent follow-up); however, an active foot problem in any category requires a more immediate referral. The specific referral policy is developed by the PACT team at each facility, to meet the requirements of the directive within the resources of the medical centre.

LIMB SALVAGE/REHABILITATION AND FURTHER PREVENTION

When patients with specific foot-related pathology present, the limb salvage component of the team need to act to prevent amputation and preserve functional capacity. This is accomplished via reconstructive foot surgery, vascular surgery (arterial bypass) or, in some cases, partial amputation.

Unfortunately, there are circumstances that still require amputation. When that occurs the patient receives extensive rehabilitation to regain as much functional capacity as possible and is looped back into the prevention component of the programme for the remaining limb. In this way, the PACT programme seeks to prevent further amputation.

SUMMARY

While providing a diabetes foot care service within the Department of Veteran Affairs, VHA involves interdisciplinary cooperation in order to deal with the complex issues presented by patients with diabetes. It is believed that this system of care may be responsible for the reduction of overall age-standardised amputation rates per 1000 veterans for patients with diabetes in VHA from 9.38 in 1999, to 7.29 in 2000, 6.38 in 2001, 5.33 in 2002, 5.18 in 2003 and to 4.73 in 2004 (Figure 8.2). While primary care provides foot screenings and management of the systemic disease of diabetes, podiatry service provides in-depth lower extremity examination

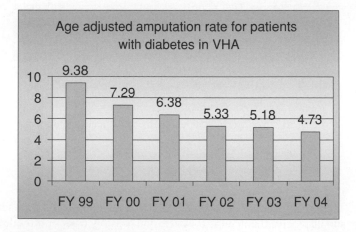

Figure 8.2   Age-adjusted amputations rates for patients with diabetes in Veterans Health Administration.

and diagnosis, surveillance of chronic foot conditions, management of acute foot diabetic problems (i.e. ulcers and infections), and reconstructive foot surgery and amputation, when necessary. As a member of the health care team, podiatry service supports primary care by reinforcing tight glycaemic control, proper nutrition, weight control and exercise, smoking cessation and follow-up foot inspections. This interdisciplinary patient-focused system of care provides veterans with high-quality foot care designed to maintain mobility and maximum functional potential.

REFERENCES

1. Moulik PK, Mtonga R, Gill GV. Amputation and mortality in new onset diabetic foot ulcers stratified by etiology. *Diabetes Care* 2003;26:491–494.
2. Tentolouris N, Al-Sabbagh S, Walker MG, *et al*. Mortality in diabetic and non-diabetic patients after amputations performed from 1990 to 1995. *Diabetes Care* 2004;27:1598–1604.
3. *Veterans Medical Programs Amendments of 1992*. Public Law 102–405.
4. Department of Veteran Affairs. *Preservation Amputation Care and Treatment*. Washington DC: Veterans Health Administration; May 11, 2001. (VHA Directive 2001–030).
5. Nelson EC, Batalden PB, Huber TP, *et al*. Microsystems in health care, Part 1: learning from high-performing front line clinical units. *Jt Comm J Qual Improv* 2002;28:472–493.
6. Lavery LA, Armstrong DG, Vela Sa, *et al*. Practical criteria for screening patients at high risk for diabetic foot ulceration. *Arch Intern Med* 1998;158:157–162.
7. Peters EJ, Lavery LA. Effectiveness of the diabetic foot risk classification system of the international working group on the diabetic foot. *Diabetes Care* 2001;24:1442–1447.
8. Abbott CA, Carrington AL, Ashe H, *et al*. The North-West Diabetes Foot Care Study. Incidence of, and risk factors for, new diabetic foot ulceration in a community-based patient cohort. *Diabet Med* 2002;19:377–384.
9. Boulton AJ, Vileikyte L. The diabetic foot: the scope of the problem. *J Fam Pract* 2000;49:S3–S8.
10. Mayfield JA, Reiber GE, Sanders LJ, *et al*. Preventive foot care in people with diabetes (technical review). *Diabetes Care* 1998;21:2161–2177.
11. Edelman D, Sanders LJ, Pogach L. Reproducibility and accuracy among primary care providers of a screening examination for foot ulcer risk among diabetic patients. *Prev Med* 1998;27:274–278.
12. Boyko EJ, Ahroni JH, Stensel V, *et al*. A prospective study of risk factors for diabetic foot ulcer. The Seattle Diabetic Foot Study. *Diabetes Care* 1999;22:1036–1042.
13. Adler AJ, Boyko EJ, Ahroni JH, *et al*. Lower-extremity amputation in diabetes. The Independent effects of peripheral vascular disease. *Diabetes Care* 1999;22:1029–1035.
14. Litzelman DK, Slemenda CW, Langefeld CD. Reduction of lower extremity clinical abnormalities in patients with non-insulin-dependent diabetes mellitus. *Ann Intern Med* 1993;119:36–41.
15. Reiber GE, Pecoraro RE, Koepsell TD. Risk factors for amputation in patients with diabetes mellitus: a case controlled study. *Ann Intern Med* 1992;117:97–105.
16. Ramsey SD, Newton K, Blough D, *et al*. Incidence, outcomes and cost of foot ulcers in patients with diabetes. *Diabetes Care* 1999;22:382–387.
17. American Diabetes Association. Preventive foot care in diabetes. *Diabetes Care* Jan 2004;27:S63–S64.
18. Lavery LA, Armstrong DG, Wunderlich RP, Boulton AJM, Tredwell JL. Diabetic foot syndrome: evaluating the prevalence and incidence of foot pathology in Mexican Americans and non-Hispanic Whites from a diabetes disease management cohort. *Diabetes Care* 2003;26:1435–1438.
19. Ortegon MM, Redekop WK, Niessen LW. Cost-effectiveness of prevention and treatment of the diabetic foot. A Markov analysis. *Diabetes Care* 2004;27;901–907.

20. Singh N, Armstrong DA, Lipsky BA. Preventing foot ulcers in patients with diabetes. *JAMA* 2005;293:217–228.
21. Driver VR, Madsen J, Goodman RA. Reducing amputations rates in patients with diabetes at a military medical centre: the limb preservation service model. *Diabetes Care* 2005;28:248–253.
22. Pogach LM, Brietzke SA, Cowan CL, *et al.* Development of evidence-based clinical practice guidelines for diabetes: The Department of Veterans Affairs/Department of Defense Guidelines Initiative. *Diabetes Care* 2004;27:B82–B89.
23. VHA/Department of Defence. *Clinical Practice Guideline for the Management of Diabetes Mellitus: Module F – Foot Care.* Available at: http://vaww.visn15.med.va.gov/clinical/clinguide/diabetes/html/contents.htm.
24. Louis Stokes Cleveland VA Medical Centre. *Preservation Amputation Care and Treatment (PACT)Programme.* March 5, 2004 (Medical Centre Policy 011-057).

9 Providing a Diabetic Foot Care Service: The Exeter Integrated Diabetic Foot Project

Mollie Donohoe, Roy Powell and John Tooke

INTRODUCTION

The Exeter Diabetic Foot Care Team no longer provides a 'Cinderella service'. In this chapter, we outline the improvements that we have made to our service, which is now fully integrated across the primary care–secondary care interface.

It is well recognised that diabetic foot ulceration, in spite of being potentially preventable, places a heavy burden on health care resources.[1] Foot ulceration represents a major cause of hospital bed occupancy for people with diabetes, who undergo between 40 and 70% of all non-traumatic, lower limb amputations.[2] Furthermore, an amputation – in addition to resulting in considerable personal loss for patients – costs in excess of £11 000.

The National Service Framework (NSF)[3] aims to foster major improvements in the care of people with diabetes over the next 10 years. It recommends that those with at-risk feet should participate in foot care programmes providing education, podiatry and footwear advice. The Exeter diabetes service, being aware that 75% of diabetic patients in the area are managed primarily in the community, has collaborated closely with primary care in attempting to provide a seamless, districtwide service. Despite this, in a regional audit, we found the rates of amputation in diabetic patients were high compared to national averages (mean 16.5/100 000 population 1994–1996 inclusive) in the health districts served by The Royal Devon and Exeter hospital. We also found in a district survey of diabetic patients attending general practices that 52% possessed one or more major risk factors for diabetic foot ulceration; yet only 51% of those declared at high risk were receiving podiatry. Conversely, 33% of low-risk patients were receiving podiatry, suggesting an inappropriate use of this resource.[4] A parallel study of the podiatrists serving this patient population showed that health professionals' understanding of risk status was suboptimal, with imperfect conception of high-risk foot status and confused referral patterns to both primary and secondary care.[5] There was, however, no coordinated postgraduate education regarding diabetic foot complications.[4] We suggest that if professional staff were confused, then the person with diabetes, who plays a fundamental part in any preventative strategy, is likely to have been unclear as to his or her role.

The Foot in Diabetes, 4th Edition. Editors Andrew J.M. Boulton, Peter R. Cavanagh and Gerry Rayman.
© 2006 John Wiley & Sons, Ltd.

THE INTEGRATED CARE PATHWAY

To combat these barriers to good care, we proposed that an integrated approach would be essential, particularly if the NSF milestones related to chronic diabetic foot complications were to be attained. This would require involvement by health professionals in primary care as the key professionals who can ensure that those at risk of diabetic foot disease receive care appropriate to their level of risk of future disease. The principal strategy for change was to introduce an integrated care pathway for diabetic foot care aimed at improving identification and management of the foot at risk of ulceration.

Initial Evaluation

This integrated care pathway incorporated a package of supportive and complementary educational initiatives aimed at clarifying management of the diabetic foot, referral criteria and professional responsibilities (Figure 9.1). The initial introduction to five practices was part of a randomised controlled trial (RCT) in 1997.[6] This was undertaken with matched cluster randomisation of practices from ten towns drawn from mid and east Devon, responsible for the care of 1939 people with diabetes (age > 18 years). Outcome measures were patients' attitudes regarding the value and importance of foot care, patients' foot care knowledge, health care professionals' foot care knowledge and pattern of service utilisation. We showed that patients' and health professionals' knowledge of, and attitudes towards, foot care improved significantly in the group exposed to the model of care.

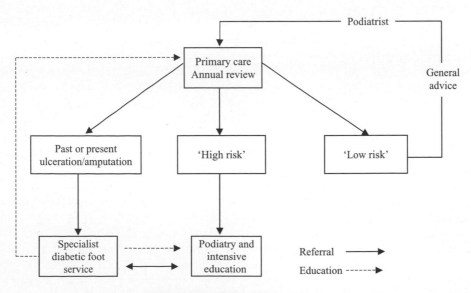

Figure 9.1   Integrated care pathway.

Table 9.1   Criteria for referral to the specialist foot clinic

Ulcer with evidence of spreading infection, cellulitis, digital necrosis or gangrene: a same-day
 referral
Ulceration involving subdermal tissues, which does not respond after 1 week's treatment
Suspected Charcot arthropathy
Patients with high-risk feet, for advice, assessment and provision of appropriate footwear

Roll out of the Model

Given the success of the initiative, a working party was set up to introduce this model of care to
all primary care centres in Exeter, mid Devon and east Devon. Referral pattern pathways and
documented guidelines were distributed to all primary care centres in the three trusts described
(Figure 9.1, Table 9.1). All health professionals actively involved in foot care had access
to a Semmes–Weinstein monofilament (Owen Mumford Ltd, Oxon, cost £10) and patient
educational leaflets (£6/100). Annual educational sessions concerning the management of the
at-risk diabetic foot were organised for podiatrists, and for district and practice nurses. Regular
updates on diabetic foot care were made available on the Internet[7] and sent to all practices.
Three diabetic liaison podiatrists were appointed and re-graded with cost implications of
approximately £2000 per podiatrist per annum. Their role was to coordinate diabetic clinics,
ensure effective prioritisation of caseloads, audit care and provide expert advice for lower grade
podiatrists. This addressed the problem of the professional isolation of community podiatrists,
which was identified in the described RCT[6] as one of the major barriers to seamless integration
of diabetic foot care. Every fortnight they undertook to conduct a community diabetic clinic
and every 3 months participated in a shared clinic with the principal podiatrist in secondary
care. They visited each practice twice over a 2-year period in 2001 and 2002 and audited
the uptake by practice nurses of the model of integrated foot care, including assessment of
neuropathy, ischaemia, footwear and referral patterns.

The Impact of the Model of Care

Five years after the roll out of the model, we evaluated its impact through a combination of
assessment of health professionals' knowledge, their clinical practice and the appropriateness
of referrals. Health professionals' knowledge increased significantly from baseline (66.6 to
79.6%; $p = 0.015$). This was most marked among practice nurses (64.3%, increasing to 82.6%,
Figure 9.2), the health professional primarily responsible for undertaking the patients' annual
review in the community. Patients' knowledge scores were unchanged but their satisfaction
with and attitudes towards foot care services remained favourable.

Prior to the programme, no practices had been using monofilaments to assess peripheral
neuropathy. An audit performed by the diabetic liaison podiatrists indicated that more practice
nurses were using the monofilament confidently (36/52 (69%) vs 44/49 (90%); $p = 0.02$) and
that their confidence remained high in checking foot pulses (43/52 (80%) vs 42/49 (86%);
$p = 0.68$) and advising on footwear (45/52 (87%) vs 42/49 (86%); $p = 0.90$).

The percentage of patients referred to community podiatry clinics with at-risk feet increased
from 89% in 1997 to 97% in 2002, $p = 0.028$, indicating a more appropriate use of this stretched

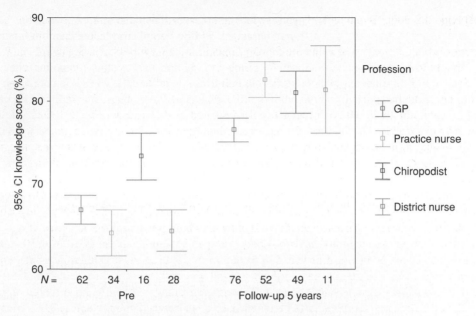

Figure 9.2 Change in knowledge score by profession

resource. Furthermore, there was a significant increase in the proportion of appropriate referrals to the foot clinic, between baseline (67%) and at 5 years (81%), $p = 0.026$.

CONCLUSIONS

We propose that the introduction of an integrated care pathway with clear guidelines can lead to improved patient and health professional awareness of the diabetic foot. We were encouraged to show that nurses, who play a major role in the routine management of diabetes, had the greatest increase in knowledge (Figure 9.2). They also demonstrated, during the roll-out period, increased confidence in using the monofilament and sustained expertise in checking for foot pulses. Patients' attitudes towards their foot care and satisfaction with foot care services remained high. Assuming that the patients have a close relationship with their practice nurse, we maintain that there will be an enhanced recognition of potential foot problems, which will lead to more appropriate use of acute specialist services.

Both primary and secondary care foot services are overstretched and likely to be more so with the rising prevalence of diabetes and increasing pressures on the workforce. We have demonstrated a more appropriate use of skills and the creation of a new role of diabetic liaison podiatrist, which we propose will build strong relations between the primary care and podiatrists, and ensure that clear guidelines regarding management are available.

To meet the challenging targets within the Diabetes NSF, it is essential to ensure that the skills and knowledge to manage the diabetic foot are focused on primary care with rapid access to specialist services when appropriate. An integrated approach is crucial if this goal is to be secured.

ACKNOWLEDGEMENTS

The authors thank Shirley Brooks for secretarial support, John Fletton for his research input and Ian Robinson for facilitating the new posts of diabetic liaison podiatrists.

REFERENCES

1. Bild DE, Selby JV, Sinnock PA, Browner WS, Braueman P, Showstack JA. Lower extremity amputation in people with diabetes: epidemiology and prevention. *Diabetes Care* 1989;12:24–31.
2. The LEA Study Group. Comparing the incidence of lower extremity amputations across the world: the Global Lower Extremity Amputation Study. *Diabet Med* 1995;12:14–18.
3. Department of Health. *National Service Framework (2001) on Standards.* http://www.dh.gov.uk/PolicyAndGuidance/HealthAndSocialCareTopics/Diabetes/fslen.
4. Fletton JA, Perkins J, Jaap AJ, *et al.* Is community chiropodial/podiatric care appropriately targeted at the 'at-risk' diabetic foot? *Foot* 1995;5:176–179.
5. Fletton JA, Robinson IM, Tooke JE. Community chiropodial podiatric care and the 'at risk' diabetic foot: a case for professional updating? *J Br Podiatr Med* 1996;51:4.
6. Donohoe ME, Fletton JA, Hook A, *et al.* Improving foot care for people with diabetes mellitus – randomized controlled trial of an integrated care approach. *Diabet Med* 2000;17:581–587.
7. http://www.rdehospital.nhs.uk/diabetes/home.htm.

10 The Diabetic Foot in Primary Care: A UK Perspective

Roger Gadsby

INTRODUCTION

Traditionally, most people with diabetes in the United Kingdom had their care supervised by hospital doctors, but there was no organised system of care for those who did not attend hospital clinics. In the 1970s, a few systems of 'shared care' between hospital clinics and general practitioners (GPs) were developed, and by the 1980s a number of GPs who had a particular interest in, and enthusiasm for, diabetes care began to develop diabetes clinics within their practices.[1] Published evidence suggested that these clinics provided a standard of care equivalent to that provided by hospital clinics.[2]

In 1990, a new contract for the provision of care in general practice introduced incentive payments for the provision of 'chronic disease management programmes', which included diabetes care. The payments were fairly small, but encouraged more GPs to introduce diabetes clinics in their practices. In 1999, in a national questionnaire survey, 71% of practices questioned were running diabetes clinics, providing most of the routine care for 75% of their patients with diabetes.[3]

In the year 2000, a report from the audit commission reviewing secondary diabetes care in England and Wales found that many hospital diabetes services were overstretched with long waiting times for outpatient appointments. The report concluded that hospital diabetes services were already under considerable strain, that little was taking place in the way of strategic planning and that options for coping with future demand needed to be explored urgently. It suggested that one way forward is for primary care to provide more routine care for people with diabetes, leaving hospitals to concentrate on specialist care and professional support and training, while allowing patients to receive continuity of their diabetes care closer to home.[4]

Since then, the shift of routine diabetes care from secondary to primary care has been encouraged by a number of government initiatives and policy documents. These have included the Diabetes National Service Framework (NSF) and the new General Practitioner Contract Quality and Outcomes Framework, underpinned by clinical guidelines from the National Institute of Clinical Excellence (NICE). The impact of these on diabetic foot care will now be discussed.

The Foot in Diabetes, 4th Edition. Editors Andrew J.M. Boulton, Peter R. Cavanagh and Gerry Rayman.
© 2006 John Wiley & Sons, Ltd.

DIABETES NATIONAL SERVICE FRAMEWORK

National Service Frameworks (NSFs) are statements of health standards and developments published by the Department of Health. The Diabetes NSF was published in two parts. The first was 'Standards'[5] published in December 2001. The second 'Delivery Strategy'[6] was published in December 2002. They contained few specific milestones and targets, unlike previous NSFs for other conditions. The Standards document states that diabetes is the second commonest cause of lower limb amputation. The Diabetes NSF is unique in having a specific standard around patient empowerment. Standard 3 states that

All children, young people and adults with diabetes will receive a service that encourages partnership in decision-making, supports them in managing their diabetes and helps them to adopt and maintain a healthy lifestyle. This will be reflected in an agreed and shared care plan in an appropriate format and language. Where appropriate, parents and carers should be fully engaged in the process.

There is little specific mention of foot care in the document, but Standard 10 states that

all young people and adults with diabetes will receive regular surveillance for the long term complications of diabetes.

Under this standard, the document states that diabetic foot problems are the most frequent manifestations of diabetic neuropathy. Foot ulceration and lower limb amputation can be reduced if people who have sensory neuropathy affecting their feet are identified and offered foot care education, podiatry services and, where required, protective footwear. Prompt treatment of foot ulcers can reduce the risk of amputation. For those who require amputation, their rehabilitation can be optimised through the provision of care by integrated, multidisciplinary, rehabilitation, prosthetic and social support teams.

The Delivery document has virtually nothing specific to foot care. It develops the concept of diabetes networks across the primary–secondary care interface to integrate diabetes care, but does not specifically mention how foot care fits into this model.

THE NEW GENERAL PRACTITIONER CONTRACT QUALITY AND OUTCOMES FRAMEWORK

In the supporting documentation for the new GP contract,[7] the authors note that under the old contract, volume rather than quality was the main emphasis. The new contract addresses this imbalance through introducing a quality and outcomes framework based on best evidence. High achievement against these quality standards is encouraged and will result in substantial financial rewards to practices.

The Department of Health states that the quality and outcomes framework represents, for the first time for any large health system in any country, that GP practices will be systematically rewarded on the basis of the quality of care delivered to patients.

The framework contains four domains. Each domain contains a range of areas described by key indicators. The indicators describe different aspects of performance. The four domains are

– clinical;

– organisational;

– additional services;

– patient experience.

There are a maximum of 1050 points in the whole of the four domains that are available to attain. The clinical domain contains ten disease areas, for which there are a maximum of 550 points. The diabetes area has a maximum of 99 points (approximately 10% of the total points available), spread across 18 clinical indicators. The diabetes quality targets cover structure, process and outcome. The 99 diabetes points are distributed between these as follows: structure (6 points) – practice diabetes register; process (35 points) – completing various tasks of clinical management; outcome (58 points) – demonstrating that people with diabetes achieve good standards of care.[8]

There are 2 of the 18 clinical indicators that refer specifically to foot care. These are as follows: diabetes quality indicator 9 (DM9) – the percentage of patients with diabetes with a record of the presence or absence of peripheral pulses in the previous 15 months (minimum threshold $= 25\%$, maximum threshold to earn full available 3 points $= 90\%$); and diabetes quality indicator 10 (DM10) – the percentage of patients with diabetes with a record of neuropathy testing in the previous 15 months (minimum threshold $= 25\%$, maximum threshold to earn full available 3 points $= 90\%$).

This means that if a practice can demonstrate that 90% of the patients on the practice diabetes register have a record of foot pulses and neuropathy testing within the past 15 months, they will score the full 6 points. Each point for the average practice of about 7500 patients with an average prevalence of diabetes is worth about £120 for 2005–2006, so diabetes foot care can earn up to $6 \times £120 = £720$; and scoring the full 99 points of the diabetes clinical indicators gives an income of $99 \times £120 = £11\,880$. These methods of giving financial incentives for demonstrating good-quality evidence-based clinical care seem to be working. The government was expecting that the average attainment would be around 850 out of the maximum 1050 points. Many practices in the United Kingdom are on target to achieve around 1000 points. The quality and outcome scores were published in Autumn 2005, and so this information will be in the public domain. The average score for diabetes was 93 points out of 99 maximum.

NICE GUIDELINE: TYPE 2 DIABETES

Prevention and Management of Foot Problems

The National Institute of Clinical Excellence (NICE) published an updated guideline in January 2004.[9] A previous foot care guideline had been published in the year 2000 under the auspices of the Royal College of General Practitioners, Royal College of Physicians, Royal College of Nursing and British Diabetic Association (now Diabetes UK). It was developed utilising the NICE methodology for guideline development.

A number of research studies published since the previous guideline have informed the conclusions for the new guideline. It can be downloaded from the NICE Web site www.nice.org.uk, and is available in a full version, a patient version and a quick reference guide. The quick reference guide was sent to all GPs in England and Wales.

The main recommendations have gradings of level A to level D. Level A is directly based on category 1 evidence (meta-analysis of randomised controlled trials (RCTs), or at least one RCT). Level B is directly based on category 2 evidence (at least one study without randomisation or at least one other type of quasi-experimental study) or extrapolated from category 1 evidence. Level C is directly based on category 3 evidence (evidence from non-experimental descriptive studies, such as comparative studies, correlation studies and case–control studies) or extrapolated from category 1, 2 or 3 evidence. Level D is directly based on category 4 evidence (evidence from expert committee reports or opinions and/or clinical experience of respected authors).

Some of the recommendations concerning education are drawn from the NICE 2003 appraisal of patient education models for diabetes. *The initial recommendations* are for a simple screening examination for risk factors for diabetic foot ulceration as part of the annual review process for everyone with diabetes. The recommendation is (1) examination of the feet and lower legs for any foot deformity; (2) palpation of foot pulses; (3) testing of foot sensation using 10-g nylon monofilament or vibration; and (4) inspection of footwear.

The evidence level for this recommendation is given as level A. These items link to indicators 9 and 10 of the diabetes quality framework of the new GP contract, in which quality points are awarded for the percentage of people with diabetes with a record of the presence or absence of foot pulses, and the percentage of people with a record of neuropathy testing in their records. The guidelines state that patients who have any of the above abnormalities detected, and do not have an active foot ulcer, should be referred to the local foot protection team for further assessment. This team with expertise in protecting the foot would typically contain podiatrists, orthotists and foot care specialists. They would assess patients as being either at high risk or at increased risk of foot ulcers. Those found to be at high risk need management and frequent review (1–3 monthly).

The following items are included in each review: (1) inspection of the patient's feet; (2) a review of the need for vascular assessment; (3) an evaluation of the provision and appropriateness of intensified foot care education, specialist footwear and insoles, and skin and nail care.

Those found to be at increased risk of foot ulceration should be reviewed every 3–6 months as follows: (1) review the need for vascular assessment; (2) evaluate footwear; (3) provide enhanced foot care education.

In most practices, about one third of people with diabetes will have some abnormality giving them some degree of increased foot ulcer risk. These individuals need referral to the foot protection programme. The remaining approximately two thirds of the practice population will have no at-risk features, and just need re-screening at their next annual review.

The other major recommendations of relevance to primary care are those dealing with the management of someone newly presenting with foot care emergencies. These are defined as new ulceration, swelling and discolouration. Such emergencies need to be referred to a multidisciplinary foot care team within 24 h. This is defined as a team of highly trained specialist podiatrists and orthotists, nurses with training in dressing diabetic foot wounds and diabetologists with expertise in lower limb complications. The evidence level for this recommendation is given as level D.

The expectation would be that as a minimum the team should (1) investigate and treat vascular insufficiency; (2) initiate and supervise wound management, using dressings and debridement and systemic antibiotics for cellulitis or bone infection as indicated; (3) ensure an effective means of distributing foot pressures, including specialist footwear, orthotics and casts; and (4) try to achieve optimal blood glucose levels and control of risk factors for cardiovascular disease.

IMPLICATIONS OF THE NICE GUIDELINES FOR PRIMARY CARE

It used to be said that all people with diabetes needed referral for podiatric assessment. This resulted in many people with diabetes and normal feet attending the podiatry services, which often became overwhelmed. The recommendations of the new guideline mean that the one third of people with diabetes who need the expertise of the podiatry service should be able to get it, and those who have normal feet can have basic foot care advice in the practice and can cut their own toenails or have them cut by a carer. It may require a reorganisation of local podiatry services, but many already are providing a community-based foot protection programme. This guideline provides support to get them developed in areas where it is not yet happening. Some hospitals already have multidisciplinary foot care teams. Others as yet do not. The guideline should encourage and provide impetus for their development.

If the NICE guideline is followed, it seems highly likely to improve the outcome for patients in the primary care setting. The messages of the guideline are simple. It outlines a brief screening examination in primary care, the fulfilment of which will earn quality points in the new GP contract; patients who screen positive should be referred for further assessment and education to a foot protection programme; anyone newly presenting with a foot emergency should be referred to a multidisciplinary foot care team within 24 h. The guideline should also provide support for service improvement in areas where foot care services are underdeveloped. The quick reference guide version of the guideline contains a clear and helpful 'pathway of care' algorithm which outlines the clinical decisions that need to be made at each stage of the pathway. There is also a patient guide that can be used by people with diabetes to help understand foot problems and what sort of care they should expect for their feet.

The guideline development process involved the critical review of over 300 papers and studies to underpin the evidence base for the recommendations. The full draft guideline of nearly 200 pages (including appendices)[9] provides a wealth of information and analysis for those with a special interest. However, the quick reference guide contains all the simple messages that if fully implemented across the country would undoubtedly reduce the number of amputations in people with diabetes.

Testing Neuropathy in Primary Care

The quality and outcomes framework of the new GP contract does not specify which method of testing for neuropathy should be used in primary care, but only that a patient should have a record of a neuropathy test. The NICE report states that there is a good evidence base for the use of the biothesiometer and the 10-g nylon monofilament to detect neuropathy.[9] The monofilament is easy to use, light, reproducible[10] and cheap compared to the biothesiometer, which often weighs 2.5 kg, requires a power source and costs around £400.[11] The assessment of vibration using the 128-Hz tuning fork is much less reliable as a test for neuropathy. The NICE report states that identification of neuropathy, based on insensitivity to a 10-g nylon monofilament, is convenient and appears cost-effective[9] (recommendation level C). The 10-g nylon monofilament seems to have become the neuropathy test that is used in foot care screening in primary care in the United Kingdom. Not all 10-g nylon monofilaments generate 10 g of force, and so it important to use the most reliable ones. All current monofilaments do

Table 10.1 The procedure for testing neuropathy with the 10-g monofilament

- Bend the monofilament a couple of times at the beginning of each clinic before you use it. This removes any residual stiffness.
- Explain what you are doing to the patient and apply the monofilament on a sensitive area of the skin, e.g. inside the forearm.
- Ask the patients to close their eyes and say 'yes' every time they feel you touch their feet no matter how lightly they perceive the touch.
- Place the monofilament at 90° to the skin surface and slowly push the monofilament until it has bent approximately 1 cm. This should take 0.5 s. Do not jab the skin with the monofilament.
- Hold the monofilament in position for 1–2 s and then slowly release the pressure over 1–2 s, until the monofilament is straight. At this point remove the monofilament from contact with the skin.
- Repeat the procedure for all testing sites on both feet and record the findings.
- If during this test you obtain areas where the patient does not respond, repeat the test at the same site twice more, and if there is still no response record a negative response.

have a life expectancy and get fatigued if used repeatedly for long periods without allowing the nylon to recover.[12] The preferred method of using the monofilament is shown in Table 10.1.

The literature is equivocal about the definitive sites that must be tested for determining ulcer risk, and papers reporting 1–14 sites on each foot have been published.[13] However, there are sites that are common to virtually all publications, namely the plantar surface of the metatarsal heads and the big toe. The rationale is that these sites most frequently ulcerate. When testing, areas of scar tissue or callus should be avoided.[14] There is no clear evidence on how many negative response sites implies an 'at-risk' foot. However, some papers show that even one site with a negative response on each foot may indicate 'at-risk' status.[13] Clearly, the more negative responses there are, the greater the risk.

In summary, when considering neuropathy screening in a busy general practice diabetes clinic, the sites that should be tested are the plantar surfaces of the big toe and a minimum of three metatarsal heads (four sites/foot). Neuropathy is determined by the inability to detect the monofilament at one or more sites on each foot.

WHO SHOULD DO FOOT CARE SCREENING?

Anyone with the skills and competency to perform the testing safely should do foot care screening. In most general practice diabetes clinics, a practice nurse involved in diabetes care will do the screening. In some practices, testing is being performed by health care assistants who have had appropriate training and supervision. In some parts of the United Kingdom, local podiatry services have contracted to provide a screening service for primary care. In this model, podiatrists either attend the practice to do foot screening and provide basic foot education or send invitations for patients to attend the local podiatry department for this work. In another model, foot screening is done at the same time as digital retinal photography in a mobile screening programme.[15]

One potential difficulty of involving trained podiatrists in primary screening in the community is shortage of podiatrists. The author estimates that approximately half of the available hours of all trained podiatrists could be consumed in the process of primary care diabetic foot screening. However, the expertise of trained podiatrists is vitally needed in the education and follow-up of people with 'at-risk' feet, and in the care of people with ulcers in multidisciplinary foot teams. Thus, it is in these areas that podiatry expertise should be concentrated, rather than in primary screening, which is a fairly routine process that less qualified personnel can effectively perform.

ACTIONS TO BE TAKEN AFTER FOOT EXAMINATION

In this section, the actions to be taken, depending on the outcome of the foot examination, will be discussed.

If the foot is normal and, therefore, at low current risk of ulceration, the practitioner should reinforce general foot care education and advice (Table 10.2). The patient should return for a repeat examination annually.

Patients who are determined to have at-risk feet must be referred to the specialist team. The NICE guideline[9] states that 'Implementing a screening and foot protection programme for patients with risk factors for ulceration reduces morbidity and is cost effective' and recommends that the following actions be performed: (1) inspect patients' feet every 3–6 months; (2) enhance foot care education (Table 10.3); (3) evaluate footwear; (4) review the need for further vascular assessment. All these statements are given as evidence level D.

Table 10.2 General foot care and advice to be given to diabetic patients

---

Self-care and self-monitoring, including
- daily examination of the feet for problems (colour change, swelling, breaks in the skin, pain or numbness);
- footwear (the importance of well-fitting shoes and hosiery);
- hygiene (daily washing and careful drying);
- nail care;
- dangers associated with practices such as skin removal (including corn removal);
- methods to help self-examination/monitoring (e.g. the use of mirrors if mobility is limited).

When to seek advice from a health care professional?

- if any colour change, swelling, breaks in the skin, pain or numbness is found;
- if self-care and -monitoring is not possible or difficult (e.g. because of reduced mobility).

Possible consequences of neglecting the feet:

- foot problems can often be prevented by good diabetes overall management as well as specific foot care;
- prompt detection and management of any problems is important, and thus the importance of seeking help as soon as the problem is noticed;
- complications of diabetes such as neuropathy and ischaemia can lead to foot problems such as ulcers, infections and, in extreme cases, gangrene and amputation.

From the NICE clinical guideline.[9] Copyright, the National Institute for Health and Clinical Excellence.

Table 10.3   Foot care advice and education to be given to patients with at-risk feet

---

If neuropathy is present, the resulting numbness means that problems may not be noticed, so extra care and vigilance is needed, and the following advice/precautions to keep the feet protected should be given:
- not walking barefoot;
- seeking help to deal with corns and callus;
- dangers associated with over-the-counter preparations for foot problems (e.g. the corn cures);
- potential burning of numb feet, checking bath temperatures, avoiding hot water bottles, electric blankets, foot spas and sitting too close to fires;
- moisturise areas of dry skin.

Footwear advice to be given:

- regular checking of footwear for areas that will cause friction or trauma;
- seeking help from a health care professional if footwear causes difficulties or problems;
- wearing specialist footwear that has been prescribed or supplied.

Additional advice about foot care on holiday:

- not wearing new shoes;
- planning adequate rest periods to avoid additional stress on feet;
- if flying, walk up and down aisles;
- use of sun block on feet especially on dry skin;
- take a first-aid kit and cover any sore places with sterile dressing;
- seek help if problems develop;
- holiday insurance issues (ensure diabetes cover).

From the NICE clinical guideline.[9] Copyright, the National Institute for Health and Clinical Excellence.

If the above review identifies patients at 'high risk', then the following actions are recommended: (1) frequent review every 1–3 months; (2) intensified foot care education; (3) specialist footwear and insoles; (4) skin and nail care; (5) review of need for vascular assessment; (6) ensuring special arrangements for those people with disabilities or immobility.

One study has demonstrated the potential effectiveness of the above approach. McCabe and colleagues describe a strategy for screening and intervention based on a trial of 2001 patients attending a hospital clinic.[16] Patients were randomised to a control group ($n = 1000$), which continued to receive standard care in the routine diabetes clinic, and an index group ($n = 1001$). The index group was screened for risk factors and patients found to be at increased risk ($n = 259$) were recalled. Following a second assessment, 193 patients with foot deformities, vascular disease or a history of ulceration were entered into a foot protection programme with eligibility for weekly clinics providing chiropody and hygiene maintenance, hosiery and protective footwear. When compared to the control group, the index group demonstrated non-significant trends in reduced ulceration and minor amputations, and statistically significant reductions in overall and major amputations. Of those presenting with ulcers, significantly fewer progressed to amputation in the index group. The foot protection programme was cost-effective in terms of major amputations prevented. (Cost of clinic £100 372; savings from avoiding 11 major amputations estimated at £12 000 each = £13 2000.) It is possible that broader inclusion criteria and increased compliance in the above study might have further improved the cost-effectiveness.

REFERRAL FOR PEOPLE NEWLY PRESENTING WITH A FOOT ULCER AND/OR CELLULITIS OF THE FOOT

In this case, the NICE guidelines[9] recommend referral to a specialised foot care team within 24 h. The guidelines suggest that as a minimum the team should perform the following actions: (1) investigate and treat vascular insufficiency; (2) initiate and supervise wound management; (3) use dressings and debridement as indicated; (4) use systemic antibiotic for cellulitis or bone infection as indicated; (5) ensure an effective means of distributing foot pressures, including specialist footwear, orthotics and casts; (6) try to achieve optimal glucose levels and control of risk factors for cardiovascular disease. These recommendations are mostly given at evidence level D.

Although most areas of the United Kingdom have such a multidisciplinary foot care team based in a local hospital, gaining access to the team within the 24-h timeframe, especially during the evenings and weekends, can be problematic. There are also sometimes difficulties in getting the necessary foot experts in the team to work together. These teams need clear leadership, each member needs clearly defined roles and responsibilities and the GP needs to know whom to speak with about the referral. These details need to be clear for referrals both within 'office' hours, and for out-of-hour emergencies. The development of consultant podiatrists who can lead the foot care team would be one way of resolving some of these potential difficulties.

The message about prompt urgent referral for newly presenting foot ulceration in someone with diabetes represents somewhat of a paradigm shift for many GPs. There may be a temptation to follow a traditional management plan whereby the GP referred the patient to the practice nurse for a dressing with a prescription to the patient for a broad-spectrum antibiotic to be taken orally if infection was suspected. The practice nurse then arranged to see the patient every few days to change the dressings. Such a 'wait-and-see' policy often continued for several weeks before referral was contemplated. Such a policy can prove disastrous. In a study of 669 ulcers presenting to a specialist foot team,[17] the median time between ulcer onset and first professional review was 4 days (range 0–247). The median time from first professional review and first referral to the specialist team was 15 days (range 0–608). Only 30% of patients were referred to the team within 1 week of onset, 48% within 2 weeks of onset and 78% within 6 weeks of onset. It was considered that the condition of 25 ulcers may have deteriorated as a result of delayed referral to the specialist team. This study confirms that in the United Kingdom in the 1990s, the message about prompt urgent referral had still to impact many in general practice. It is to be hoped that the message from the NICE guideline is getting through and that prompt urgent referral is now usual.

FOOT CARE IN TYPE 1 DIABETES

National clinical guidelines for the diagnosis and management of type 1 diabetes in adults[18] and in children and young people[19] were published by NICE in 2004.

The development group for the guidelines for adults noted that foot care had been examined by other quality guideline groups internationally in type 2 diabetes, and that consistency with prior statements would be desirable. An annual foot review was thought to be desirable for reasons of both foot surveillance and education. The simple and effective utility of the monofilament was noted.[18] The development group for the guidelines for children and young people noted that clinical neuropathy is rare in children and young people with good glycaemic control, but recommended that all children and young people with type 1 diabetes should be offered an annual foot care review.[19]

EDUCATION OF STAFF IN PRIMARY CARE

Few primary care physicians or nurses are likely to have had much in-depth teaching on diabetes foot care as part of their initial training. There are now a number of excellent diabetes education and training programmes available in the United Kingdom that enable a health care professional to gain skills in diabetes care (including foot care) at certificate, diploma and masters level. These include the Warwick Diabetes Care, Certificate in Diabetes Care (CIDC) at the University of Warwick, where there is also a Diabetes Masters programme with a foot care module that can be taken as a stand-alone post-graduate award.[20]

Health care professionals working to deliver good-quality diabetes care in the community need to keep themselves up-to-date and need to support each other. To this end, a primary care diabetes society (PCDS) is being set up, dedicated to support primary care professionals to deliver high-quality clinically effective care in order to improve the lives of people living with diabetes. It has a Web site, pages in the journal *Diabetes and Primary Care* and is running a national conference.[21] Diabetes UK, the patient and professional group, also provides information and support for health care professionals.[22] Podiatrists with a special interest in diabetes have set up a support group, Podiatry Diabetes United Kingdom (PDUK), that runs a very successful Web chat forum in which members can e-mail questions, concerns and requests for information, which are answered by other members.[23]

SUMMARY

There is currently a rapid increase in the United Kingdom, as in many countries, in the number of people developing diabetes. A shift in diabetes care delivery from the secondary (hospital) sector to the primary (general practice) sector is happening. This has been facilitated by government policy (Diabetes NSFs) and through the quality and outcomes framework of the new general practice contract. Clinical recommendations on diabetes foot care in the United Kingdom that are up-to-date and evidence based have been published by NICE to underpin management. There is still much to be done to ensure that good-quality primary foot care screening is performed on everyone on an annual basis, and that those with at-risk feet get referred and properly managed in foot protection clinics. Patients newly presenting with a foot ulcer and/or cellulitis also need to receive appropriate care within 24 h from a multidisciplinary foot care team. The principles are in place, which should translate into reduced numbers of people with diabetes experiencing ulcers and amputations, and future research is likely to demonstrate that such improved clinical outcomes will be cost-effective.

REFERENCES

1. Moor MJ, Gadsby R. Non insulin dependant diabetes mellitus in general practice. *Practitioner* 1984;228:675–679.

2. Greenhalgh P. *Shared Care for Diabetes – A Systematic Review.* London: Royal College of General Practitioners; Oct 1994. (Occasional Paper 67)

3. Pierce M, Agarwal G, Rideout D. A survey of diabetes care in general practice in England and Wales. *Br J Gen Pract* 2000;50:542–545.

4. *Testing Times: A Review of Diabetes Services in England and Wales.* London: Audit Commission; Apr 2000.

5. Department of Health. *National Service Framework for Diabetes. Standards.* London: Department of Health; Dec 2001.

6. Department of Health. *National Service Framework for Diabetes. Delivery Strategy.* London: Department of Health; Dec 2002.

7. BMA and NHS Confederation. *New GMS Contract 2003.* London: BMA and NHS Confederation; 2003. Available at: www.bma.org. Accessed Jun 27, 2005.

8. Gadsby R. *Delivering Quality Diabetes Care in General Practice.* London: Royal College of General Practitioners; March 2005.

9. National Institute of Clinical Excellence (NICE). *NICE Clinical Guideline 10. Type 2 Diabetes: Prevention and Management of Foot Problems.* London: NICE; Jan 2004. Available at: www.nice.org.uk. Accessed Mar 13, 2006.

10. Smieja M, Hunt DL, Edelman D, Etchells E, Cornuj J, Simel DL. Clinical examination for the detection of proactive sensation in the feet of diabetic patients. International Cooperative Group for Clinical Examination Research. *J Gen Intern Med* 1999;14:418–424.

11. Kumar S, Fernando DJS, Veves A, *et al.* Semmes–Weinstein monofilaments: a simple, effective and inexpensive screening device for identifying diabetic patients at risk of foot ulceration. *Diabetes Res Clin Pract* 1991;13:63–68.

12. Booth J, Young MJ. Differences in performance of commercially available nylon monofilaments. *Diabetes Care* 2000;23:984–988.

13. Baker N, Murali-Krishan S, Rayman G. A user's guide to foot screening, Part 1: peripheral neuropathy. *Diabet Foot* 2005;8:28–37.

14. Perkins BA, Olaleye D, Zinman B, Bril V. Simple screening tests for peripheral neuropathy in the diabetes clinic. *Diabetes Care* 2001;24:250–256.

15. Sampson MJ, Barrie P, Dozio N, *et al.* A mobile screening programme for the cardiovascular and microvascular complications of type 2 diabetes in primary care. *Diabet Med* 2005;22:256–257.

16. McCabe CJ, Stevenson RC, Dolan AM. Evaluation of a diabetic foot screening and protection programme. *Diabet Med* 1998;15:80–84.

17. Macfarlane RM, Jeffcoate WJ. Factors contributing to the presence of diabetic foot ulcers. *Diabet Med* 1997;14:867–870.

18. NICE. *Type 1 Diabetes in Adults. National Clinical Guideline for Diagnosis and Management in Primary and Secondary Care.* London: NICE; 2004.

19. NICE. *Type 1 Diabetes. Diagnosis and Management of Type 1 Diabetes in Children and Young People.* London: NICE; 2004.

20. www.diabetescare.warwick.ac.uk. Accessed Mar 13, 2006.

21. www.pcdsociety.org. Accessed Mar 13, 2006.

22. www.diabetes.org.uk. Accessed Mar 13, 2006.

23. www.pduk.org.uk. Accessed Jun 27, 2005.

11 Psychological and Behavioural Issues in Diabetic Foot Ulceration

Loretta Vileikyte

Foot ulceration in persons with diabetes is an increasing problem worldwide,[1] with over 80% of amputations preceded by foot ulcers,[2] and there is little evidence of reduction in amputation rates.[3] There is a need to better understand both the psychosocial factors involved in the development of diabetic foot ulcers and the ways by which foot ulceration influences an individual's functioning. There has been a steady increase in publications in this field over the past 5 years. The present chapter summarises the key findings from recently conducted and ongoing studies into how patients adapt to diabetic foot ulceration, by focusing on two areas: the role of psychological factors in guiding adherence to preventive foot self-care and foot ulcer treatment; and the impact of diabetic foot ulceration on an individual's emotional state and quality of life (QoL).

The chapter opens with an overview of the earlier educational and behavioural studies in this area, highlighting the limitations of previous research, which include a paucity of studies, poor methodological quality of many reports and the lack of a theory-driven, patient-centred approach when studying adherence to foot self-care. Subsequently, it introduces a novel approach to the study of psychological factors influencing adherence behaviours and demonstrates how patients' lay beliefs about foot complications combine with medical information and foot ulcer experience in shaping adherence to foot self-care. Next, studies linking diabetic foot ulceration to depressive symptoms are reviewed. Finally, by comparing and contrasting the generic (non-specific to foot ulceration) approach to QoL assessment with patient-centred, foot-problem-focused investigations, it describes the ways by which foot ulceration impacts an individual's functioning and QoL.

REVIEW OF EDUCATIONAL/BEHAVIOURAL STUDIES OF FOOT ULCER PREVENTION

Three systematic reviews of educational and behavioural studies have been conducted to evaluate the role of patient's foot care education in the prevention of foot ulceration.[4–6] The

The Foot in Diabetes, 4th Edition. Editors Andrew J.M. Boulton, Peter R. Cavanagh and Gerry Rayman.
© 2006 John Wiley & Sons, Ltd.

reviews were unanimous in their main conclusion: due to the poor methodological quality of the studies, the available evidence is 'generally unsatisfactory', 'inconclusive' or 'needs confirmation'. For example, the results of the eight randomised controlled trials (RCTs),[7–14] selected for the most recent review by Valk et al.,[6] though conflicting, suggest that although education seems to have a short-term positive effect on foot care knowledge and behaviours, whether it can prevent foot ulceration and amputations remains uncertain. Most of these studies were insufficiently powered to detect clinically important effects of patient education on the hard end points (foot ulceration and amputation) and had inadequate follow-up to assess the potential for prevention of foot complications. Moreover, the eligibility criteria with regard to risk for foot ulceration were described adequately in only one of the RCTs,[10] and monitoring of adherence to the intervention and outcomes was largely unacceptable (only three studies assessed both adherence to foot care and ulceration/amputation rates).[9,13,14]

One of the most commonly cited studies conducted by Litzelman et al.[13] introduced a system of reminders and assessed the effect of this intervention on the prevalence of risk factors for lower extremity amputation in type 2 diabetic subjects. This 12-month intervention was multifaceted and aimed at both the patient and the health care provider. Patients received foot care education and entered into a behavioural contract for foot self-care, which was reinforced through telephone and postcard reminders. In addition, the folders for intervention patients had special identifiers that prompted health care providers to (1) ask that patients remove their footwear; (2) perform foot examinations; (3) provide foot care education; and (4) refer to specialist care (podiatric, vascular and/or orthopaedic) when appropriate. This important study demonstrated that foot self-care and professional foot care matter in reducing foot ulcer rates. Patients receiving the intervention were more likely to report appropriate foot self-care behaviours than were control patients, and were less likely to have serious foot lesions. However, it is unknown whether these behaviours were retained or faded out after the intervention ended. It is conceivable that the behavioural change might not have been sustained, as it was not intrapersonally generated, i.e. it was not determined by an individual's understanding and beliefs about foot complications; rather, it was imposed by researchers.

The other commonly cited study by Malone et al.[10] randomised diabetic patients presenting with severe foot complications (foot infection, ulceration or prior amputation) into those receiving basic foot care education and those with no education. A brief 1-h education session consisted of fear-inducing communication (review of slides depicting infected diabetic feet and amputated diabetic limbs) and a provision of a simple set of instructions for patients regarding foot self-care. After 2 years follow-up, the ulceration and amputation rates were three times lower in the intervention than in the control group. This study included only patients who had already experienced severe foot complications and it is, therefore, not clear whether the behavioural change took place in response to the intervention or whether it was the development of a foot ulcer that impacted foot self-care, as it is known that foot ulcer experience is predictive of better foot self-care.[15] Thus, while education may well be more effective in this group, generalisation to patients who have never experienced diabetic foot complications remains questionable.

Importantly, all the aforementioned trials were designed to provide patients with an action plan, i.e. a list of preventive foot self-care behaviours, and/or enhancement of their behavioural skills, and none of the studies attempted to understand the psychological factors that might be implicated in patients' foot care routine. This, at least in part, could explain why the behavioural change was short lived[11,14] or not achieved.[9,12]

PREVIOUS STUDIES OF PSYCHOLOGICAL FACTORS AFFECTING FOOT SELF-CARE

The literature examining psychological factors underlying adherence to foot self-care is sparse and is mainly restricted to published abstracts.[16,17] Vileikyte et al.,[16] using the Health Belief Model (HBM),[18] investigated the perceived severity of, and vulnerability to, foot complications and perceived barriers to and benefits of foot care. Intriguingly, patients diagnosed as having neuropathy and no evidence of peripheral vascular disease, despite the fact that the researchers explained the results of the tests, perceived themselves as significantly more vulnerable to gangrene of the feet (a vascular complication) than to foot ulceration (primarily a consequence of having neuropathy). Although this was an interesting finding, the researchers were unable to explain, within the HBM framework, why neuropathic patients rated their vulnerability to vascular complications as significantly greater than to foot ulceration. This may be due to the limitations of the HBM outlined by Leventhal and Nerenz[19]: although the HBM provides global evaluations of vulnerability to health threats, it lacks content and thus explanatory power for how vulnerability judgments are made.

The study of McKay et al.[17] tested the role of personality traits in predicting a series of relatively independent self-management behaviours (diet, exercise, blood glucose testing and foot care) in a sample of 221 users of an Internet-based diabetes support system. They found that the conscientiousness score was an independent predictor of adherence to foot care. However, this observation needs to be treated with caution because it was made in a highly self-selected group of patients. Additionally, the role of personality might have been more fully understood if it had been assessed using the self-regulatory framework, that is, by introducing illness cognition as a potential mediator of the association between conscientiousness and adherence. Nevertheless, it is an interesting finding and supports a commonly held belief by practitioners that patient's personality influences adherence to treatment recommendations.

Several other reports, though not explicitly assessing the psychological factors influencing adherence to foot care, point to the possibility that such factors are at play when patients make behavioural decisions respecting preventive foot self-care. When comparing two groups of high-risk neuropathic patients with and without foot ulcer history, Vileikyte et al.[20] reported that although both groups had a sufficient amount of knowledge regarding preventive foot care, scores for self-reported foot care practice were significantly higher in those patients who had experienced a foot ulcer, in comparison to those with no ulcer history. It could be speculated that the development of a foot ulcer resulted in reappraisal of the health threat, making it more relevant to the 'self', more threatening and thus resulting in better foot care practice. Similarly, Breuer[21] showed that adherence to protective footwear was significantly higher in those patients who perceived the health status of their feet as less favourable than those who did not wear the recommended shoes. These observations indicate that patients' behavioural decisions are influenced by their representation of the health threat and point to the need for an examination of how diabetic patients at high risk for developing a neuropathic foot ulcer understand their neuropathy and control their risks of developing a foot ulcer.

THE COMMON SENSE MODEL OF ILLNESS BEHAVIOUR

The Common Sense Model (CSM) of Illness Behaviour provides a framework for exploring how people give meaning and make decisions to take specific actions in response to the diagnosis and symptoms associated with chronic illness.[22] The CSM postulates that patients process health-threatening information by constructing common sense disease models or understanding about illness in terms of symptoms and diagnostic labels, antecedent conditions believed to cause illness, expected duration, possibility of cure or prevention and anticipated impact of illness. Two types of information are integrated when patients construct 'common sense' views of their health status: verbal information from other persons, including physicians, other patients and family members, and concrete experience of symptoms and physical dysfunction.

Guided by the CSM, studies of patient adherence to treatment for chronic conditions such as hypertension and congestive heart failure indicate that inconsistencies between information provided by practitioners and the patients' common sense interpretation of medical diagnoses and symptom experience result in non-adherence to treatment recommendations.[23,24] Baumann and Leventhal, for example, showed that people with hypertension tend to believe that they can tell when the blood pressure is elevated and use symptoms as indicators as to whether or not to take anti-hypertensive medication.[23] More recently, Horowitz and colleagues demonstrated that patients with chronic heart failure perceive it to be an acute medical condition and, as a result, do not manage symptoms on a regular basis and fail to prevent exacerbations.[24]

The main concept of the CSM can be further illustrated by a clinical example of a patient with painful neuropathy and no evidence of peripheral vascular disease (Figure 11.1). His common sense understanding or 'folk' model that the painful sensations in his feet were caused by poor circulation led him to set as a goal the improvement of the blood supply to his feet: he therefore decided to cut the toe box off the shoes thereby enabling him to 'wiggle' his toes, which he believed would improve the circulation. His actions alleviated pain, thereby confirming his 'diagnosis' of poor circulation, and so this individual continued to engage in

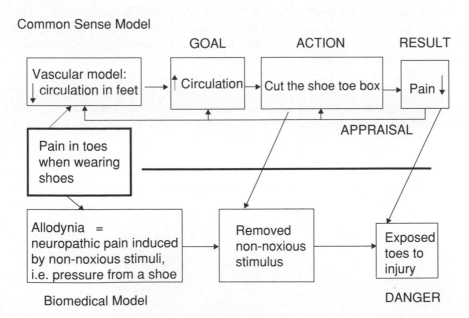

Figure 11.1 Patient's Common Sense versus Health Care Provider's Model of neuropathic pain experience (see text for further discussion)

potentially damaging behaviours (wearing open-toed shoes). From the medical perspective, his symptoms could be described as allodynia, which improved when the non-noxious stimulus, i.e. the pressure from the shoes, was removed, which then, of course, exposed his toes to potential injury. This case demonstrates that patients respond to foot complications by constructing their own images or models that may be inconsistent with the biomedical processes underlying the disease.

In the context of neuropathy, it is therefore important to determine whether a patient's understanding and perception of neuropathy capture the features of this medical disorder that are critical for his/her participation in foot self-care. For example, do patients understand the nature of neuropathy, i.e. that the absence of symptoms does not indicate that the feet are healthy? Do they understand how neuropathy may result in foot ulceration and why, for example, it is important to have their feet measured when buying shoes or why regular removal of callus reduces their risk for foot ulceration? Thus, uncovering the patients' representations of diabetic foot complications and understanding how patients merge 'folk' beliefs with information from practitioners may hold the key to understanding patients' participation in foot self-care.

PATIENTS' COMMON SENSE MODELS IN THE INTERPRETATION OF DIABETIC FOOT COMPLICATIONS AND FOOT SELF-CARE

The combination of the CSM with clinical experience and evidence from interviews with patients at high risk for foot ulceration has informed the development of the Neuropathy Psychosocial Inventory, NPI, an instrument that assesses patients' representations of neuropathy and foot ulceration.[25] A large UK and US study employed the NPI to describe the ways in which the patients' 'folk' beliefs combine with medical information to predict engagement in preventive foot self-care.[25] Additionally, it examined the role of foot ulcer history in shaping the patients' beliefs about diabetic foot complications and foot self-care behaviours. The results of this prospective study indicate that the majority of patients diagnosed with diabetic neuropathy believe that the development of a foot ulcer would be accompanied by pain. Additionally, patients anticipate that any foot damage from diabetes would be vascular and that vascular damage should be reflected in poor circulation and 'cold feet'. These 'folk' beliefs falsely reassure the patient that his or her feet are healthy, leading to a failure to engage in preventive foot self-care and resulting in similar behaviours to those practised by an individual with intact sensation in the feet (e.g. relying on feeling the fit of the shoes rather than having the feet measured when buying a new pair). In contrast, patients who accurately interpret the health care provider's diagnosis, 'neuropathy', and realise that it is possible to have a serious medical condition even if the feet are warm and asymptomatic report higher levels of preventive foot self-care. Furthermore, our results showed that ulcer causal beliefs are among the strongest predictors of preventive foot self-care. That is, patients who have a coherent picture of how various neuropathic risk factors may lead to foot ulceration are more likely to engage in foot self-care actions that reduce the impact of these risk factors. Having had a foot ulcer motivates actions to avoid risks and prevent recurrence. It teaches patients that 'folk' beliefs – such as that good circulation means healthy feet – may be inaccurate and that pain is not a necessary feature of foot ulcers. Moreover, a foot ulcer experience facilitates better understanding of how foot ulcers occur. This could be simply a reflection of 'learning by experience process', e.g.

an individual who develops a painless foot ulcer while wearing a new pair of shoes realises that footwear, in combination with reduced feeling in the feet, results in ulceration. As demonstrated by Del Aguila et al.,[26] it is also possible that practitioners are more likely to provide information about the health threats when confronted with a patient presenting with a foot ulcer, rather than the risk factors alone. It is most likely, however, that foot ulcer experience interacts with medical information processing in shaping the patients' perceptions about diabetic foot complications. Interestingly, beliefs about the nature of neuropathy were independent of foot ulcer history,[25] suggesting that foot ulcer experience is not sufficient to teach patients that neuropathy is a core problem underlying diabetic foot complications and that this fact requires additional explanation by the health care provider.

Contrary to the belief commonly held by clinicians that their patients ignore the risks because they use denial as a protective mechanism from being emotionally overwhelmed, Vileikyte[25] did not find evidence for curvilinearity: that is, higher levels of fear of amputation were associated with better foot self-care. It is important to note that it is not the intensity of fear but the source of fear or the nature of beliefs underlying emotion that is critical. For example, while fear of complications may lead someone who has poorly controlled diabetes on tablets alone to seek medical care, fear may result in avoidance behaviours if it is the potential treatment (e.g. insulin) that is feared. Moreover, while specific emotion of worry about foot ulcers and amputation appears to motivate preventive actions, generalised (non-specific, not related to illness) anxiety does not seem to affect foot self-care actions. These observations are consistent with increasing research evidence that emotional responses that are attached to specific aspects of illness (fear of threatening outcomes such as cancer, AIDS) are important predictors of health care behaviours in contrast to the weak and inconsistent relationships of illness behaviours with measures of generalised distress.[27,28] Finally, of the five personality traits (neuroticism, conscientiousness, intellect, extraversion and agreeableness) and personality-like characteristics (hostility), only conscientiousness was significantly associated with better foot self-care.[25] It appears that conscientiousness affects foot self-care actions both directly and indirectly; that is, conscientious individuals are likely to have more accurate understanding about neuropathy and foot ulceration.

These findings strongly suggest that the patients' common sense beliefs about foot complications are important determinants of a lack of foot self-care and that the health care provider's ability to identify these misperceptions and correct them, by communicating clear messages about the nature of neuropathy, is pivotal for insuring effective patient foot self-care.

Finally, loss of pain sensation not only impacts adherence to preventive foot self-care, but also results in a lack of adherence to prescribed foot ulcer treatment (wearing a foot ulcer offloading device to reduce mechanical stress) and contributes significantly to non-healing of foot ulcers.[29] Whereas persons with foot lesions in the absence of neuropathy avoid walking on such wounds because of pain, patients with insensitive feet continue to walk on plantar ulcers. This, in turn, prolongs the patients' physical and psychosocial dysfunction, including restrictions in activities of daily living and associated emotional distress.[30]

FOOT ULCERATION AND DEPRESSION: IS THERE A LINK?

Foot-ulcer-specific emotional responses are prominent and include fear of potential consequences and anger directed at health care providers as a result of a perceived lack of timely and clear explanation about foot complications.[25] However, there is no evidence in the literature for the association between foot ulceration and depressive symptoms. Vileikyte and colleagues have investigated both cross-sectionally[31] and prospectively[32] the relationship between active foot ulcers, the development of a new ulcer during the18-month follow-up and depression scores and found no association between foot ulceration and depression. Similarly, Ismail and colleagues have examined the role of depression in recurrence and healing of foot ulcers over the 18-month period in patients presenting with the first episode of foot ulceration and showed that depression is not predictive of foot ulcer recurrence or healing.[33] Furthermore, Willrich et al., using the Zung Self-Rating Depression Scale and the Short-Form (SF)-36 questionnaire, have demonstrated that while foot ulcers and Charcot neuroarthropathy have negative effects on patients' physical and mental functioning, this does not seem to be associated with clinical depression.[34] Moreover, Lin et al. have examined the relationship between depression and various diabetes self-care activities and have found that depression was associated with poorer exercise, diet and medication adherence but not with preventive foot selfcare.[35]

The lack of a link between foot ulceration and depression is somewhat unexpected, in view of the evidence that foot ulcers are associated with severe restrictions in mobility, loss of work time and other disruptions in activities of daily living. A possible explanation for this could be that the levels of physical disruptions caused by foot ulceration do not reach those needed to produce depression. It could also be possible that patients affected by foot ulceration receive sufficient social (family and medical) support, which may act as a buffer against depression.Additionally, other psychosocial variables, such as a perceived lack of treatment control and chronic duration of illness, known to be important determinants of depression may not be sufficiently pronounced in patients experiencing foot ulceration to cause depression. Although foot ulcers are difficult to treat and do take a long time to heal, they usually are curable and thus of limited duration. It is important to remember, however, that even though foot ulceration is not associated with depressive symptoms, other experiences of neuropathy such as pain and unsteadiness are important predictors of depression in this group of patients. Therefore, persons with diabetic neuropathy have an increased risk for depressive symptoms and should be carefully monitored to determine whether they are depressed and provided with treatment or referral as necessary.

DIABETIC FOOT ULCERATION AND QUALITY OF LIFE: STUDIES THAT EMPLOYED GENERIC APPROACH

Studies into the effects of foot ulceration on patients' physical functioning, psychosocial functioning and QoL have made clear that foot ulcers can be a source of severe disability, which in turn has a negative impact on QoL.

One of the first studies in this area was conducted in Manchester, United Kingdom, by Carrington and associates.[36] Using a battery of self-report psychological instruments, the investigators have compared the psychological status among diabetic people with chronic foot ulcers, unilateral lower limb amputations and diabetic control subjects with no history of foot ulceration. Psychological assessment included the Psychosocial Adjustment to Illness Scale, the Hospital Anxiety and Depression Scale, a foot questionnaire specifically designed to assess the attitudes and feelings diabetic persons have towards their feet and a QoL ladder. The study reported that patients with both chronic foot ulcers and unilateral amputations had poorer psychosocial adjustment to diabetes than did the control subjects. Specifically, these two groups had made significantly poorer psychosocial adjustments to their situations in the domains of domestic and social environment and reported poorer overall QoL. In addition, foot ulcer patients reported significant problems with their employment and more psychological stress than did the control subjects. Interestingly, no significant differences in psychosocial adjustment were observed between the ulcer and the amputee groups. This could, in part, be due to patient selection bias as pointed out by the authors of this paper: while all subjects with foot ulceration had recurrent, non-healing foot ulcers of at least 3 months duration, all but one of the amputee patients had a below-knee amputation and were mobile with no ulcers on the remaining foot at the time of the interview. It was therefore concluded that future studies should include patients with varying amputation levels, i.e. minor (e.g. toe) and major (below knee/above knee), and varying duration of foot ulceration.

A study from Sweden by Ragnarson Tennvall and Apelqvist did exactly that by comparing the health status in 457 diabetes patients with current foot ulcers, to those with primary healed ulcers, and those who had undergone minor or major amputations.[30] The researchers used a 5-item generic measure of health status, the EQ-5D. Each item in this instrument assesses separate health-related dimensions: mobility, self-care, usual activities, pain/discomfort and anxiety/depression with the response choice of *no problems*, *some problems* and *severe problems*. A single numeric index of health status was then generated from the five dimensions. In addition, this instrument contains a visual analogue scale (VAS) where patients are asked to rate their present health on a scale from 0 to 100. The results of this study demonstrated that subjects with current ulcers had lower health status than both patients who had healed primarily without any amputation and those who had undergone a minor amputation. Patients who had undergone a major amputation had poorer health status than both patients who healed primarily and patients who had undergone a minor amputation. Interestingly, this study also failed to demonstrate significant differences between the current foot ulcer and major amputation groups, as did the study by Carrington and colleagues. This could indicate that (a) either the two groups do not differ in terms of their health status, or (b) the generic questionnaires are not sensitive enough to pick up more subtle differences that exist between these groups of patients.

The results of the following reports cast further doubt as to the appropriateness of generic questionnaires when examining the health status of patients with foot ulceration, especially in the domain of mental functioning. A study by Meijer *et al.*, using the SF-36, compared the health status and mobility between diabetic patients with either past or present foot ulceration and diabetic individuals without a history of foot ulcers.[37] The results of the study demonstrated that the presence or history of foot ulceration had a negative impact on physical (physical role, physical functioning and mobility) but not mental functioning. Similar results were obtained by Ahroni *et al.*, who demonstrated prospectively that the development of neuropathic complications including foot ulceration and amputation was associated with a decline in four out of eight SF-36 scales representing physical functioning (general health, physical functioning, physical role and vitality).[38] In contrast, a recent study, which compared the performance of the generic SF-12 and a neuropathy and foot-ulcer-specific questionnaire, the Neuropathy and Foot-Ulcer-Specific Quality of Life instrument (NeuroQoL; described below), demonstrated that while the mental functioning scale from the SF-12 was not associated with foot ulcer presence, a foot-problem-specific emotional burden scale from the NeuroQoL showed a strong association with the presence of foot ulceration and was the most important link between foot ulceration and reduced QoL.[39] These findings point to the importance of using condition-specific questionnaires when studying the effects of foot ulceration on individual's health status and QoL.

DIABETIC FOOT ULCERATION AND QUALITY OF LIFE: ADDRESSING THE PATIENT'S PERSPECTIVE

The studies described above used generic questionnaires, the content of which was imposed by the investigators and did not emerge from patients affected by foot ulcers. Thus, the findings from these studies left a gap between foot ulceration as abstractly defined and the patient's experience of foot ulceration that is essential for framing effective interventions. It is increasingly recognised that QoL, rather than being a mere rating of health status, is actually a uniquely personal experience, representing the way that individuals perceive and react to their health status.[40] This recognition emphasises the importance of addressing the patient's perspective rather than the researcher's views when measuring QoL. In an attempt to overcome these shortcomings, several questionnaires assessing QoL from the perspective of an individual affected by foot ulceration were recently developed. Examples include the Diabetic Foot Ulcer Scale (DFS)[41] and the NeuroQoL.[39] A series of interviews with foot ulcer patients and their caregivers were conducted to elicit life domains affected by foot ulceration that are important to an individual's QoL. These interviews demonstrated that the loss of mobility caused by non-weight-bearing treatment is central to foot ulcer experience. It results in severe restrictions in activities of daily living, including daily tasks, leisure activities and employment. Brod, for example, reported that approximately half of the interviewed patients had either retired early or lost time from work, and career opportunities were sometimes missed.[42] Moreover, limited mobility causes problems with social and interpersonal relationships and perceptions of diminished value of the self due to inability to perform social and family roles.

A recent study employed the NeuroQoL to investigate the impact of diabetic neuropathy (symptoms and foot ulceration) on QoL.[39] Findings from this investigation were largely consistent with the main themes that have emerged from prior qualitative studies. Patients experiencing neuropathic symptoms (pain, lost or reduced feeling in the feet and unsteadiness) and foot ulcers reported severe restrictions in daily activities (e.g. leisure, paid work and daily tasks), problems with interpersonal relationships and changes in self-perception (e.g. being treated differently from other people). This study demonstrated that among the psychosocial variables, changes in self-perception as a result of foot complications have most devastating effects on an individual's QoL.

In summary, diabetic foot ulceration is a source of severe physical dysfunction, emotional distress and poor QoL. While foot ulceration is not predictive of depressive symptoms, it is a source of ulcer-specific emotional responses, which either facilitate (fear of potential consequences) or inhibit (anger at health care providers) preventive foot self-care actions. Patients respond to diabetic foot complications by creating their own models or understanding about this medical disorder, which is largely inconsistent with the practitioner's view (the biomedical view), resulting in a lack of foot self-care. The health care provider's ability to understand and share the patients' common sense perspective is therefore central to effective health care provider–patient communication and should potentially lead to better foot self-care and fewer foot ulcers and amputations.

REFERENCES

1. Boulton AJM, Vileikyte L. Diabetic foot problems and their management around the world. In: Bowker JH, Pfeifer MA, eds. *The Diabetic Foot.* 6th edn. Philadelphia: WB Saunders; 2001:261–273.

2. Pecoraro R, Reiber GE, Burgess EM. Pathways to diabetic limb amputation. *Diabetes Care* 1990;13:513–521.

3. Trautner C, Haastert B, Spraul M, Giani G, Berger M. Unchanged incidence of lower-limb amputations in a German city 1990–1998. *Diabetes Care* 2001;24:855–859.

4. Mazzuca SA, Moorman NH, Wheeler ML. The diabetes education study: a controlled trial of the effects of diabetes patient education. *Diabetes Care* 1986;9:1–10.

5. O'Meara S, Cullum N, Majid M, Sheldon T. Systematic reviews of wound care management: diabetic foot ulceration. *Health Technol Assess (Rockv)* 2000;21:113–238.

6. Valk GD, Kriegsman DM, Assendelft WJJ. Patient education for preventing diabetic patient ulceration: a systematic review. *Endocrinol Metab Clin N Am* 2002;31:633–658.

7. Mazzuca SA, Moorman NH, Wheeler ML. The diabetes education study: a controlled trial of the effects of diabetes patient education. *Diabetes Care* 1986;9:1–10.

8. Rettig BA, Shrauge DG, Recker RR. A randomized study of the effects of a home diabetes education program. *Diabetes Care* 1986;9:173–178.

9. Bloomgarden ZT, Karmally W, Metzger MJ. Randomized controlled trial of diabetic patient education: improved knowledge without improved metabolic status. *Diabetes Care* 1987;10:263–272.

10. Malone JM, Snyder M, Anderson G, Bernhard VM, Holloway GA Jr, Bunt TJ. Prevention of amputation by diabetic education. *Am J Surg* 1989;158:520–523.

11. Barth R, Campbell LV, Allen S, Jupp JJ, Chisholm DJ. Intensive education improve knowledge, compliance, and foot problems in type 2 diabetes. *Diabet Med* 1991;8:111–117.

12. Kruger S, Guthrie D. Foot care: knowledge retention and self-practices. *Diabetes Educ* 1992;18:487–490.

13. Litzelman DK, Slemenda CW, Langefeld CD, *et al.* Reduction of lower extremity clinical abnormalities in patients with non-insulin-dependent diabetes mellitus. *Ann Intern Med* 1993;119:36–41.

14. Ronnemaa T, Hamalainen H, Toikka T. Evaluation of the impact of podiatrist care in the primary prevention of foot problems in diabetic subjects. *Diabetes Care* 1997;20:1833–1837.

15. Vileikyte L, Rubin RR, Leventhal H. Psychological aspects of diabetic neuropathic foot complications: an overview. *Diabetes Metab Res Rev* 2004;20:S13–S18.

16. Vileikyte L, Shaw JE, Boulton AJM. Diabetic foot: patients' perceptions of risks and barriers to foot care may be the final determinants of ulceration (abstract). *Diabetes* 1997;46:A147.

17. McKay HG, Boles SM, Glasgow RE. Personality (conscientiousness) and environmental (barriers) factors related to diabetes self-management and quality of life (abstract). *Diabetes* 1998;47:A44.

18. Rosenstock IM. The health belief model and preventive health behavior. *Health Educ Monogr* 1974;2:354–386.

19. Leventhal H, Nerenz D. The assessment of illness cognition. In: Karoly P, ed. *Measurement Strategies in Health.* New York: Wiley; 1985:517–554.

20. Vileikyte L. Psychological aspects of diabetic peripheral neuropathy. *Diabetes Rev* 1999;7:387–394.

21. Breuer U. Diabetic patients' compliance with bespoke footwear after healing of neuropathic foot ulcers. *Diabetes Metab* 1994;20:415–419.

22. Leventhal H, Meyer D, Nerenz D. The common sense representation of illness danger. In: Rachman S, ed. *Contributions to Medical Psychology.* Vol 2. New York: Pergamon; 1980:7–30.

23. Baumann LJ, Leventhal H. I can tell when my blood pressure is up, can't I? *Health Psychol* 1985;4:203–218.

24. Horowitz CR, Stephanie BR, Leventhal H. A story of maladies, misconceptions and mishaps: effective management of heart failure. *Soc Sci Med* 2004;58:631–643.

25. Vileikyte L. *Psychological Aspects of Diabetic Peripheral Neuropathy and Its Late Sequelae* (PhD thesis). University of Manchester; 2004.

26. Del Aguila MA, Reiber GE, Koepsell TD. How does provider and patient awareness of high risk status for lower extremity amputation influence foot-care practice? *Diabetes Care* 1994;17:1050–1054.

27. Diefenbach MA, Miller SM, Daly MB. Specific worry about breast cancer predicts mammography use in women at risk for breast and ovarian cancer. *Health Psychol* 1999;18:532–536.

28. Mora PA, Robitaille C, Leventhal H, Swigar M, Leventhal EA. Trait negative affect relates to prior weak symptoms, but not to reports of illness episodes, illness symptoms and care seeking. *Psychosom Med* 2002;64:436–449.
29. Boulton AJM, Armstrong DG. Clinical trials in plantar neuropathic diabetic foot ulcers: time for a paradigm shift? *Diabetes Care* 2003;26:2689–2690.
30. Ragnarson Tennvall G, Apelqvist J. Health-related quality of life in patients with diabetes mellitus and foot ulcers. *J Diabetes Complications* 2000;14:235–241.
31. Vileikyte L, Leventhal H, Gonzalez JS, *et al.* Diabetic peripheral neuropathy and depressive symptoms: the association revisited. *Diabetes Care* 2005;28:2378–2383.
32. Vileikyte L, Gonzalez JS, Leventhal H, *et al.* Predictors of depression in subjects with diabetic peripheral neuropathy: a longitudinal study. *Ann Behav Med* 2004;11:P62.
33. Ismail K, Winkley K, Chalder T, Edmonds ME. Is depression associated with a worse prognosis following the first onset of a diabetic foot ulcer? *Diabetes* 2005;54:1969P.
34. Willrich A, Pinzur M, McNeil M, Juknelis D, Lavery L. Health related quality of life, cognitive function, and depression in diabetic patients with foot ulcer or amputation. A preliminary study. *Foot Ankle Int* 2005;26:128–134.
35. Lin EH, Katon W, Von Korff M, *et al.* Relationship of depression and diabetes self-care, medication adherence, and preventive care. *Diabetes Care* 2004;26:2154–2160.
36. Carrington AL, Mawdsley SK, Morley M, Kincey J, Boulton AJ. Psychological status of diabetic people with or without lower limb disability. *Diabetes Res Clin Pract* 1996;32:19–25.
37. Meijer JW, Trip J, Jaegers SM, *et al.* Quality of life in patients with diabetic foot ulcers. *Disabil Rehabil* 2001;23:336–340.
38. Ahroni JH, Boyko EJ. Responsiveness of the SF-36 among veterans with diabetes mellitus. *J Diabetes Complications* 2000;14:31–39.
39. Vileikyte L, Peyrot M, Bundy EC, *et al.* The development and validation of a neuropathy and foot ulcer specific quality of life instrument. *Diabetes Care* 2003;26:2549–2555.
40. Gill TM, Feinstein AR. A critical appraisal of the quality of quality-of-life measurements. *JAMA* 1994;272:619–625.
41. Abetz L, Sutton M, Brady L, McNulty P, Gagnon DD. The Diabetic Foot Ulcer Scale (DFS): a quality of life instrument for use in clinical trials. *Pract Diabetes Int* 2002;19:167–175.
42. Brod M. Quality of life issues in patients with diabetes and lower extremity ulcers: patients and care givers. *Qual Life Res* 1998;7:365–372.

12 Education in the Management of the Foot in Diabetes

Kate Radford, Susan Chipchase and William Jeffcoate

INTRODUCTION

It is invariably recommended that people with diabetes should be offered education about preventive foot care, and this should be repeated at intervals – most frequently for those at greatest risk. While there is no disputing this principle, it is based on a number of assumptions. Thus, it assumes that such education will result in a significant change in behaviour and that this in turn will lead to a reduction in the incidence of foot problems. It also assumes that the content of the information to be taught is established, as well as its optimal mode of delivery. In practice, the evidence base is extremely thin and the only aspect of education that is beyond dispute is that people with diabetes should be told that foot ulcers may occur, and that they should do their best to look after their feet in order to prevent them. There is a pressing need for further work to be done in order to establish the structure and content of educational programmes, as well as their cost-effectiveness. Such work should determine the extent to which education is best directed at the patient or at the professional. It should also investigate who should do the teaching, how often, what is taught and what methods should be used. The question of educating the educators should be addressed. Without formal evaluation, the implementation of detailed prevention programmes may consume resources that might be better directed at the more effective management of the established foot ulcer.

EVIDENCE FOR THE EFFECTIVENESS OF EDUCATION

Education might be used in primary prevention (in those who have never had a foot problem), in secondary prevention (prevention of recurrence) and in the management of established ulcers. Evidence of effectiveness might be either direct (reduction in incidence of ulcers or amputation) or indirect (using surrogate end points such as knowledge and foot care behaviour).

The Foot in Diabetes, 4th Edition. Editors Andrew J.M. Boulton, Peter R. Cavanagh and Gerry Rayman.
© 2006 John Wiley & Sons, Ltd.

Primary Prevention

Reduced incidence of ulcers and amputation

Intensive education with follow-up contact and reminders over 12 months led to a weakly significant reduction (OR 0.41; CI 0.16–1.00) in incidence of new ulcers in a relatively socially disadvantaged, predominantly female, group of patients with type 2 diabetes in Indianapolis, although the study was not large enough to demonstrate an equivalent effect on amputations.[1] McCabe and colleagues[2] undertook a larger, but incompletely randomised study (in the sense that all those at high risk were allocated to the intervention group) in Liverpool, United Kingdom, and found that the introduction of an integrated foot care programme did not reduce new foot ulcers in high-risk patients, although there was a significant reduction ($p < 0.01$) in the incidence of major amputation. In two randomised studies of educational interventions covering multiple aspects of diabetes care, neither Rettig and colleagues[3] nor Bloomgarden et al.[4] found any reduction in the incidence of foot problems after 12 and 18 months, respectively. Similarly, Ronnemaa et al.[5] found that education did not lead to a reduction in ulcer incidence after 12 months, while Hamalainen and colleagues[6] found no benefit of education in low-risk patients in a study involving 7-year follow-up

Surrogate end points

Of those studies listed above, which were also designed to assess foot care knowledge and behaviour, there was a significant improvement in the intervention group in three,[3,5,6] while there was no change in one.[4] Corbett[7] reported that one-to-one education resulted in a significant improvement in knowledge ($p < 0.03$) and foot care behaviour ($p < 0.01$) at 3 months, while Mazzuca et al.[8] found no effect at 1 year. In a small study comparing a low-intensity (1-h foot care advice) with a high-intensity (general diabetes education programme followed by 9-h foot care teaching over 4 weeks) programme, there was marked ($p < 0.001$) difference in foot care knowledge and behaviour over the succeeding 6 months.[9] This was associated with a fall ($p < 0.001$) in the incidence of active foot 'problems requiring treatment' – although almost all of these 'problems' appear to have been abnormalities of nail and skin other than ulceration. In a study exploring different educational interventions, Kruger and Guthrie[10] reported improved health care behaviour at 6 months in both intervention groups. Pieber and colleagues also reported a reduced prevalence of callus and nail abnormalities following general diabetes education of low-risk patients managed in the community.[11]

Secondary Prevention

Reduced incidence of ulcers and amputation

Malone and colleagues[12] randomised 203 patients who had been admitted to hospital with foot problems (ulcer, infection or amputation) to either receive or not a single, hour-long education session that included display of graphic visual images. They found that the intervention group had a threefold and highly significant reduction in both new ulceration (OR 0.28; CI 0.13–0.59) and amputation (OR 0.32; CI 0.14–0.71). We have been unable to identify any other studies of education in secondary prevention.

Management of Established Ulcers

A recent (and very large) study from Chennai reported that of 1259 patients at previous high risk and who presented with foot ulcers, healing occurred in 82% who were judged (retrospectively and in an unspecified way) to have adhered to foot and ulcer care advice, compared to 50% of those who did not.[13] There have been no other specific studies of the effect of education on established ulcers, although it could be assumed that one benefit of a pre-emptive education programme might be that those who later develop an ulcer would be empowered to seek expert help earlier. Early self-referral may be associated with an improved outcome, and this may be the explanation for the reduced incidence of amputation in the otherwise neutral study by McCabe *et al.*,[2] as well as the apparently startling reduction in amputation reported by Malone and colleagues[12] and the reduced healing time reported by Griffiths and Wieman.[14]

CONCLUSIONS CONCERNING THE PUBLISHED LITERATURE

A recent Cochrane systematic review[15] drew attention to the paucity of good-quality research in the area. Published trials of interventions were often poorly designed and described. The content and style of the education delivered varied widely. Even the better designed studies were too small and therefore insufficiently powered to detect true effects. There is, therefore, a danger of both a Type I error (concluding that an intervention is effective when it is not) and a Type II error (concluding that is not effective when it is). There is also a very real risk of a Type III error[16] – whereby an intervention that is shown to be ineffective when evaluated in isolation and as part of a formal trial may yet be effective in practice when it is delivered as part of a coordinated multidisciplinary programme. Moreover, it should be recognised that the effectiveness of any education programme is critically dependent on the availability of complementary clinical services. Thus, a programme that emphasises the importance of seeking immediate expert advice will be ineffective if such advice is not available.

Valk *et al.*[15] concluded that the evidence to suggest that patient education *per se* reduces the incidence of both foot ulcers and amputations was weak and inconclusive. While an education programme may increase knowledge or awareness, this does not necessarily result in changes in foot care skills or behaviour, or in clinically significant benefit. Moreover, the effectiveness of educational measures appears to be generally short term.[6,9] It is clear that there is a need for more high-quality randomised controlled trials, based on modern concepts of educational practice. These trials should explore the content and methodology of education programmes, as well as seek to define both their effectiveness and cost benefit.[17]

ISSUES TO BE ADDRESSED IN PLANNING AN EDUCATION PROGRAMME

Aim

The aim of the intervention is to induce a change of behaviour, which will result in a lower incidence of, or improved outcome from, diabetic foot disease.

Who Is to Be Educated?

Professionals

If improved outcome of ulcers – rather than reduced incidence – is the principal aim, then it is most likely that this will be best achieved by improving the knowledge, skills and coordination of professionals. This aspect of the topic has not yet received much attention, although Connelly and colleagues demonstrated that much of the variation in the incidence of major amputation for diabetes in three towns in northern England could be attributed to differences in professional attitudes and beliefs concerning ulcer management.[18] A change in behaviour of professionals may also have a significant impact on the incidence of new ulcers. Del Aguila and colleagues[19] have shown that health care providers have limited awareness of the potential for protective management in patients whose feet are at risk from either neuropathy or vascular disease, and this has been echoed in a recent report by Lawrence and colleagues.[20] Others have judged that action or inaction by professionals is twice as likely to result in the presentation of a foot ulcer than anything that the patient does or does not do.[21]

There is evidence that education of health care professionals is associated with improved clinical practice with regard to preventive foot care (as opposed to actual ulcer incidence). In an attempt to determine the effects of educating physicians, Bruckner et al.[22] ran 1-day statewide workshops on diabetes foot care. When reviewing, after an interval of 9 months, the records of the patients of the 560 clinicians who took part, they found better documentation of education, improved self-care and a trend towards reduced lower limb amputation. O'Brien et al.[23] also showed that lectures given to primary care physicians in Texas, United States – when combined with the instruction that clinic support staff should remove the socks and shoes of all diabetes patients who were placed in exam rooms – resulted in a significant increase in performance and documentation at 6 months of proper foot examination, from 14 to 62% and from 33 to 73%, respectively. This confirms the observations made by Cohen, 20 years earlier.[24] However, as with educational interventions for patients, no professional education programme has yet been shown to have a significant impact on either ulcer incidence or ulcer outcome[22] – unless it was undertaken as part of a comprehensive programme of improving medical support in previously deprived communities with a particularly high baseline incidence of amputation.[25] This is in contrast to the results of Plank and colleagues[26] who demonstrated that the simple strategy of implementing routine podiatric supervision of those at greatest risk, independent of specific education, was associated with a significant reduction in ulcer recurrence.

There is a clear need for more research in this area. Such work should probably acknowledge that it is inappropriate to require professionals in primary care to have detailed knowledge of ulcer aetiology and assessment – because non-specialists actually encounter relatively few ulcers in any one year. They do, however, need to be able to identify the patient 'at risk' (see below) and all professional staff need to understand the importance and potential urgency of any newly presenting ulcer. There should be agreed pathways for assessment and care, with appropriate early referral to specialist hospital clinics.

Patients

Educational initiatives for patients need to be considered under three headings: those with no special increase in risk, those at increased risk and those at much increased risk. Those at

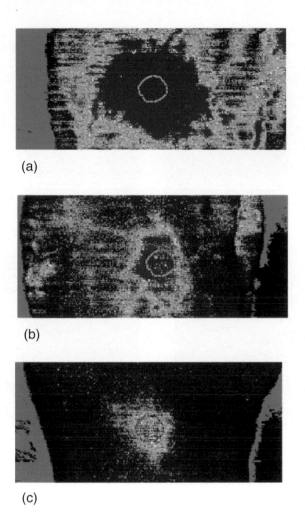

(a)

(b)

(c)

Plate 1 Examples of LDIflare: (a) control subject; (b) subject with diabetes but no neuropathy; (c) subject with diabetes and neuropathy (Adapted from Krishnan *et al.*[39])

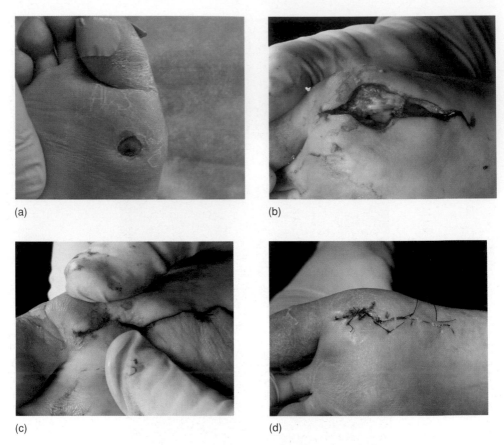

(a)

(b)

(c)

(d)

Plate 2 (a) Chronic ulceration under the first metatarso-phalangeal joint. The medial sesamoid is palpable at base of ulcer; (b) the sesamoid has been excised, the metatarsal head is visible at the depth of the wound just prior to suturing the tendon of the flexor hallucis brevis and the inter-sesamoid ligament; (c) just prior to suturing the skin, showing approximation of the skin flaps for primary closure; (d) 1-month post-operative, demonstrating healing of incision

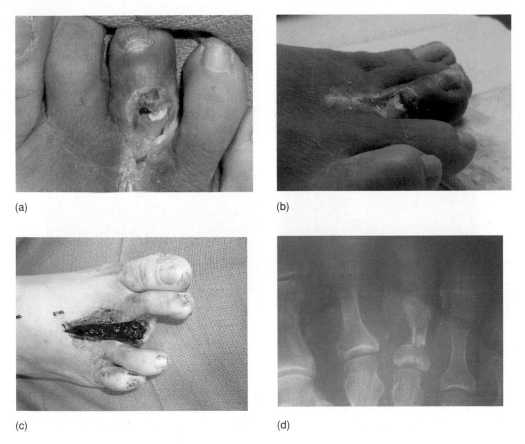

(a)

(b)

(c)

(d)

Plate 3 (a) Chronic dorsal ulceration of toe exposing deep tissue; (b) phalanx is visible in the wound; (c) web-splitting incision for debridement of deep infection, including resection of third metatarsal; (d) osteomyelitis of the second ray on oblique radiograph

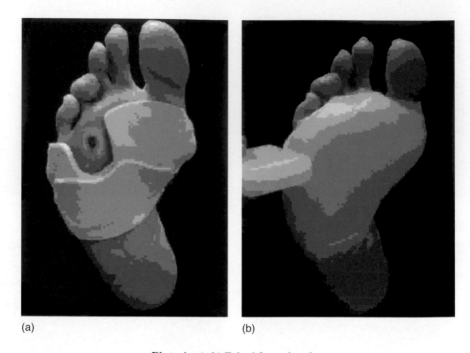

(a)   (b)

Plate 4   (a,b) Felted foam dressing

increased risk are those with one identified risk factor (neuropathy or ischaemia or deformity), while those at greatly increased risk are those with two or more risk factors or those who have had a previous foot ulcer. The educational methods used will depend on the level of individual risk, and studies designed to determine the effectiveness of such interventions must take this into account.

Education of Patients with no Increased Risk

Prevention of neuropathy, ischaemia and deformity

Information imparted might include advice on the undisputed importance of maintaining good glycaemic control, and minimising vascular risk by not smoking, by taking exercise, dietary modification and, when appropriate, taking aspirin and lipid-lowering therapy. Education will not minimise the effects of any deformity that is congenital, or acquired as a complication of diabetes (such as neuropathy and Achilles tendon shortening), but patients should learn the importance of accommodating the deformed foot in appropriate footwear. Education given to younger people about pointed-toed shoes may in theory reduce the incidence of bunions in later life, but in practice it is likely to be ignored.

General foot care

Recommendations can be given concerning the general care of feet but it is unlikely that they will lead to a change in behaviour in the majority of those without special risk. Thus, those with intact peripheral circulation and sensation are unlikely to perceive the need to, for instance, inspect their feet carefully every day, to dry carefully between their toes or to adhere to any of the other (often unsubstantiated) advice that might be found in educational leaflets on foot care which are available. Similarly, it is very unlikely that any study will ever be possible that will prove the utility or futility of such aspects of general advice – because the incidence of new ulceration is so low and the numbers needed to study would be prohibitive. It seems, therefore, that the answer to this question will never be available.

Given that detailed information on foot care is unlikely to have a major impact on ulcer incidence in this group (and since the healing of any accidental injury is also unlikely to be a problem), professionals should bear in mind the potential adverse effects of giving instruction that is of limited use to the patient. If the guidance is sufficiently far removed from the patient's own foot care beliefs and health expectations, it may induce unnecessary alienation.

Particular thought should be given to the seemingly non-controversial advice that a patient should never go barefoot. There is no reason why this advice should be given to someone whose circulation and sensation are intact. There is, for instance, little point in advising young persons with uncomplicated type 1 diabetes not to go barefoot when they are about to go to a beach resort in the sun. Not only are they at no increased risk if their sensation and circulation are intact, but they would not take any notice anyway. Similarly, consideration should also be given to the validity of advice that people with uncomplicated diabetes should not go barefoot in their own home. It should be borne in mind that the incidence of foot ulceration is very much lower in South Asian individuals living in the United Kingdom than it is in Caucasians,[27] despite the fact that walking barefoot in the home is not uncommon in this group. If the floor covering is good and uncluttered, it is possible (albeit unsubstantiated) that walking barefoot in the home may actually be beneficial (for those without either peripheral vascular disease or neuropathy) in the long term, by reducing any adverse effects of footwear.

Surveillance

People without any particular increase in risk should, however, be advised to ask their doctor or nurse to examine their feet for signs of neuropathy or ischaemia on a regular basis, in order to ensure that they remain complication free and without increased risk. It is recommended (but without evidence and mainly for ease of administration) that this be done annually. While there is no evidence that regular examination results in a short-term reduction in ulcer incidence,[28] the practice will serve to emphasise the importance of foot care in later life.

Education of Patients at Increased Risk

Those at increased risk (because of neuropathy or ischaemia or deformity) need to be advised that they are 'at risk'. Evidence from the United Kingdom suggests that although the incidence of new ulceration in the total population with diabetes is of the order of 2% per year,[29] the incidence in those with neuropathy exceeds 7%.[30] More detailed information (such as the need for regular podiatry, appropriate footwear, avoidance of accidental injury) will depend on the individual problem and particular liability.

Surveillance

The persons with feet at risk should ideally examine their feet each day – if they are able to. They should be encouraged to look for sores or unexpected changes and if they find them, they should seek professional help sooner rather than later. If it is not possible for them to examine their feet themselves (for example, because of poor vision or limited mobility), it may be appropriate to ask them to enlist the help of a family member or friend. It should, however, be borne in mind that neither the patients nor their helpers may like this idea.

The 'at-risk' foot also needs to be reviewed by the patient's professional carer at intervals. The length of the interval varies according to feasibility and need, but it is not always either necessary or desirable to insist (as some do) that the person's feet should be inspected by the doctor or nurse at every visit. While unsuspected (or undisclosed) ulcers will occasionally be detected, the primary purpose of such regular inspection is to reinforce the fact that the foot is 'at risk', and to emphasise the need for both appropriate protective behaviour and urgent assessment if any new lesion arises. Foot inspection at every visit in this group will certainly do no harm and may be beneficial. Nevertheless, a single study designed to document the benefit of more frequent foot examinations failed to demonstrate any benefit in terms of reduced incidence of amputation in a high-risk population.[28]

Advising other professional carers that the feet are at risk

The patients should be encouraged to advise all professionals involved in their care that their feet have been designated 'at risk'. In an ideal world, this would then ensure that preventive measures were taken whenever the person was put at extra risk by, for instance, being confined to bed by intercurrent illness. Sadly, there is currently little sign that other professionals have anything other than minimal awareness of the implications of foot risk factors in people with diabetes.[20]

Action to be taken if a new problem occurs

The final element of education for the patients with 'at-risk' feet concerns action to be taken if they have a new lesion. In brief, they should be encouraged to contact the medical professional who deals with them most closely as soon as possible, preferably by phone. It goes without saying that those who might take such phone calls should be aware of the urgency with which they should be handled.

Education of Patients at Greatly Increased Risk

The principles of education for this group are very similar to those for the 'at-risk' group. The differences relate to frequency of review and to relative degrees of urgency, rather than to matters of substance. In general, this group might be expected to remain under long-term care by a multidisciplinary foot team and it is to this team that they might be advised to turn to in case of need.

THE EFFECT OF EDUCATION ON BEHAVIOUR CHANGE

Factors other than the degree of risk must be taken into consideration when planning the content and presentation of educational material to be made available to an individual.[31] New information does not generally result in the desired change in behaviour unless it is relevant to the persons and their lifestyle. For instance, it would serve no purpose to instruct persons to wash their feet regularly when they already do it five times each day as part of their usual religious observance. Advice on footwear must take into account the persons' normal practice, including their mobility, employment and their culture.

Adherence and Non-compliance

It is normal for people to express their independence by either doing what they think is best for themselves or doing what they want. It is not normal to follow instruction without question. On the other hand, people will follow instruction if they perceive the need for behaviour change, if the instruction is compatible with their own wishes and intentions and if they trust, for whatever reason, the person doing the instructing. To that extent, it is counterproductive if instructors or educators express surprise when people display non-compliance (or non-adherence), and if they blame them for it.

The common sense model of illness behaviour[32] provides an appropriate structure for considering factors underlying variation in adherence to self-care in diabetes, and with respect to foot care in particular.[33] Patients hold implicit beliefs and apprehensions concerning the nature of their disease and the threat it poses, and these influence both their behaviour and their response to education. People's understanding of their disease is affected by social and cultural contexts, as well as the quality of their communication with their health care professional.[34] The implication is that adherence will be improved if professionals involved in patient education explore the patient's understanding, beliefs and fears, and use these as a basis for choosing the advice that is given.

Depression

It has been estimated that some 14% of patients with diabetes have clinical depression – two to three times that in the general population,[35,36] and this has been shown to be associated with both poor glycaemic control and chronic complications of diabetes.[37,38] It therefore follows that a significant proportion of those at risk of foot complications will be depressed, and depression is associated with poor self-care behaviour, poor participation in education programmes for diabetes[39] and reduced confidence in their ability to care for their feet.[38] Those planning educational programmes might therefore consider the option of screening for depression with a view to instituting specific therapy.[40,41] Vileikyte et al.[38] commented that one reason for the inconclusive nature of the results of trials of education in this field might relate to the absence of any assessment of adherence to the intervention in half of the studies, and to failure to explore people's understanding of the factors involved or their emotional reactions to them.

Transtheoretical Model of Behavioural Change

The transtheoretical model of behaviour change – which deals with the evolution of behaviour change into a new habit – has been explored in a variety of clinical settings.[42–44] Behaviour change may be regarded as being in one of the five stages: pre-contemplation, contemplation, preparation, action and maintenance. With this in mind, educational interventions can be designed and tailored to facilitate transition from one stage to the next. Thus, a technique such as motivational interviewing[45] might be used to help a person who is in the pre-contemplative and contemplative stages (merely thinking about changing) to move to the stage of adopting new foot care practices.

In the preparative stage, information about foot care may be enough to trigger change in some people, while others may remain ambivalent. This ambivalence may be the result of perceived barriers, such as insufficient time, money, other priorities and the attitudes of family and friends.[45] If these barriers are significant, then they will obstruct the attempts of a professional to induce behaviour change. Moreover, persons who believe that the advised health behaviour challenges their personal freedom or standards may react by exaggerating their problem behaviour. For example, if prescribed footwear is regarded as unattractive by a woman because it has implications for the selection of other items of clothing (e.g. trousers rather than a skirt), then she may start to demonstrate a preference for the clothing with which the footwear is incompatible. This has been termed 'psychological reactance'.[45] It follows that it is essential to base the structure of the education programme on the preferences and obligations of the patient, and these will not be perceived unless there is some form of initial assessment.

INITIAL ASSESSMENT

The initial assessment is based on the understanding that the process of education is one that is directed at an individual, and interventions should be tailored to help people change their behaviour in order to meet their personal needs. The assessment involves determination of the degree of risk, exploration of the extent to which their current behaviour might enhance this risk, barriers to the adoption of improved foot care behaviour and consideration of which form of educational intervention might have the greatest impact.

The degree of risk can be assessed most simply from the presence of ischaemia, neuropathy or deformity and from whether or not the patient has had a previous foot problem. Co-morbidities – such as those that result in immobilisation – may also increase the risk to the foot. Assessment of current foot care behaviour involves assessment of patients' usual daily activities and the extent to which they choose, or are required, to be on their feet each day. It also involves looking at their shoes and using this to explore their preferences and preconceptions concerning the choice of footwear. It is then necessary to define the extent to which physical, social and cultural factors might act as barriers to any change in foot care behaviour that is thought to be necessary. Physical factors include the extent to which foot care might be limited by poor vision or other incapacity. Social factors would include employment details and inescapable responsibilities to their family and other contacts. Cultural issues would include those that influence the use of footwear and include those exerted by society, as well as the sometimes very powerful influence of people's perception of the importance of their choice of footwear as an expression of their self-image.

THE STRUCTURE OF AN EDUCATIONAL PROGRAMME

Integration with Other Facets of Diabetes Education

There is a danger that foot care may be considered in isolation when it would be better integrated into other aspects of education about a person's diabetes management. In practice, it may often be better delivered as part of a general education package, which has the advantages of tailoring the package to the requirements of an individual as well as improving coordination between different members of the multidisciplinary team. New models of care need to be adopted which help address the personal, social and environmental factors that condition the persons' health and their capacity for self-care. These factors influence both the content of the education programme and the way in which it is delivered.

Content

There is an outstanding need to define which aspects of foot care behaviour are definitely associated with a reduction in ulcer incidence. We have some preliminary evidence that professionals from different specialty subgroups (e.g. doctors, nurses, podiatrists) differ in how they rank the importance of different aspects of foot care behaviour. Much of the advice to be found in different foot care leaflets (and which is presumably similar to that which is delivered verbally) has no grounding in science, and may occasionally be inconsistent. Is there evidence, for instance, that drying carefully between toes after washing (any more than people would anyway) results in decreased incidence of *tinea pedis*, or that the use of moisturising cream has a specific benefit on the incidence of foot cracks or ulcers? Is it known that the application of moisturising cream between toes causes any harm? Thus, it could be argued that some foot care advice may currently be too detailed and may be no better than that which simply relies on general principles. It could also be argued that the use of detailed guidelines, with lists of prescriptive instructions, may sometimes have a potential adverse effect – if failure to follow them induces a sense of guilt in the patient who goes on to get an ulcer. Guilt may lead to delayed self-referral and the ulcer may worsen as a result.

Delivery

The scientific basis of foot care education for people with diabetes is in its infancy but there is relevant experience in other fields. Similar issues have been addressed in the management of rheumatoid arthritis, for instance, and it has been shown that behavioural interventions (such as those providing skills practice, goal setting and home programmes) have significant positive effects on functional ability, mood and morbidity.[46] However, these reviewers also reported that the greatest benefit in rheumatoid arthritis was observed in response to behavioural interventions, while those based simply on didactic measures (such as information giving and attempts at persuasion) and counselling (enhancing social support and discussion of problems) had little effect. Even so, the responses to behavioural therapy were only modest and their clinical relevance was unclear.[47]

Kruger and Guthrie[10] compared the effect on foot care behaviour of two different educational interventions: didactic alone versus didactic combined with a 'hands-on' practical demonstration. There was no difference in knowledge between the two groups at 6 months, but those receiving the practical programme had better foot care behaviour. Barth *et al.*[9] showed that an intensive education programme had a greater short-term effect on knowledge and foot care behaviour, but it was not associated with any reduction in the incidence of new foot problems.

Media and resources

There are no data relevant to foot care available to help determine whether education is best delivered simply in person or combined with materials and technologies such as interactive Web site, video, CD-ROM, audiotape or foot care leaflet. Television facilities are now commonplace in hospital waiting areas and could be used to present a foot care video, featuring an influential member of the professional team (or a patient), running intermittently. The content need not be complex and could comprise a simple explanation of the main risk factors for ulcer development and a demonstration of good foot care practice. There would be an inherent danger, however, that repeated delivery might lead to annoyance, and some may resent being treated as a captive audience in this way, with the associated intrusion into their thoughts and privacy. It might be better for such a facility to be simply available in a separate area rather than being imposed on all.

Leaflets

Most would feel that the provision of educational leaflets was an essential part of routine care – the evidence from other fields is that the impact of educational leaflets on behaviour is not great,[46] and is very dependent on both content and design. Content is inevitably based on the beliefs and practice of the author(s), and our own unpublished data indicate that these may vary between different professional groups. Design is also important: texts that are easy to read can increase the reader's motivation and interest.[48] Readability depends on many factors including print legibility, use of illustrations and the complexity of words or sentence structure. Tests of readability and comprehension tests – such as Flesh Reading Ease Scores[49] and the Cloze procedure[50] – can be simply and easily applied. Evaluation of leaflets in this way indicated that readability, comprehension and usefulness were the biggest overall predictors of whether UK National Health Service nurses intended to follow safe manual handling practices.[48]

Group Versus Individual Education

Groups allow for interaction and shared learning[31] and Malone and colleagues used group teaching to effect a major reduction in amputation.[12] However, the delivery format will be influenced to a large extent by the client group. Younger people at risk of ulceration are a high priority for education and may respond better to individually tailored sessions, which are timed to suit them, although it is also possible that some would prefer the informality of group teaching and would find it less intimidating. It follows that if both group and individual sessions are available, the opportunity to join a group should be offered to all. Group education sessions might be held at the hospital, general practitioner's surgery, community-based clinics or local sports and community centres – provided the venue has a suitable room with the required audiovisual equipment, is easily accessible and can accommodate people with disabilities. People with persisting wounds, who are unable to drive, are wheelchair dependent or who live alone may require special transport arrangements to be made, and this will affect participation and attendance and, hence, choice of venue. Those with diabetes-related or other medical problems may be already committed to multiple hospital attendances and may be unwilling to attend. Flexible arrangements will be needed to accommodate those who are working.

Individual education

Individual education has some advantages. The session speed and content can be tailored to suit the person's needs and abilities, and information about foot care can be specific to what is known about his/her particular problem. There may be greater scope to employ motivational or cognitive behavioural techniques. Individual sessions also provide an opportunity for goal setting and review, and so may be used to target those who have difficulty in embracing behaviour change for whatever reason. Individual education may also be more suited to people with impaired mobility and who are less able to travel with ease, since it will be associated with more options for where the education might take place. Superficially, individual education may appear more time consuming and expensive, but this is justified if it is shown that the benefit is greater.[51]

Timing and Intensity

Optimal timing of foot care education is not known, and nor is its ideal intensity – the number and duration of separate sessions. In the absence of specific information, the format adopted will vary with the group or individual being educated, and the availability of educational resources.

People's response to education diminishes over time,[6,9] and this means that whatever the content and the mode of delivery, the process should involve systematic repetition and reinforcement.

EDUCATING THE EDUCATORS

It would be wrong to assume that any health care professional (such as podiatrist, nurse or doctor) has the skills necessary to deliver effective patient education simply by virtue of his/her title and knowledge. The delivery of diabetes education requires specialist skills and training.[31] This is recognised in the United States, for example, by the Registered Diabetes Educator qualification that is held by a wide range of health professionals. Health care professionals may, therefore, require additional training in psychological skills (e.g. active listening), teaching skills (e.g. theories of learning, managing groups), psychosocial skills (interactions between diabetes and the social environment), team building and organisation of care (multidisciplinary team work) and in evaluating behaviour and the impact of treatment. Training staff in new or specialist skills also means that they may need support to apply what they have learned, by freeing up time and releasing them from some of their existing duties.[52] The need for such special training may, however, limit the extent to which effective education can be implemented in clinical practice.

ASPECTS OF TRIAL DESIGN IN EVALUATING FOOT CARE EDCUATION

One main reason for the lack of evidence concerning the effectiveness of education is the problem posed by trial design in this field.

Choice of Intervention

The criticism which can be levelled at any study that fails to show a positive effect is that the choice, or delivery, of the intervention was at fault. There is no answer to this, other than to say that the value of any programme lies in the extent to which it can be extrapolated to larger populations. Although education is best delivered by those with special training, skills and resources, the focus of research in the foreseeable future should be on the evaluation of interventions that are simple and capable of being implemented on a large scale.

Consideration should, however, be given to whether or not education should be studied in isolation or as part of an integrated package of improved care. There is good evidence that its incorporation as part of a package of care is associated with improved clinical outcomes in populations that are socially disadvantaged or that otherwise have access to limited medical surveillance. There may be a better case for studying education in isolation in communities that already have equitable access to good primary health care services.

Outcome Measures

The aim is to demonstrate that education induces behaviour change and that behaviour change induces an improved clinical outcome. The demonstration of the effect of an intervention on behaviour change is easier to achieve (although relevant disease-specific and validated measures of behaviour do not currently exist) and would mean more in terms of likely clinical benefit than the demonstration of increased knowledge. However, the induction of behaviour change is itself of no value unless it is proved that it improves clinical well-being. There are two main clinically relevant end points: reduction in ulcer incidence and improved outcome of ulcers (or other foot problems) that arise. Measures of patient well-being, emotion, function and satisfaction are appropriate secondary end points, as are measures of cost.

Sample Size

Ragnarson Tennvall and Apelqvist[53] have calculated that if any intervention is to be cost-effective, it should reduce incidence by at least 25%. The number of people needed for study is determined by the outcome measure chosen. The size of the population is also determined by the level of risk and the size of the hoped-for benefit. Studies of specific behaviour change can be relatively small, whereas studies with outcomes of direct clinical relevance have to be very much larger. Since the incidence of new ulceration is only of the order of 2% per year (even when the younger population is excluded), the size of studies that use either ulcer incidence or ulcer outcome as their primary end point may require such large populations that they are either logistically impossible or prohibitively expensive – even when very simple interventions are used. Any study designed to assess the effect of education in ulcer prevention would require something of an order of 10 000 relatively older subjects in order to have 200 incident events in 1 year. However, the incidence of new ulcers is higher in those who are known to be at increased risk (e.g. those with neuropathy) and the study size in this group would be commensurately (approximately three times) smaller. The highest incidence is observed in those who have had ulcers that have only recently healed, and if this population was chosen for study, the population needed may be only of the order of 200.

CONCLUSION

There needs to be a systematic approach to foot care education that ensures that appropriate foot care advice and information is available to all people with diabetes. Those identified as being at increased risk of developing ulcers should receive education designed to change behaviour with the result that there is reduced ulcer incidence and improved ulcer outcome. The programme adopted should address the needs of the individuals being targeted, and those delivering it require special training. None of this can, however, be properly implemented until further research has been undertaken. This research is needed to define with greater precision the extent to which any educational strategy is accompanied by behaviour change, the extent to which this change in behaviour achieves the desired clinical effect and whether the magnitude of the benefit would justify the cost of implementation.

REFERENCES

1. Litzelman DK, Slemenda CW, Langeveld CD, *et al.* Reduction of lower extremity clinical abnormalities in patients with non-insulin-dependent diabetes mellitus. *Ann Intern Med* 1993;119:36–41.

2. McCabe CJ, Stevenson RC, Dolan AM. Evaluation of a diabetic foot screening and protection programme. *Diabet Med* 1998;15:80–84.
3. Rettig BA, Shrauger DG, Recker RR, Gallagher TF, Wiltse H. A randomized study of the effects of a home diabetes education program. *Diabetes Care* 1986;9:173–178.
4. Bloomgarden ZT, Karmally W, Metzger MJ, *et al.* Randomized, controlled trial of diabetic patient education: improved knowledge without improved metabolic status. *Diabetes Care* 1987;10:263–272.
5. Ronnemaa T, Hamalainen H, Toikka T, Liukonen I. Evaluation of the impact of podiatrist care in the primary prevention of foot problems in diabetic subjects. *Diabetes Care* 1997;20:1833–1837.
6. Hamalainen H, Ronnemaa T, Toikka T, Liukkonen I. Long-term effects of one year of intensified podiatric activities on foot-care knowledge and self-care habits in patients with diabetes. *Diabetes Educ* 1998;24:734–740.
7. Corbett CF. A randomized pilot study of improving foot care in home health patients with diabetes. *Diabetes Educ* 2003;29:273–282.
8. Mazzuca KB, Farris NA, Mendenhall J, Stoupa RA. Demonstrating the added value of community health nursing for clients with insulin-dependent diabetes. *J Community Health Nurs* 1997;14:211–224.
9. Barth R, Campbell LV, Allen S, Jupp JJ, Chisholm DJ. Intensive education improves knowledge, compliance and foot problems in type 2 diabetes. *Diabet Med* 1991;8:111–117.
10. Kruger S, Guthrie D. Foot care: knowledge retention and self-care practices. *Diabetes Educ* 1992;18:487–490.
11. Pieber TR, Hollwe A, Siebenhofer A, *et al.* Evaluation of a structured teaching and treatment programme for type 2 diabetes in general practice in a rural area of Austria. *Diabet Med* 1995;12:349–354.
12. Malone JM, Snyder M, Anderson G, Bernhard VM, Holloway GA, Bunt TJ. Prevention of amputation by diabetic education. *Am J Surg* 1989;158:520–524.
13. Viswanathan V, Mhahavan A, Rajasekar S, Chamukuttan S, Ambady R. Amputation prevention in South India: positive impact of foot care education. *Diabetes Care* 2005;28:1019–1021.
14. Griffiths GD, Wieman TJ. Meticulous attention to foot care improves the prognosis in diabetic ulceration of the foot. *Surg Gynecol Obstet* 1992;174:49–51.
15. Valk GD, Kriegsman DM, Assendelft WJ. Patient education for preventing diabetic foot ulceration (Cochrane Review). In: *The Cochrane Library*. Issue 2. Oxford: Update Software; 2005.
16. Wade D. Research into the black box of rehabilitation: the risks of a Type III error. *Clin Rehabil* 2001;15:1–4.
17. Singh N, Armstrong DG, Lipsky BA. Preventing foot ulcers in patients with diabetes. *JAMA* 2005;293:217–228.
18. Connelly J, Airey M, Chell S. Variation in clinical decision making is a partial explanation for geographical variation in lower extremity amputation rates. *Br J Surg* 2001;88:1265–1266.
19. Del Aguila MA, Reiber GE, Koepsell TD. How does provider and patient awareness of high-risk status for lower-extremity amputation influence foot-care practice? *Diabetes Care* 1994;17:1050–1054.
20. Lawrence SM, Wraight PR, Campbell DA, Colman PG. Assessment and management of inpatients with acute diabetes-related foot complications: room for improvement. *Intern Med J* 2004;34:229–233.
21. Fletcher EM, Macfarlane R, Jeffcoate WJ. Can foot ulcers be prevented by education? *Diabet Med* 1992;9:S41–S42.
22. Bruckner M, Mangan M, Godin S, Pogach L. Project LEAP of New Jersey: lower extremity amputation prevention in persons with type 2 diabetes. *Am J Manag Care* 1999;5:609–616.
23. O'Brien KE, Chandramohan V, Nelson DA, Fischer JR, Stevens G, Poremba JA. Effect of a physician-directed educational campaign on performance of proper diabetic foot exams in an outpatient setting. *J Gen Intern Med* 2003;18:258–265.

24. Cohen SJ. Potential barriers to diabetes care. *Diabetes Care* 1983;6:499–500.
25. Rith-Najarian S, Branchaud C, Beaulieu O, Gohdes D, Simonson G, Mazze R. Reducing lower-extremity amputations due to diabetes. Application of the staged diabetes management approach in a primary care setting. *J Fam Pract* 1998;47:127–132.
26. Plank J, Haas W, Rakovac I, *et al*. Evaluation of the impact of chiropodist care in the secondary prevention of foot ulcerations in diabetic subjects. *Diabetes Care* 2003;26:1691–1695.
27. Chaturvedi N, Abbott CA, Whalley A, Widdows P, Leggetter SY, Boulton AJ. Risk of diabetes-related amputation in South Asians vs Europeans in the UK. *Diabet Med* 2002;19:99–104.
28. Mayfield JA, Reiber GE, Nelson RG, Greene T. Do foot examinations reduce the risk of diabetic amputation? *J Fam Pract* 2000;49:499–504.
29. Abbott CA, Carrington AL, Ashe H, *et al.*, and the North-West Diabetes Foot Care Study. The North-West Diabetes Foot Care Study: incidence of, and risk factors for, new diabetic foot ulceration in a community-based patient cohort. *Diabet Med* 2002;19:377–384.
30. Abbott CA, Vileikyte L, Williamson S, Carrington AL, Boulton AJ. Multicenter study of the incidence of and predictive risk factors for diabetic neuropathic foot ulceration. *Diabetes Care* 1998;21:1071–1075.
31. Assal JP, Mühlhauser I, Pernet A, Gfeller R, Jörgens V, Berger M. Patient education as the basis for diabetes care in clinical practice and research. *Diabetologia* 1985;28:602–613.
32. Meyer D, Leventhal H, Gutmann M. Common-sense models of illness: the example of hypertension. *Health Psychol* 1985;4:115–135.
33. Vileikyte L. Diabetic foot ulcers: a quality of life issue. *Diabetes Metab Res Rev* 2001;17:246–249.
34. Vileikyte L. Psychological aspects of diabetic peripheral neuropathy. *Diabetes Rev* 1999;7:387–394.
35. Gavard JA, Lustman PJ, Clouse RE. Prevalence of depression in adults with diabetes: an epidemiological evaluation. *Diabetes Care* 1993;16:1167–1178.
36. Anderson RJ, Freedland KE, Clouse RE, Lustman PJ. The prevalence of comorbid depression in adults with diabetes: a meta-analysis. *Diabetes Care* 2001;24:1069–1078.
37. Lustman PJ, Anderson R, Freedland K, De Groot M, Carney R, Clouse R. Depression and poor glycemic control: a meta-analytic review of the literature. *Diabetes Care* 2000;23:934–942.
38. Vileikyte L, Rubin RR, Leventhal H. Psychological aspects of diabetic neuropathic foot complications: an overview. *Diabetes Metab Res Rev* 2004;20:S13–S18.
39. Park H, Hong Y, Lee H, Ha E, Sung Y. Individuals with type 2 diabetes and depressive symptoms exhibited lower adherence to self-care. *J Clin Epidemiol* 2004;57:978–984.
40. Lustman PJ, Griffith L, Freedland K, Kissel S, Clouse R. Cognitive behaviour therapy for depression in type 2 diabetes: a randomised controlled trial. *Ann Intern Med* 1998;129:613–621.
41. Lustman PJ, Freedland K, Griffith L, Clouse R. Effects of fluoxetine on depression and glycemic control in diabetes: a double-blind, placebo-controlled trial (abstract). *Ann Behav Med* 1999;21:S158.
42. Prochaska JO, DiClemente CC. Stages of change in the modification of problem behaviors. *Prog Behav Modif* 1992;28:183–218.
43. Marshall SJ, Biddle SJ. The transtheoretical model of behavior change: a meta-analysis of applications to physical activity and exercise. *Ann Behav Med* 2001;23:229–246.
44. Littell JH, Girvin H. Stages of change. A critique. *Behav Modif* 2002;26:223–273.
45. Miller WR, Rollnick S. *Motivational Interviewing: Preparing People for Change*. New York: Guilford Press; 2002.
46. Riemsma R, Kirwan J, Taal E, Rasker JJ. Patient education for adults with rheumatoid arthritis. *Cochrane Database Syst Rev* 2002;3:CD003688.
47. Riemsma R, Kirwan J, Taal E, Rasker JJ. Patient education programmes for adults with rheumatoid arthritis. *BMJ* 2002;325:558–559.
48. Ferguson E, Bibby PA, Leaviss J, Weyman A. *Effective Design of Workplace Risk Communications*. Norwich, UK: Health and Safety Executive; 2003.
49. Singer H, Donlan D. *Reading and Learning from Text*. 2nd edn. Hilldale, NJ: Lawrence Erlbaum Associates; 1989.

50. Taylor WL. 'Cloze procedure': A new tool for measuring readability. *JQ* 1953;30:415–433.
51. Rickheim PL, Weaver TW, Flader JL, Kendall DM. Assessment of group versus individual diabetes education: a randomized study. *Diabetes Care* 2002;25:269–274.
52. Doherty Y, Hall D, James PT, Roberts SH, Simpson J. Change counselling in diabetes: the development of a training programme for the diabetes team. *Patient Educ Couns* 2000;40:263–278.
53. Ragnarson Tennvall G, Apelqvist J. Prevention of diabetes-related foot ulcers and amputations: a cost-utility analysis based on Markov model simulations. *Diabetologia* 2001;44:2077–2087.

13 Infection of the Foot in Persons with Diabetes: Epidemiology, Pathophysiology, Microbiology, Clinical Presentation and Approach to Therapy

Benjamin A. Lipsky and Anthony R. Berendt

Foot infections occur frequently in persons with diabetes, and the occurrence of infection is an event that most often leads to more serious sequelae, particularly hospitalisation and amputation.[1] In this chapter, we will discuss the recognition and evaluation of infected foot wounds and the selection of appropriate antimicrobial therapies.

BACKGROUND

Epidemiology

A retrospective computer search survey in a US Veterans Affairs medical centre found that the rate of lower extremity cellulitis or osteomyelitis ranged from 1.5/1000 to 4.3/1000 patient discharges between 1994 and 2000.[2] A recent prospective trial found that the annual incidence of foot infection in a closely followed cohort of diabetic persons was 36.5/1000.[3] Among these infections, 63% affected only the soft tissue, while 22% involved bone as well.[3] Diabetic patients are over ten times more likely than non-diabetics to be hospitalised for soft tissue and bone infections of the foot.[4] An infected foot ulcer precedes about 60% of lower extremity amputations in diabetic patients[5,6] and only gangrene surpasses infection as a cause of diabetic foot amputations.[7] Diabetic patients who develop a foot infection are almost 30 times more likely to require an amputation than those who do not, and bone involvement increases the amputation risk eightfold over just soft tissue infection.[3]

The Foot in Diabetes, 4th Edition. Editors Andrew J.M. Boulton, Peter R. Cavanagh and Gerry Rayman.
© 2006 John Wiley & Sons, Ltd.

Pathophysiology

Foot infections usually occur in a site of trauma or ulceration.[3,8] Thus, patients with peripheral neuropathy or foot deformity are at increased risk for infection. Once the protective epidermal envelope is disrupted, bacteria that colonise the skin can enter the dermal and subcutaneous tissues. When the invading organisms are particularly virulent, the bacterial inoculum especially large or the patient sufficiently immunocompromised (locally or systemically), infection can ensue. Factors that may increase the risk of infection in diabetic patients include their high rate of anterior nasal colonisation with *Staphylococcus aureus*[9,10] and their more frequent encounters with the health care system.

Local problems that may predispose to infection include lower extremity ischaemia, venous or lymphatic insufficiency, obesity, poor foot care practices and fungal infections of the skin or nails. Diabetes itself causes a systemically immunocompromised state in many patients.[11–13] The exact mechanisms leading to the increased infection risk are not well understood, but diabetic persons do have diminished activity of leucocytes and some aspects of cell-mediated immunity. Both systemic and local factors may account for the fact that many diabetic patients with foot infections fail to show classic signs of inflammation, mount a fever or develop leucocytosis.[14–19] When infection is not adequately addressed, it can progress to involve deeper foot structures, including tendons, joints and bone.

MICROBIOLOGY

Culture Techniques

Selecting appropriate antimicrobial therapy for a diabetic foot infection usually requires knowing the causative organisms.[20] One exception to this rule may be patients with acute cellulitis without an associated open wound; in this situation it is difficult to obtain a specimen for culture and the organisms are predictably aerobic Gram-positive cocci, especially streptococci.[21] In most other instances, the results of wound culture and sensitivity testing will help guide therapy. Unfortunately, clinicians often fail to obtain wound cultures, including in half the cases of infections severe enough to warrant hospitalisation.[22] Before obtaining a specimen for culture, one must cleanse and debride the wound of any superficial necrotic or foreign material. Most clinicians obtain cultures by rolling a swab over the wound. While the results of some studies suggest these types of specimens give results similar to those of deep tissue biopsies,[23] most investigations have found swabs to be less sensitive and specific,[24–27] especially for deep (e.g. bone) infections.[28,29] Obtaining a specimen for culture from an open wound by tissue curettage (usually with a scalpel) is more accurate than by swabbing. Aspiration with a needle and syringe may be useful for obtaining specimens of purulent secretions or for cellulitis. Blood cultures are indicated in systemically ill patients; bacteraemia is infrequent, but the most commonly isolated pathogen is *S. aureus*, or occasionally *Bacteroides* spp.[30] For patients with osteomyelitis, bone is the optimal specimen for culture (Chapter 14).

Fungi

While bacteria cause most infections, diabetic patients appear to have a higher rate of fungal infections of the foot than do non-diabetics.[31–33] These include both skin infections (tinea or dermatophytosis) and nail infections (onychomycosis). In one recent study of adult type 1 diabetic patients, over 80% had evidence of fungal foot infection.[34] Problems directly related to these fungal diseases are occasionally sufficient to warrant treatment, but more importantly they serve to disrupt the skin envelope and thereby increase the risk of bacterial infections. Thus, patients should be taught proper foot hygiene in order to minimise the likelihood of these infections, and they may need antifungal therapy if they develop dermatophytosis.

Bacteria

Because most diabetic foot infections are caused by skin flora, it is not surprising that aerobic Gram-positive cocci are the most common aetiological agents.[35-41] *S. aureus* is the most important pathogen, followed by coagulase-negative staphylococci and streptococci (especially group B and other non-group-A species).[42] This is particularly true for patients presenting with acute infections, especially those who have not recently received antibiotic therapy. Chronic infections, or those that have failed to respond to antibiotic therapy, often have aerobic Gram-negative rods as well as the Gram-positives.[43] With optimal microbiological techniques, most of these infections are noted to be polymicrobial, with three to five isolates per specimen. Cultures from a substantial minority of infections, especially those accompanied by necrosis or gangrene, yield obligate anaerobes. These are almost always found in a mixed infection with aerobes, and the clinical importance of these isolates is unclear.[44] Some organisms, e.g. enterococci and *Pseudomonas aeruginosa*, are often colonisers rather than pathogens, and antimicrobial therapy specifically targeted against them may not be required.[45] On the other hand, organisms often considered non-pathogens, e.g. corynebacteria and coagulase-negative staphylococci, can cause infections in the diabetic foot.[46]

CLINICAL PRESENTATION

Only about half the patients who present with a foot ulcer have clinical signs of infection.[3] Infection is generally defined clinically by the presence of purulent secretions or at least two of the classic signs of inflammation (redness, warmth, swelling or induration, tenderness or pain).[47,48] These findings can, however, be both obscured and mimicked by the consequences of peripheral neuropathy, lower extremity ischaemia, immunological dysfunction or metabolic perturbations.[49] Thus, some advocate considering other findings in diagnosing infection, such as wound malodour, poor granulation tissue or delayed healing response.[17,50] Some evidence suggests that wounds progress from uninfected to infected along a continuum, with an increasing 'bacterial bioburden' leading to 'critical colonisation' (often defined as the presence of at least 100 000 bacteria per gram of tissue) and ultimately overt infection.[51] The new onset of foot pain or tenderness, particularly in a patient who has previously had neuropathy-induced loss of sensation, should suggest the possibility of infection. Similarly, clinicians should consider a foot infection in any diabetic patient presenting with fever, leucocytosis or sudden worsening of glycaemic control.

Why is the definition of infection important? Because most authorities advocate providing antibiotic therapy only to patients with infected wounds.[47,52] If uninfected wounds do not require antibiotic therapy, there is usually no reason to culture them, unless the clinician is looking for an epidemiologically significant organism (e.g. methicillin-resistant *S. aureus* (MRSA)). Unfortunately, there are few studies upon which to base this judgment,[53] and some preliminary data support better outcomes when clinically uninfected wounds are treated with antibiotics.[17] Since all antibiotics may cause adverse effects, cost money and have the potential for driving antibiotic resistance, it is best to withhold therapy in uninfected wounds.

THERAPY OF DIABETIC FOOT INFECTIONS

General Approach

When a patient presents with a foot wound, the clinician should embark on a systematic evaluation to determine whether or not it is infected and, if infected, how severely. This starts with an overview of the patient, checking vital signs and mental status, and then examining the limb and finally the foot, to determine whether there is neuropathy or ischaemia. The wound should be probed to determine its depth and to look for any foreign material. Most patients should have a plain X-ray of the foot to look for evidence of gas, a foreign body or osteomyelitis. Further diagnostic tests, e.g. nuclear medicine or particularly magnetic resonance imaging,[54] may be needed in some cases. Blood tests are useful for a patient with a moderate or severe infection; these would include a complete blood count, basic chemistries and possibly an erythrocyte sedimentation rate or C-reactive protein level.[19,55]

These investigations contribute to helping the clinician classify the infection as mild, moderate or severe (see Table 13.1). Some refer to more severe infections as being

Table 13.1 Clinical classification of a diabetic foot infection

Clinical manifestations of infection	Infection severity	PEDIS grade[a]
Wound lacking purulence or any manifestations of inflammation	Uninfected	1
Presence of ≥2 manifestations of inflammation (purulence, or erythema, pain, tenderness, warmth or induration), but any cellulitis/erythema extending ≤2 cm around the ulcer, and infection limited to the skin or superficial subcutaneous tissues; no other local complications or systemic illness	Mild	2
Infection (as above) in a patient who is systemically well and metabolically stable but which has ≥1 of the following characteristics: cellulitis extending >2 cm, lymphangitic streaking, spread beneath the superficial fascia, deep tissue abscess, gangrene and involvement of muscle, tendon, joint or bone	Moderate	3
Infection in a patient with systemic toxicity or metabolic instability (e.g. fever, chills, tachycardia, hypotension, confusion, vomiting, leucocytosis, acidosis, severe hyperglycaemia or azotaemia)	Severe	4

Note: Foot ischaemia may increase the severity of any infection, and the presence of critical ischaemia often makes the infection severe. PEDIS perfusion, extent/size, depth/tissue loss, infection, sensation.
[a]International Consensus on the Diabetic Foot.

'limb-threatening',[56] but this term could aptly be applied to almost all foot infections in a diabetic patient. Classifying by severity helps to decide which patients may need to be hospitalised or be treated with parenteral and broad-spectrum antibiotic therapy. Hospitalisation is the most costly aspect of caring for a patient with a diabetic foot infection; potential indications include severe infections, need for diagnostic tests or surgical interventions that are not available on an ambulatory basis and psychosocial issues that preclude the patient receiving proper care as an outpatient. Types of diabetic foot infection include the following: paronychia (nail-bed infection); cellulitis; infected ulcer; deep soft tissue infection (ranging from a mild subcutaneous extension to necrotising fasciitis), septic arthritis and osteomyelitis. Infections can be quite indolent, persisting for days or weeks, or can progress surprisingly rapidly, often in a matter of hours. Most diabetic foot infections require some surgical intervention, if only a bedside debridement or incision and drainage.[57] For deep tissue infections it is crucial to involve a clinician with surgical training to determine whether or not the patient needs an operative procedure.[58–64] In most cases, it is better to move ahead with any needed surgical debridement quickly, rather than to delay it to provide prolonged antibiotic therapy.

Antibiotic Therapy

Virtually all diabetic foot infections require antimicrobial therapy, but it is important to remember that while this is a *necessary* step, it is rarely *sufficient*.[65] Several factors help the clinician determine which agent to select.[66] The first is the likely microbiology of the wound; when known, the choice is relatively easy. In most cases, however, the initial therapy is empiric, as culture results are not yet available. For severe infections it is best to cover most possible pathogens, as the consequences of failing to treat adequately may be dire. With mild, and many moderate, infections, it is often reasonable to use relatively narrow-spectrum therapy. Factors such as recent antimicrobial therapy, exposure to health care settings and local antibiotic susceptibility patterns may help guide the choice of agents.

The second issue to consider is the route of therapy. For severe infections, parenteral therapy is usually preferable, but for many moderate and most mild infections, this is unnecessary. The availability of highly bioavailable antibiotic agents, e.g. fluoroquinolones and oxazolidinones, makes selecting the oral route of therapy more often appropriate.[67,68] In some cases, it is wise to start with parenteral therapy and then switch to oral in a few days, when culture results have returned and the patient is clinically improving. For mildly infected ulcers, topical antimicrobial therapy is another option, although this approach has been less well studied. The third issue to consider is the duration of antibiotic therapy. Most mild infections require only a week or two of treatment, while more severe infections may require up to 3–4 weeks. Bear in mind that antibiotics are being used for treating the infection, not healing the wound, which is likely to take considerably longer. The therapy of osteomyelitis will be discussed in Chapter 14.

The final consideration is the selection of a specific agent or combination. There have been many published studies of antibiotic therapy of diabetic foot infection.[47] Many are retrospective case series, but several are well-designed randomised trials. The studied agents have all been found to be reasonably effective, and no single agent or combination has emerged as the treatment of choice. Selection of a regimen is thus based mostly on the principles discussed above, as well as on any patient-specific conditions (e.g. renal dysfunction, allergies), formulary restrictions, convenience and cost considerations. A general approach is outlined in Table 13.2.

Table 13.2   Suggested empirical antibiotic regimens, based on clinical severity, for diabetic foot infections

Route and agent(s)	Mild	Moderate	Severe
Advised route	Oral for most	Oral or parenteral, based on clinical situation and agent(s) selected	Intravenous, at least initially
Dicloxacillin	Yes	—	—
Clindamycin	Yes	—	—
Cephalexin	Yes	—	—
Trimethoprim–sulfamethoxazole	Yes	Yes	—
Amoxicillin–clavulanate	Yes	Yes	—
Levofloxacin	Yes	Yes	—
Cefoxitin	—	Yes	—
Ceftriaxone	—	Yes	—
Ampicillin–sulbactam	—	Yes	—
Linezolid[a] (with or without aztreonam)	—	Yes	—
Daptomycin[a] (with or without aztreonam)	—	Yes	—
Ertapenem	—	Yes	—
Cefuroxime with or without metronidazole	—	Yes	—
Ticarcillin/clavulanate	—	Yes	—
Piperacillin/tazobactam	—	Yes	Yes
Levofloxacin or ciprofloxacin with clindamycin	—	Yes	Yes
Imipenem–cilastatin	—	—	Yes
Vancomycin[a] and ceftazidime (with or without metronidazole)	—	—	Yes

Note: Definitive regimens should consider results of culture and susceptibility tests, as well as the clinical response to the empirical regimen. Similar agents of the same drug class may be substituted. Some of these regimens may not have US Food and Drug Administration approval for complicated skin and skin structure infections, and only linezolid Ertapenem and Piperacillin/tazobactam are currently specifically approved for diabetic foot infections.
[a]For patients in whom methicillin-resistant *Staphylococcus aureus* infection is proven or likely.

Adjunctive Treatments

An optimal outcome when treating a diabetic foot infection requires attention to principles of good wound care, i.e. adequate (and often repeated) debridement, incision and drainage and offloading of pressure from the infected site; these are discussed in detail elsewhere in this book.(Chapters 6, 25 and 30). Many types of non-antimicrobial treatments have been advocated for diabetic foot infections. Only two have been the subject of sufficient investigation to merit comment.

Granulocyte-colony-stimulating factors (G-CSFs) have been used as adjunctive therapy in five studies of patients with diabetic foot infections. A recent meta-analysis of these studies[69] found that G-CSF preparations did not appear to hasten the resolution of diabetic foot infection or ulceration but were associated with a reduced rate of amputation and other surgical procedures. The small number of patients who needed to be treated (4.5–8.6 NNT) to gain these benefits suggests that using G-CSF should be considered, especially in patients with limb-threatening infections.

Hyperbaric oxygen (HBO) therapy has also been used in many studies of infected foot wounds. While most of the studies are anecdotal or retrospective case series, several randomised controlled trials have been published. The overall quality of the studies is poor but the results suggest that HBO may be beneficial as an adjunctive therapy for chronic non-healing diabetic wounds.[70] Based on the results of four trials with diabetic foot ulcers, a Cochrane review concluded that HBO significantly reduced the risk of major amputation and may improve the chance of healing at 1 year. Using HBO may be justified where the facilities and financing are available. In view of the modest number of patients, methodological shortcomings and poor reporting, however, the result should be interpreted cautiously.[71]

REFERENCES

1. Reiber GE, Vileikyte L, Boyko EJ, *et al.* Causal pathways for incident lower-extremity ulcers in patients with diabetes from two settings. *Diabetes Care* 1999;22:157–162.
2. Schwartzman WA. Identifying practice changes in diabetic lower limb infections by automated data retrieval in large VA system. In: *Abstracts of the 41st Annual Meeting of IDSA*. San Diego, CA: Infectious Dieseases Society of America; 2003.
3. Lavery LA, Armstrong DG, Wunderlich RP, Tredwell J, Boulton AJ. Diabetic foot syndrome: evaluating the prevalence and incidence of foot pathology in Mexican Americans and non-Hispanic whites from a diabetes disease management cohort. *Diabetes Care* 2003;26:1435–1438.
4. Boyko EJ, Lipsky BA. Infection and diabetes mellitus. In: Harris MI, ed. *Diabetes in America.* Bethesda, MD: National Institutes of Health; 1995:485–496.
5. Pecoraro RE, Reiber GE, Burgess EM. Pathways to diabetic limb amputation. Basis for prevention. *Diabetes Care* 1990;13:513–521.
6. Reiber GE, Pecoraro RE, Koepsell TD. Risk factors for amputation in patients with diabetes mellitus. A case–control study. *Ann Intern Med* 1992;117:97–105.
7. Fylling CP, Knighton DR. Amputation in the diabetic population: incidence, causes, cost, treatment, and prevention. *J Enterostomal Ther* 1989;16:247–255.
8. Peters EJ, Lavery LA, Armstrong DG. Diabetic lower extremity infection: influence of physical, psychological, and social factors. *J Diabetes Complications* 2005;19:107–112.
9. Lipsky BA, Peugeot RL, Boyko EJ, Kent DL. A prospective study of *Staphylococcus aureus* nasal colonization and intravenous therapy-related phlebitis. *Arch Intern Med* 1992;152:2109–2112.
10. Boyko EJ, Lipsky BA, Sandoval R, *et al.* NIDDM and prevalence of nasal *Staphylococcus aureus* colonization. San Luis Valley Diabetes Study. *Diabetes Care* 1989;12:189–192.
11. Joshi N, Caputo G, Weitekamp M, Karchmer A. Infections in patients with diabetes mellitus. *N Engl J Med* 1999;341:1906–1912.
12. Geerlings SE, Hoepelman AIM. Immune dysfunction in patients with diabetes mellitus (DM). *FEMS Immunol Med Microbiol* 1999;26:259–265.
13. Rajagopalan S. Serious infections in elderly patients with diabetes mellitus. *Clin Infect Dis* 2005;40:990–996.

14. Armstrong DG, Lavery LA, Sariaya M, Ashry H. Leukocytosis is a poor indicator of acute osteomyelitis of the foot in diabetes mellitus. *J Foot Ankle Surg* 1996;35:280–283.
15. Armstrong DG, Perales TA, Murff RT, Edelson GW, Welchon JG. Value of white blood cell count with differential in the acute diabetic foot infection. *J Am Podiatr Med Assoc* 1996;86:224–227.
16. Edmonds ME. The diabetic foot, 2003. *Diabetes Metab Res Rev* 2004;20:S9–S12.
17. Edmonds M, Foster A. The use of antibiotics in the diabetic foot. *Am J Surg* 2004;187:25S–28S.
18. Eneroth M, Apelqvist J, Stenstrom A. Clinical characteristics and outcome in 223 diabetic patients with deep foot infections. *Foot Ankle Int* 1997;18:716–722.
19. Eneroth M, Larsson J, Apelqvist J. Deep foot infections in patients with diabetes and foot ulcer: an entity with different characteristics, treatments, and prognosis. *J Diabetes Complications* 1999;13:254–263.
20. Carvalho CB, R MN, Aragao LP, Oliveira MM, Nogueira MB, Forti AC. [Diabetic foot infection: bacteriologic analysis of 141 patients.]. *Arq Bras Endocrinol Metabol* 2004;48:406–413.
21. Caputo G. The rational use of antimicrobial agents in diabetic foot infection. In: Boulton AJM, Connor H, Cavanagh PR, eds. *The Foot in Diabetes*. London: Wiley; 2000:143–151.
22. Edelson GW, Armstrong DG, Lavery LA, Caicco G. The acutely infected diabetic foot is not adequately evaluated in an inpatient setting. *J Am Podiatr Med Assoc* 1997;87:260–265.
23. Pellizzer G, Strazzabosco M, Presi S, *et al.* Deep tissue biopsy vs superficial swab culture monitoring in the microbiological assessment of limb-threatening diabetic foot infection. *Diabet Med* 2001;18:822–827.
24. Wheat LJ, Allen SD, Henry M, *et al.* Diabetic foot infections. Bacteriologic analysis. *Arch Intern Med* 1986;146:1935–1940.
25. Sapico FL, Canawati HN, Witte JL, Montgomerie JZ, Wagner FW Jr., Bessman AN. Quantitative aerobic and anaerobic bacteriology of infected diabetic feet. *J Clin Microbiol* 1980;12:413–420.
26. Sharp CS, Bessmen AN, Wagner FW Jr., Garland D, Reece E. Microbiology of superficial and deep tissues in infected diabetic gangrene. *Surg Gynecol Obstet* 1979;149:217–219.
27. Lipsky BA, Pecoraro RE, Larson SA, Hanley ME, Ahroni JH. Outpatient management of uncomplicated lower-extremity infections in diabetic patients. *Arch Intern Med* 1990;150:790–797.
28. Slater RA, Lazarovitch T, Boldur I, *et al.* Swab cultures accurately identify bacterial pathogens in diabetic foot wounds not involving bone. *Diabet Med* 2004;21:705–709.
29. Perry CR, Pearson RL, Miller GA. Accuracy of cultures of material from swabbing of the superficial aspect of the wound and needle biopsy in the preoperative assessment of osteomyelitis. *J Bone Joint Surg Am* 1991;73:745–749.
30. Sapico FL, Bessman AN, Canawati HN. Bacteremia in diabetic patients with infected lower extremities. *Diabetes Care* 1982;5:101–104.
31. Tan JS, Joseph WS. Common fungal infections of the feet in patients with diabetes mellitus. *Drugs Aging* 2004;21:101–112.
32. Chincholikar DA, Pal RB. Study of fungal and bacterial infections of the diabetic foot. *Indian J Pathol Microbiol* 2002;45:15–22.
33. Gupta AK, Humke S. The prevalence and management of onychomycosis in diabetic patients. *Eur J Dermatol* 2000;10:379–384.
34. Mayser P, Hensel J, Thoma W, *et al.* Prevalence of fungal foot infections in patients with diabetes mellitus type 1 – underestimation of moccasin-type tinea. *Exp Clin Endocrinol Diabetes* 2004;112:264–268.
35. Lipsky BA, Pecoraro RE, Wheat LJ. The diabetic foot. Soft tissue and bone infection. *Infect Dis Clin North Am* 1990;4:409–432.
36. Borrero E, Rossini M Jr. Bacteriology of 100 consecutive diabetic foot infections and in vitro susceptibility to ampicillin/sulbactam versus cefoxitin. *Angiology* 1992;43:357–361.
37. Goldstein EJ, Citron DM, Nesbit CA. Diabetic foot infections. Bacteriology and activity of 10 oral antimicrobial agents against bacteria isolated from consecutive cases. *Diabetes Care* 1996;19:638–641.

38. Jones EW, Edwards R, Finch R, Jeffcoate WJ. A microbiological study of diabetic foot lesions. *Diabet Med* 1985;2:213–215.

39. Urbancic-Rovan V, Gubina M. Bacteria in superficial diabetic foot ulcers. *Diabet Med* 2000;17:814–815.

40. Viswanathan V, Jasmine JJ, Snehalatha C, Ramaohandran A. Prevalence of pathogens in diabetic foot infection in South Indian type 2 diabetic patients. *J Assoc Physicians India* 2002;50:1013–1016.

41. Ge Y, MacDonald D, Hait H, Lipsky B, Zasloff M, Holroyd K. Microbiological profile of infected diabetic foot ulcers. *Diabet Med* 2002;19:1032–1034.

42. Reyzelman AM, Lipsky BA, Hadi SA, Harkless LB, Armstrong DG. The increased prevalence of severe necrotizing infections caused by non-group A streptococci. *J Am Podiatr Med Assoc* 1999;89:454–457.

43. Pathare NA, Bal A, Talvalkar GV, Antani DU. Diabetic foot infections: a study of microorganisms associated with the different Wagner grades. *Indian J Pathol Microbiol* 1998;41:437–441.

44. Gerding DN. Foot infections in diabetic patients: the role of anaerobes. *Clin Infect Dis* 1995;20: S283–S288.

45. Cunha BA. Antibiotic selection for diabetic foot infections: a review. *J Foot Ankle Surg* 2000;39: 253–257.

46. Bessman AN, Geiger PJ, Canawati H. Prevalence of *Corynebacteria* in diabetic foot infections. *Diabetes Care* 1992;15:1531–1533.

47. Lipsky BA, Berendt AR, Deery HG, 2nd, *et al.* IDSA Guidelines: Diagnosis and treatment of diabetic foot infections. *Clin Infect Dis* 2004;39:885–910.

48. Lipsky BA. A report from the international consensus on diagnosing and treating the infected diabetic foot. *Diabetes Metab Res Rev* 2004;20:S68–S77.

49. Williams DT, Hilton JR, Harding KG. Diagnosing foot infection in diabetes. *Clin Infect Dis* 2004;39:S83–S86.

50. Schultz GS, Sibbald RG, Falanga V, *et al.* Wound bed preparation: a systematic approach to wound management. *Wound Repair Regen* 2003;11:S1–S28.

51. Edwards R, Harding KG. Bacteria and wound healing. *Curr Opin Infect Dis* 2004;17:91–96.

52. Lipsky BA, Berendt AR, Embil J, De Lalla F. Diagnosing and treating diabetic foot infections. *Diabetes Metab Res Rev* 2004;20:S56–S64.

53. Chantelau E, Tanudjaja T, Altenhofer F, Ersanli Z, Lacigova S, Metzger C. Antibiotic treatment for uncomplicated neuropathic forefoot ulcers in diabetes: a controlled trial. *Diabet Med* 1996;13:156–159.

54. Schweitzer ME, Morrison WB. MR imaging of the diabetic foot. *Radiol Clin North Am* 2004;42: 61–71, vi.

55. Kaleta JL, Fleischli JW, Reilly CH. The diagnosis of osteomyelitis in diabetes using erythrocyte sedimentation rate: a pilot study. *J Am Podiatr Med Assoc* 2001;91:445–450.

56. Grayson ML, Gibbons GW, Habershaw GM, *et al.* Use of ampicillin/sulbactam versus imipenem/cilastatin in the treatment of limb-threatening foot infections in diabetic patients. *Clin Infect Dis* 1994;18:683–693.

57. Rauwerda JA. Foot debridement: anatomic knowledge is mandatory. *Diabetes Metab Res Rev* 2000;16:S23–S26.

58. Scher KS, Steele FJ. The septic foot in patients with diabetes. *Surgery* 1988;104:661–666.

59. Bose K. A surgical approach for the infected diabetic foot. *Int Orthop* 1979;3:177–181.

60. Gould JS, Erickson SJ, Collier BD, Bernstein BM. Surgical management of ulcers, soft-tissue infections, and osteomyelitis in the diabetic foot. *Instr Course Lect* 1993;42:147–158.

61. Steffen C, O'Rourke S. Surgical management of diabetic foot complications: the Far North Queensland profile. *Aust N Z J Surg* 1998;68:258–260.

62. Tan JS, Friedman NM, Hazelton-Miller C, Flanagan JP, File TM Jr. Can aggressive treatment of diabetic foot infections reduce the need for above-ankle amputation? *Clin Infect Dis* 1996;23:286–291.

63. Chaytor ER. Surgical treatment of the diabetic foot. *Diabetes Metab Res Rev* 2000;16:S66–S69.
64. van Baal JG. Surgical treatment of the infected diabetic foot. *Clin Infect Dis* 2004;39:S123–S128.
65. Lipsky BA. Evidence-based antibiotic therapy of diabetic foot infections. *FEMS Immunol Med Microbiol* 1999;26:267–276.
66. Grayson ML. Diabetic foot infections. Antimicrobial therapy. *Infect Dis Clin North Am* 1995;9: 143–161.
67. Lipsky BA, Itani K, Norden C. Treating foot infections in diabetic patients: a randomized, multicenter, open-label trial of linezolid versus ampicillin–sulbactam/amoxicillin–clavulanate. *Clin Infect Dis* 2004;38:17–24.
68. Lobmann R, Ambrosch A, Seewald M, *et al.* Antibiotic therapy for diabetic foot infections: comparison of cephalosporines with chinolones. *Diabetes Nutr Metab* 2004;17:156–162.
69. Cruciani M, Lipsky BA, Mengoli C, de Lalla F. Are granulocyte colony-stimulating factors beneficial in treating diabetic foot infections?: a meta-analysis. *Diabetes Care* 2005;28:454–460.
70. Wang C, Schwaitzberg S, Berliner E, Zarin DA, Lau J. Hyperbaric oxygen for treating wounds: a systematic review of the literature. *Arch Surg* 2003. 138:272–279, discussion 280.
71. Kranke P, Bennett M, Roeckl-Wiedmann I, Debus S. Hyperbaric oxygen therapy for chronic wounds. *Cochrane Database Syst Rev* 2004:CD004123.

14 Challenges in the Infected Diabetic Foot: Osteomyelitis and Methicillin-Resistant *Staphylococcus aureus*

Anthony R. Berendt and Benjamin A. Lipsky

OSTEOMYELITIS INTRODUCTION

The preceding chapter provided a systematic framework for the evaluation and treatment of soft tissue infections of the diabetic foot. There is a range of outcomes for an acute soft tissue infection. A common and important complication, which most often arises if ulceration leads to prolonged soft tissue loss and unresolved local infection, is contiguous focus osteomyelitis of the underlying bone.[1] Although bone can be infected haematogenously, osteomyelitis in the diabetic foot is overwhelmingly caused by destruction of soft tissue overlying bone or joint.[2] This disrupts the periosteum and/or the joint capsule, and permits access of pathogenic bacteria to the surface of the bone or to the joint cavity. *Staphylococcus aureus* has a particular predilection for bone and joint, possessing numerous cell-wall-anchored receptors that mediate adherence to the extracellular matrix components of these tissues.[3,4] Adhesion is followed by proliferation and the production of density-dependent chemical regulators, through the phenomenon of quorum sensing. This leads to the orchestrated production of numerous tissue-damaging exocellular toxins.

Infection triggers an acute inflammatory response that usually includes the production of pus.[5] In the rigid mechanical environment within bone, acute inflammation may simultaneously control infection, to the benefit of the host, while harmfully compromising blood supply through excessive intra-osseous pressures and the effects of procoagulant cytokines. The result may be avascular necrosis of areas of bone in the infected field. These areas of dead bone (sequestra) are typical features of chronic osteomyelitis; their formation marks the transition between an acute and a chronic infection. Sequestra provide a focus for bacteria to adhere in physiological states, conferring substantial phenotypic resistance to antibiotics. This phenomenon, and the fact that dying osteoblasts are capable of releasing viable *S. aureus*, permits recurrence of infection after treatment with antibiotic regimens that would otherwise have been curative.[6] Dead bone impedes soft tissue healing, as granulation tissue forms over it only slowly, while ongoing infection leads to inflammatory wound drainage that also impairs wound closure. The result of this sequence is a chronic draining ulcer or sinus, at the base of which dead, infected bone may be visible or palpable. Sequestra may be spontaneously discharged if the inflammatory response, which triggers resorption of surrounding living bone, can separate them for subsequent fragmentation and passage down the sinus or out of the wound. If this process can contain the infection within the remaining living bone, it can lead to 'self-cure', with resolution of the infection and subsequently the ulcer. All too often, however, a rolling progression of the infection through the bone occurs, with the development of additional sinuses or sequestra distant from the original focus.

Osteomyelitis therefore poses a number of challenges to all who manage the diabetic foot. Without its successful resolution, failure of wound healing is predictable. Progressive or re-current soft tissue infection is also highly likely, placing the patient at risk for lower extremity amputation. The foot may also be threatened if enough bone destruction occurs to compromise irremediably the biomechanics of the foot. Furthermore, uncertainties remain over the optimal approach to diagnosis and treatment of osteomyelitis in the diabetic foot. Adding the increasing prevalence of multi-resistant pathogens, notably MRSA, introduces additional practical and financial complexities. We shall now consider these aspects in turn.

Diagnosis

The diagnostic process is often considered a binary one: a patient does, or does not, have the condition in question. In the case of diabetic foot osteomyelitis, there are particular difficulties in attempting to apply such a 'yes–no' process. In diagnosing osteomyelitis elsewhere in the skeleton, [5] we would focus on:

- those aspects of the history that suggest infection, notably wound drainage and pain;
- the findings of clinical examination, including bone tenderness and purulence;
- the presence of radiographic evidence of rapidly progressive and mixed destructive and reparative responses, notably bone lucency, cortical destruction, sclerosis and periosteal reaction;
- the findings on more sophisticated imaging, particularly magnetic resonance imaging (MRI), of marrow oedema, or sinus tracts;
- ultimately, as the criterion standard, the combination of culturing microorganisms and seeing histological features of infection in samples of bone obtained in circumstances that minimise the risk of false-positive or false-negative results. This means obtaining samples at surgery after thorough debridement or by percutaneous biopsy through an uninvolved field. Culture results are best if the patient has not been on antibiotics for at least a week prior to the biopsy.

In the diabetic foot, however, one or more of the following situations complicate diagnosis:[7]

- The typical symptoms of bone infection may be masked by peripheral neuropathy.
- The radiological features are confounded by the possibility of diabetic neuro-osteoarthropathy, especially in florid cases of Charcot neuroarthropathy.

- There is often no local expertise in obtaining bone samples through uninfected parts of the foot without recourse to surgery.

- Empiric antibiotic therapy has usually been started before the diagnosis has been made.

- The reality or threat of foot ischaemia or serious soft tissue loss makes the withholding or withdrawing of antibiotics unattractive to clinicians.

These circumstances have made it difficult to define rigorous criterion standards for the diagnosis of osteomyelitis in the diabetic foot.[8,9] This also makes it difficult to compare, or aggregate, the numerous studies performed to evaluate different diagnostic tests.[10] Allowing for this, however, the evidence does support the following synthesis of the diagnostic process.[11]

Clinical features

Osteomyelitis almost always arises in the context of a pre-existing neuropathic ulceration, or occasionally an acute penetrating injury.[2] Bony changes that occur in the non-ulcerated foot should raise suspicion of Charcot changes. Ulcers that overlie a bony prominence, and are of longer duration, have an increased risk of being complicated by osteomyelitis.[12] Similarly, the presence of previously undiagnosed osteomyelitis may be contributing to poor ulcer healing. Deeper ulcers are more likely to have compromised the periosteum or joint capsule. Peripheral vascular disease of the lower extremity increases the risk of osteomyelitis.[13] Ulcers that have failed to heal despite optimal offloading (e.g. total contact casting) for at least 2 months, in the presence of adequate perfusion, should arouse suspicion of underlying osteomyelitis. The discharge of bone fragments or the ability to see or palpate exposed bone virtually assures that osteomyelitis is present. The 'probe to bone' test, in which a sterile metal probe is inserted into the wound in search of gritty, palpable bone, has moderate predictive value in populations of patients with infected foot ulcers.[14] The visual appearances at surgery of purulence within bone, and dead bone, are highly suggestive of infection. Fever, leucocytosis and a left-shifted differential white blood cell count are each infrequent in diabetic foot infections,[15] even with osteomyelitis, but a highly elevated erythrocyte sedimentation rate[16] or C-reactive protein[17] suggests osteomyelitis.

Plain radiology

X-rays are of limited value except for the observation of serial changes over a period of weeks.[18–20] In acute infection, it takes up to 2 weeks for changes visible on plain film to develop; in chronic infection the changes are similar to those of Charcot neuroarthropathy.[21] Bone destruction immediately beneath an ulcer is suggestive of infection, as is rapid progression of lucency and periosteal reaction. The anatomic location of changes in the foot may be helpful; osteomyelitis is most commonly localised to an area of the forefoot underlying an ulcer, whereas Charcot changes are typically in the midfoot and produce large areas of fragmentation and destruction. In the calcaneum, both infection and osteoarthropathy can occur, sometimes simultaneously. Published sensitivities and specificities range from 23 to 93%, and 40 to 94%, respectively.

Isotope bone scans

[99]Technetium (^{99}Tc) bone scans are sensitive but non-specific, and cannot distinguish osteoarthropathy from infection, or active from recently cured infection. Indium-labelled white cell scans have been disappointing even combined with technetium bone scanning, though ^{99}Tc-labelled hexamethylpropyleneamine oxime (HMPOA) white cell scans have a high sensitivity and specificity, at least in the hands of experts.[22] The value of various new scanning techniques, including labelled immunoglobulins or anti-white cell antibodies, and positron emission tomography (PET) scans remains unproven.[23–29] Published sensitivities and specificities range from 50 to 100% and 7 to 83% respectively for ^{99}Tc bone scan, and 33 to 100% and 29 to 89% for Indium-labelled white cell scan.

MRI scanning

This has become the favoured imaging modality for the diagnosis of osteomyelitis.[30–32] It produces images of anatomic quality (Figure 14.1), showing cortical destruction, soft tissue collections and sinus tracts, that are based on physiological information (water and fat content, and thus bone marrow oedema, the hallmark of infection). MRI has high sensitivity and specificity, but requires an expert in interpretation to distinguish infection from Charcot changes.[33] The combination of the type of changes and their anatomic site is diagnostically most valuable; sensitivities and specificities range from 29 to 100% and from 40 to 100%, respectively.

Histology

The pattern of bone death accompanied by acute inflammatory and reparative responses is highly suggestive of infection, but can also be seen in acute Charcot neuroarthropathy. Thus, clinical correlation is needed when interpreting the results. It is difficult to assess sensitivity or specificity of histology, as it is usually one of the criterion standards used to assess other tests.

Culture

Although it is a criterion standard for diagnosing osteomyelitis, culture is difficult to evaluate; yet cases of strongly suspected infection may sometimes be culture negative. This may be

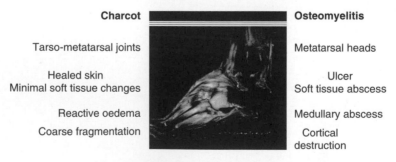

Figure 14.1   Interpretation of MRI to differentiate between Charcot neuroarthropathy and osteomyelitis. (Courtesy of Dr. E. McNally, Nuffield Orthopaedic Centre, Oxford)

explained by the small samples usually taken with non-surgical specimens and the frequent prior use of antibiotics, both of which can lead to false-negative results. In addition, using histology as the criterion standard may be misleading if cases of Charcot neruoarthropathy, in which negative cultures would be expected, are misdiagnosed as osteomyelitis. Culture has the major advantage of providing the causative organism and its antibiotic susceptibilities.[34] The results of bone cultures and simultaneously obtained soft tissue cultures often differ substantially.[35]

A Diagnostic Algorithm

The algorithm shown in Figure 14.2 recognises the difficulties in using a single test, on a single occasion, to diagnose osteomyelitis.[11] It also incorporates the controversies in the treatment of osteomyelitis, which we discuss further below.

Treatment of Osteomyelitis

Successfully treating chronic osteomyelitis has generally been thought to require the combination of surgical and antimicrobial therapy.[36-39] Increasingly, it is also recognised that specialised techniques may be needed to manage the soft tissues and avoid the slow-healing

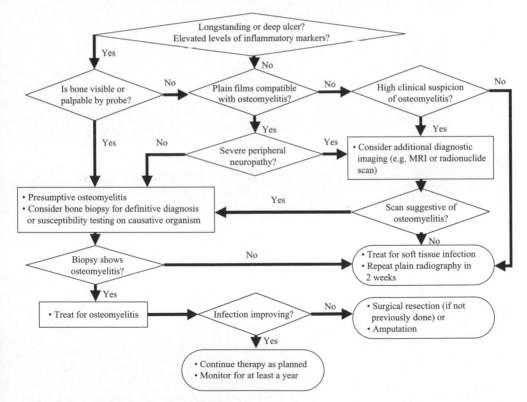

Figure 14.2 A diagnostic algorithm for osteomyelitis of the foot in a diabetic patient[11]

wounds that pose a risk of secondary infection.[40] In the diabetic foot, however, views on treatment have evolved over time to a current state of uncertainty. Initial therapeutic nihilism, coupled with a lack of reconstructive methods to overcome vascular disease, frequently led to major limb amputation as the outcome of osteomyelitis. That surgical debridement of non-ischaemic diabetic foot infection led to rapid healing encouraged a view that osteomyelitis could be expediently treated with minor amputation of digit(s), ray excision or transmetatarsal amputation.[41] In patients with osteomyelitis and ischaemia, vascular reconstruction with angioplasty or distal bypass can accompany surgery for infection.[42-45] More recently, surgeons have recognised the secondary effects of minor amputation in causing post-amputation transfer ulcerations.

Because of these and other problems associated with surgery, attention has recently been focused on prolonged antibiotic therapy alone.[46,47] 'Conservative' therapy, as this has come to be known, involves prolonged duration of antibiotics, accompanied by appropriate podiatric care of the foot. The latter includes regular wound care, debridement and pressure offloading. Some centres also remove accessible sequestra during curettage of the ulcer base.[48] In over 500 cases described from 11 centres, the success rate in arresting infection was nearly 70%.[49] Most studies lacked clear criteria for likely success or failure and did not explain how patients were selected. This approach is controversial, however, and some strongly believe that delaying surgery can be associated with inferior outcomes.[50-52] Major prospective studies are needed either to test the outcomes of standardised protocols employed across a wide range of centres, or to conduct a randomised controlled trial comparing the two strategies.

Where surgery is needed, the priority is to remove any necrotic bone or soft tissue, drain pus and to promote a healing environment for remaining tissues.[50] At the same time, the surgeon must consider the foot as a biomechanical platform. Little is gained by preserving a non-functional foot, or one at extreme risk of recurrent ulceration. A multidisciplinary (medical, surgical and ancillary services) team approach can produce excellent outcomes with chronic osteomyelitis.[53]

Duration and Route of Administration of Therapy

Historically, osteomyelitis was deemed to routinely require prolonged antibiotic therapy. Anatomically defining the infection (Figure 14.3), however, allows rational choices about the duration of therapy. Recommendations (Table 14.1) focus on the extent of residual infected bone, the viability of that bone and the presence of accompanying soft tissue infection.[11]

The advent of highly bioavailable oral antibiotics has also allowed increasing confidence in this route of therapy.[54,55] Appropriately selected oral agents have logistical, safety and financial advantages over intravenous therapy. Prolonged parenteral therapy, when needed, can safely be provided outside the hospital with an established programme.[56] No single drug, or route of administration, has proven to be superior over others in the treatment of osteomyelitis.[57] There are surprisingly few studies by which to judge the efficacy of most antibiotics and few have a specific approval for bone and joint infection. It is unclear if determining the bone penetration of an antibiotic helps to predict its efficacy for treating osteomyelitis. A range of antimicrobials have been found to be effective, provided the pathogen is sensitive to the drug used, the treatment is of sufficient duration (see above) and the drug can be delivered in doses sufficient to give high tissue levels.[58]

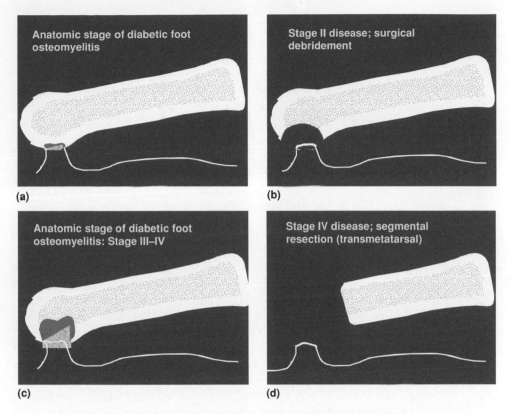

Figure 14.3 Anatomic staging of osteomyelitis of the diabetic foot

For localised lesions amenable to resection, some clinicians implant antibiotic-loaded polymethylmethacrylate (PMMA) beads, collagen fleece or calcium sulfate (plaster of Paris), all of which elute high levels of selected antibiotics.[59–62] Locally implanted antibiotics are rational only when dead bone is resected, given the limited penetration into the bone surrounding the cavity into which the antibiotic-loaded carrier is placed. These various approaches to therapy must be taken in the context of high failure rates, even with apparently appropriate therapy. The goal is not merely to arrest infection within the bone, but to preserve that

Table 14.1 Recommendations for antibiotic therapy

Residual infected bone?	Residual infected soft tissue?	Recommended duration of antibiotic therapy
None (ablative therapy, whole bone removed)	None	2–3 days
None (ablative therapy, whole bone removed)	Yes	7–14 days
Yes (viable bone only)	Yes or no	4–6 weeks
Yes (dead bone present)	Yes or no	Minimum 3 months

bone and heal the overlying ulcer. This approach should help prevent future major or minor amputations. In one survey of attitudes of infectious diseases experts to therapy of diabetic foot osteomyelitis, the Emerging Infections Network concluded that failure rates of over 30% were 'acceptable', a likely reflection of the difficulties generally experienced in managing this condition.[63]

METHICILLIN-RESISTANT *STAPHYLOCOCCUS AUREUS*

Historical Introduction

A discussion about antimicrobial resistance in the context of the diabetic foot inevitably focuses on methicillin-resistant *S. aureus* (MRSA). *S. aureus*, whether methicillin-sensitive (MSSA) or resistant, is a central pathogen in all manifestations of diabetic foot infection, including osteomyelitis,[64] and in all settings and countries.[65,66] From the early days of the antibiotic era, it became clear that certain organisms rapidly acquired resistance. Penicillin resistance was identified among *S. aureus* isolates within a few years of its widespread use (Figure 14.4). It became so prevalent that outbreaks of resistant 'hospital Staph' led to ward and, sometimes institutional, closures.

This penicillin resistance problem was resolved only with the development of methicillin and the other parenteral and oral penicillinase-resistant penicillins. These drugs remained the mainstays of anti-staphylococcal therapy until resistance (MRSA) was encountered in the 1960s. The isolation of MRSA remained sporadic for nearly two decades, and there was debate as to its virulence and clinical significance. During the 1980s, however, epidemic strains of MRSA emerged that were transmissible in the hospital environment and capable of causing severe disease. Since then, MRSA has become endemic in the health care setting in the majority of (but not all) countries worldwide.

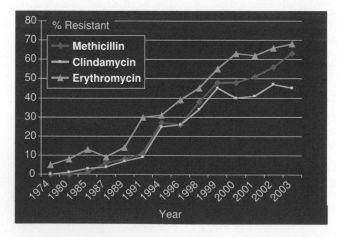

Figure 14.4 Timeline of resistance of *Staphylococcus aureus* isolates (from inpatient and outpatient settings) to three commonly used anti-staphylococcal antibiotics (methicillin, clindamycin and erythromycin) at the Veterans Affairs Puget Sound Health Care System (1974 to 2003)

The MRSA rate for a medical centre is the proportion of clinically significant *S. aureus* isolates from blood or soft tissue specimens that are MRSA. Data from many centres demonstrated rates rising from under 5% to over 50% in the 1990s (Figure 14.4).

This was accompanied by an increasing pool of individuals infected or colonised with MRSA, not only within, but also outside the hospital environment. Patients particularly at risk for MRSA colonisation and infection are nursing home residents and others (like diabetic persons) having frequent contact with health care institutions.

Mechanisms and Consequences

In *S. aureus* organisms, penicillin resistance is due to an enzyme called penicillinase, which destroys the antibiotic before it can act. The penicillinase is encoded by a small piece of genetic material borne on a highly mobile plasmid. Methicillin resistance, by contrast, is the result of a very large piece of DNA containing multiple genes involved in the expression and control of a protein known as PBP2'. To understand the significance of this, we must understand something of the mechanism of action of penicillin and related antibiotics. These agents (including cephalosporins and carbapenems) act to disrupt bacterial cell wall synthesis. Because of a common essential core structure, the β-lactam ring, these drugs are called β-lactam antibiotics. β-Lactams bind to and inhibit the proteins that build the bacterial cell wall, which are therefore known as penicillin-binding proteins (PBPs). Different classes of β-lactams have been developed to deal with the natural diversity of PBPs. PBP2' is a penicillin-binding protein that is novel to the staphylococcal genome. While related to other PBPs, it is not inhibited by any of the β-lactam antibiotics. Thus, rather than destroying the antibiotic, as in penicillin resistance mediated by penicillinase, methicillin-resistant organisms have acquired a novel pathway that bypasses the antibiotic target.

Epidemiology

The epidemiology of MRSA is in many respects the same as the epidemiology of all *S. aureus* strains.[67] Colonisation of the anterior nares is associated with secondary colonisation of the skin, including the hairline, axillae, groins and sometimes the throat. Wounds are especially prone to become colonised with *S. aureus*, and they can then become infected when the organisms proliferate and overwhelm local defences.[68]

Transmission of MRSA is mainly via person-to-person contact. When MRSA was confined to hospitals, spread was almost entirely through patient—health care worker–patient pathways. Some can occur by environmental contamination, for example by shedding of skin scales from a colonised patient with an exfoliative skin condition, such as eczema or psoriasis. Distinctive epidemiological characteristics of MRSA compared with MSSA concern risk factors for acquisition. *S. aureus* colonisation is long term in ~30% of individuals, and intermittent in another further 30–40%. Patients with frequent contact with hospitals generally have higher levels of colonisation. Unlike MSSA, MRSA colonisation has until recently been restricted to hospitalised patients, and is directly related to time in hospital and antibiotic exposure. More recently, non-hospitalised patients with major exposure to health care environments, such as nursing home residents, have been found to have high rates of MRSA carriage. Now, advances in the evolution of MRSA have led to transmission in environments unrelated to health care institutions.[69]

New Developments: Vancomycin Resistance and Community-Acquired MRSA

Vancomycin resistance

Vancomycin, a glycopeptide antibiotic, has been the major agent used for treating MRSA infections for decades. It has also been used via the oral pathway for treating *Clostridium difficile* associated diarrhoea. A closely related drug, avoparcin, has been widely used in the livestock industry as a growth promoter. Not surprisingly, vancomycin-resistant strains of enterococci have arisen and spread, apparently from the animal reservoir, to become noso-comial pathogens in the most compromised hosts. Scientists had been watching closely for the acquisition of vancomycin resistance in *S. aureus*, and had even conducted experiments to demonstrate that the genes encoding vancomycin resistance could be transferred from entero-cocci to staphylococci.[70] The first natural indication of resistance came with the identification of strains of MRSA with intermediate sensitivity to vancomycin. These glycopeptide-intermediate *S. aureus* (GISA) strains have alterations in the thickness of the cell wall providing excess quan-tities of target to which vancomycin could bind, ensuring some cell wall synthesis.[71] GISA strains have become widespread in North America, Australia and Europe.[72,73]

More recently, *in vivo* genetic transfer of enterococcal vancomycin resistance genes has occurred, as predicted by the animal experiments. Three patients, in different places, who were infected with vancomycin-resistant *S. aureus* (VRSA) have now been reported. Of note, two of these cases were diabetic patients with foot ulcers who had been treated with multiple courses of antibiotics.[74,75] This emphasises the way in which the diabetic foot can contribute to the genesis and spread of antimicrobial resistance, providing a niche for polymicrobial colonisation in the face of extensive antimicrobial pressure.

Community-acquired MRSA

This epidemiological complexity of staphylococcal infections has been further increased by the emergence of new strains of MRSA with several distinctive features. These strains have been described in community-dwelling populations, such as children, athletes involved in contact sports and incarcerated prisoners.[76–82] The strains are associated with aggressive soft tissue infection and the production of abscesses, sometimes complicated by more severe illness.[83] Although resistant to methicillin, these strains lack the co-resistance to a wide range of other antibiotics, which is a feature of the epidemic hospital strains.

Molecular analysis of these strains, designated community-acquired MRSA or CA-MRSA, shows a smaller genetic element conferring methicillin resistance in comparison with the earlier strains. This has novel features, including a strong genetic linkage to a toxin previously associated with severe soft tissue infection, the Panton–Valentin leucocidin.[84] CA-MRSA fearfully links genetic fitness, methicillin resistance and microbial virulence. It remains to be seen whether the strains will remain confined to the younger age risk groups, or diversify to involve other members of the community, including the diabetic population and diabetic foot ulcers.

Clinical Implications

There are relatively few studies specifically concerning MRSA in the diabetic foot. A number of studies have demonstrated rises in MRSA rates among *S. aureus* isolates from diabetic foot clinics, in parallel with the global epidemiological trends set out above.[85–88] Based on available data and past experience, it is likely that MRSA rates in diabetic foot clinics will at least mirror rates in leg ulcer and wound clinics, and in bloodstream isolates, for the geographic area under consideration.

Even fewer reports have specifically studied the effect of MRSA on diabetic foot outcomes, but it appears that MRSA colonisation and infection is associated with longer times to healing and worse outcomes.[89,90] Because MRSA is a marker for hosts with poorer wound status, slower healing and so a higher amputation risk, cause and effect cannot be separated in these studies. In light of data from other infections, such as bacteraemia and pneumonia, the balance of opinion is that MRSA is directly associated with worse outcomes than MSSA. We believe it is worth expending the effort to prevent MRSA from becoming resident in medical centres where it is not already common, and try to reduce the prevalence and spread where it is already a problem.

Treatment Implications

MRSA strains are resistant to all β-lactam antibiotics, meaning that alternative anti-staphylococcal agents must be used instead.[91] For intravenous therapy the mainstay of treatment is vancomycin, and outside the United States (where it remains unlicensed), teicoplanin.[92] A number of well-established, orally available drugs are active against some strains of MRSA, including clindamycin, macrolides (e.g. erythromycin), tetracyclines, rifamp(ic)in, fusidic acid (in Europe) and trimethoprim/sulphamethoxazole.[67,93] In practice, co-resistance to other, non-β-lactam antibiotics is common in MRSA, especially hospital-acquired strains, reducing the number of available options.

Several newer antibiotics for MRSA are either now available or in development.[94] Most established, and with a specific license indication for diabetic foot infection (but not for diabetic foot osteomyelitis *per se*), is linezolid, an oxazolidinone antibiotic active against both methicillin- and vancomycin-resistant organisms.[95,96] In addition to the encouraging results in a large randomised diabetic foot study,[97] linezolid has performed well for other complicated skin and soft tissue infections[98] and in a number of case series and case reports of bone infection[54] While the availability of both oral and parenteral formulations is convenient, its high cost is likely to limit its worldwide use for diabetic foot osteomyelitis involving MRSA.

Other drugs that are less well studied for treating diabetic foot infections include the marketed agents Synercid (quinupristin–dalfopristin)[99] and daptomycin,[100] and the still investigative agents dalbavancin[101] and oritavancin[102] (newer glycopeptides), telavancin (a lipoglycopeptide)[103] and tigecycline (a novel tetracycline).[104] What places these will find in the armamentarium for treating diabetic foot osteomyelitis remains to be seen, but it is likely that at least some will be employed in treating MRSA soft tissue infections.[105]

Prevention and Future Developments

The experience with MRSA has suggested that with careful attention to hand hygiene, the behaviors of health care workers and the cleanliness of the hospital environment, transmission can be substantially reduced.[106–108] Indeed, in a number of institutions worldwide, successful infection control programmes have reduced transmission by half or more. The advent of transmission outside health care institutions raises the possibility that cases of MRSA in the diabetic foot clinic may, in the future, be less attributable to the infection control practices of health care workers, than to the increased prevalence of methicillin resistance in the population. For now, proper hand hygiene, avoiding procedures that disseminate bacteria (e.g. pressure-device debridement, grinding nails or calluses), cleaning of the physical environment (especially after its use by colonised patients with desquamating skin) and adopting 'universal precautions' for patient contact are mandatory. These, combined with rational and time-limited antibiotic use, remain the cornerstones of the struggle against MRSA colonisation and subsequent infection. Those treating the diabetic foot, and in particular diabetic foot osteomyelitis, would do well to remember that antibiotic strategies should, whenever possible, focus on treatments with the minimum ecological impact (through use of narrow-spectrum regimens) given for the minimum possible time.

REFERENCES

1. Lipsky BA. Osteomyelitis of the foot in diabetic patients. *Clin Infect Dis* 1997;25:1318–1326.
2. Berendt AR, Lipsky BA. Bone and joint infections in the diabetic foot. *Curr Treat Options Infect Dis* 2003;5:345–360.
3. Mandal S, Berendt AR, Peacock SJ. *Staphylococcus aureus* bone and joint infection. *J Infect* 2002;44:143–151.
4. Ciampolini J, Harding KG. Pathophysiology of chronic bacterial osteomyelitis. Why do antibiotics fail so often? *Postgrad Med J* 2000;76:479–483.
5. Lew DP, Waldvogel FA. Osteomyelitis. *Lancet* 2004;364:369–379.
6. Ellington JK, Harris M, Webb L, *et al.* Intracellular *Staphylococcus aureus*. A mechanism for the indolence of osteomyelitis. *J Bone Joint Surg Br* 2003;85:918–921.
7. Berendt AR, Lipsky B. Is this bone infected or not? Differentiating neuro-osteoarthropathy from osteomyelitis in the diabetic foot. *Curr Diabetes Rep* 2004;4:424–429.
8. Snyder RJ, Cohen MM, Sun C, Livingston J. Osteomyelitis in the diabetic patient: diagnosis and treatment, Part 1: Overview, diagnosis, and microbiology. *Ostomy Wound Manage* 2001;47:18–22, 25–30; quiz 31–32.
9. Bonham P. A critical review of the literature, part I: diagnosing osteomyelitis in patients with diabetes and foot ulcers. *J Wound Ostomy Continence Nurs* 2001;28:73–88.
10. Wrobel JS, Connolly JE. Making the diagnosis of osteomyelitis. The role of prevalence. *J Am Podiatr Med Assoc* 1998;88:337–343.
11. Lipsky BA, Berendt AR, Deery HG, II, *et al.* IDSA Guidelines: Diagnosis and treatment of diabetic foot infections. *Clin Infect Dis* 2004;39:885–910.
12. Newman LG, Waller J, Palestro CJ, *et al.* Unsuspected osteomyelitis in diabetic foot ulcers. Diagnosis and monitoring by leukocyte scanning with indium in 111 oxyquinoline. *JAMA* 1991;266:1246–1251.
13. Hill SL, Holtzman GI, Buse R. The effects of peripheral vascular disease with osteomyelitis in the diabetic foot. *Am J Surg* 1999;177:282–286.
14. Grayson ML, Gibbons GW, Balogh K, Levin E, Karchmer AW. Probing to bone in infected pedal ulcers: a clinical sign of underlying osteomyelitis in diabetic patients. *JAMA* 1995;273:721–723.
15. Armstrong DG, Lavery LA, Sariaya M, Ashry H. Leukocytosis is a poor indicator of acute osteomyelitis of the foot in diabetes mellitus. *J Foot Ankle Surg* 1996;35:280–283.

16. Kaleta JL, Fleischli JW, Reilly CH. The diagnosis of osteomyelitis in diabetes using erythrocyte sedimentation rate: a pilot study. *J Am Podiatr Med Assoc* 2001;91:445–450.

17. Upchurch GR Jr, Keagy BA, Johnson G Jr. An acute phase reaction in diabetic patients with foot ulcers. *Cardiovasc Surg* 1997;5:32–36.

18. Crim JR, Seeger LL. Imaging evaluation of osteomyelitis. *Crit Rev Diagn Imaging* 1994;35:201–256.

19. Becker W. Imaging osteomyelitis and the diabetic foot. *Q J Nucl Med* 1999;43:9–20.

20. Shults DW, Hunter GC, McIntyre KE, Parent FN, Piotrowski JJ, Bernhard VM. Value of radiographs and bone scans in determining the need for therapy in diabetic patients with foot ulcers. *Am J Surg* 1989;158:525–529, discussion 529–530.

21. Dutronc H, Bocquentin F, Dupon M. [Radiographic diagnosis in bone and joint infection management]. *Med Mal Infect* 2004;34:257–263.

22. Blume PA, Dey HM, Daley LJ, Arrighi JA, Soufer R, Gorecki GA. Diagnosis of pedal osteomyelitis with Tc-99m HMPAO labeled leukocytes. *J Foot Ankle Surg* 1997;36:120–126, discussion 160.

23. Palestro CJ, Caprioli R, Love C, et al. Rapid diagnosis of pedal osteomyelitis in diabetics with a technetium-99m-labeled monoclonal antigranulocyte antibody. *J Foot Ankle Surg* 2003;42: 2–8.

24. Sarikaya A, Aygit AC, Pekindil G. Utility of 99mTc dextran scintigraphy in diabetic patients with suspected osteomyelitis of the foot. *Ann Nucl Med* 2003;17:669–676.

25. Poirier JY, Garin E, Derrien C, et al. Diagnosis of osteomyelitis in the diabetic foot with a 99mTc-HMPAO leucocyte scintigraphy combined with a 99mTc-MDP bone scintigraphy. *Diabetes Metab* 2002;28:485–490.

26. Harwood SJ, Valdivia S, Hung G-L, Quenzer RW. Use of sulesomab, a radiolabeled antibody fragment, to detect osteomyelitis in diabetic patients with foot ulcers by leukocintigraphy. *Clin Infect Dis* 1999;28:1200–1205.

27. Devillers A, Garin E, Polard JL, et al. Comparison of Tc-99m-labelled antileukocyte fragment Fab' and Tc-99m-HMPAO leukocyte scintigraphy in the diagnosis of bone and joint infections: a prospective study. *Nucl Med Commun* 2000;21:747–753.

28. Keidar Z, Militianu D, Melamed E, Bar-Shalom R, Israel O. The diabetic foot: initial experience with 18F-FDG PET/CT. *J Nucl Med* 2005;46:444–449.

29. Rubello D, Casara D, Maran A, Avogaro A, Tiengo A, Muzzio PC. Role of anti-granulocyte Fab' fragment antibody scintigraphy (LeukoScan) in evaluating bone infection: acquisition protocol, interpretation criteria and clinical results. *Nucl Med Commun* 2004;25:39–47.

30. Schweitzer ME, Morrison WB. MR imaging of the diabetic foot. *Radiol Clin North Am* 2004;42:61–71, vi.

31. Chatha DS, Cunningham PM, Schweitzer ME. MR imaging of the diabetic foot: diagnostic challenges. *Radiol Clin North Am* 2005;43:747–759, ix.

32. Gil HC, Morrison WB. MR imaging of diabetic foot infection. *Semin Musculoskelet Radiol* 2004;8:189–198.

33. Dogan BE, Sahin G, Yagmurlu B, Erden I. Neuroarthropathy of the extremities: magnetic resonance imaging features. *Curr Probl Diagn Radiol* 2003;32:227–232.

34. Khatri G, Wagner DK, Sohnle PG. Effect of bone biopsy in guiding antimicrobial therapy for osteomyelitis complicating open wounds. *Am J Med Sci* 2001;321:367–371.

35. Zuluaga AF, Galvis W, Jaimes F, Vesga O. Lack of microbiological concordance between bone and non-bone specimens in chronic osteomyelitis: an observational study. *BMC Infect Dis* 2002;2:8.

36. Lipsky BA, Berendt AR. Principles and practice of antibiotic therapy of diabetic foot infections. *Diabetes Metab Res Rev* 2000;16:S42–S46.

37. Mader JT, Ortiz M, Calhoun JH. Update on the diagnosis and management of osteomyelitis. *Clin Podiatr Med Surg* 1996;13:701–724.

38. Bonham P. A critical review of the literature, Part II: antibiotic treatment of osteomyelitis in patients with diabetes and foot ulcers. *J Wound Ostomy Continence Nurs* 2001;28:141–149.

39. Senneville E. Antimicrobial interventions for the management of diabetic foot infections. *Expert Opin Pharmacother* 2005;6:263–273.
40. Snyder RJ, Cohen MM, Sun C, Livingston J. Osteomyelitis in the diabetic patient: diagnosis and treatment, Part 2: Medical, surgical, and alternative treatments. *Ostomy Wound Manage* 2001;47:24–30, 32–41; quiz 42–43.
41. Van Damme H, Rorive M, Martens De Noorthout BM, Quaniers J, Scheen A, Limet R. Amputations in diabetic patients: a plea for footsparing surgery. *Acta Chir Belg* 2001;101:123–129.
42. Chang BB, Darling RC, III, Paty PS, Lloyd WE, Shah DM, Leather RP. Expeditious management of ischemic invasive foot infections. *Cardiovasc Surg* 1996;4:792–795.
43. Akbari CM, Pomposelli FB, Jr, Gibbons GW, *et al.* Lower extremity revascularization in diabetes: late observations. *Arch Surg* 2000;135:452–456.
44. Holstein PE, Sorensen S. Limb salvage experience in a multidisciplinary diabetic foot unit. *Diabetes Care* 1999;22:B97–B103.
45. Rauwerda JA. Surgical treatment of the infected diabetic foot. *Diabetes Metab Res Rev* 2004;20:S41–S44.
46. Pittet D, Wyssa B, Herter-Clavel C, Kursteiner K, Vaucher J, Lew PD. Outcome of diabetic foot infections treated conservatively: a retrospective cohort study with long-term follow-up. *Arch Intern Med* 1999;159:851–856.
47. Venkatesan P, Lawn S, Macfarlane RM, Fletcher EM, Finch RG, Jeffcoate WJ. Conservative management of osteomyelitis in the feet of diabetic patients. *Diabet Med* 1997;14:487–490.
48. Piaggesi A, Schipani E, Campi F, *et al.* Conservative surgical approach versus non-surgical management for diabetic neuropathic foot ulcers: a randomized trial. *Diabet Med* 1998;15:412–417.
49. Jeffcoate WJ, Lipsky BA. Controversies in diagnosing and managing osteomyelitis of the foot in diabetes. *Clin Infect Dis* 2004;39:S115–S122.
50. Ha Van G, Siney H, Danan JP, Sachon C, Grimaldi A. Treatment of osteomyelitis in the diabetic foot. Contribution of conservative surgery. *Diabetes Care* 1996;19:1257–1260.
51. Tan JS, File TM Jr. Diagnosis and treatment of diabetic foot infections. *Baillieres Best Pract Res Clin Rheumatol* 1999;13:149–161.
52. Henke PK, Blackburn SA, Wainess RW, *et al.* Osteomyelitis of the foot and toe in adults is a surgical disease: conservative management worsens lower extremity salvage. *Ann Surg* 2005;241:885–892, discussion 892–894.
53. Salvana J, Rodner C, Browner BD, Livingston K, Schreiber J, Pesanti E. Chronic osteomyelitis: results obtained by an integrated team approach to management. *Conn Med* 2005;69:195–202.
54. Rao N, Ziran BH, Hall RA, Santa ER. Successful treatment of chronic bone and joint infections with oral linezolid. *Clin Orthop Relat Res* 2004;427:67–71.
55. Lew DP, Waldvogel FA. Quinolones and osteomyelitis: state-of-the-art. *Drugs* 1995;49:100–111.
56. Tice A, Hoaglund P, Shoultz DA. Outcomes of osteomyelitis among patients treated with outpatient parenteral antimicrobial therapy. *Am J Med* 2003;114:723–728.
57. Lazzarini L, Lipsky BA, Mader JT. Antibiotic treatment of osteomyelitis: what have we learned from 30 years of clinical trials? *Int J Infect Dis* 2005;9:127–138.
58. Berendt AR, Lipsky BA. Should antibiotics be used in the treatment of the diabetic foot? *Diabetic Foot* 2003;6:18–28.
59. Yamashita Y, Uchida A, Yamakawa T, Shinto Y, Araki N, Kato K. Treatment of chronic osteomyelitis using calcium hydraxyapatite ceramic implants impregnated with antibiotic. *Int Orthop* 1998;22:247–251.
60. Roeder B, Van Gils CC, Maling S. Antibiotic beads in the treatment of diabetic pedal osteomyelitis. *J Foot Ankle Surg* 2000;39:124–130.
61. Becker PL, Smith RA, Williams RS, Dutkowsky JP. Comparison of antibiotic release from polymethylmethacrylate beads and sponge collagen. *J Orthop Res* 1994;12:737–741.

62. Armstrong DG, Lipsky BA. Advances in the treatment of diabetic foot infections. *Diabetes Technol Ther* 2004;6:167–177.

63. Perencevich EN, Kaye KS, Strausbaugh LJ, Fisman DN, Harris AD. Acceptable rates of treatment failure in osteomyelitis involving the diabetic foot: a survey of infectious diseases consultants. *Clin Infect Dis* 2004;38:476–482.

64. Lipsky BA, Pecoraro RE, Wheat LJ. The diabetic foot. Soft tissue and bone infection. *Infect Dis Clin North Am* 1990;4:409–432.

65. Abbas ZG, Gill GV, Archibald LK. The epidemiology of diabetic limb sepsis: an African perspective. *Diabet Med* 2002;19:895–899.

66. Viswanathan V, Jasmine JJ, Snehalatha C, Ramachandran A. Prevalence of pathogens in diabetic foot infection in South Indian type 2 diabetic patients. *J Assoc Physicians India* 2002;50:1013–1016.

67. Cunha BA. Methicillin-resistant *Staphylococcus aureus*: clinical manifestations and antimicrobial therapy. *Clin Microbiol Infect* 2005;11:33–42.

68. Eady EA, Cove JH. Staphylococcal resistance revisited: community-acquired methicillin resistant *Staphylococcus aureus* – an emerging problem for the management of skin and soft tissue infections. *Curr Opin Infect Dis* 2003;16:103–124.

69. Favero MS. Outbreaks of community-associated methicillin-resistant *Staphylococcus aureus* skin infections. *Infect Control Hosp Epidemiol* 2003;24:787.

70. Tenover FC, McDonald LC. Vancomycin-resistant staphylococci and enterococci: epidemiology and control. *Curr Opin Infect Dis* 2005;18:300–305.

71. Sieradzki K, Markiewicz Z. Mechanism of vancomycin resistance in methicillin resistant *Staphylococcus aureus*. *Pol J Microbiol* 2004;53:207–214.

72. Cartolano GL, Cheron M, Benabid D, Leneveu M, Boisivon A. Methicillin-resistant *Staphylococcus aureus* (MRSA) with reduced susceptibility to glycopeptides (GISA) in 63 French general hospitals. *Clin Microbiol Infect* 2004;10:448–451.

73. Apfalter P. [MRSA/MRSE-VISA/GISA/VRSA-PRP-VRE: current gram positive problem bacteria and mechanism of resistance, prevalence and clinical consequences]. *Wien Med Wochenschr* 2003;153:144–147.

74. Chang S, Sievert DM, Hageman JC, *et al.* Infection with vancomycin-resistant *Staphylococcus aureus* containing the vanA resistance gene. *N Engl J Med* 2003;348:1342–1347.

75. Vancomycin-resistant *Staphylococcus aureus* – Pennsylvania, 2002. *MMWR Morb Mortal Wkly Rep* 2002;51:902.

76. Methicillin-resistant *Staphylococcus aureus* skin or soft tissue infections in a state prison – Mississippi, 2000. *MMWR Morb Mortal Wkly Rep* 2001;50:919–922.

77. Methicillin-resistant *Staphylococcus aureus* infections in correctional facilities – Georgia, California, and Texas, 2001–2003. *MMWR Morb Mortal Wkly Rep* 2003;52:992–996.

78. Methicillin-resistant *staphylococcus aureus* infections among competitive sports participants – Colorado, Indiana, Pennsylvania, and Los Angeles County, 2000–2003. *MMWR Morb Mortal Wkly Rep* 2003;52:793–795.

79. Centers for Disease Control and Prevention. Public health dispatch: outbreaks of community-associated methicillin-resistant *Staphylococcus aureus* skin infections – Los Angeles County, California, 2002–2003. *JAMA* 2003;289:1377.

80. Community-associated methicillin-resistant *Staphylococcus aureus* infections in Pacific Islanders – Hawaii, 2001–2003. *MMWR Morb Mortal Wkly Rep* 2004;53:767–770.

81. Barrett TW, Moran GJ. Update on emerging infections: news from the Centers for Disease Control and Prevention. Methicillin-resistant *Staphylococcus aureus* infections among competitive sports participants – Colorado, Indiana, Pennsylvania, and Los Angeles County, 2000–2003. *Ann Emerg Med* 2004;43:43–45, discussion 45–47.

82. Kazakova SV, Hageman JC, Matava M, *et al.* A clone of methicillin-resistant *Staphylococcus aureus* among professional football players. *N Engl J Med* 2005;352:468–475.

83. Fridkin SK, Hageman JC, Morrison M, *et al.* Methicillin-resistant *Staphylococcus aureus* disease in three communities. *N Engl J Med* 2005;352:1436–1444.
84. Baggett HC, Hennessy TW, Rudolph K, *et al.* Community-onset methicillin-resistant *Staphylococcus aureus* associated with antibiotic use and the cytotoxin Panton–Valentine leukocidin during a furunculosis outbreak in rural Alaska. *J Infect Dis* 2004;189:1565–1573.
85. Tentolouris N, Jude EB, Smirnof I, Knowles EA, Boulton AJ. Methicillin-resistant *Staphylococcus aureus*: an increasing problem in a diabetic foot clinic. *Diabet Med* 1999;16:767–771.
86. Dang C, Prasad Y, Bouton A, Jude EB. Methicillin-resistant *Staphylococcus aureus* in the diabetic foot clinic: a worsening problem. *Diabet Med* 2003;20:159–61.
87. Fejfarova V, Jirkovska A, Skibova J, Petkov V. [Pathogen resistance and other risk factors in the frequency of lower limb amputations in patients with the diabetic foot syndrome]. *Vnitr Lek* 2002;48:302–306.
88. Grimble SA, Magee TR, Galland RB. Methicillin resistant *Staphylococcus aureus* in patients undergoing major amputation. *Eur J Vasc Endovasc Surg* 2001;22:215–218.
89. Mantey I, Hill RL, Foster AV, Wilson S, Wade JJ, Edmonds ME. Infection of foot ulcers with *Staphylococcus aureus* associated with increased mortality in diabetic patients. *Commun Dis Public Health* 2000;3:288–290.
90. Wagner A, Reike H, Angelkort B. [Highly resistant pathogens in patients with diabetic foot syndrome with special reference to methicillin-resistant *Staphylococcus aureus* infections]. *Dtsch Med Wochenschr* 2001;126:1353–1356.
91. Chopra I. Antibiotic resistance in *Staphylococcus aureus*: concerns, causes and cures. *Expert Rev Anti Infect Ther* 2003;1:45–55.
92. Marone P, Concia E, Andreoni M, Suter F, Cruciani M. Treatment of bone and soft tissue infections with teicoplanin. *J Antimicrob Chemother* 1990;25:435–439.
93. Paradisi F, Corti G, Messeri D. Antistaphylococcal (MSSA, MRSA, MSSE, MRSE) antibiotics. *Med Clin North Am* 2001;85:1–17.
94. Raghavan M, Linden PK. Newer treatment options for skin and soft tissue infections. *Drugs* 2004;64:1621–1642.
95. Batts DH. Linezolid – a new option for treating gram-positive infections. *Oncology (Williston Park)* 2000;14:23–29.
96. Cepeda JA, Whitehouse T, Cooper B, *et al.* Linezolid versus teicoplanin in the treatment of Gram-positive infections in the critically ill: a randomized, double-blind, multicentre study. *J Antimicrob Chemother* 2004;53:345–355.
97. Lipsky BA, Itani K, Norden C. Treating foot infections in diabetic patients: a randomized, multicenter, open-label trial of linezolid versus ampicillin–sulbactam/amoxicillin–clavulanate. *Clin Infect Dis* 2004;38:17–24.
98. Weigelt J, Itani K, Stevens D, Lau W, Dryden M, Knirsch C. Linezolid versus vancomycin in treatment of complicated skin and soft tissue infections. *Antimicrob Agents Chemother* 2005;49:2260–2266.
99. Rubinstein E, Keller N. Future prospects and therapeutic potential of streptogramins. *Drugs* 1996;51:38–42.
100. Lipsky BA, Stoutenburgh U. Daptomycin for treating infected diabetic foot ulcers: evidence from a randomized, controlled trial comparing daptomycin with vancomycin or semi-synthetic penicillins for complicated skin and skin-structure infections. *J Antimicrob Chemother* 2005;55:240–245.
101. Lin G, Credito K, Ednie LM, Appelbaum PC. Antistaphylococcal activity of dalbavancin, an experimental glycopeptide. *Antimicrob Agents Chemother* 2005;49:770–772.
102. Mercier RC, Hrebickova L. Oritavancin: a new avenue for resistant Gram-positive bacteria. *Expert Rev Anti Infect Ther* 2005;3:325–332.
103. Stryjewski ME, O'Riordan WD, Lau WK, *et al.* Telavancin versus standard therapy for treatment of complicated skin and soft-tissue infections due to gram-positive bacteria. *Clin Infect Dis* 2005;40:1601–1607.

104. Bradford PA, Weaver-Sands DT, Petersen PJ. In vitro activity of tigecycline against isolates from patients enrolled in phase 3 clinical trials of treatment for complicated skin and skin-structure infections and complicated intra-abdominal infections. *Clin Infect Dis* 2005;41:S315–S332.

105. Appelbaum PC, Jacobs MR. Recently approved and investigational antibiotics for treatment of severe infections caused by Gram-positive bacteria. *Curr Opin Microbiol* 2005.

106. Raboud J, Saskin R, Simor A, *et al*. Modeling transmission of methicillin-resistant *Staphylococcus aureus* among patients admitted to a hospital. *Infect Control Hosp Epidemiol* 2005;26:607–615.

107. Johnston P, Norrish AR, Brammar T, Walton N, Hegarty TA, Coleman NP. Reducing methicillin-resistant *Staphylococcus aureus* (MRSA) patient exposure by infection control measures. *Ann R Coll Surg Engl* 2005;87:123–125.

108. Boyce JM, Havill NL, Kohan C, Dumigan DG, Ligi CE. Do infection control measures work for methicillin-resistant *Staphylococcus aureus*? *Infect Control Hosp Epidemiol* 2004;25:395–401.

15 Dressings: Is There an Evidence Base?

Ann Knowles

For an obstinate ulcer, sweet wine and a lot of patience should be enough
                                                    – Hippocrates (460–377BC)

INTRODUCTION

Wounds have existed since time began. The use of dressings to protect flesh wounds can be traced back to the ancient Egyptians who used plasters of honey, grease and lint, or mud, clay and herbs.[1] The ancient Greeks were greatly influenced by the Egyptians and used wine or vinegar to wash wounds and as dressings.[1] Neither the Greeks nor the Egyptians understood the scientific basis for the benefits of these dressings. Wound care has evolved since then and has been influenced by the work in the mid-nineteenth century of Joseph Lister and Louis Pasteur who helped to establish a scientific basis for wound management. Conflicts and war have also necessitated the development of new ways of managing wounds.[2]

Dressings are designed to keep the wound clean and free from contamination while promoting wound healing.[3] They can also absorb exudate and insulate the wound, and should be non-adherent and non-toxic. Choosing the right dressing is important and will depend on the stage of healing and the condition of the wound. An ulcer with a black eschar or slough may need a dressing which is different from that for a granulating or epithelialising wound. However, dressings must never be used in isolation in the treatment of diabetic foot ulcers; if pressure relief is forgotten, a neuropathic ulcer is unlikely to heal, however expensive the dressing.

Wound care products account for a significant proportion of general practitioner prescriptions in England, and in 1997, cost over $80 million.[4] Many dressings are expensive and add to the financial burden of the health care system. The advent of nurse prescribing has encouraged nurses to participate in the development of wound care guidelines in their own trust or health authority.[5] With the abundant choice of wound care products on the market, dressing choice can be influenced by cost, efficacy, availability, safety and evaluation of new products. Practitioners therefore need to choose carefully a dressing that is both efficacious and practical. The cost of topical wound treatment can be related to the severity of the ulcer, wound-healing time, frequency of dressing change, transport and staff costs.[6]

The Foot in Diabetes, 4th Edition. Editors Andrew J.M. Boulton, Peter R. Cavanagh and Gerry Rayman.
© 2006 John Wiley & Sons, Ltd.

FACTORS INFLUENCING DRESSING CHOICE

Scrutinising the enormous amount of available literature may influence dressing choice, but much of this information is anecdotal and not evidence based. Sussman suggests that evidence-based practice is a 'practice based on proof from scientific research, applied with clinical judgement'.[7] Once the evidence has been gathered, practitioners should appraise its value and decide whether or not a change in practice is warranted.[8] Unfortunately, evidence-based practice in wound care has not kept pace with the vast number of products on the market,[9] and there is little motivation for manufacturers to fund comparative studies of their own products against those of competitors.[10]

Cullum *et al.*, in a comprehensive review of dressing trials of diabetic foot ulcers, found that the sample sizes of the studies they looked at were small with insufficient evidence of effect.[11] So, while evidence-based prescribing is the ideal, in practice many of the wound care companies rely on anecdotal case reports or small studies to promote their products, leaving nurses and podiatrists with the dilemma of what to use. Clinicians should therefore question the validity of end point studies in wound-healing experiments.[2]

A lot of the available information on wound healing refers to acute and experimental ulcers and may therefore not be relevant.[11] Which dressing to choose can be difficult, and practitioners may select a particular dressing because it is cheap, readily available or familiar to them.

Care of the diabetic foot requires a team effort involving input from the podiatrist, specialist nurse, doctor, orthotist and patient. Wound management must be integrated into an effective programme of multidisciplinary care.[12] Dressing choice is not usually the first consideration when treating a diabetic foot ulcer, as in addition to pressure relief, other measures including callus debridement, infection control and an adequate blood supply must be addressed if the ulcer is to heal. Ulcer classification such as the University of Texas wound classification system, which grades ulcer depth, infection and ischaemia, can predict the likelihood of healing.[13]

The mid-1990s saw many new dressing products added to the drug tariff following the introduction of hydrocolloid, iodine and seaweed dressings in the 1980s.[9] Since then, wound care manufacturers have regularly introduced new products. Popular at the moment are the silver, iodine and honey products that are promoted as agents to help eradicate bacteria, including methicillin-resistant *Staphylococcus aureus* (MRSA). The multiple resistances to oral and intravenous antibiotics of organisms such as MRSA have encouraged the use of alternative topical treatments.

HONEY PRODUCTS

Honey, Pooh Bear's favourite food, is now increasingly popular for the treatment of wounds and ulcers due to its antimicrobial properties. Although honey has been used for over 2000 years,[14] it went out of fashion when antibiotics were introduced.[9] Molan suggests that in addition to having an antimicrobial action, honey provides a moist wound-healing environment that rapidly clears infection, deodorises and reduces inflammation, oedema and exudates.[15] The antibacterial action of honey is due to the release of low levels of hydrogen peroxide, the phytochemicals from the nectar of particular plant species and its osmolality created by its high sugar content.[16,17]

The antibacterial action of honey[18] has encouraged its use on wounds infected with MRSA and other organisms. *In vitro* studies show that honey has proven antibacterial activity against

Pseudomonas aeruginosa,[19] MRSA and vancomycin-sensitive cocci (VSE).[20] The antibacterial action of the Manuka honey (Nature's Nectar Ltd, Ash, UK) was double that of the pasture honey.[21] Honey derived from particular floral sources in New Zealand and Australia, such as the Manuka honey, tends to have enhanced antibacterial activity[22] but its potency can vary.[21] Anecdotal evidence shows rapid healing and eradication of MRSA,[23] but Fox suggests that the evidence is weak and should be interpreted with caution.[24]

There are a variety of medical-grade honey products for wound care, which are marketed as impregnated dressings and actual honey. In a study of 60 patients with complicated surgical, acute traumatic and chronic wounds, Ahmed *et al.* found that honey-medicated dressings were easy to apply to all but one patient.[18] Honey can be messy and this may stop some practitioners from using it; it should therefore be applied to a dressing first.[25] There is concern that secondary infections may be caused by contamination of the honey with microorganisms;[18] therefore, in order to safeguard patient safety only the medical-grade honey, which is sterilised for use on wounds, should be used.[26]

Mesitran (Medlock Medical, Oldham, UK), a new hydroactive range of honey dressings that are available in a variety of easy-to-use preparations, was recently introduced and is claimed to provide a complete solution for all stages of wound healing. It is available as an ointment, hydrogel-coated mesh and semipermeable wound dressing. Other ingredients in the ointment include lanolin, sunflower oil, cod liver oil, calendula and vitamins C and E. Anecdotal case studies show promising results with this product.

A large study in India of 900 patients with partial-thickness burns in less than 40% of the body surface area compared honey ($n = 450$) with conventional dressings of Vaseline gauze, Opsite film, an antibiotic dressing, sterile linen or sterile gauze (90 subjects in each group).[27] The mean wound-healing time was less in the honey-treated subjects (9 days) compared to the conventionally treated subjects (13.5 days). The same author later randomised a further 100 subjects in a study comparing honey dressings ($n = 50$) to sulphadiazine dressings ($n = 50$) and found improved healing times in the honey group with reduced hospital inpatient stays.[28]

In a systematic review of seven randomised trials of the use of honey in the treatment of superficial burns and wounds, Moore *et al.* found that although healing time was significantly shorter for honey dressings, the quality of the studies was low.[29] Comparators included polyurethane foam, silver sulphadiazine[29] and boiled potato peel.[30] A comprehensive literature search of honey dressings in 2004 also found only seven randomised controlled studies, a multitude of case reports and observational studies.[26] There were no trials in the use of honey on diabetic foot wounds and research mainly concentrated on wounds with superficial burns. Well-constructed clinical trials are needed to compare honey with other therapies on which to base clinical use,[30] particularly in diabetic foot wounds.

SILVER-CONTAINING DRESSINGS

Silver is a topical antiseptic that is also gaining popularity and is marketed in the form of a variety of silver-release products such as films, foams, hydrocolloids and hydrofibre dressings. The use of silver on chronic wounds dates back as early as the seventeenth century[31]; dilute solutions of silver nitrate were used in the nineteenth century to treat burns and eye infections.[32] Silver is effective against a broad range of organisms including yeast, fungi, viruses and methicillin and vancomycin strains.[33]

Silver is included in wound care products as elemental silver, inorganic compounds or organic complexes.[33] Silver-containing dressings are designed to release free silver ions into the wound site,[34] or wound exudates.[35] Some bacteria can develop a resistance to silver[36] but as most preparations can deliver sustained silver-ion release, no resistant strains have been found clinically.[37]

A small safety study of Contreet foam (Coloplast, Humlebaek, Denmark), a sustained silver-releasing foam dressing in 27 patients with diabetic foot ulcers (Wagner grade 1 and 2), showed it to be a safe, easy-to-use dressing.[38] Contreet is available as a foam or a hydrocolloid and therefore does not require a secondary dressing. Punch biopsy wounds in rats demonstrated with this dressing, the importance of wound moisture in releasing the active silver ions.[35]

In another small study to evaluate the patterns of silver release from selected sustained silver-release dressings, sequential microbiological examinations of wound swabs from seven patients with chronic wounds were used to measure the silver content using atomic absorption spectrometry.[35] Samples of wound exudate and wound scale were also examined. All were found to be safe for use on chronic wounds, and although the bacterial burden was controlled it was not eliminated. Excess silver ions were found to be bound by wound exudates and scales. The author suggests that further studies are needed to examine any potential silver resistance.

An *in vitro* study[32] was used to compare the antimicrobial effects of four silver dressings on three microorganisms (*S. aureus*, *Escherichia coli* and *Candida albicans*). Analysis of the silver content of each dressing showed varied release of the highly active silver ions in three of the dressings. In another *in vitro* study, the silver content and antimicrobial properties of ten silver-containing dressings were compared.[39] Highly significant differences were found in the distribution of silver within the different dressings, its chemical and physical form (metallic bound or ionic state) and the dressing's affinity to moisture, which is needed to release the silver ions. Additional research confirmed that the presence of sodium ions can influence the antimicrobial activity of different dressings in different ways.[40]

The safety of silver dressings and the possibility of systemic absorption and toxicity were looked at by Lansdown and Williams, who suggested 'research is needed to find out the minimal concentration of silver needed to achieve bacteriostasis without causing toxicity'.[34] The silver in a dressing should be released over a number of days rather than a short period[41] to avoid bolus dosing and minimising the possibility of systemic toxicity.[42] Silver dressings have an important role in the treatment of infected exuding wounds but their value has not been determined in the presence of slough and necrosis.[42]

White[43] looked at the results of seven studies (five randomised and controlled; two non-comparative) in patients with chronic wounds, using Actisorb (a charcoal dressing with silver (Johnson & Johnson Medical Ltd, Ascot, UK)). He concluded that the dressing was a safe and effective product for infected and malodorous wounds. Masson[44] suggests that for surface wounds a sustained release silver dressing is more appropriate than iodine, which is rapidly inactivated.

IODINE DRESSINGS

Iodine is one of the longest established antiseptics.[45] It is commonly available as povidone iodine and cadexomer iodine. The original iodine preparations used in the early eighteenth century often caused local pain and tissue irritation, which would have limited their use.[45]

Povidone iodine, 'the tamed iodine', is a safer form of iodine that was introduced about 40 years ago[46] and is commonly used as a skin disinfectant for operation sites and surgeons' hands. It is also available as a dressing, an example of this being inadine (Johnson & Johnson Medical Ltd, Ascot, UK), a knitted viscose fabric impregnated with a polyethylene glycol base containing 10% povidone iodine which is water soluble.

Cadexomer iodine was introduced over 20 years ago[45] and has a highly absorptive capacity. Iodine is slowly released when exudate is absorbed from the wound. Iodosorb ointment is one such preparation that contains 0.9% of elemental iodine.

Both iodine products require a secondary dressing.

There is an anecdotal case report of iodine-induced hyperthyroidism in two elderly patients, after the treatment of small leg ulcers.[47] Aronoff *et al.*[48] also found increased levels of serum iodide in patients treated with topically applied povidone iodine and suggest measurement of serum iodide in patients with impaired renal function. There is also minimal risk of thyroid gland disturbances[49] and patients with thyroid disorders should be closely monitored and treatment should not exceed 3 months.[50]

A review of 11 small studies of cadexomer iodine in venous leg ulcers found that it helped to reduce wound exudate, with superior healing in the iodine group when compared to standard wound healing.[51] A larger study of leg ulcers ($n = 153$) found a significantly better healing rate in the cadexomer iodine group compared to hydrocolloid dressings and paraffin gauze.[52]

An economic analysis of deep diabetic foot ulcers found considerably lower weekly treatment costs in the cadexomer iodine group compared to the standard treatment group.[53] In a study in pigs with wounds, which were inoculated with a known amount of MRSA,[54] cadexomer-iodine-dressed wounds had a significantly reduced MRSA and total bacteria count compared to the control group.

HYDROCOLLOID DRESSINGS

Hydrocolloid dressings are occlusive dressings that create a moist wound-healing environment when wound exudate forms a gel in the dressing. As hydrocolloids do not absorb large amounts of exudate, they should not be used in heavily exuding wounds. Their occlusive nature can prevent bacteria outside the dressing from contaminating the wound. In a small study of six patients with MRSA, the use of a hydrocolloid dressing prevented its spread to other inpatients.[55]

Hydrocolloids are popular with nurses and podiatrists,[56] as they do not require a secondary dressing and can be left in place for a week. There is controversy about the use of hydrocolloid dressings in diabetic foot ulcers[57] and there are anecdotal reports of adverse events. Eight cases of wound deterioration were reported by Foster *et al.* when the dressing was left in place for 5–7 days and dressings applied to some ulcers that were already infected.[58] A further two anecdotal cases were reported in Sweden of infection under hydrocolloid dressings[59] that were again inappropriately used. A retrospective review comparing the use of Granuflex (Convatec Ltd, Clwyd, UK) with other dressings (250 ulcers) found no increase in infection in the hydrocolloid group.[60] Care should be taken when using hydrocolloid dressings on diabetic foot ulcers, and dressings should be changed at least twice a week. Their use should be avoided on infected wounds. Deciding the interval between dressing changes is a skill that has to be learnt[61] and comes with experience.

Aquacell (Convatec Ltd, Clwyd, UK) is a hydrofibre dressing made of a hydrophilic non-woven sheet composed of hydrocolloid fibres. It is ideal for exuding wounds and is also available impregnated with silver (Aquacell Ag).

ALGINATE DRESSINGS

Alginate dressings are derived from seaweed and have the capacity to absorb large amounts of exudate. Kaltostat (Convatec Ltd, Clwyd, UK) is also marketed as a haemostat. If used incorrectly, alginates can form a plug restricting the exit of wound exudate. There are anecdotal reports of the plugging of four ulcers due to blockage of exudate.[62,63] If alginates are used in deep wounds they should not be tightly packed or allowed to dry out.[64]

HYDROGELS

Hydrogels are in the form of an aqueous gel that can be used to aid the rehydration of a hard eschar and to remove slough. They promote autolytic debridement in dry wounds and can absorb exudate in moist wounds, and are available as sheets and gels. In a review of trials of hydrogels, Jones[65] found that the main comparator was saline gauze, with most studies conducted on leg ulcers and few on diabetic foot ulcers.

Purilon gel (Coloplast, Humlebaek, Denmark) is the only hydrogel that is recommended for use prior to larva therapy, as it contains no propylene glycol, a preservative commonly used in other hydrogels. Granugel (Convatec Ltd, Clwyd, UK) is a gel that combines the features of a hydrogel with a hydrocolloid, which also maintains a moist wound-healing environment and promotes the debridement of slough.[66] Care should always be taken with ischaemic ulcers, as debridement may not always be appropriate.

SECONDARY DRESSINGS

The control of exudate is particularly important in managing chronic wounds,[67] as it can cause excoriation of the surrounding skin. Strike through and staining of the dressing will allow infection to reach the wound. Alginate and hydrofibre dressings will absorb exudate but both require a secondary dressing. Absorbent foam sheets such as Allevyn (Smith & Nephew, Hull, UK) can be used as primary or secondary dressings and will absorb exudate. Allevyn is also available as a heel cup. Other examples of foam dressings are Tielle (Johnson & Johnson Medical Ltd, Ascot, UK), Biatain (Coloplast, Humblebaek, Denmark), Mepilex (Molnlylcke Health Care, Gothenburg, Sweden) and Lyofoam (Medlock Medical, Oldham, UK). These dressings are available in different sizes.

Hypergranulation can be a problem in some wounds, and a study of Lyofoam showed that it was successful in reducing the height of over-granulation tissue within 2 weeks.[68]

OTHER DRESSINGS

Promogran (Smith & Nephew, Hull, UK) is a freeze-dried preparation that is made from a collagen (55%) and oxidised regenerated cellulose (45%). It is available as a hexagonal-shaped sheet that is stored at room temperature and is easy to apply. It forms a gel in the

Table 15.1 Practical use of dressings

Dressing	Function	Caution/contraindications
Honey products	Moist wound-healing environment Antibacterial action Desloughs	Only use medical-grade honey
Silver dressings	Antibacterial action	Saline can deactivate action of silver. Needs moist wound to activate silver ions
Charcoal dressings	Malodourous wounds	Treat cause of odour
Iodine dressings	Antibacterial action	Check if sensitive to iodine Caution with patients with renal and thyroid conditions
Hydrocolloid dressings	Moist wound-healing environment Occlusive dressing	Do not use on infected wounds Change at least twice a week Do not absorb exudate
Alginates	Exuding wounds Haemostat	Can plug wound and prevent drainage
Hydrogels	Debridement	
Foam dressings	Primary and secondary absorbent dressing	Change if strike through
Promogran and Hyalofill	Difficult to heal wounds	Wounds should be free of necrotic and sloughy tissue
Kerraboot	Moist wound-healing environment Easy to change	Can view wound without disturbing dressing
Living skin equivalents	Difficult to heal wounds	Do not use on infected wounds Expensive

presence of wound exudate and binds the naturally occurring growth factors and protects against degradation by proteases. It is ideal for chronic wounds that are free from necrotic tissue and infection.

A multicentre, randomised controlled trial of Promogran versus standard treatment in diabetic foot ulcers[69] failed to demonstrate superior efficacy to standard care (moistened gauze). Pressure relief was not standardised but was left to individual centres, which may partially explain the negative result of this trial.

A cost-effective study in four European countries looked at the healing of deep diabetic foot ulcers after the use of Promogran over a 3-month period.[70] Slightly more ulcers in the Promogran group (26%) healed than in the good wound care group (20.7%) but the results were not significant.

HYALOFILL

Hyalofill (Convatec Ltd, Clwyd, UK) contains hyaff, a derivative of hyaluronic acid, which is naturally present in body tissue and is associated with tissue repair.[71] It is manufactured as a cream-coloured fleece that is available as a flat sheet or rope and should be used on clean wounds. In a study of indolent neuropathic diabetic foot ulcers ($n = 30$) comparing hyaff ($n = 15$) with standard treatment ($n = 15$), the hyaff group had improved healing of ulcers and a higher degree of closure of sinuses.[72] A study of 36 patients with diabetic foot ulcers also showed improved healing with a Hyalofill dressing.[73] However, in neither of the above studies was a statistical improvement demonstrated due to the relatively small numbers of patients in each group.

THE KERRABOOT

The Kerraboot (Ark Therapeutics Ltd, London, UK) is a novel device for the healing of leg and foot ulcers that is available on drug tariff. It is a clear plastic, boot-shaped dressing with an absorbent pad incorporated into the base. It is designed to create a warm, moist wound-healing environment and manage wound exudate. The clear plastic allows the wound to be viewed without disturbing the dressing, and its ease of application can save nurses time and dressing materials.[74] Trials are very limited and include a randomised controlled study of the Kerraboot versus Allevyn in diabetic foot ulcers,[75] which resulted in a reduction of dressing time with the Kerraboot with patients being able to change their own dressings. Another small study of 14 diabetic patients who used the Kerraboot for 28 days also confirmed its ease of application and removal.[76]

THIRD GENERATION DRESSINGS

Cavanagh refers to active wound-healing products as third-generation wound-healing agents such as growth factors and bioengineered skin substitutes, which may hold the future for wound healing.[10]

LIVING SKIN EQUIVALENTS

Living skin equivalents such as Dermagraft (Smith & Nephew, Largo, FL, USA) or Graftskin (Organogenesis, Canton, MA, USA) may be useful in certain cases such as difficult-to-heal ulcers. In a multicentred study of Graftskin, patients were randomly assigned to either Graftskin ($n = 112$) or saline-moistened gauze ($n = 96$).[77] The Graftskin was applied weekly for a maximum of 4 weeks or earlier if complete healing occurred. After 12 weeks, 56% of the Graftskin group had healed compared to 38% of the standard treatment group. There were no significant side effects and the authors conclude that although Graftskin may a useful adjunct for resistant foot ulcers, due to its considerable cost, it should be reserved for chronic non-healing ulcers.

In a multicentre study of Dermagraft, 50 patients with diabetic foot ulcers were treated over a 12-week period.[78] Three groups were randomised to three different dosage regimes of Dermagraft and the fourth, the control group, treated with the same dressing but no living skin equivalent. In the group with the highest number of applications of Dermagraft (one piece weekly for 8 weeks) 50% healed compared to 8% in the control group. The authors found that after a mean of 14 months (11–22) follow-up, there were no re-ulcerations in the

Dermagraft-treated group. Due to the small numbers in this study, statistical significance was not demonstrated.

Dermagraft was also used in a large multicentre study, in the United States, of 314 patients with diabetic foot ulcers[79] in which 30% of the Dermagraft patients had healed by week 12 compared to 18.3% of the control group. The Dermagraft group also experienced fewer ulcer-related adverse events.

Living skin equivalents can be time consuming to apply and this and their cost could limit their use. However, in a recent review Pham *et al.*[80] suggest that they could have a significant role in the management of diabetic foot ulcers.

CONCLUSION

Although there is a lack of evidence to support the use of dressings in the healing of wounds, there is a considerable amount of clinical experience in the use of new treatments that are proving beneficial and acceptable to patients on account of their ability to reduce pain, odour or leakage.[1] A small number of studies do exist but there is no compelling evidence to favour any particular dressing. Wound care is often based on tradition rather than current research,[81] and it is important to understand the general and specific properties of modern dressing materials.[82]

As practitioners, we have a responsibility to ensure that our practice is based on sound clinical evidence and that the care we deliver is of a high quality.[8] Unfortunately, there is still little evidence to indicate which dressings or topical agents are most effective in the treatment of chronic wounds.[3]

Dressings must never be seen as an isolated treatment of a wound; rather, they should be considered as part of the multifaceted approach to wound care. It is essential to remember the words of Dr Paul Brand: 'dressings have the potential to deceive both the doctor and patient into thinking that by covering a wound they were curing it'.

REFERENCES

1. Cohen IK. *A brief history of wound healing.* Oxford Clinical Communications Inc; 1998.
2. Harding KG, Jones V, Price P. Topical treatment: which dressing to choose. *Diabetes Metab Res Rev* 2000;16:S47–S50.
3. Bradley M, Cullum N, Nelson EA, Petticrew M, Sheldon T, Torgeson D. Systematic reviews of wound care management: (2). Dressings and topical agents used in the healing of chronic wounds. *Health Technol Assess* 1999;3:1–35.
4. *Prescription Cost Analysis, England 1997.* Department of Health, Government Statistical Service Branch SD1E. 1997.
5. Modern wound management dressings. *Prescrib Nurs Bull* 1999;1:5–8.
6. Apelqvist J, Ragnarson-Tennvall G, Larsson J. Topical treatment of diabetic foot ulcers: an economic analysis of treatment alternatives and strategies. *Diabet Med* 1995;12:123–128.
7. Sussman C. Expanding wound care products. *Interdisciplin J Rehabil* 2001.
8. Baxter R, Baxter H. Clinical governance, I: Evidence-based practice. *J Wound Care* 2002;11:7–12.
9. Morgan D. Wounds – what should a dressing formulary include? *Hosp Pharm* 2002;9:261–266.
10. Cavanagh P. Making diabetic foot care evidence based: what is missing? Part 2: treatment. *Diabet Foot* 2002;7:108–112.

11. Cullum C, Majid M, O'Meara S, Sheldon T. Use of dressings: is there an evidence base? In: Boulton AJM, Connor H, Cavanagh PR, eds. *The Foot in Diabetes*. 3rd edn. Chichester: Wiley; 2000:153–168.

12. Jeffcoate WJ, Price P, Harding KG, for the International Working Group on Wound Healing and Treatments for People with Diabetes. *Diabetes Metab Res Rev* 2004;20:S78–S89.

13. Armstrong DG, Lavery LA, Harkless LB. Validation of the diabetic wound classification: the contribution of depth, infection and vascular disease to the risk of amputation. *Diabetes Care* 1998;21:855–859.

14. Dunford C, Cooper R, Molan P, White R. The use of honey in wound management. *Nurs Stand* 2000;5:63–68.

15. Molan PC. Re-introducing honey in the management of wounds and ulcers – theory and practice. *Ostomy Wound Manage* 2002;48:28–40.

16. Molan PC. Potential of honey in the treatment of wounds and burns. *Am J Clin Dermatol* 2001;2:13–19.

17. Molan PC, Betts JA. Clinical usage of honey as a wound dressing: an update. *J Wound Care* 2004;13:353–356.

18. Ahmed AK, Hoekstra MJ, Hage JJ, Karim RB. Honey-medicated dressing: transformation of an ancient remedy into modern therapy. *Ann Plast Surg* 2003;50:143–147.

19. Cooper RA, Halas E, Molan C. The efficacy of honey in inhibiting strains of *Pseudomonas aeruginosa* from infected burns. *J Burn Rehabil* 2002;23:366–370.

20. Cooper RA, Molan PC, Harding KG. The sensitivity of honey to gram-positive cocci of clinical significance isolated from wounds. *J Appl Microbiol* 2002;93:857–863.

21. Allen KL, Hutchinson G, Molan PC. The potential for using honey to treat wounds infected with MRSA and VRE. Paper presented at: the First World Wound Healing Congress; 2000;20:878–889. Melbourne, Australia. Paper presented on 10th–13th September 2000 and is online.

22. Lusby PE, Coombes A, Wilkinson JM. Honey: a potent agent for wound healing. *J Wound Ostomy Continence Nurs* 2002;29:295–300.

23. Natarajan S, Williamson D, Grey J, Harding KG, Cooper RA. Healing of an MRSA-colonised, hydroxyurea-induced leg ulcer with honey. *J Dermatol Treat* 2001;10:530–534.

24. Fox C. Honey as a dressing for chronic wounds in adults. *Br J Community Nurs* 2002;10:530–534.

25. Molan PC. *Selection of Honey for Use on Wounds*. Handout for the Infection Control Conference, New Zealand; 1999.

26. Gethin G. Is there enough clinical evidence to use honey to manage wounds? *J Wound Care* 2004;13:275–287.

27. Subrahmanyam M. Honey dressings for burns – an appraisal. *Ann Burns Fire Disaster* 1996;1X:33–35.

28. Subrahmanyam M, *et al*. Effect of topical application of honey on burn wound healing. *Ann Burns Fire Disaster* 2001;XIV:143–145.

29. Moore OA, Smith LA, Campbell F, Seers K, McQuay HJ, Moore RA. Systematic review of the use of honey as a wound dressing. *BMC Compl Altern Med* 2001;1:2.

30. Subrahmanyan M. Honey dressings versus boiled potato peel in the treatment of burns: a prospective randomised study. *Burns* 1996;22:491–493.

31. Klasen HJ. Historical review of the use of silver in the treatment of burns, 1: early uses. *Burns* 2000;26:117–130.

32. Thomas S, McCubbinn P. A comparison of the antimicrobial effects of four silver-containing dressings on three organisms. *J Wound Care* 2003;12:101–107.

33. Dowsett C. The use of silver-based dressings in wound care. *Nurs Stand* 2004;19:56–60.

34. Lansdown ABG, Williams A. How safe is silver in wound care? *J Wound Care* 2004;13:131–136.

35. Lansdown ABG, Williams A, Chandler S, Benfield S. Silver absorption and antibacterial efficacy of silver dressings. *J Wound Care* 2005;14:155–160.

36. Lansdown ABG. Silver 1: its antibacterial properties and mechanisms of action. *J Wound Care* 2002;11:125–130.

37. Russell AD, Hugo WB. Antimicrobial activity and action of silver. In: Ellis GP, Luscombe DK, eds. *Progress in Medical Chemistry.* Elsevier Science; 1994:351–369.
38. Rayman G, Rayman A, Baker NR, *et al.* Sustained silver-releasing dressing in the treatment of diabetic foot ulcers. *Br J Nurs* 2005;14:109–114.
39. Thomas S, McCubbin P. An in vitro analysis of the antimicrobial properties of 10 silver containing dressings. *J Wound Care* 2003;12:305–308.
40. Thomas S, Ashman P. In-vitro testing of silver containing dressings. *J Wound Care* 2004;13:392–393.
41. White RJ. An historical overview on the use of silver in modern wound management. *Br J Nurs* 2002;15(silver suppl, pt 1):3–8.
42. Thomas S. MRSA and the use of silver dressings: overcoming bacterial resistance. *World Wide Wounds.Com.* 2004;1–21. Online journal.
43. White RJ. A charcoal dressing with silver in wound infection: clinical evidence. *Br J Nursing* 2002 (silver suppl, pt 2):4–11.
44. Masson E. Silver dressings: healing is a matter of time, and sometimes opportunity. *Diabet Foot* 2005;8:12–17.
45. Lawrence JC. The use of iodine as an antiseptic agent. *J Wound Care* 1998;7:421–425.
46. Higgins DG. Povidine iodine: the tamed iodine. *Chemist Druggist,* Aug 30, 1975;274–275.
47. Michanek A, Hansson C, Berg G, Maneskold-Claes A. Iodine-induced hyperthyroidism after cadexomer iodine treament of leg ulcers. *Lakartidningen* 1998;9:5755–5756.
48. Aronoff GR, Friedman SJ, Doedens DJ, Lavelle KJ. Increased serum iodide absorption through wounds treated topically with povidone iodine. *Am J Med Science* 1980;279:173–176.
49. Sundberg J, Mellor R. A retrospective review of the use of cadexomer iodine in the treatment of chronic wounds. *Wounds* 1997;9:68–86.
50. Gibson H. Iodoflex in the management of chronic wounds. *Diabet Foot* 2001;4:44–46.
51. Bianchi J. Cadexomer-iodine in the treatment of venous leg ulcers: what is the evidence. *J Wound Care* 2001;10:225–229.
52. Hansson C, and the Cadexomer Iodine Study Group. The effects of cadexomer iodine paste in the treatment of venous leg ulcers compared with hydrocolloid dressing and paraffin gauze dressing. *Int J Dermatol* 1998;37:390–396.
53. Apelqvist J, Ragnarson Tennvall G. Cavity foot ulcers in diabetic patients: a comparative study of cadexomer iodine ointment and standard treatment. An economic analysis alongside a clinical trial. *Acta Derm Venereol* 1996;25:89–93.
54. Mertz PM, Oliveira-Gandia MF, Davis SC. The evaluation of a cadexomer iodine wound dressing on methicillin resistant *Staphylococcus aureus* (MRSA) in acute wounds. *Dermatol Surg* 1999;25:89–93.
55. Wilson P, Burroughs D, Dunn LJ. Methicillin-resistant *Staphylococcus aureus* and hydrocolloid dressings. *Pharm J* Dec 1988;787–788.
56. Fisken RA, Digby M. Which dressing for diabetic foot ulcers? *J Br Podiatr Med* 1997;2:20–22.
57. Jones V, Gill D. Hydrocolloid dressings and diabetic foot lesions. *Diabet Foot* 1998;1:127–134.
58. Foster AVM, Spencer S, Edmonds ME. Deterioration of diabetic foot lesions under hydrocolloid dressings. *Pract Diabetes Int* 1997;14:62–64.
59. Lithner F. Adverse effects on diabetic foot ulcers of highly adhesive hydrocolloid occlusive dressings. *Diabetes Care* 1990;13:814–815.
60. Knowles EA, Westwood B, Young MJ, Boulton AJM. A retrospective study of the use of Granuflex and other dressings in the treatment of diabetic foot ulcers. In:*Proceedings of the 3rd European Conference on Advances in Wound Management.* London: Macmillan; 1993:117–120.
61. Gill D. The use of hydrocolloid dressings in the treatment of diabetic foot. *J Wound Care* 1999;8:204–206.
62. Foster AVM, Greenhill MT, Edmonds ME. Comparing two dressings in the treatment of diabetic foot ulcers. *J Wound Care* 1994;3:224–228.

63. Lawrence IG, Lear JT, Burden AC. Alginate dressings and the diabetic foot ulcer. *Pract Diabetes Int* 1997;14:61–62.
64. Jones V. Alginate dressings and diabetic foot lesions. *Diabet Foot* 1999;2;8–14.
65. Jones V. Use of hydrogels and iodine in diabetic foot lesions. *Diabet Foot* 1999; 2:47–54.
66. Williams C. Granugel. Hydrocolloid dressing. *Br J Nurs* 1996;5:188–189.
67. White R. Managing exudate. *Nurs Times 97* 2001;9:X1–X11.
68. Harris A, Rolstad BS. Hypergranulation tissue: a non-traumatic method of management. In: *The 3rd European Conference on Advances in Wound Management Proceedings*. London: Macmillan Magazines; 1992.
69. Veves A, Sheehan P, Pham HT. A randomised controlled trial of promogran vs standard treatment in the management of diabetic foot ulcers. *Arch Surg* 2002;137:822–827.
70. Ghanekar O, Willis M, Persson U. Cost-effectiveness of treating deep diabetic foot ulcers with Promogran in four European countries. *J Wound Care* 2002;11:70–74.
71. Edmonds M, Foster A. Hyalofill: a new product for chronic wound management. *Diabet Foot* 2000;3:29–30.
72. Foster AM, Bates M, Doxford M, Edmonds ME. The treatment of indolent neuropathic ulceration of the diabetic foot with Hyaff. *Diabet Med* 1999;16:94.
73. Vazquez JR, Short B, Findlow AH. Outcomes of hyaluronan therapy in diabetic foot wounds. *Diabetes Res Clin Pract* 2003;59:123–127.
74. Ashton J. Managing leg and foot ulcers: the role of the Kerraboot. *Br J Community Nurs* 2004;9:S26–S30.
75. Edmonds M, Foster A, Jemmott T, *et al*. Randomised study of Kerraboot vs standard wound care in the management of diabetic neuropathic foot ulcers. Presented at: Wounds UK Conference; November 15–17, 2004; Harrogate.
76. Leigh R, Barker S, Murray N, Hurel SJ. The Kerraboot: a novel wound dressing device for the management of leg and foot ulcers. *Pract Diabetes* 2004;21:27–30.
77. Veves A, Falanga V, Armstrong DG, Sabonlinski ML. Apligraf diabetic food Graftskin, a human skin equivalent, is effective in the management of noninfected neuropathic diabetic foot ulcers: a prospective randomised multicenter clinical trial. *Diabetes Care* 2001;24:290–295.
78. Gentzkow G, Iwasaki SD, Horshon KS, *et al*. Use of dermagraft, a cultured human dermis, to treat diabetic foot ulcers. *Diabetes Care* 1996;4:350–354.
79. Williams A, Marston MD. The efficacy and safety of Dermagraft in improving the healing of chronic diabetic foot ulcers. *Diabetes Care* 2003;26:1701–1705.
80. Pham HT, Rich J, Veves A. Using living skin equivalents for diabetic foot ulceration. *Int J Low Extrem Wounds* 2002;1:27–32.
81. Flanagan M. Variables influencing nurses' selection of wound dressings. *J Wound Care* 1992;1:33–34.
82. Jones V. Selecting a dressing for the diabetic foot: factors to consider. *Diabet Foot* 1998;1:48–52.

16 New and Alternative Treatments for the Diabetic Foot: Stem Cells and Gene Transfer

Jeffrey M. Davidson

INTRODUCTION

Advances in molecular and cell biology promise to help us both understand and treat many of the clinical problems in wound healing. The normal progression of events in repair following haemostasis – inflammation, proliferation and remodelling – require the coordinated and sequential activation and inactivation of gene expression programmes in response to signals from the cellular environment. Although it is a major health problem, there are few genetic defects that are directly linked to altered wound healing. The reverse genetic approach in recombinant mice and other species has identified many genes whose over- or under-expression leads, in part, to a wound-healing phenotype.[1,2] These studies, together with detailed, descriptive studies of patterns of gene expression in normal and abnormal healing,[3] have lead to the selection of leading candidates for potential therapeutic application. The first part of this chapter will discuss the rationale, advances and prospects for using gene transfer as a method for wound therapy.

The mention of the stem cell immediately conjures up an image of regeneration, and the concept has been refined over more than one and one-half centuries to include both *totipotential* cells from embryos and other sources that have the capability of developing into all adult tissues, as well as *pluripotential* cells from adult tissues that provide a renewable resource for replacement of select tissues.[4] The first mammalian stem cells to be studied in detail were those of the haematopoietic system, and much is understood about conditions that cause these marrow precursors to differentiate along different pathways in order to maintain appropriate concentrations of a variety of cell populations in circulating blood. Characteristically, these marrow stem cells divide much more slowly than their surrounding, derived cell population, and they remain in a relatively undifferentiated state as long as they reside in an appropriate environment (niche).[5] Similarly, more recent research has refined the concept of the resident stem cell, a subpopulation in various tissues and organs that can potentially be

The Foot in Diabetes, 4th Edition. Editors Andrew J.M. Boulton, Peter R. Cavanagh and Gerry Rayman.
© 2006 John Wiley & Sons, Ltd.

called upon to restore solid tissue after depletion due to damage or disease. The third type of precursor cell to be considered is the marrow-derived tissue progenitor that circulates in the bloodstream, waiting to be called into sites of injury, to participate in the repair process.[6] The second part of this chapter will consider the known and potential role of pluripotential cells in the wound.

GENE TRANSFER TO WOUNDS

By 1990, many investigators had clearly established both an intrinsic and a therapeutic role for peptide growth factors in wound healing, and many biotechnology groups had succeeded in expressing the recombinant proteins as potential therapeutic agents.[7] However, as clinical trials with agents such as epidermal growth factor (EGF), fibroblast growth factor 2 (FGF-2), platelet-derived growth factor (PDGF) and transforming growth factor β (TGF-ß) proceeded, it was quickly appreciated that very high levels of exogenous peptides would be needed in chronic, human wounds to mimic the effects of very small amounts of similar or identical proteins expressed by the resident cells.[8-19] Thus, several groups developed strategies to augment the putative deficiencies of peptide growth factors by introducing cDNA copies of the growth factor genes into target cells at the wound site. There were several supporting principles: (1) the growth factor molecules would be expressed by resident cells rather than being applied to the exterior of a hostile, degradative wound environment; (2) the active principle, regardless of the end product, was DNA; (3) several techniques were available to ensure local delivery and action of the genes in question; (4) unless otherwise desired, the action of the introduced gene would be transient, thus denoting the technique as *gene transfer*, as opposed to the correction of an underlying genetic defect by gene therapy.

There are several potential methods to transfer genes into skin or wounds.[20,21] Physical methods involve driving the DNA vector (a purified bacterial plasmid) into tissue cells with mechanical or electrical force. Successful introduction of biologically active DNA into wounds has been achieved with the 'gene gun', a device that propels small, DNA-coated gold/tungsten particles into the tissue in a shotgun pattern,[22] a needle array that functions much like a tattooing instrument[23] and an electrode array that uses a train of high-voltage pulses to create temporary pores in nearby cells.[24,25] Chemical methods of DNA delivery are less efficient but less expensive, and they have included liposomes, nanoparticles, dried methylcellulose discs and collagen gels or scaffolds. Viruses are natural gene delivery systems.[26] DNA viruses, such as adenovirus, do not insert viral DNA into the host genome, and so they act as transient gene delivery systems. Adenovirus does express proteins that can incite an inflammatory response, and newer vectors have been engineered to minimise this reaction, albeit a minor consideration for wound infection. Adeno-associated virus produces less inflammatory response, although it has limitations in the amount of genetic material it can carry and the cell types that can be infected.[27,28] RNA viruses (retroviruses) such as Moloney sarcoma virus and the lentiviruses act by stable insertion of their genome into the host genome; thus they are more useful for gene therapy applications, in combination with a tissue engineering substitute that has a limited lifespan in the host, or by placing the gene under regulation of a drug. Traditional retroviruses infect only dividing cells, but derivatives of HIV-like lentiviruses are able to infect a wide variety of cell types.[29] Transient transformation of wounds with candidate genes can result in 1–3 weeks of expression, depending on the delivery method and the choice of DNA regulatory sequence. In practice, most current protocols for wound gene transfer employ a strong, promiscuous promoter of gene expression that is derived from cytomegalovirus (CMV). Greater selectivity of gene action can readily be achieved by using gene regulation sequences that are tissue specific or that respond to a drug/hormone such as RU-486 or tamoxifen.[30-32]

Gene transfer has achieved a successful outcome in many pre-clinical models, using cDNAs for EGF, TGF-ß1, PDGF, FGF-2, vascular endothelial growth factor (VEGF), hepatocyte growth factor (HGF) and other peptides in the delivery systems described above.[21] A potentially attractive aspect of gene transfer is the ease of combining two genes into one DNA vector. This may be a way to develop, with a less complicated regulatory pathway, a therapy that capitalises upon the synergistic effects of growth factor or cytokine combinations.[33-35] As another strategy, gene transfer studies have also shown that (wound) cells may benefit from added expression of not only the stimulus, but the receptor for that stimulus and the machinery that transmits signals from the receptor to other cellular machinery. For example, wound healing is enhanced by transfection of the EGF receptor, and wounds expressing higher levels of EGF receptor are more responsive to exogenous EGF.[36] Perhaps, chimaeric vectors that expressed both the factor and its receptor would be far more potent than those that expressed either alone. Gene transfer has recently taken on a role in drug development, since it is a relatively efficient method to screen for genes that have wound-healing properties, independent of a requirement that they act on cells from the outside. Indeed, nuclear transcription factors such as HoxA3,[37] Smads 3 and 7,[38,39] Egr-1,[40] engineered zinc finger proteins[41,42] and cardiac ankyrin repeat protein (CARP)[43] as well as signal transduction molecules such as eps8, which act inside of cells (Y. Shi J.M. Davidson, unpublished), are active in wounds of either normal or diabetic animal, after gene transfer. Gene transfer is thus a powerful screening method for the most effective therapeutic genes.

Two gene therapy clinical trials for wound healing are underway. One is a National Institutes of Health (NIH)-sponsored trial of PDGF-BB delivered by an adenovirus in diabetic foot ulcers.[44] A second, phase I trial has been completed by Tissue Repair Company (formerly Selective Genetics), which administers adenoviral PDGF to diabetic foot ulcers. Positive findings of the latter trial were recently reported at the 2005 annual meeting of the Wound Healing Society. There are also many efforts to use FGF-2 and VEGF[42,45,46] in gene transfer experiments to improve (lower extremity) circulation. It is likely that success in these trials would have an important influence on the management and prognosis of the diabetic foot ulcer. Additional trials with FGF-2 and VEGF genes or proteins for the development of collateral circulation (usually cardiovascular) may eventually have an impact on improving collateral circulation in the diabetic limb.

STEM CELLS

There has been an explosive growth of information and speculation regarding the therapeutic potential of stem cells derived from adult and embryonic tissues.[47] A more conservative perspective focuses on the role of adult stem cells in wound repair. The present concept of stem cell differentiation is evolving, however, since progenitor cells from many tissues seem to be able to transdifferentiate into other cell types when placed in an appropriate environment. DNA transfer must be carefully ruled out to validate these findings. There are three categories of bone-marrow-derived cells that participate in the repair of connective tissue: (1) the angioblast or endothelial precursor cell (EPC); (2) the fibrocyte; (3) the marrow/mesenchymal stem cell (MSC). Epithelial layers, in general, harbour resident stem cells.

The EPC is derived from a primitive haematopoietic cell in the bone marrow, prior to differentiation into the leucocyte lineage. It was first reported in 1997 as a cell type that could be isolated from circulating blood, cultivated *in vitro*, transplanted into a syngeneic host and localised to vascular structures.[48] Further work has decisively demonstrated that EPCs are recruited from the bloodstream at many sites of vasculogenesis, that is the *de novo* formation of new capillaries. EPCs are recruited to sites of repair or vessel growth by VEGF[49] and stromal-cell-derived factor (SDF).[50,51] These factors may also be involved in the mobilisation of the precursors from the marrow.[52] EPCs are not true stem cells, since they are apparently committed to the endothelial lineage while in circulation. For this reason, such cells can be purified from whole blood, based on their expression of the VEGF receptor 2 (flk-1) and the angiopoietin 1 receptor (tie-2). The haemangioblast and a more primitive progenitor, the multipotent adult progenitor cell (MAPC), have been suggested as the marrow-based precursors.[53]

The fibrocyte, first described in 1994, is a leucocyte-like cell that infiltrates wounds during the inflammatory phase, produces collagen and has many characteristics of the antigen-presenting, dendritic cell.[54–56] This cell type can produce many cytokines, collagen and growth factors, and its presence has been associated with fibrotic conditions. Adoptive bone marrow transplantation confirms that these cells arrive in the circulation from the bone marrow.

The MSC is another circulating, marrow-derived cell that was initially described by Friedenstein in 1976 in the marrow space.[57,58] It is a pluripotential stem cell, in that it can be isolated from marrow and grown for many generations *in vitro*, and MSC can be induced to differentiate into many types of mesodermal derivatives, including bone, cartilage, skeletal muscle and adipose.[59] MSCs traffic to many different connective tissues,[60–63] and recent studies in a mouse model from this laboratory have shown that MSCs constitute a significant proportion of the collagen-producing, fibroblastic population in a healing wound.[64]

At present, it is not known whether these circulating sources of stem/precursor cells may be rate limiting for wound-healing processes. Patients undergoing immunosuppressive therapy are certainly at risk for healing problems due to infection, but marrow-derived mesenchymal cells may be more resistant. Ageing may affect the availability and regenerative capacity of stem cells. It is conceivable that we will be able to identify the factors that mobilise stem/precursor cells from the marrow and that stimulate their recruitment to sites of injury.[65] There is not a great deal of evidence that these marrow-derived cells take up *permanent* residence in tissues. They may be largely important during phases of acute repair where local proliferation cannot meet tissue needs.[64,66] It has recently come to light that many connective tissues do harbour pluripotential stem cell populations, including dermis,[67,68] adipose[69–73] and skeletal muscle.[74] These may be alternative sources of stem cells for therapeutic applications.

Many epithelial tissues have much higher rates of cellular turnover and renewal, and resident stem cells are localised to specific areas. In the epidermis, stem cell populations have been identified in the bulge region of the hair follicle [75] and in the interfollicular zone.[76] The interfollicular cells represent a subset of the epidermal basal cells that undergo differentiation as they detach from the basal lamina and move towards the stratum corneum. While it has been difficult to identify specific surface characteristics that could aid in epidermal stem cell purification,[77,78] it is likely that these cells provide a significant fraction of the dividing keratinocytes in cultures that have been used to generate skin substitutes. There are several reports that indicate that these stem cells may be multipotent, and there are also reports that marrow-derived cells can be recruited through the bloodstream and participate in epidermal structure.[79]

The clinical application of stem cells is well advanced for the treatment of corneal stem cell deficiency, chemical burns and several disease states.[80,81] This procedure uses a population of epithelial stem cells from the corneal limbus for engraftment. Both unfractionated bone marrow as well as purified MSC from marrow and connective tissue sources have been evaluated in many forms of tissue repair: skin, bone, teeth, cartilage and tendon. There have been only a few attempts to apply MSC to wounds: one study simply used whole marrow populations on three non-healing wounds with a favourable outcome[82]; another study reported improved healing on systemic injection of a dermal MSC population[67]; there is also a report of MSC effects in deep burn wounds in rats. The principal development of the MSC has been in the context of tissue engineering devices, frequently combined with gene transfer to the cells, to convert the device into a drug delivery system. Favourable repair results have been obtained in bone and cartilage, and there is every reason to expect that living skin equivalents so engineered could enhance wound healing. It is as yet unclear whether MSC *per se* will be valuable for wound therapy. Strategies that improve their recruitment or growth may be effective.

Since the vascular supply is often rate limiting for repair, EPCs also offer therapeutic potential.[83] Agents that recruit EPC, such as VEGF,[52] also increase vascularity and other aspects of wound healing.[49] EPCs are readily purified from whole blood by apheresis techniques. Pre-clinical studies suggest that these cells and the factors that recruit them can reverse tissue ischaemia. A recent study reports that purified human EPCs enhanced wound repair in the athymic nude mouse, increased vascularity and macrophage influx and occasionally became incorporated into patent, hCD-31 positive vessels.[84]

SUMMARY

Gene transfer and applications of progenitor cells are two advanced technologies with great promise in wound healing and tissue repair applications. Safety issues have slowed the commercial development of gene transfer, but active trials are underway. This strategy is likely to overcome many of the drawbacks of recombinant proteins at potentially lower cost. Stem cell therapies with autologous grafting are likely to be accepted more easily by the medical and regulatory communities. Factors that regulate the mobilisation, recruitment and differentiation of progenitors will also play an important role. Many of these findings will find their way into the development of more effective tissue engineering devices. The combination of these two strategies has even greater potential, since it would lead to the design of medical devices that contained multipotential cells that were capable of delivering specific gene products.

REFERENCES

1. Grose R, Werner S. Wound-healing studies in transgenic and knockout mice. *Mol Biotechnol* 2004;28:147–166.
2. Grose R, Werner S. Wound healing studies in transgenic and knockout mice. A review. *Methods Mol Med* 2003;78:191–216.
3. Werner S, Grose R. Regulation of wound healing by growth factors and cytokines. *Physiol Rev* 2003;83:835–870.
4. Conrad C, Huss R. Adult stem cell lines in regenerative medicine and reconstructive surgery. *J Surg Res* 2005;124:201–208.
5. Li L, Xie T. Stem cell niche: Structure and function. *Annu Rev Cell Dev Biol* 2005;21:605–631.

6. Hennessy B, Korbling M, Estrov Z. Circulating stem cells and tissue repair. *Panminerva Med* 2004;46:1–11.
7. Martin P, Hopkinson-Woolley J, McCluskey J. Growth factors and cutaneous wound repair. *Prog Growth Factor Res* 1992;4:25–44.
8. Finch PW, Rubin JS. Keratinocyte growth factor/fibroblast growth factor 7, a homeostatic factor with therapeutic potential for epithelial protection and repair. *Adv Cancer Res* 2004;91:69–136.
9. Sibbald RG, Torrance G, Hux M, Attard C, Milkovich N. Cost-effectiveness of becaplermin for nonhealing neuropathic diabetic foot ulcers. *Ostomy Wound Manage* 2003;49:76–84.
10. Landi F, *et al.* Topical treatment of pressure ulcers with nerve growth factor: a randomized clinical trial. *Ann Intern Med* 2003;139:635–641.
11. Shackelford DP, Fackler E, Hoffman MK, Atkinson S. Use of topical recombinant human platelet-derived growth factor BB in abdominal wound separation. *Am J Obstet Gynecol* 2002;186:701–704.
12. Mandracchia VJ, Sanders SM, Frerichs JA. The use of becaplermin (rhPDGF-BB) gel for chronic nonhealing ulcers. A retrospective analysis. *Clin Podiatr Med Surg* 2001;18:189–209, viii.
13. Payne WG, *et al.* Long-term outcome study of growth factor-treated pressure ulcers. *Am J Surg* 2001;181:81–86.
14. Kallianinen LK, Hirshberg J, Marchant B, Rees RS. Role of platelet-derived growth factor as an adjunct to surgery in the management of pressure ulcers. *Plast Reconstr Surg* 2000;106:1243–1248.
15. Fu X, *et al.* Randomised placebo-controlled trial of use of topical recombinant bovine basic fibroblast growth factor for second-degree burns. *Lancet* 1998;352:1661–1664.
16. Piascik P. Use of Regranex gel for diabetic foot ulcers. *J Am Pharm Assoc (Wash)* 1998;38:628–630.
17. Fricker J. Keratinocyte growth factor on trial for wound repair. *Mol Med Today* 1998;4:229.
18. Rieck P, *et al.* Recombinant human basic fibroblast growth factor (Rh-bFGF) in three different wound models in rabbits: corneal wound healing effect and pharmacology. *Exp Eye Res* 1992;54:987–998.
19. Brown GL, *et al.* Enhancement of wound healing by topical treatment with epidermal growth factor. *N Engl J Med* 1989;321:76–79.
20. Petrie NC, Yao F, Eriksson E. Gene therapy in wound healing. *Surg Clin North Am* 2003;83:597–616, vii.
21. Eming SA, Krieg T, Davidson JM. Gene transfer in tissue repair: status, challenges and future directions. *Expert Opin Biol Ther* 2004;4:1373–1386.
22. Davidson JM, Krieg T, Eming SA. Particle-mediated gene therapy of wounds. *Wound Repair Regen* 2000;8:452–459.
23. Eriksson E, *et al.* In vivo gene transfer to skin and wound by microseeding. *J Surg Res* 1998;78:85–91.
24. Marti G, *et al.* Electroporative transfection with KGF-1 DNA improves wound healing in a diabetic mouse model. *Gene Ther* 2004;11:1780–1785.
25. Byrnes CK, *et al.* Electroporation enhances transfection efficiency in murine cutaneous wounds. *Wound Repair Regen* 2004;12:397–403.
26. Crombleholme TM. Adenoviral-mediated gene transfer in wound healing. *Wound Repair Regen* 2000;8:460–472.
27. Lu Y. Recombinant adeno-associated virus as delivery vector for gene therapy – a review. *Stem Cells Dev* 2004;13:133–145.
28. Flotte TR. Gene therapy progress and prospects: recombinant adeno-associated virus (rAAV) vectors. *Gene Ther* 2004;11:805–810.
29. Brenner S, Malech HL. Current developments in the design of onco-retrovirus and lentivirus vector systems for hematopoietic cell gene therapy. *Biochim Biophys Acta* 2003;1640:1–24.
30. Siprashvili Z, Khavari PA. Lentivectors for regulated and reversible cutaneous gene delivery. *Mol Ther* 2004;9:93–100.
31. Cao T, Longley MA, Wang XJ, Roop DR. An inducible mouse model for epidermolysis bullosa simplex: implications for gene therapy. *J Cell Biol* 2001;152:651–656.
32. Arin MJ, Longley MA, Wang XJ, Roop DR. Focal activation of a mutant allele defines the role of stem cells in mosaic skin disorders. *J Cell Biol* 2001;152:645–649.

33. Lynch SE, *et al.* Effects of the platelet-derived growth factor/insulin-like growth factor-I combination on bone regeneration around titanium dental implants. Results of a pilot study in beagle dogs. *J Periodontol* 1991;62:710–716.

34. Ono I, *et al.* Combined administration of basic fibroblast growth factor protein and the hepatocyte growth factor gene enhances the regeneration of dermis in acute incisional wounds. *Wound Repair Regen* 2004;12:67–79.

35. Broadley KN, *et al.* The diabetic rat as an impaired wound healing model: stimulatory effects of transforming growth factor-beta and basic fibroblast growth factor. *Biotechnol Ther* 1989;1:55–68.

36. Nanney LB, *et al.* Boosting epidermal growth factor receptor expression by gene gun transfection stimulates epidermal growth in vivo. *Wound Repair Regen* 2000;8:117–127.

37. Mace KA, Hansen SL, Myers C, Young DM, Boudreau N. HOXA3 induces cell migration in endothelial and epithelial cells promoting angiogenesis and wound repair. *J Cell Sci* 2005;118:2567–2577.

38. Saika S, *et al.* Transient adenoviral gene transfer of Smad7 prevents injury-induced epithelial-mesenchymal transition of lens epithelium in mice. *Lab Invest* 2004;84:1259–1270.

39. Flanders KC. Smad3 as a mediator of the fibrotic response. *Int J Exp Pathol* 2004;85:47–64.

40. Bryant M, *et al.* Tissue repair with a therapeutic transcription factor. *Hum Gene Ther* 2000;11:2143–2158.

41. Rebar EJ, *et al.* Induction of angiogenesis in a mouse model using engineered transcription factors. *Nat Med* 2002;8:1427–1432.

42. Romano Di Peppe S, *et al.* Adenovirus-mediated VEGF(165) gene transfer enhances wound healing by promoting angiogenesis in CD1 diabetic mice. *Gene Ther* 2002;9:1271–1277.

43. Shi Y, *et al.* CARP, a cardiac ankyrin repeat protein, is up-regulated during wound healing and induces angiogenesis in experimental granulation tissue. *Am J Pathol* 2005;166:303–312.

44. Margolis DJ, *et al.* Clinical protocol. Phase I trial to evaluate the safety of H5.020CMV.PDGF-b and limb compression bandage for the treatment of venous leg ulcer: trial A. *Hum Gene Ther* 2004;15:1003–1019.

45. Fujihara Y, Koyama H, Nishiyama N, Eguchi T, Takato T. Gene transfer of bFGF to recipient bed improves survival of ischemic skin flap. *Br J Plast Surg* 2005;58:511–517.

46. Caron A, *et al.* Human FGF-1 gene transfer promotes the formation of collateral vessels and arterioles in ischemic muscles of hypercholesterolemic hamsters. *J Gene Med* 2004;6:1033–1045.

47. Weissman IL. Translating stem and progenitor cell biology to the clinic: barriers and opportunities. *Science* 2000;287:1442–1446.

48. Asahara T, *et al.* Isolation of putative progenitor endothelial cells for angiogenesis. *Science* 1997;275:964–967.

49. Galiano RD, *et al.* Topical vascular endothelial growth factor accelerates diabetic wound healing through increased angiogenesis and by mobilizing and recruiting bone marrow-derived cells. *Am J Pathol* 2004;164:1935–1947.

50. Ceradini DJ, Gurtner GC. Homing to hypoxia: HIF-1 as a mediator of progenitor cell recruitment to injured tissue. *Trends Cardiovasc Med* 2005;15:57–63.

51. Vandervelde S, van Luyn MJ, Tio RA, Harmsen MC. Signaling factors in stem cell-mediated repair of infarcted myocardium. *J Mol Cell Cardiol* 2005;39:363–376.

52. Young PP, Hofling AA, Sands MS. VEGF increases engraftment of bone marrow-derived endothelial progenitor cells (EPCs) into vasculature of newborn murine recipients. *Proc Natl Acad Sci USA* 2002;99:11951–11956.

53. Verfaillie CM. Multipotent adult progenitor cells: an update. *Novartis Found Symp* 2005;265:55–61; discussion 61–65, 92–97.

54. Quan TE, Cowper S, Wu SP, Bockenstedt LK, Bucala R. Circulating fibrocytes: collagen-secreting cells of the peripheral blood. *Int J Biochem Cell Biol* 2004;36:598–606.

55. Abe R, Donnelly SC, Peng T, Bucala R, Metz CN. Peripheral blood fibrocytes: differentiation pathway and migration to wound sites. *J Immunol* 2001;166:7556–7562.

56. Bucala R, Spiegel LA, Chesney J, Hogan M, Cerami A. Circulating fibrocytes define a new leukocyte subpopulation that mediates tissue repair. *Mol Med* 1994;1:71–81.

57. Friedenstein AJ. Marrow stromal fibroblasts. *Calcif Tissue Int* 1995;56:S17.

58. Friedenstein AJ, Gorskaja JF, Kulagina NN. Fibroblast precursors in normal and irradiated mouse hematopoietic organs. *Exp Hematol* 1976;4:267–274.

59. Pittenger MF, *et al.* Multilineage potential of adult human mesenchymal stem cells. *Science* 1999;284:143–147.

60. Abedin M, Tintut Y, Demer LL. Mesenchymal stem cells and the artery wall. *Circ Res* 2004;95:671–676.

61. Roufosse CA, Direkze NC, Otto WR, Wright NA. Circulating mesenchymal stem cells. *Int J Biochem Cell Biol* 2004;36:585–597.

62. Kuwana M, *et al.* Human circulating CD14+ monocytes as a source of progenitors that exhibit mesenchymal cell differentiation. *J Leukoc Biol* 2003;74:833–845.

63. Hayakawa J, Migita M, Ueda T, Shimada T, Fukunaga Y. Generation of a chimeric mouse reconstituted with green fluorescent protein-positive bone marrow cells: a useful model for studying the behavior of bone marrow cells in regeneration in vivo. *Int J Hematol* 2003;77:456–462.

64. Opalenik SR, Davidson JM. Fibroblast differentiation of bone marrow-derived cells during wound repair. *FASEB J* 2005;19:1561–1563.

65. Neuss S, Becher E, Woltje M, Tietze L, Jahnen-Dechent W. Functional expression of HGF and HGF receptor/c-met in adult human mesenchymal stem cells suggests a role in cell mobilization, tissue repair, and wound healing. *Stem Cells* 2004;22:405–414.

66. Borue X, *et al.* Bone marrow-derived cells contribute to epithelial engraftment during wound healing. *Am J Pathol* 2004;165:1767–1772.

67. Chunmeng S, *et al.* Effects of dermal multipotent cell transplantation on skin wound healing. *J Surg Res* 2004;121:13–19.

68. Shi C, *et al.* Transplantation of dermal multipotent cells promotes survival and wound healing in rats with combined radiation and wound injury. *Radiat Res* 2004;162:56–63.

69. Cao Y, *et al.* Human adipose tissue-derived stem cells differentiate into endothelial cells in vitro and improve postnatal neovascularization in vivo. *Biochem Biophys Res Commun* 2005;332:370–379.

70. Rodriguez AM, Elabd C, Amri EZ, Ailhaud G, Dani C. The human adipose tissue is a source of multipotent stem cells. *Biochimie* 2005;87:125–128.

71. Gimble JM, Guilak F. Differentiation potential of adipose derived adult stem (ADAS) cells. *Curr Top Dev Biol* 2003;58:137–160.

72. Gimble J, Guilak F. Adipose-derived adult stem cells: isolation, characterization, and differentiation potential. *Cytotherapy* 2003;5:362–369.

73. Zuk PA, *et al.* Human adipose tissue is a source of multipotent stem cells. *Mol Biol Cell* 2002;13:4279–4295.

74. Peng H, *et al.* Synergistic enhancement of bone formation and healing by stem cell-expressed VEGF and bone morphogenetic protein-4. *J Clin Invest* 2002;110:751–759.

75. Lavker RM, *et al.* Hair follicle stem cells. *J Investig Dermatol Symp Proc* 2003;8:28–38.

76. Watt FM. The stem cell compartment in human interfollicular epidermis. *J Dermatol Sci* 2002;28:173–180.

77. Benitah SA, Frye M, Glogauer M, Watt FM. Stem cell depletion through epidermal deletion of Rac1. *Science* 2005;309:933–935.

78. Watt FM. Role of integrins in regulating epidermal adhesion, growth and differentiation. *Embo J* 2002;21:3919–3926.

79. Badiavas EV, Abedi M, Butmarc J, Falanga V, Quesenberry P. Participation of bone marrow derived cells in cutaneous wound healing. *J Cell Physiol* 2003;196:245–250.

80. Agrawal VB, Tsai RJ. Corneal epithelial wound healing. *Indian J Ophthalmol* 2003;51:5–15.

81. Lavker RM, Tseng SC, Sun TT. Corneal epithelial stem cells at the limbus: looking at some old problems from a new angle. *Exp Eye Res* 2004;78:433–446.

82. Badiavas EV, Falanga V. Treatment of chronic wounds with bone marrow-derived cells. *Arch Dermatol* 2003;139:510–516.

83. Hristov M, Weber C. Endothelial progenitor cells: characterization, pathophysiology, and possible clinical relevance. *J Cell Mol Med* 2004;8:498–508.

84. Suh W, *et al.* Transplantation of endothelial progenitor cells accelerates dermal wound healing with increased recruitment of monocytes/macrophages and neovascularization. *Stem Cells* 2005;23:1571–1578.

17 An Introduction to Larval Therapy

Stephen Thomas

Maggots are living chemical factories that produce a complex mixture of biologically active molecules. Clinical experience with maggots over hundreds of years has generally been positive, and the wealth of recorded observations concerning the ability of these creatures to debride wounds, combat infection and stimulate healing is gradually beginning to be substantiated by structured clinical investigations.

Although larval therapy has been used for all types of chronic wounds, the technique is of particular value in the treatment of the diabetic foot. In many cases, the maggots are able to remove all traces of necrotic tissue and eliminate wound infections in a fraction of the time taken by conventional therapies. The procedure may often be carried out in the patient's own home thus reducing or eliminating the need for hospitalisation, with important implications for overall treatment costs.

INTRODUCTION

Wound bed preparation, including the removal of infected and necrotic tissue, is a key stage in the management of all types of wounds,[1] but nowhere is this process more important than in the treatment of the diabetic foot.

If surgical intervention is not an option, an alternative method of wound debridement must be adopted that should meet certain key performance requirements. Specifically, the selected technique should be rapid, painless and easily employed with minimal training. It should also not damage healthy or peri-wound tissue, or pose a health or infection risk to the patient, the operator or others in the vicinity. The chosen technique should also not impact significantly upon a patient's mobility or quality of life.

Within the last decade, sterile maggots have become accepted as a valuable resource for the debridement of all types of infected and necrotic wounds, including the diabetic foot, as they appear to meet most or all of the requirements of the ideal wound-cleansing therapy identified above.[2]

The clinical use of maggots is not new, as they were widely used in the first half of the twentieth century as a treatment for osteomyelitis and soft tissue infections, but the popularity

The Foot in Diabetes, 4th Edition. Editors Andrew J.M. Boulton, Peter R. Cavanagh and Gerry Rayman.

of the technique declined in the 1940s with the introduction of antibiotics that appeared to offer an easier and more aesthetically acceptable form of treatment for serious wound infections.

The revival of maggot therapy (also known as larval therapy) began in the United States in 1983 when Sherman *et al.* used maggots for treating pressure ulcers in persons who had suffered spinal cord injuries.[3] This was followed by further reports of the use of larval therapy in podiatry[4] and recurrent venous ulceration.[5] Sterile maggots under the brand name of *LarvE* were reintroduced into Europe in 1995 by the Biosurgical Research Unit, now ZooBiotic Ltd.[6] Since that time, over 50 000 containers of maggots have been supplied to an estimated 20 000 patients in some 2000 centres throughout the United Kingdom.

FREQUENTLY ASKED QUESTIONS CONCERNING MAGGOT THERAPY

What Type of Maggots Are Used for Larval Therapy

The maggots generally employed are those of *Lucilia sericata,* a member of the family Calliphoridae.[7] The adult insects are a metallic coppery green colour, hence the common name 'greenbottles'.

How Do Maggots Function?

Maggots remove dead tissue by the production of a complex mixture of proteolytic enzymes that break down dead tissue to a semi-liquid form that is subsequently ingested by the creatures. It has also been demonstrated that maggots produce a natural 'growth factor' that has been shown to stimulate fibroblast growth *in vitro,*[8] and secrete a natural antibiotic-like molecule that inhibits the growth of many microorganisms. Furthermore, it has been shown that bacteria that are not killed by the maggots' secretions are ingested by feeding larvae,[9] and killed as they pass through the insects' guts.[10,11]

Although larvae are generally applied to cleanse wounds in order to promote healing, they have also been used to improve the quality of life of patients for whom healing is not a realistic option. In such situations, it has been reported that they can eliminate odour and reduce wound-related pain.[12]

It has also been suggested that the use of maggots effectively prepares the wound bed for grafting or the application of other sophisticated preparations or dressing treatments.

Can Maggot Damage Healthy Tissues?

It is believed that in human wounds, the proteolytic enzymes produced by *Lucilia sericata* are inactivated by enzyme inhibitors in the living tissue that are not present in necrotic tissue or slough. This means that although the maggots' secretions can rapidly degrade dead or devitalised material such as necrotic tissue or keratinised epidermis, they will not harm healthy living tissue.

How Are Maggots Applied?

Maggots can be either placed directly into a wound and allowed to wander freely in search of food, or contained in a bag made from fine net or foam that facilitates both application and removal. Although confining the maggots in this way enhances their clinical acceptability, available evidence strongly suggests that this method of application also markedly reduces their clinical effectiveness and increases the time taken to achieve successful debridement.

Various techniques have been described for retaining free-range maggots within a wound.[5,13,14] In the main, these rely upon the use of a piece of sterile net anchored to a suitable substrate applied to the area surrounding the wound to form a simple enclosure, or the use of a net boot or sleeve for more extensive wounds. A piece of moist gauze is then applied over the net to prevent the young maggots from drying out in the early stages of treatment, followed by a simple absorbent pad to complete the dressing system.

The adhesive substrate, which may consist of a hydrocolloid dressing, a zinc paste bandage or some other suitable alternative, fulfils three important functions. It provides a sound base for the net, protects the skin from the potent proteolytic enzymes produced by the maggots and prevents any tickling sensation caused by the creatures wandering over the intact skin surrounding the area of the wound. If maggots are applied to the toes, or between them, it is prudent to protect the adjacent toes with a suitable barrier cream, pieces of zinc paste bandage or small amount of alginate fibre to absorb any excess secretions.

How Long Should Maggots Be Left on the Wound?

Maggots are generally left in place for about 3 days by which time they are normally fully grown, but some centres leave them *in situ* longer than this, particularly if the patient is insensate. Because the retention net is partially transparent, the activity of the larvae can be monitored without removing the primary dressing, but the outer absorbent dressing can be changed as often as required.

How Many Applications of Maggots Are Generally Required?

Treatment duration varies according to the severity of the wound and the number of larvae applied. A small wound may require only one application lasting 3 days, but extended treatment times may be required for more extensive wounds containing large amounts of necrotic tissue. Experience suggests that the continued application of maggots to a chronic or indolent wound following complete debridement will help to prevent further infection and may actually promote healing.

Is Maggot Activity Adversely Affected by the Concurrent Use of Antibiotics or Other Treatments?

Studies have shown that maggots are unaffected by the concurrent administration of most systemic antibiotics,[15] but unconfirmed observations suggest that they do not appear to survive well in patients receiving topical or systemic metronidazole. Residues of some hydrogel dressings within the wound may also have an adverse effect upon maggot development.[16] Unpublished studies have shown that larvae appear to be unaffected by X-rays and therefore do not need to be removed from a wound for this purpose.

What Clinical Evidence Is Available to Support the Use of Maggots

Although the literature contains a wealth of evidence that describes the clinical effectiveness of maggots across a range of wound types, much of this is anecdotal or limited to case reports or small uncontrolled studies. Nevertheless in many of these studies, the speed of debridement reported with maggot therapy is often quite remarkable and undoubtedly much faster than is generally achieved using autolytic techniques. A comprehensive review of the subject area has been published previously.[17]

Are Any Side Effects Associated with the Use of Maggots?

A review of the literature has revealed no significant risks causally linked to the clinical application of sterile maggots of *L. sericata* when used as directed, although increased wound pain has been reported in some instances, particularly in the case of ischaemic leg ulcers.

Can Maggots Combat Wound Odour?

Slough and necrotic tissue support the proliferation of proteolytic bacteria that produce volatile amines which are responsible for the unpleasant smell associated with some types of wounds. Maggots, like any other effective debridement technique that removes the necrotic material and associated bacteria, will help to reduce or eliminate wound odour.

Can You Feel Maggots Moving in a Wound?

Most people are unaware of the presence of maggots within their wound, although a small number of patients claim that they can feel them. If full-grown maggots are allowed to get onto intact skin surrounding a wound they may tickle, but this can be easily prevented by the application of an appropriate dressing system.

Will Maggots Burrow into Healthy Tissue?

The maggots of *L. sericata* will not attack or burrow into healthy tissue, although the proteolytic enzymes that they produce can occasionally cause irritation to unprotected skin.

Will Maggots Turn into Flies Within a Wound?

It takes about 10–14 days for a newly hatched maggot to complete its life cycle and turn into a fly. Dressings should be changed every 3–4 days so that the fully grown larvae are removed well before they are ready to pupate. Furthermore, the larvae like somewhere dry to pupate and so they will attempt to leave the moist environment of the wound in order to do so.

Will Maggots Lay Eggs in the Wound?

Only adult flies can reproduce or lay eggs.

Can Maggots Be Used Under Compression Bandages?

In most instances, the application of a compression bandage should not interfere with the action of maggots, provided they receive sufficient air to breathe.

When Should I Stop Using Maggots?

Most practitioners stop when the wound is clean and free of necrotic tissue, but there is some evidence to suggest that, for chronic wounds, it may be beneficial to continue the treatment, possibly with smaller numbers of maggots, until granulation is well established.

Do I Have to Count the Maggots into and out of the Wound?

Some practitioners have suggested that maggots should be counted into and out of a wound to ensure that they have all been removed. This is totally unnecessary. Furthermore, it is not uncommon for a proportion of the maggots that are applied to a wound to fail to survive. This means that even if it were possible to count large numbers of maggots into a wound, an almost impossible task, this number would not correlate with the number of full-grown maggots that were recovered after several days of treatment.

Do I Need to 'Water' the Maggots on a Daily Basis?

Some practitioners recommend that the completed dressing should be moistened on a daily basis to prevent the maggots from drying out, as described previously. Although very young maggots are quite delicate and susceptible to desiccation, after about the first 24 h they become much more resistant to dehydration and generally do not require the application of any additional liquid.

Are There Any Activities That Should Be Avoided During Treatment with Maggots?

Patients undergoing treatment with maggots should not immerse their wound in water or sit with the affected area too close to a source of heat, particularly in the first 24 h after application, as there is a possibility that the maggots might dry out and die. Care should also be taken when maggots are applied to weight-bearing areas such as the feet or buttocks. Ambulant patients receiving maggot therapy on a leg ulcer, for example, may continue to live normally and go about their daily business as usual.

Do Maggots Affect Wound Pain?

In some instances, it has been reported that wound pain is reduced following the application of maggots, probably due to the elimination of infection, which is responsible for the formation of inflammatory mediators. In some wounds, however, pain may be *increased* by the presence of maggots. Patients who have leg ulcers with a significant arterial component sometimes report that their wounds become more painful on the second or third day of therapy. The reason for this is not certain, but it may be associated with pH changes within the wound. In such situations, it is recommended that the maggots be removed after 2 days instead of 3, and that the patient's analgesia be reviewed.

Are Maggots Effective Against All Types of Wound Infections?

Maggots appear to be effective in most types of infected wounds, although their secretions appear to more effective against Gram-positive than Gram-negative organisms.[18] Published data also suggest that they are even effective against antibiotic-resistant strains such as methicillin-resistant *Staphylococcus aureus*.[19–21] Wounds containing large numbers of *Pseudomonas* sp. may require a higher density of maggots to eliminate infections caused by these microorganisms.

REFERENCES

1. Falanga V. Classifications for wound bed preparation and stimulation of chronic wounds. *Wound Repair Regen* 2001;8:347–352.
2. Thomas S. Sterile maggots and the preparation of the wound bed. In: Cherry G, Harding KG, Ryan TJ, eds. *Wound bed preparation*. London: Royal Society of Medicine Press; 2001:59–65.
3. Sherman RA, Wyle F, Vulpe M. Maggot therapy for treating pressure ulcers in spinal cord injury patients. *J Spinal Cord Med* 1995;18:71–74.
4. Stoddard SR, Sherman RM, Mason BE, Pelsang DJ. Maggot debridement therapy – an alternative treatment for nonhealing ulcers. *J Am Podiatr Med Assoc* 1995;85:218–221.
5. Sherman RA, My-Tien-Tran J, Sullivan R. Maggot therapy for venous stasis ulcers. *Arch Dermatol* 1996;132:254–256.
6. Thomas S, Jones M, Andrews A. The use of fly larvae in the treatment of wounds. *Nurs Stand* 1997;12:54–59.

7. Crosskey RW. Introduction to the Diptera. In: Lane RP, Crosskey RW, eds. *Medical Insects and Arachnids*. London: Chapman & Hall; 1995.
8. Prete P. Growth effects of *Phaenicia sericata* larval extracts on fibroblasts: mechanism for wound healing by maggot therapy. *Life Sci* 1997;60:505–510.
9. Lerch K, Linde HJ, Lehn N, Grifka J. Bacteria ingestion by blowfly larvae: an in vitro study. *Dermatology* 2003;207:362–366.
10. Robinson W, Norwood VH. Destruction of pyogenic bacteria in the alimentary tract of surgical maggots implanted in infected wounds. *J Lab Clin Med* 1934;19:581–586.
11. Mumcuoglu KY, Miller J, Mumcuoglu M, Friger M, Tarshis M. Destruction of bacteria in the digestive tract of the maggot of *Lucilia sericata* (Diptera: Calliphoridae). *J Med Entomol* 2001;38:161–166.
12. Evans H. A treatment of last resort. *Nurs Times* 1997;93:62–64, 65.
13. Armstrong DG, Mossel J, Short B, Nixon BP, Knowles EA, Boulton AJM. Maggot debridement therapy A primer. *J Am Podiatr Med Assoc* 2002;92:398–401.
14. Thomas S, Jones M, Andrews AM. The use of larval therapy in wound management. *J Wound Care* 1998;7:521–524.
15. Sherman RA, Wyle FA, Thrupp L. Effects of seven antibiotics on the growth and development of *Phaenicia sericata* (Diptera: Calliphoridae) larvae. *J Med Entomol* 1995;32:646–649.
16. Thomas S, Andrews AM. The effect of hydrogel dressings on maggot development. *J Wound Care* 1999;8:75–77.
17. Sherman RA, Hall MJ, Thomas S. Medicinal maggots: an ancient remedy for some contemporary afflictions. *Annu Rev Entomol* 2000;45:55–81.
18. Steenvoorde P, Jukema GN. The antimicrobial activity of maggots: in-vivo results. *J Tissue Viability* 2004;14:97–101.
19. Thomas S, Jones M. *Maggots and the Battle Against MRSA*. Bridgend: The Surgical Material Testing Laboratory; 2000.
20. Bexfield A, Nigam Y, Thomas S, Ratcliffe NA. Detection and partial characterisation of two antibacterial factors from the excretions/secretions of the medicinal maggot *Lucilia sericata* and their activity against methicillin-resistant *Staphylococcus aureus* (MRSA). *Microbes Infect* 2004;6:1297–304.
21. Armstrong J, Zhang L, McClellan AD. Axonal regeneration of descending and ascending spinal projection neurons in spinal cord-transected larval lamprey. *Exp Neurol* 2003;180:156–166.

18 New and Alternative Treatments for Diabetic Foot Ulcers: Hormones and Growth Factors

Matthew J. Hardman and Gillian S. Ashcroft

In diabetic patients, the major underlying causal changes that lead to foot ulcers are neuropathy and ischaemia. Impaired pain sensation often leads to patients inadvertently injuring their foot, whilst changes in local circulation increase the risk of infection and reduce tissue oxygenation. These and other local changes are responsible for converting an acute wound into a chronic non-healing ulcer. Current best practice involves wound assessment/classification, offloading of pressure, debridement and control of infection. However, despite these measures, a significant proportion of wounds fail to heal, ultimately leading to amputation, highlighting the need for new and improved therapies. This chapter will outline the role of hormones and growth factors during normal and perturbed wound healing. The current use of hormones and growth factors will be summarised and future prospects for treatments of non-healing diabetic wounds discussed.

INTRODUCTION

Under normal circumstances an acute wound heals via a carefully orchestrated series of overlapping events, involving multiple cell types. These complex and diverse local cellular changes are controlled by an equally complex extracellular milieu of locally synthesised cytokines, growth factors and newly deposited extracellular matrix (ECM). Specific cell types exhibit changes in morphology, function and gene expression, in response to a range of extracellular factors (Table 18.1). A healing wound represents a delicate balance between matrix deposition and inflammation-associated matrix remodelling, with subtle signals leading to the resolution of inflammation and formation of a mature scar. Non-healing wounds, such as diabetic ulcers, generally arise from an imbalance between these key processes. In diabetic patients, changes in the microvasculature circulation predispose to poor oxygenation (ischaemia), whilst high blood glucose levels retard inflammatory cell function leading to increased incidence of

The Foot in Diabetes, 4th Edition. Editors Andrew J.M. Boulton, Peter R. Cavanagh and Gerry Rayman.
© 2006 John Wiley & Sons, Ltd.

Table 18.1 Growth factors and cytokines in the wound environment

Growth factor	Main cellular source	Effects on healing
PDGF family	Platelets, macrophages	Promotes neutrophil/fibroblast chemotaxis. Induces myofibroblast differentiation
FGF family	Fibroblasts, endothelial cells	Stimulates angiogenesis. Broad mitogenic spectrum
FGF-7 (KGF)	Fibroblasts	Promotes keratinocyte chemotaxis
EGF	Platelets, keratinocytes	Mitogenic for keratinocytes and fibroblasts
TGF-α	Macrophages, keratinocytes	Mitogenic for inflammatory cells and fibroblasts
TGF-β isoforms	Multiple	Stimulate fibroblast differentiation and matrix deposition. Inhibit proliferation
VEGF family	Keratinocytes, macrophages	Stimulates angiogenesis
IGF-I	Keratinocytes, macrophages	Potent mitogenic factor involved in survival of many cell types
Activin	Keratinocytes, fibroblasts	Increases granulation tissue deposition, promotes re-epithelialisation
GM-CSF	Monocytes, fibroblasts	Stimulates neutrophil function and endothelial migration. Keratinocyte mitogen
HGF/SF	Fibroblasts, keratinocytes	Stimulates keratinocyte migration/MMP production and angiogenesis
NGF	Keratinocytes, fibroblasts	Stimulates nerve growth, keratinocyte proliferation and myofibroblast differentiation
MCP-1	Monocytes, keratinocytes	Major monocyte/macrophage chemoattractant
IL-6	Neutrophils, macrophages	Regulates immune cell activation, fibroblast chemotaxis, keratinocyte activation
IL-10	Keratinocytes, neutrophils	Terminates inflammation, regulates keratinocyte and endothelial cell growth
MIF	Keratinocytes, macrophages	Promotes inflammation and matrix degradation
SLPI	Macrophages, keratinocytes	Inhibits proteases and activates leucocytes to accelerate healing

PDGF, platelet-derived growth factor; FGF-7, fibroblast growth factor 7; KGF, keratinocyte growth factor; EGF, epidermal growth factor; TGF-α, transforming growth factor α; TGF β, transforming growth factor β; VEGF, vascular endothelial growth factor; IGF-I, insulin-like growth factor I; GM-CSF, granulocyte-monocyte colony-stimulating factor; HGF/SF, hepatocyte growth factor/scatter factor; NGF, nerve growth factor; MCP-1, monocyte chemotactic protein 1; IL-6, interleukin 6; IL-10, interleukin 10; MIF, macrophage migration inhibitory factor; SLPI, secretory leucocyte protease inhibitor.

infection. These changes result in impaired tissue repair, susceptibility to ulcers and a poor long-term prognosis, with wounds that are non-responsive to current treatment often leading to amputation. Diabetic ulcers are characterised by prolonged and excessive inflammation, in conjunction with impaired inflammatory cell chemotaxis/function, and reduced ECM deposition. Interestingly, these general changes are common to many types of impaired cutaneous repair, e.g. venous ulcer, and hormonally associated delayed healing. In diabetic patients changes in the microvasculature circulation predispose to poor oxygenation (ischemia) and high blood glucose levels retard inflammatory cell function leading to increased incidence of infection. These changes are responsible for converting an acute wound into a chronic non-healing ulcer. Current best practice involves wound assessment/classification, offloading of pressure, debridement and control of infection. However, a significant proportion of wounds fail to heal, ultimately leading to amputation, highlighting the need for new and improved therapies. This chapter will outline the role of hormones and growth factors during normal and perturbed wound healing. The current use of hormones and growth factors will be summarized and future prospects for treatments of non-healing wounds discussed.

ROLE OF HORMONES

The authors have previously demonstrated a clear inverse correlation between age and efficiency of acute wound healing. Elderly subjects heal more slowly, with an excessive local inflammatory response. In females, this shift in healing ability precisely correlates with the dramatic reduction in sex steroids, which occurs as a result of the menopause. Systemic hormone replacement therapy (HRT) significantly accelerates acute wound healing in the elderly, as does topical oestrogen treatment[1–2] (Figure 18.1). Using genetically null animals, we have recently identified macrophage migration inhibitory factor (MIF) as a downstream mediator of oestrogen's effects on wound healing.[3] *In vitro* oestrogen directly regulates MIF by an oestrogen-receptor-mediated mechanism. MIF levels are high in chronic non-healing ulcers,

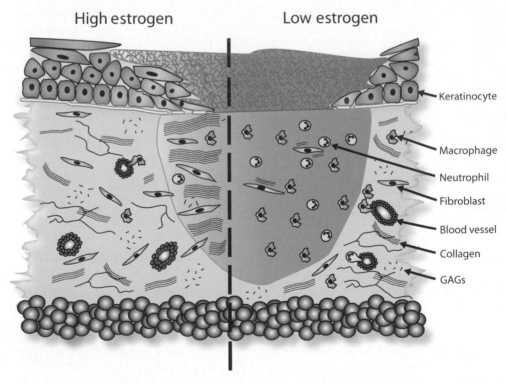

High estrogen   Low estrogen

Keratinocyte
Macrophage
Neutrophil
Fibroblast
Blood vessel
Collagen
GAGs

Figure 18.1 Diagrammatic representation of the effects of estrogen on cutaneous wound healing. Estrogen promotes healing (compare left with right). Reduced estrogen leads to substantially increased granulation tissue area, increased inflammation resulting in enhanced proteolysis, reduced fibroblast-derived matrix deposition and retarded reepithelialization. GAGs, Glycosaminoglycans.

Table 18.2 Effects of hormones on wound healing

Process	Oestrogens	Androgens
Inflammation	↓	↑
Cytokine expression	↓	↑
Re-epithelialisation	↑	↔
Angiogenesis	???	???
Matrix deposition	↑	↓
Wound contraction	↑	???
Overall rate of healing	↑	↓

and then fall with successful healing (Hardman M.J. and Ashcroft G.S., unpublished). In addition, MIF regulates a plethora of wound-healing-associated genes, indicating a fundamental regulatory role for this cytokine (Hardman M.J. and Ashcroft G.S., unpublished). There is now considerable evidence that oestrogen treatment, either topical or systemic, will accelerate healing. Moreover, Margolis *et al.* in a recent case–cohort study identified reduced risk of developing a venous leg or pressure ulcers in elderly females undergoing HRT.[4] Nevertheless, the possible detrimental effect of oestrogen treatment on other systems is problematic, highlighted by oestrogen's addition to the federal list of cancer-causing agents in the United States. For this reason, the authors are actively pursuing downstream genes/factors that mediate oestrogen's effects, such as MIF. Clinical manipulation of these factors should aid healing of ulcers without the detrimental effects of systemic oestrogen treatment on other physiological processes (Table 18.2).

In contrast to oestrogen, androgens inhibit healing. Castrated mice, with reduced systemic testosterone, display accelerated healing.[5] Unlike oestrogen, androgens appear to modulate healing by a direct action on wound cell populations, and cytokine profiles, thereby enhancing the inflammatory response. The role of androgens in human healing is highlighted by neural network studies indicating that elderly males are more likely to develop non-healing ulcers than are elderly females.[6]

ROLE OF GROWTH FACTORS

Growth factors play a critical role, regulating all aspects of wound healing[7] (Table 18.1). In clinical trials, both epidermal growth factor (EGF) and fibroblast growth factor 2 (FGF-2) were found to accelerate healing of acute wounds by several days.[8–9] Chronic wounds provide a more complex challenge, characterised by fluxes in the local non-healing wound environment in which growth factors can quickly become trapped within, or degraded by, the proteolytic extracellular milieu.[10] Protein levels of platelet-derived growth factor (PDGF), EGF, FGF-2 and transforming growth factor β (TGF-β) are all reportedly reduced in chronic wounds.[11] Furthermore, certain growth factors are selectively inhibited in the ulcer environment; for example, specific heparin-like factors expressed by non-healing wounds inhibit FGF activity.[12] Numerous growth factors have been employed for the treatment of chronic wounds. Nearly 20 years ago, Knighton *et al.* reported successful treatment of chronic ulcers with platelet wound-healing formula (PDWHF, an autologous platelet-derived product containing among other factors PDGF, EGF, FGF and TGF-β).[13] This was soon followed by successful studies

Table 18.3 Current and potential exogenous agents for treatment of delayed healing

Factor	Animal studies	Human studies	Therapeutic use
PDGF	Reduced expression in delayed-healing wounds of diabetic mice	Reduced in non-healing ulcers. Topically accelerates ulcer healing	Current treatment for diabetic foot ulcers
FGF-2	Delayed healing in null mice	Mixed results from clinical trials	
		Effective in several ulcer studies	Good clinical trials. Approved for use in ulcers
EGF	Topical treatment accelerates wound strength and re-epithelialisation	Topical treatment accelerates healing. Limited effect on venous ulcers	Limited clinical trials Approved for use in ulcers
KGF	Normal healing in null mice. Topically accelerates healing of porcine wounds	Liposomal KGF cDNA gene transfer accelerates healing	No clinical trials
TGF-α	Topical application accelerates healing of acute wounds	Topical application accelerates healing of acute wounds	No clinical trials
TGF-β	Multiple with complex findings	Topical TGF-β3 accelerates healing of pressure ulcers	Promising TGF-β3 trials
VEGF	Delayed wound healing/angiogenesis in null/inhibitor treated.	VEGF neutralisation strongly impairs angiogenic activity of wound fluid	Stimulates blood vessel formation in arterial disease
GM-CSF	Transgenic over-expression directly accelerates healing of acute wounds	Promising acceleration of ulcer healing in several studies	Initial studies with infected diabetic ulcers
IGF-I	Accelerates cutaneous healing in a diabetic mouse model	Markedly reduced at the edge of diabetic foot ulcers	No clinical trials
HGF/SF	Over-expression results in increased angiogenesis and granulation deposition	Decreased biologically active HGF in chronic ulcers	No clinical trials
NGF	Accelerated healing in healing-impaired diabetic mice	Promotes healing of pressure ulcers	No clinical trials
MCP-1	Significantly delayed wound healing in null mice	Upregulated in human excisional wounds	No clinical trials
IL-6	Up to threefold delayed healing in null mice, with greatly delayed re-epithelialisation	Elevated in non-healing ulcers	No clinical trials

(Continued)

Table 18.3   (*Continued*)

Factor	Animal studies	Human studies	Therapeutic use
MIF	MIF neutralisation accelerates wound repair.	MIF levels are elevated in chronic non-healing wounds	No clinical trials
Oestrogen	In ovariectomised mice acute wound healing is delayed. Topical or systemic oestrogen accelerates delayed healing	Topical or systemic oestrogen accelerate age-associated delayed healing	Initial studies with acute wounds only
Testosterone	Accelerated acute wound healing in castrated mice or following AR blockade	None	No clinical trials

using PDWHF to specifically treat diabetic ulcers.[14] Several subsequent studies have shown recombinant human PDGF alone to be effective in treating a range of non-healing wounds; of particular relevance is the combined analysis of multiple studies involving diabetic ulcer patients.[15] In clinical trials, FGF-2 has been shown to be effective in accelerating healing of a range of chronic cutaneous wounds, such as pressure sores[16] and diabetic ulcers.[17] The outcome in patients with pressure sores was particularly impressive where 91% of FGF-treated wounds healed after 4 weeks, compared to 0% of untreated wounds. EGF also accelerates healing of diabetic ulcers, in one study increasing 12-week healing rates from 42% in control patients to 95% in those topically treated with EGF.[18] Increasing evidence points to an essential role for exogenous growth factors in non-healing wounds (see Table 18.3 for current factors and novel candidates). Whether these exogenous factors exert their effects by binding their respective surface receptors directly or also act indirectly by inducing further endogenous growth factors is at present largely unknown. Encouragingly for future treatment prospects, fibroblasts from wounds of patients with diabetes, with characteristically reduced proliferation, are particularly responsive to exogenous growth factors.[19]

TREATMENT METHODS

In early trials, growth factors were applied in a liquid vehicle or via multiple injections around the ulcer margin. The most common current methods of growth factor treatment are still via direct topical application generally in the form of a cream. To overcome the possibility of degradation in the wound environment, several researchers have employed time release technology with varying success.[20] Gene therapy provides an interesting proposition. Adenovirus-mediated transfection provides the prospect of continuous production of large quantities of growth factors within the wound environment.[21] However, gene transfer technology is only in early-stage clinical trials and may be very difficult to introduce into the clinical practice. A recent transgenic model, in which the secretory leucocyte protease inhibitor (*SLPI*) gene is deleted, suggests an alternative approach. It appears that SLPI is a potent anti-proteolytic and antibacterial agent, which could be applied alone or in combination with other growth factors to prevent destruction of the latter and to accelerate healing.

RISKS

Growth factors and hormones regulate the balance between proliferation and differentiation in not only the healing wound, but also numerous other biological processes including the deregulated proliferation observed in cancer cells, n.[22] The main candidates for acceleratory wound-healing treatments, such as EGF, FGFs and PDGF, either are directly involved in the signalling events that lead to malignant transformation or are upregulated in neoplastic cells.[23] Moreover, concern has been expressed over the use of supraphysiological doses. Reassuringly, there has been absolutely no evidence from any clinical trials of an increased incidence of malignant cutaneous changes even after substantial follow-up periods. In addition, no trial to date has reported increased incidence of hypertrophic scar formation.

CONCLUSIONS

Early experiments using PDWHF highlighted the potential benefits of exogenous growth factors and hormones in the treatment of non-healing wounds.[13-14] The past decade has seen the production, clinical testing and approval of several recombinant growth factors for the treatment of non-healing wounds. In both the United Kingdom and the United States, PDGF has been specifically approved for the treatment of diabetic foot ulcers, and in China, EGF and FGF-2 have been approved for the treatment of both acute and chronic wounds. However, specific dosing and treatment regimens have yet to be standardised for many types of non-healing wounds. The use of growth factors as adjunct therapy to skin grafts or by incorporation into a range of artificial skin substitutes is yielding promising results for treating wounds that are very large (i.e. burns) or persistently non-healing (i.e. diabetic ulcers). Whilst no single exogenously applied growth factor is currently able to eliminate scarring or regenerate the diverse array of structures present in normal integument, such as sweat gland and hair follicles, with recent advances in our understanding of cutaneous lineage determination,[24] we are entering an era where this goal may soon be attainable. Equally, single growth factors need not be employed in isolation; a combination of growth factors can be used to compliment both the existing treatment regimes, e.g. SLPI plus EGF/FGF-2, etc. In addition, a more detailed understanding of the role of hormones in age-related healing will allow us to use specific topical applications of oestrogen receptor agonists or downstream gene targets. The scene is set for many exciting advances over the next decade, where a more detailed understanding of the molecular and cellular changes that lead to delayed healing will lead to the generation of more effective treatments.

REFERENCES

1. Ashcroft GS, Green-Wild T, Horan MA, Wahl SM, Ferguson MW. Topical estrogen accelerates cutaneous wound healing in aged humans associated with an altered inflammatory response. *Am J Pathol* 1999;155:1137–1146.
2. Ashcroft GS, Dodsworth J, van Boxtel E, *et al.* Estrogen accelerates cutaneous wound healing associated with an increase in TGF-β1 levels. *Nat Med* 1997;3:1209–1215.

3. Ashcroft, GS, Mills SJ, Lei K, *et al*. Estrogen modulates cutaneous wound healing by downregulating macrophage migration inhibitory factor. *J Clin Invest* 2003;111:1309–1318.

4. Margolis DJ, Knauss J, Bilker W. Hormone replacement therapy and prevention of pressure ulcers and venous leg ulcers. *Lancet* 2002;359:675–677.

5. Ashcroft GS, Mills SJ. Androgen receptor-mediated inhibition of cutaneous wound healing. *J Clin Invest* 2002;110: 615–624.

6. Taylor RJ, Taylor AD, Smyth JV. Using an artificial neural network to predict healing times and risk factors for venous leg ulcers. *J Wound Care* 2002;11:101–105.

7. Werner S, Grose R. Regulation of wound healing by growth factors and cytokines. *Physiol Rev* 2003;83:835–870.

8. Brown GL, Nanney LB, Griffen J, *et al*. Enhancement of wound healing by topical treatment with epidermal growth factor. *N Engl J Med* 1989;321:76–79.

9. Fu X, Shen Z, Chen Y, *et al*. Randomized placebo-controlled trial of use of topical recombinant bovine basic fibroblast growth factor for second-degree burns. *Lancet* 1998;352:1661–1664.

10. Trengove NJ, Stacey MC, MacAuley S, *et al*. Analysis of the acute and chronic wound environments: the role of proteases and their inhibitors. *Wound Repair Regen* 1999;7:442–452.

11. Tarnuzzer RW, Schultz GS. Biochemical analysis of acute and chronic wound environments. *Wound Repair Regen* 1996;4:321–325.

12. Landau Z, David M, Aviezer D, Yayon A. Heparin-like inhibitory activity to fibroblast growth factor-2 in wound fluid of patients with chronic skin ulcers and its modulation during wound healing. *Wound Repair Regen* 2001;9:323–328.

13. Knighton DR, Ciresi KF, Fiegel VD, Austin LL, Butler EL. Classification and treatment of chronic nonhealing wounds. Successful treatment with autologous platelet-derived wound healing formula (PDWHF). *Ann Surg* 1986;204:322–330.

14. Holloway GA, Steed DL, DeMarco MJ. A randomised controlled dose response trial of activated platelet supernatant topical CT-102 (ASPT) in chronic non-healing wounds in patients with diabetes mellitus. *Wounds* 1993;5:198–206.

15. Smiell JM, Wieman TJ, Steed DL, Perry BH, Sampson AR, Schwab BH. Efficacy and safety of Beclapermin (recombinant platelet-derived growth factor-BB) in patients with non-healing, lower extremity diabetic ulcers: a combined analysis of four randomised studies. *Wound Repair Regen* 1999;7:335–346.

16. Robson MC, Phillips LG, Lawrence WT, *et al*. The safety and effect of topically applied recombinant basic fibroblast growth factor on the healing of chronic pressure sores. *Ann Surg* 1992;216:401–406.

17. Fu X, Shen Z, Chen Y, *et al*. Recombinant bovine basic fibroblast growth factor accelerates wound healing in patients with burns, donor sites and chronic dermal ulcers. *Chin Med J (Engl)* 2000;113:367–371.

18. Tsang MW, Wong WK, Hung CS, *et al*. Human epidermal growth factor enhances healing of diabetic foot ulcers. *Diabetes Care* 2003;26:1856–1861.

19. Grazul-Bilska AT, Luthra G, Reynolds LP, *et al*. Effects of basic fibroblast growth factor (FGF-2) on proliferation of human skin fibroblasts in type II diabetes mellitus. *Exp Clin Endocrinol Diabetes* 2002;110:176–181.

20. Slavin J, Hunt JA, Nash JR, Williams DF, Kingsnorth AN. Recombinant basic fibroblast growth factor in red blood cell ghosts accelerates incisional wound healing. *Br J Surg* 1992;79:918–921.

21. Andree C, Swain WF, Page CP, *et al*. In vivo transfer and expression of a human epidermal growth factor gene accelerates wound repair. *Proc Natl Acad Sci USA* 1994;91:12188–12192.

22. Favoni RE, Cupis AD. The role of polypeptide growth factors in human carcinomas: new targets for a novel pharmacological approach. *Pharmacol Rev* 2000;52:179–205.

23. Kawai T, Hiroi S, Torikata C. Expression in lung carcinomas of platelet-derived growth factor and its receptor. *Lab Invest* 1997;77:431–436.

24. Watt FM, Brigid LM. Out of eden: stem cell and their niches. *Science* 2000;287:1427–1430.

19 Radiology and Magnetic Resonance Imaging of the Diabetic Foot

Richard W. Whitehouse

Clinicians managing diabetic patients' foot problems make frequent use of the radiology department, particularly where trauma or infection is suspected. Whilst this chapter emphasises the imaging appearances of diabetic foot complications, this should be tempered with the realisation that many articles (this chapter included) illustrate the imaging of the complications with 'textbook' examples. The true value of a diagnostic test in practice should be based on a Bayesian statistical approach. For infection, for example, a clinical finding of an ulcer that can be probed to bone is as predictive of the presence of osteomyelitis as any imaging test, whilst a warm, well-perfused, swollen foot with intact skin is much more likely to be neuropathic than osteomyelitic. Imaging tests would need extremely high specificity to significantly alter the pre-test probability in each of these scenarios. Thus, a plain film examination might confirm neuropathic changes in the latter case but may be inappropriate to confirm superadded osteomyelitis.[1]

Current literature tends to underemphasise the plain radiograph in the assessment of the foot in patients with diabetes, nuclear medicine scans utilising a variety of radiopharmaceuticals, computed tomography, angiography and magnetic resonance (MR) imaging (and MR angiography) being at the fore. These latter techniques are powerful tools in the evaluation of the diabetic foot; they are, however, time consuming to perform and interpret, expensive, of limited availability and, for nuclear medicine in particular, of relatively high radiation dose.

Plain radiographs are relatively cheap, quick, widely available and usually can be provided immediately to the requesting clinician, rather than awaiting a radiologist's report. They have also undergone considerable technological development in the last decade. Computerised radiography (CR) and direct digital radiography (DDR) both produce electronic renditions of the radiographic image. The image data from such acquisitions undergo computer manipulation to optimise the greyscale, widen the latitude and emphasise tissue planes before being presented to the viewer. If viewed at an appropriate workstation rather than a hardcopy (film), then further image manipulation is possible. This technology markedly reduces the effect of radiographic overexposure and also allows a degree of underexposure to provide acceptable images. Many of the limitations of conventional radiography do, however, remain. Limited soft tissue contrast

The Foot in Diabetes, 4th Edition. Editors Andrew J.M. Boulton, Peter R. Cavanagh and Gerry Rayman.
© 2006 John Wiley & Sons, Ltd.

resolution, superimposition of complex structures and adequate evaluation of cortical bone being restricted to those bone edges depicted in profile are the main limitations of radiography. In addition, visible changes on radiographs tend to lag behind the evolution of disease, both in its progression and in its resolution. The computer manipulations that 'bring out' soft tissue appearances in the image also tend to reduce the contrast of bony structures; consequently, the assessment of bone density, already subjective on conventional films, is even more difficult.

In practice, radiographs remain valuable for the initial diagnosis and day-to-day management of most diabetic patients' foot pathology, and most primary care physicians rely heavily on radiographic findings, despite the known limitations of sensitivity and specificity for this technique.[2] It is recommended that plain radiography should be the initial imaging procedure for suspected osteomyelitis in the diabetic patient.[3] Further imaging investigations are then appropriate in the minority of patients where radiography and other clinical tests have not provided sufficient information for satisfactory clinical management.

The role of a radiologist in providing interpretation of the radiograph, along with suggestion of further imaging where appropriate, is valuable, but prior to this, the need for interested and motivated radiographers cannot be overemphasised. Conventional radiography of the foot includes the routine dorsi-plantar and oblique views, but many more specialised views, such as lateral views, weight-bearing views, views of the toes, sesamoids (Figure 19.1), forefoot, subtalar joint, heel and ankle, can be performed. These views, when appropriate, have the advantage of placing the region of greatest clinical interest into the most appropriate projection for the suspected pathology; they allow the radiographic exposure to be optimised to that specific region. The smaller imaged volume from these views results in reduced X-ray dose and consequently also reduced X-ray scatter, which improves image quality. Whilst originally developed in the absence of any alternative imaging technique, these views are still useful when appropriately performed. Despite the value of an initial radiograph and of serial follow-up radiographs where appropriate, as described in this chapter, it is concerning that even hospital admission for infected diabetic foot ulceration may not precipitate a radiographic examination, with 33% of such patients not being radiographed in one study.[4]

Radiological manifestations of diabetes in the foot are due to a combination of trauma, neuropathy, infection and vascular disease, which between them affect all the tissues of the foot (bone, muscle, blood vessels, connective tissues and skin). Neuropathy and vascular disease can be thought of as intrinsic complications of diabetes, whilst infection requires ingress of an extrinsic component (microorganisms), usually through a skin ulcer or perforation but also

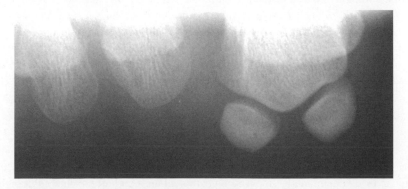

Figure 19.1   Sesamoid view, demonstrating the sesamoid bones beneath the great toe metatarsal head

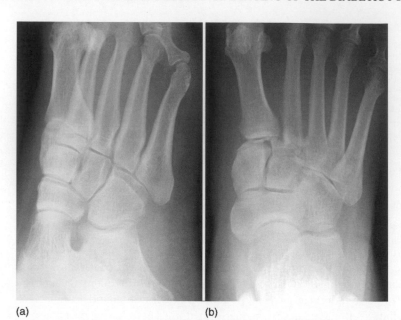

(a)   (b)

Figure 19.2   (a) Patient with a warm, swollen foot, thought to be cellulutis, is found to be radiograph-ically normal. (b) Three weeks later, repeat radiography demonstrates a neuropathic LisFranc fracture dislocation

potentially by haematogenous spread. Features of infection in the diabetic foot are almost invariably superimposed on pre-existing neuropathy and vascular disease.

Trauma to the diabetic foot may go unnoticed or its severity under-appreciated by the patient and carers. Simple fractures are common in the feet of people with diabetes and diagnosis may be delayed. In the author's view, all diabetic patients presenting with trauma or unexplained swelling or deformity of the foot, however minor, should have foot radiography performed as part of their assessment, and if this is normal, it should be repeated within 2–4 weeks (Figure 19.2).

RADIATION EXPOSURE

The consequences of ionising radiation exposure are divided into deterministic and non-deterministic (stochastic or random) effects. Deterministic effects (for example hair loss or skin erythema) always occur if a threshold dose of radiation is exceeded. Stochastic effects may or may not occur but the probability of an effect occurring does increase with increasing radiation dose, the induction of malignant disease being the best known stochastic effect. The threshold doses for significant deterministic effects are unlikely to be exceeded by foot radio-graphy, even when frequently repeated. However, there is uncertainty about a threshold dose below which there is no risk of inducing malignant disease. The 'linear no threshold' (LNT) hypothesis extrapolates the recognised and quantified risk of malignant disease induction at high radiation exposure back to a risk of zero at a dose of zero. Although there is actually epi-demiological and experimental evidence suggesting a beneficial effect (the radiation hormesis hypothesis) from low doses of ionising radiation (doses below 200 millisieverts (mSv)), the LNT hypothesis indicates that any radiation exposure, however small, carries a finite risk of causing malignant disease. Legislation for radiation protection is currently based on the LNT hypothesis. In the United Kingdom, this legislation is embodied in the Ionising Radiation (Medical Exposures) Regulations – IR(ME)R. This legislation requires all medical exposures to be justified, the justification to be provided by the person requesting the examination and based on his/her knowledge of the risks of radiation and benefit of the examination. The justification has to be accepted by the person performing the examination, who can then authorise and perform it. The typical effective radiation dose from foot radiography is less than 5 μSv, whilst the background radiation in the United Kingdom averages 2.4 mSv per annum. The effective radiation dose from foot radiography is thus less than the background radiation received in a single day from living in the United Kingdom. The radiation risk from foot radiography against which to balance the benefits of the examination should therefore be considered to be negligible.

NORMAL APPEARANCES

Variation in the appearance of the foot and ankle on radiographs due to radiographic projections and exposure, the complexities of normal anatomy, variations of normal anatomy between individuals and the sometimes gross abnormalities that may occur in diabetic feet all contribute to the challenge of interpretation of radiological images. Additional (accessory) ossicles are common in the foot and ankle (Figure 19.3), with over 20 recognised and named accessory

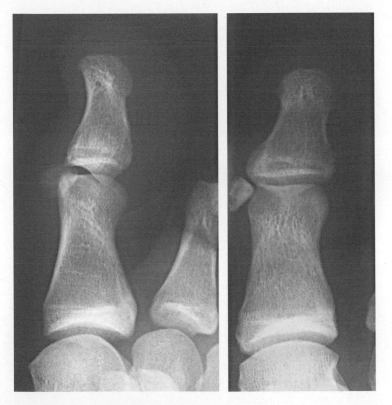

Figure 19.3 An accessory ossicle (normal variant) is present on the medial side of the great toe, adjacent to the interphalangeal joint. In people with diabetes, such bony prominences can predispose to ulceration

ossicles. Although two sesamoid bones are usually present under the great toe, these can be bi- or tripartite and sesamoids can also occur under other toes. Recognition of normal variants of radiographic appearances in the foot and ankle by reference to relevant texts is recommended.[5] Accessory ossicles or variations in the morphology or alignment of the metatarsals and pha- langes are clearly demonstrated on plain radiographs. Whilst usually considered to be normal variants, and of no clinical significance, these features may predispose to ulceration in diabetic feet, for example an interphalangeal accessory sesamoid in the great toe was present in 13 of 29 people with diabetes with great toe ulcers.[6] Such normal variants are, however, no more common in people with diabetes than in the rest of the population.[7]

TRAUMA

Plain radiography is fundamental to the diagnosis and management of fracture and dislocation in the foot and ankle. Recent fractures and dislocations, bone deformities from healed previous fractures and progressing neuropathic fracture/dislocations will all be demonstrated on radio- graphs (Figure 19.4). Although foot deformity will be clinically apparent, the radiographs can draw attention to underlying bone deformities that may predispose to soft tissue ulceration by forming pressure points. Metallic or glass radio-opaque foreign bodies may be identified in the foot[8,9] and may predispose to infection. Bone regrowth after surgical partial resection of metatarsal bone may also form pressure points and predispose to ulceration (Figure 19.5). Plain film demonstration of regrowth exceeding 3 mm was seen in 45% of such patients between 1 and 3 years after surgery.[10] Evidence of traumatic fractures, often previously unrecognised, in neuropathic diabetic feet is common, being found in 22% of neuropathic diabetic feet in one study.[7]

VASCULAR DISEASE

Peripheral vascular disease is common in diabetes. In the foot and ankle, relative sparing of the dorsalis pedis but involvement of the posterior tibial and peroneal arteries is often seen. On plain radiographs, small vessel calcification is seen throughout the foot (Figure 19.6). When completely avascular, such as in dry gangrene of the foot, the affected bones will remain unchanged, whilst the bone that is still vascularised and viable becomes demineralised, resulting in a demarcation on the plain radiograph between viable (osteopaenic) and dead (normal density) bone. Proper assessment of the vascular supply requires angiography, though contrast enhanced MR may replace conventional catheter angiography for this. The presence of radiographically demonstrated medial arterial calcinosis in diabetic feet is associated with neuropathy, ulceration, amputation and excess mortality.[11]

NEUROPATHY AND NEUROARTHROPATHY

Although originally described as the changes in the lower limb in Charcot–Marie–Tooth syn- drome, neuropathic changes in the foot are most commonly caused by diabetes and are of- ten described as Charcot neuroarthropathy. Neuroarthropathic changes in the skeleton are

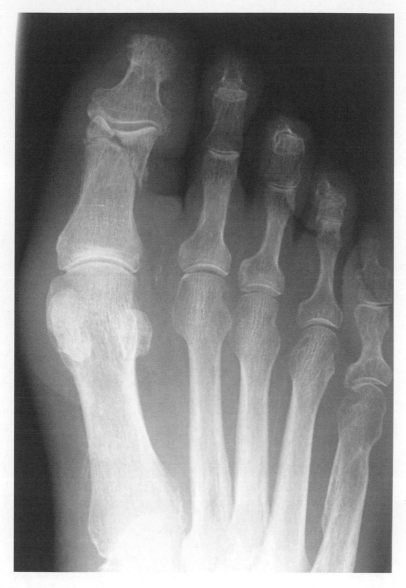

Figure 19.4 Recent intra-articular fracture of the great toe proximal phalanx. There is also a healed fracture of the fifth metatarsal

believed to be due to unnoticed repeated minor trauma, resulting in progressive joint destruction. This is superimposed on bones rendered osteopaenic from increased osteoclastic activity, driven by hyperaemia from sympathetic denervation of small blood vessels.[12] Reduced bone density directly predisposes to fracture, as bone density is a major determinant of bone strength. Consequently, neuropathic changes may manifest as arthropathy, dislocation, fracture or a combination of these features. Study of bone mineral density in diabetic feet has demonstrated peripheral osteopaenia in those patients with a fracture pattern of neuropathy,

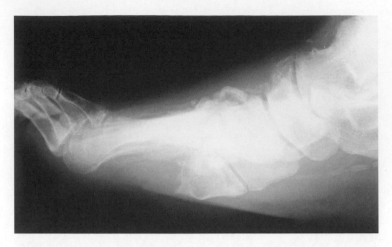

Figure 19.5 Lateral view of the foot demonstrates a bone spike projecting from the amputation stump of the great toe metatarsal; this may predispose to ulceration

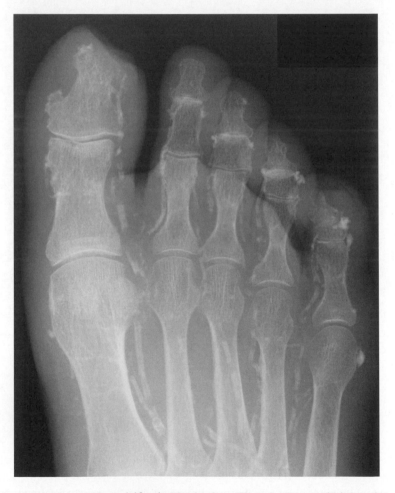

Figure 19.6 Extensive vascular calcification in the foot. There is also a soft tissue ulcer crater and underlying osteomyelitis in the great toe

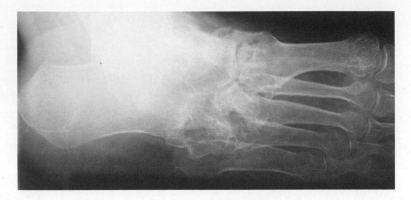

Figure 19.7 Chronic stable neuropathic foot

but relatively normal bone density in those with a dislocation pattern[13] and in those with neuropathy but no arthropathy.[14] The fracture pattern of neuropathy was commonest in the ankle and forefoot, whilst dislocations were commonest in the midfoot.[13] The Charcot foot commonly goes unrecognised until severe complications have occurred.[15] The mean delay between first clinical presentation and diagnosis of a Charcot foot in diabetes was 29 weeks in one study.[16] The changes in the Charcot foot have been divided into five stages[17]: Stage 0 is a clinical stage with a swollen, warm and often painful foot. At this stage, radiographs are normal but bone scintigraphy is positive. Stage 1 has radiographic abnormality including periarticular cysts, erosions, localised osteopaenia and diastases. Stage 2 has joint subluxations, most commonly between the middle cuneiform and base of the second metatarsal, which then spread laterally. Stage 3 has full dislocation and collapse of the longitudinal arch of the foot. The case illustrated in Figure 19.2 demonstrates the rapid progression from stage 0 to stage 3 that can occur. Stage 4 is the healed, stable end result (Figure 19.7). This description applies to neuroarthropathy involving the midfoot. Metatarso-phalangeal joint involvement by neuroarthropathy is also common (Figure 19.8), as is multiple joint involvement.[18] Neuropathic bone resorption of the phalanges can also occur, resulting in an appearance described as 'sucked candy' (Figure 19.9).

INFECTION

Almost invariably, bone infection in the diabetic foot is acquired by direct spread from an adjacent infected cutaneous ulcer, though presumed haematogenous spread of tuberculosis (TB) to involve the tarsus in a diabetic patient with pulmonary TB has been described.[19] When soft tissue infection extends to a bone, it should first affect the periosteum, causing periostitis, then the cortex of the bone, causing osteitis, and finally the marrow space, resulting in osteomyelitis. The plain film features of bone infection are periosteal reaction, cortical bone destruction and medullary bone destruction. Periosteal reaction is uncommon in osteomyelitis of tarsal bones but may be seen in metatarsal osteomyelitis (Figure 19.10). The soft tissue ulcer may contain gas, which may extend down to the bone surface or into the osteomyelitic cavity within the bone. Gas in the tissues may be in an ulcer cavity, 'pumped' into the soft tissues by the pressure of walking on an ulcer cavity or due to soft issue infection by a

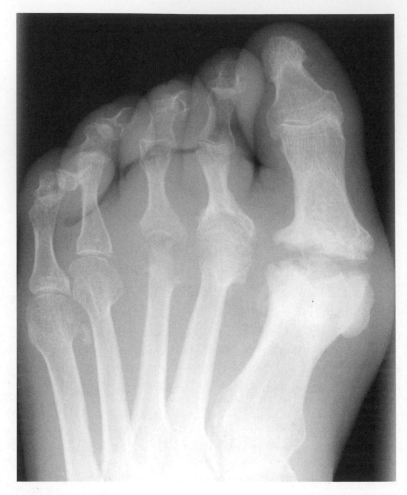

Figure 19.8   Neuropathic great toe metatarso-phalangeal joint. There is also dislocation of the second toe metatarso-phalangeal joint and osteomyelitis of the third toe metatarsal head

gas-forming organism (Figure 19.11). In necrotising fasciitis of the lower limb in diabetics, gas was seen in the soft tissues on plain radiographs in 44% of affected patients.[20] In chronic osteomyelitis, dense foci of necrotic bone may be detached from the bone of origin to form sequestra. In larger bones, these are usually within intra-osseous cavities with surrounding hypertrophic bone (the involucrum), but may be extruded through cloacae into sinus tracks or soft tissue cavities. Involucrum formation is less common in the foot. Sequestra may be extruded through the skin or removed during ulcer debridement. As treatment of cutaneous ulcers may include the use of antibiotic-releasing pellets placed within the ulcer, the appearance of these pellets should be recognised on radiographs and not confused with sequestra, particularly when the pellets become smaller, irregular and fragmented with time (Figure 19.12). Plain radiography, nuclear medicine scans, MR imaging and high-resolution ultrasound imaging of suspected osteomyelitis of the diabetic foot have all been compared. Representative figures compared with histopathology in one study give sensitivities of 69, 79, 83 and 100% for plain

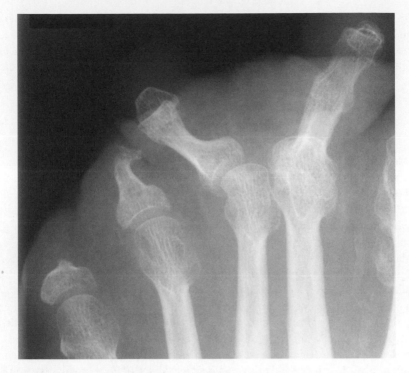

Figure 19.9 Neuropathic bone resorption resulting in a 'sucked candy' appearance to the residual phalanges of the third, fourth and fifth toes

films, ultrasound, bone scintigraphy and MR scanning respectively, with specificities of 80, 80, 75 and 75%.[21] Higher specificity can be achieved in nuclear medicine with leucocyte-labelled scanning. A suggested imaging 'cascade' in suspected osteomyelitis is therefore plain radiography, and then three-phase bone scintigraphy or MRI. If clinically neuropathy is present then infection-specific radiopharmaceuticals may be needed.[22]

MAGNETIC RESONANCE IMAGING

Whilst radiography is less sensitive than MR or nuclear medicine for the detection and evaluation of suspected osteomyelitis in the diabetic foot, it is still the most appropriate initial imaging investigation. In a complex foot infection, where deformity, previous amputations and neuropathic changes may also be present, plain films will facilitate an MR examination tailored to the individual. Plain films were found to be essential or useful in the interpretation of up to 75% of musculoskeletal MR imaging studies.[23] Many early papers on MR of the diabetic foot claimed 100% accuracy in differentiating infection from neuropathy, as fluid collections in the foot were always deemed abscesses and bone marrow oedema appeared in osteomyelitis but not in neuropathy. Whilst often helpful, these observations are not pathognomonic. More recently, it has been appreciated that bone marrow oedema on MR scanning occurs in neuropathy as well as infection.[24] The plain film appearances may assist in differentiating acute neuropathic osteoarthropathy and osteomyelitis, as bone marrow signal changes on MR in

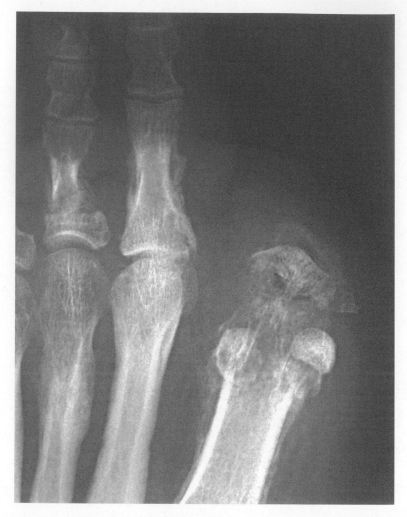

Figure 19.10 Destruction of the great toe metatarsal head, with gas within it, indicating osteomyelitis. Periosteal reaction is present along the metatarsal shaft. The great toe phalanges have been amputated and there are also old and healing fractures of the second and third toes

osteoarthropathy can mimic those in osteomyelitis.[25] The presence of fluid collections in the soft tissues on MR imaging is, however, highly suggestive of abscess formation, and its relationship to bone abnormality may then be very predictive of osteomyelitis, even in the presence of neuropathic changes.[26,27] Characteristically, bone adjacent to a neuropathic joint is of low signal intensity on both T1- and T2-weighted MR images (Figure 19.13), whilst marrow oedema is of low signal on T1-weighted but of high signal on T2-weighted images.[28] In addition to T1- and T2-weighted images, sequences that suppress the signal from fat are increasingly used. These sequences may demonstrate marrow oedema with greater sensitivity than conventional T1- or T2-weighted sequences (Figure 19.14). Availability of MR also requires the appropriate technical and interpretative skills.[29]

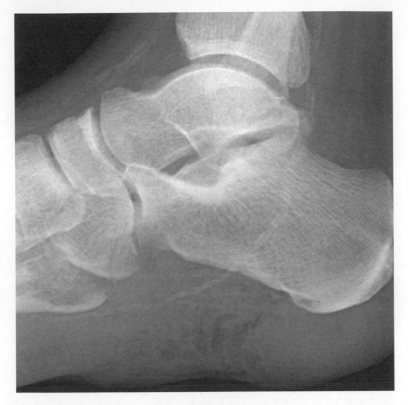

Figure 19.11 Gas in the soft tissues beneath the calcaneum, with underlying bone destruction at the base of the fifth metatarsal, indicating osteomyelitis. Note the vascular calcification

MR studies have reconfirmed the common sites of pedal osteomyelitis in the foot (fifth metatarsal, first metatarsal, and first distal phalanx in the forefoot and the calcaneus in the hindfoot), and also the usual presence of immediately adjacent cutaneous ulceration overlying osteomyelitis and the demonstration of associated septic arthritis in one third of patients with advanced pedal infection.[30]

Whilst the commonest indication for MR in the diabetic foot will be to confirm or exclude osteomyelitis, MR is the anatomic gold standard that can be used to define the extent of the pathological process in the foot,[31] an information of value in determining the amputation level where this is necessary. The frequency of tendon involvement by infection in the diabetic foot has also become more apparent with the greater use of MR imaging, the condition being present in approximately half of the patients who were scanned and then had surgery for pedal infection.[32] The MR documentation of tendon involvement influenced the surgical procedure in only 6 out of 159 patients, it being noted that proximal migration of infection along tendon sheaths was rare.

The use of intravenous enhancement with gadolinium chelate allows demonstration of tissue necrosis on MR imaging, as such regions show no enhancement. This was confirmed at surgery but it was noted that lack of enhancement in these regions could mask the coexistence of abscess and osteomyelitis.[33] MR also demonstrates marked atrophy of the intrinsic muscles in neuropathic feet, with a 73% reduction in muscle bulk compared to non-diabetic controls.[34]

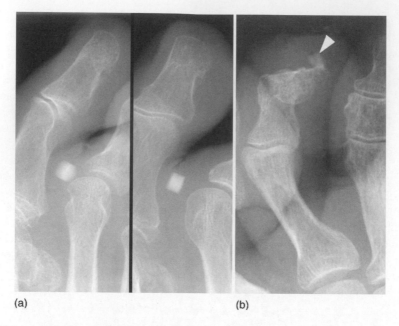

(a)   (b)

Figure 19.12   Antibiotic pellets (a) when recently implanted; (b) smaller and irregular in appearance when partially absorbed (arrowhead)

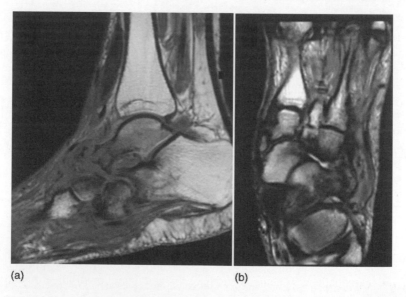

(a)   (b)

Figure 19.13   Magnetic resonance (MR) images of a neuropathic foot: (a) Sagittal T1-weighted and (b) axial T2-weighted images both show low-signal-intensity bone and marrow spaces adjacent to the abnormal articulations. (Courtesy of Dr JPR Jenkins, Consultant Radiologist, Manchester Royal Infirmary, United Kingdom)

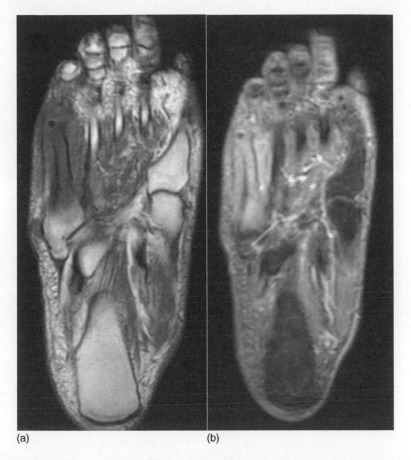

(a)   (b)

Figure 19.14   MR images of osteomyelitis: (a) T1-weighted, with low signal in the marrow space of the fifth metatarsal; (b) fat suppressed images post-contrast T1-weighted image demonstrates high signal (contrast enhancement) in the bone marrow, consistent with osteomyelitis. (Courtesy of Dr J Harris, Consultant Radiologist, Hope Hospital, Salford, United Kingdom)

CONCLUSIONS

Plain radiography and MR imaging play crucial roles in the evaluation of the diabetic foot. Prompt and repeated evaluation of the foot by plain film radiography remains valuable in the management of diabetic foot complications, supported by further studies in equivocal cases utilising nuclear medicine, MR imaging and/or angiography as appropriate to confirm or exclude infection, ischaemia or avascularity and to guide amputation where indicated.

REFERENCES

1. Wrobel JS, Connolly JE. Making the diagnosis of osteomyelitis. The role of prevalence. *J Am Podiatr Med Assoc* 1998;88:337–343.

2. Edelman D, Matchar DB, Oddone EZ. Clinical and radiographic findings that lead to intervention in diabetic patients with foot ulcers. A nationwide survey of primary care physicians. *Diabetes care* 1996;19:755–757.
3. Gold RH, Tong DJ, Crim JR, Seeger LL. Imaging the diabetic foot.*Skeletal Radiol* 1995;24:563–571.
4. Edelson GW, Armstrong DG, Lavery LA, Caicco G. The acutely infected diabetic foot is not adequately evaluated in an inpatient setting. *J Am Podiatr Med Assoc* 1997;87:260–265.
5. Keats TE, Anderson MW, eds. *Atlas of Normal Roentgen Variants That May Simulate Disease.* London: Mosby; 2001.
6. Boffeli TJ, Bean JK, Natwick JR. Biomechanical abnormalities and ulcers of the great toe in patients with diabetes. *J Foot Ankle Surg* 2002;41:359–364.
7. Cavanagh PR, Vickers KL, Young MJ, Boulton AJM, Adams JE. Radiographic abnormalities in the feet of patients with diabetic neuropathy. *Diabetes care* 1994;17:201–209.
8. Woolfrey PG, Kirby RL. Hypodermic needles in the neuropathic foot of a patient with diabetes. *CMAJ* 1998;158:765–767.
9. Arbona N, Jedrzynski M, Frankfather R, *et al.* Is glass visible on plain radiographs? A cadaver study. *J Foot Ankle Surg* 1999;38:264–270.
10. Armstrong DG, Hadi S, Nguyen HC, Harkless LB. Factors associated with bone regrowth following diabetes-related partial amputation of the foot. *J Bone Joint Surg Am* 1999;81:1561–1565.
11. Mayfield JA, Caps MT, Boyko EJ, Ahroni JH, Smith DG. Relationship of medial arterial calcinosis to autonomic neuropathy and adverse outcomes in a diabetic veteran population. *J Diabetes Complications* 2002;16:165–171.
12. Edmonds ME, Clarke MB, Newton S, Barrett J, Watkins PJ. Increased uptake of bone radiopharmaceutical in diabetic neuropathy. *Q J Med* 1985;57:843–855.
13. Herbst SA, Jones KB, Saltzman CL. Pattern of diabetic neuropathic arthropathy associated with the peripheral bone mineral density. *J Bone Joint Surg Br* 2004;86:378–383.
14. Young MJ, Selby PL, Marshall A, Boulton AJM, Adams JE. Osteopenia, neurological dysfunction, and the development of Charcot neuroarthropathy. *Diabetes Care* 1995;18:34–38.
15. Caputo GM, Ulbrecht J, Cavanagh PR, Juliano P. The Charcot foot in diabetes: six key points. *Am Fam Physician* 1998;57:2705–2710.
16. Pakarinen TK, Laine HJ, Honkonen SE, Peltonen J, Oksala H, Lahtela J. Charcot arthropathy of the diabetic foot. Current concepts and review of 36 cases. *Scand J Surg* 2002;91:195–201.
17. Sella EJ, Barrette C. Staging of Charcot neuroarthropathy along the medial column of the foot in the diabetic patient. *J Foot Ankle Surg* 1999;38:34–40.
18. Scartozzi G, Kanat IO. Diabetic neuroarthropathy of the foot and ankle. *J Am Podiatr Med Assoc* 1990;80:298–303.
19. Güttler A, Hammerschmidt S, Wirtz H, Schauer J. Unerwartete Ursache einer Fusswurzeldestruktion bei einem Diabetiker [Unexpected cause of a tarsal destruction in a diabetic patient]. *Dtsch Med Wochenschr* 2004;129:1243–1245.
20. Demirag B, Tirelioglu AO, Sarisözen B, Durak K. Bacakta diyabetik yaralara bagli nekrozitan fasiit [Necrotizing fasciitis in the lower extremity secondary to diabetic wounds]. *Acta Orthop Traumatol Turc* 2004;38:195–199.
21. Enderle MD, Coerper S, Schweizer HP, *et al.* Correlation of imaging techniques to histopathology in patients with diabetic foot syndrome and clinical suspicion of chronic osteomyelitis. The role of high-resolution ultrasound. *Diabetes care* 1999;22:294–299.
22. Becker W. Imaging osteomyelitis and the diabetic foot. *Q J Nucl Med* 1999;43:9–20.
23. Taljanovic MS, Hunter TB, Fitzpatrick KA, Krupinski EA, Pope TL. Musculoskeletal magnetic resonance imaging: importance of radiography. *Skeletal Radiol* 2003;32:403–411.
24. Tomas MB, Patel M, Marwin SE, Palestro CJ. The diabetic foot. *Br J Radiol* 2000;73:443–450.
25. Marcus CD, Ladam-Marcus VJ, Leone J, Malgrange D, Bonnet-Gausserand FM, Menanteauc BP. MR imaging of osteomyelitis and neuropathic arthropathy in the feet of diabetics. *Radiographics* 1996;16:1337–1348.

26. Eckardt A, Schöllner C, Decking J, *et al.* The impact of Syme amputation in surgical treatment of patients with diabetic foot syndrome and Charcot-neuro-osteoarthropathy. *Arch Orthop Trauma Surg* 2004;124:145–150.

27. Ledermann HP, Morrison WB, Schweitzer ME. Pedal abscesses in patients suspected of having pedal osteomyelitis: analysis with MR imaging. *Radiology* 2002;224:649–655.

28. Schweitzer ME, Morrison WB. MR imaging of the diabetic foot. *Radiol Clin North Am* 2004;42: 61–71.

29. Berendt AR, Lipsky B. Is this bone infected or not? Differentiating neuro-osteoarthropathy from osteomyelitis in the diabetic foot. *Curr Diabetes Rep* 2004;4:424–429.

30. Ledermann HP, Morrison WB, Schweitzer ME. MR image analysis of pedal osteomyelitis: distribution, patterns of spread, and frequency of associated ulceration and septic arthritis. *Radiology* 2002;22:747–755.

31. Sella EJ, Grosser DM. Imaging modalities of the diabetic foot. *Clin Podiatr Med Surg* 2003;20:729–740.

32. Ledermann HP, Morrison WB, Schweitzer ME, Raikin SM. Tendon involvement in pedal infection: MR analysis of frequency, distribution, and spread of infection. *Am J Roentgenol* 2002;179:939–947.

33. Ledermann HP, Schweitzer ME, Morrison WB. Nonenhancing tissue on MR imaging of pedal infection: characterization of necrotic tissue and associated limitations for diagnosis of osteomyelitis and abscess. *Am J Roentgenol* 2002;178:215–222.

34. Bus SA, Yang OX, Wang JH, Smith MB, Wunderlich R, Cavanagh PR. Intrinsic muscle atrophy and toe deformity in the diabetic neuropathic foot: a magnetic resonance imaging study. *Diabetes Care* 2002;25:1444–1450.

20 Interventional Radiology in the Diabetic Foot

Amman Bolia

INTRODUCTION

Over 1 million people in the United Kingdom have diabetes mellitus,[1] of whom around 7–10% will, at some point, develop a foot ulcer.[2] This becomes even more significant with the increasing age of the population and as the prevalence of diabetes increases.

Diabetic patients are particularly prone to peripheral neuropathy and peripheral atherosclerotic disease, which results in some patients getting foot ulceration and gangrene. Other contributing factors are poor glycaemic control, foot deformities associated with high mechanical pressures on overlying skin, decreased visual acuity resulting in foot trauma, limited joint mobility and also poor-fitting footwear.[3]

Foot ulceration and gangrene are important causes of morbidity in diabetic patients, and therefore it is important that measures are taken that would eventually lead to healing of the ulcers or gangrene.

Healing of such lesions requires surgical debridement of infected or necrotic tissues and restoration of pulsatile blood flow to the foot. As occlusive atherosclerotic disease of the tibial arteries is particularly common in diabetic patients, infra-popliteal revascularisation is often required. This has traditionally been accomplished by percutaneous transluminal angioplasty (PTA) or a surgical bypass, with moderately good results. More recently, subintimal angioplasty has been practised as an alternative, minimally invasive treatment to recanalise long arterial occlusions, with promising patency rates even in small vessels of the lower leg. Advanced reconstructive techniques including local or free tissue flap transfers can be used to accelerate healing of large foot wounds after successful revascularisation. Treatment of diabetic vascular disease is challenging and requires an aggressive multidisciplinary approach with cooperation between diabetologists, interventional radiologists, vascular surgeons and plastic surgeons.

BACKGROUND AND VASCULAR INVESTIGATION

There is growing evidence that the vascular contribution to diabetic foot disease is greater than was previously realised.[4] Unlike diabetic peripheral neuropathy, peripheral vascular disease

The Foot in Diabetes, 4th Edition. Editors Andrew J.M. Boulton, Peter R. Cavanagh and Gerry Rayman.
© 2006 John Wiley & Sons, Ltd.

(PVD) is more amenable to therapeutic intervention. Patients with PVD will have a low transcutaneous oxygen tension ($TcpO_2$) on the dorsum of the foot, and PVD has been demonstrated to be a greater risk factor than neuropathy in both foot ulceration and lower limb amputation in diabetic patients.[5,6]

The basic pathophysiology of atherosclerosis in patients with diabetes is probably no different from that in non-diabetic patients. However, some of the risk factors are more prevalent in the diabetic population. It has been shown that compared to non-diabetic patients with PVD, diabetic patients are twice as likely to have disease of the distal popliteal or tibial vessels.[7] However, there is no evidence that diabetic patients suffer from more macrovascular disease of the pedal vessels. Indeed, Conrad[8] demonstrated that the pedal vessels of diabetic patients were less frequently affected with atheroma than those of non-diabetic patients. Nor is there any evidence to support the widely held concept of obliterative microvascular or 'small vessel' disease of the diabetic foot.

It is therefore fortuitous that the distal tibial vessels are available and enable recanalisation of long occlusions to be achieved by subintimal angioplasty.

Non-invasive vascular imaging is normally the first-line investigation in patients with PVD. Whilst in non-diabetic patients the ankle–brachial pressure index (ABPI) is reduced in the presence of PVD, in diabetic patients it can be falsely high due to calcified and non-compliant peripheral vasculature and is therefore unreliable. Because of limitations of ABPI in diabetic patients with incompressible vessels and medial calcification, toe pressure measurements are of value. Toe pressure in patients with non-arterial symptoms are between 90 and 100 mm Hg, whereas in the presence of critical limb ischaemia, the pressure drops to below 30 mm Hg.[9]

Duplex scanning is a fast, cost-effective and non-invasive way of imaging diseased arteries in the periphery, but it is operator dependent.[10–14] The tibial arteries can sometimes be difficult to image, especially in the presence of calcification, oedema, ulceration and bandaging of the legs. Despite these limitations, it proves an extremely useful investigation and is usually sufficient to base a decision on the mode of intervention for revascularisation, either by surgery or angioplasty.

Magnetic resonance imaging has boosted the non-invasive imaging potential of patients with PVD. Excellent magnetic resonance angiographic (MRA) pictures can be produced in the majority of patients, with proximal arteries particularly well demonstrated (Figure 20.1). Accurate demonstration of tibial vessel requires a cooperative patient and a radiologist geared up to providing a good study. Patients who are incapable of keeping still and are suffering from claustrophobia may not be suitable.[15,16]

CT angiography has an application in the intra-thoracic and intra-abdominal vasculature. As multi-slice and fast scanners become more available, CT angiography may assume greater importance. Unlike duplex scanning, and like MRA, the study is non-operator dependent, and provides excellent images.

Femoral angiography or, more specifically, intra-arterial digital subtraction angiography (DSA) has been regarded as the gold standard for demonstrating the arterial tree and is particularly good at showing the foot vessels. However, nowadays, the standard practice in most departments is to use some sort of non-invasive imaging, which is then followed by a diagnostic angiogram that proceeds to an intervention at the same time.

Iodinated contrast media used in angiography are potentially nephrotoxic. The nephrotoxicity is transient, reaching a maximum at approximately 48 h, and is usually of no clinical significance in patients with normal renal function.[9] All patients should have their serum creatinine measured prior to angiography. If the creatinine is raised, but below 300 μmol/l, then

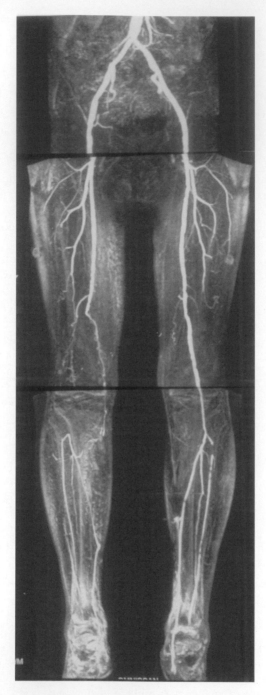

Figure 20.1 This is a composite image of an MR angiogram. It shows an occlusion of the right popliteal artery, extending up to the trifurcation

adequate hydration with intravenous fluids is recommended, commencing at least 6 h prior to the intervention. If the creatinine is more than 300 μmol/l, then serious consideration should be given as to whether an alternative modality or contrast agent should be used.

ENDOVASCULAR REVASCULARISATION

Wound healing usually requires uninterrupted pulsatile arterial blood flow into the foot. Therefore, proximal revascularisation alone, in the presence of distal disease, is insufficient and has to be combined with treatment of the distal arteries. Thus, in addition to any proximal stenotic or occlusive lesions in the aorto-iliac or femoro-popliteal segment, dilatation of stenoses or recanalisation of occlusions of one or more tibial arteries is required to provide adequate flow to the foot. The aim is to always provide a good haemodynamic result with sufficient pulsatile foot perfusion, and only under these circumstances will healing of the foot ulcers or healing of any wounds following surgery be accomplished.

PTA is usually applicable in stenotic lesions of the arteries whereby a guidewire is used to cross the lesion and the lesion dilated using a balloon catheter. Femoral artery is the usual access route for interventions in most of the arterial tree. Seldinger technique involves introduction of a guidewire through a needle puncture, and once the wire is safely into the arterial lumen, the needle is substituted with a catheter, which is fed over the wire. A formal femoral arteriogram is done using contrast injection through a pigtail catheter for outlining the whole of the peripheral arterial tree. Any aorto-iliac lesions can be treated with a retrograde puncture (where the wire through the needle advances in the caphalad direction) of the femoral artery.

When contrast injection outlines the lesion, under roadmap facility, a guidewire is passed inside the catheter lumen and is negotiated through any stenotic or occlusive lesion. An appropriate-sized balloon is placed and dilated to the desired pressure, in order to squeeze the offending atherosclerotic lesion into the wall of the artery. Dilatation results in cracking and squeezing of the atheroma into the wall as well as permanent stretching of the media, resulting in an adequate channel. A repeat inflation of balloon may be carried out if the dilatation is unsatisfactory (>30% residual stenosis). Such dilatation may require higher inflation pressure, more prolonged than before, to achieve an adequate result. Despite this, if the flow is impaired for any reason, the lesion may be stented.

Various stent types and designs are available. The two broad categories of stents are balloon expandable or self-expanding stents. Depending on the length, location and tortuosity of the lesion and whether there is calcification present, one or the other type of stent may be appropriate. Stents have the widest application in the aorto-iliac segment, and particularly for occlusive disease of the artery. Their use in the infrainguinal segment is limited.

An antegrade femoral puncture (wire heading in the caudad direction) is usually necessary to treat femoro-popliteal and/or tibial artery disease. Whilst there may be proximal disease in the aorto-iliac or femoro-popliteal segment in diabetic patients, particularly when the cause of the PVD is multifactorial, the predominant disease is present in the tibial arteries. One of the greatest advantages of PTA over surgery is that treatment can be directed at all levels at the same time, thus having maximum possibility of achieving a good pulstile flow down to the foot (Figure 20.2).

Because of the predominance of distal arterial disease in diabetic patients, any treatment capable of improving the distal arterial tree will make a substantial impact. Whilst the conventional PTA is able to treat simple stenoses or short occlusions in the tibial vessels with the help

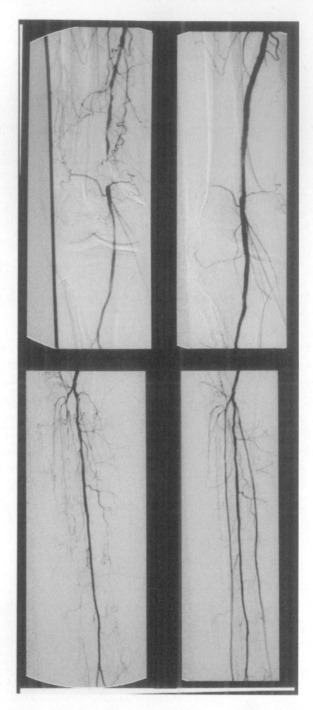

Figure 20.2   This diabetic patient has critical limb ischaemia, manifesting as foot ulceration. A short popliteal occlusion and both the anterior and posterior tibial artery occlusions were recanalised with subintimal angioplasty

of fine wires and catheter available these days, subintimal angioplasty is capable of treating a large number of cases because of the ability of the technique to treat long tibial occlusions and multiple vessels as well as to reconstitute the trifurcation.

Since the first description of subintimal angioplasty in 1989/1990,[17, 18] a number of centres have published their experience particularly in patients with critical limb ischaemia, of which diabetic patients form a large proportion. Subintimal angioplasty has been shown to make a substantial impact on the treatment of critical limb ischaemia mainly due to the fact that long superficial femoral artery (Figure 20.3) and tibial occlusions (Figure 20.2) can be tackled with this technique.

The technique has been widely described elsewhere.[19–23] Briefly, it involves traversing the occlusion not through the lumen but through the subintimal space, thus making use of the disease-free dissection space that becomes available as a conduit for blood flow. The technique utilises a deliberate but controlled arterial dissection to cross an arterial occlusion or even a segment of diffuse disease. The subintimal plane is the path of least resistance and is therefore relatively easy to cross, using a loop in a hydrophilic guidewire. After balloon dilatation, the resultant lumen is eccentric, wide and cosmetically appealing because it is disease free. Since this newly created channel is free of atheroma, good long-term patency can be expected (Figure 20.4).

RESULTS

Conventional PTA has an application in tibial arteries where there is stenotic or short occlusive disease, but the outcomes achieved at 1 year are variable and generally poor in diabetic compared to non-diabetic patients.[24–28]

There have been a number of reports from the beginning of this century that have shown that subintimal angioplasty holds promise in the treatment of critical limb ischaemia. Table 20.1 shows treatment of the femoro-popliteal segment predominantly, but also in conjunction with tibial arterial disease. Apart from the article by Florenes (diabetes incidence 9%), the incidence of diabetes in these patients with critical limb ischaemia ranges from 33 to 59%, thus constituting a substantial proportion of the patients with critical limb ischaemia.[29–34]

Despite small numbers in individual series, some important conclusions can be drawn. Firstly, subintimal angioplasty in the femoro-popliteal segment is primarily a successful

Table 20.1 This table shows the published series of subintimal angioplasty of the femoro-popliteal segments in patients with critical limb ischaemia. (Florenes showed an excellent assisted patency rates of 64% at 5 years). (Lazaris showed a limb salvage rate of 88% at 3 years)

Study	Limbs/PTS	Diabetics (%)	Primary success (%)	1-year patency (%)	1-year salvage (%)
London et al.[29]	54	49	91	78	89
Tisi et al.[30]	129	33	85	33	88
Lipsitz et al.[31]	39	59	87	74	90
Molloy et al.[32]	133	39	79	—	88
Florenes et al.[33]	116	9	87	64 (5 years)	—
Lazaris et al.[34]	112	33	89	—	88 (3 years)

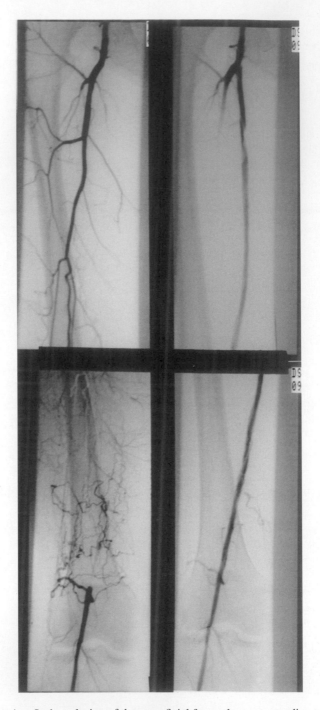

Figure 20.3   There is a flush occlusion of the superficial femoral artery extending to the mid-popliteal artery. Subintimal angioplasty achieved a successful outcome

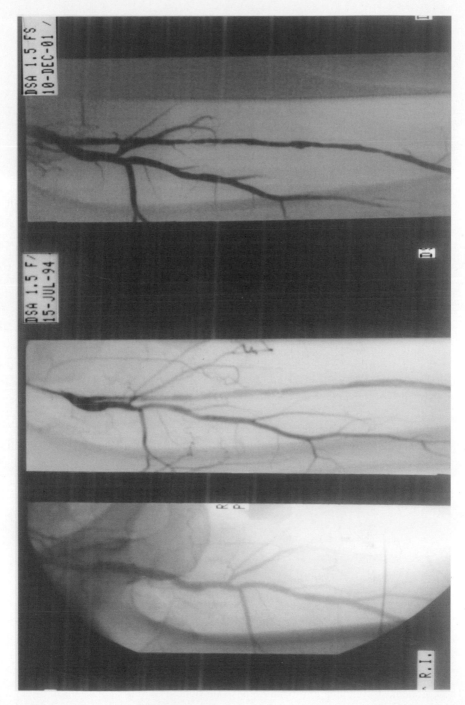

Figure 20.4   A long flush superficial femoral artery occlusion was recanalised successfully. A follow-up angiogram 7 years later shows some diffuse disease, but the artery is still patent (note the dates on the angiogram)

Table 20.2   This table shows the limb salvage rates in patients who have had subintimal angioplasty in tibial arteries only. (Ingle showed a limb salvage rate of 94% at 3 years)

Study	Limbs/PTS	Diabetics (%)	Primary success (%)	1-year patency (%)	1-year salvage (%)
Nydahl et al.[35]	28	33	80	56	85
Vraux et al.[36]	40	72	78	56	81
Ingle et al.[37]	70	46	86	—	94 (3 years)

procedure with success rates ranging from 79 to 91%. There is a learning curve to the technique, and we believe that with experience the primary success rates of recanalising occlusive disease of femoro-popliteal and tibial segment are nearer to 90%. Secondly, whilst there is variability in the patencies at 1 year, ranging from the poor 33% at 1 year, to 65% at 5 years, there is marked consistency in the limb salvage rates of around 90% at 1 year and 88% at 3 years in one of the series. It can be concluded that subintimal angioplasty even in the predominantly femoro-popliteal segment makes a significant impact on the treatment of critical limb ischaemia.

Table 20.2 shows that where the treatment has been directed exclusively to the tibial vessels alone, in patients where there was no significant supra-popliteal inflow disease, subintimal angioplasty provided equivalent results to those for the femoro-popliteal segments. The primary success rates range from 78 to 86%, and whilst patency at 1 year averages 56%, limb salvage is consistently high from 81% at 1 year to 94% at 3 years.

The incidence of diabetes ranges from 33 to 72%[35–37] between the two sites of treatment, femoro-popliteal or tibial (Tables 20.1 and 20.2), and it can be concluded that subintimal angioplasty is an effective treatment and makes a substantial impact on the treatment of critical limb ischaemia. Since a significant proportion of patients with critical limb ischaemia have diabetes, over 33% except for one series, it is not difficult to see that subintimal angioplasty is a highly effective mode of minimally invasive treatment for patients with diabetes with foot ulcers/gangrene and PVD generally.

COMPLICATIONS

Angioplasty is not without morbidity or mortality although the incidence of the latter is very small.

In a large study by Axisa,[38] 1377 procedures were reviewed. Emergency surgical intervention was required in 2.3%. The overall amputation rate following angioplasty was 0.6%, but it was 2.2% for patients with critical limb ischaemia. There was a 1.3% mortality at 30 days, the commonest cause being bronchopneumonia. In patients with critical limb ischaemia, the mortality was higher at 4.9%.

The commonest complication of angioplasty is puncture site haematoma, the incidence of which has been reported up to 10%. The vast majority of these are self-limiting, though occasionally the patient may require transfusion or even surgery, the incidence being less than 1%. A more serious complication is when bleeding from the puncture site, usually from a high puncture, tracks in the retroperitoneal space. Such an occurrence is not easily evident at the puncture site and may come to light only when the patient demonstrates symptoms of significant hypotension due to substantial blood loss. Urgent attention is necessary to prevent mortality. Rapid replacement of fluid/blood and surgical repair is warranted in these situations. Fortunately, nowadays, closure devices are available that can be used to seal the puncture site when a high puncture has been made.

Peripheral embolisation following angioplasty occurs in less than 5% of patients; the majority of the emboli can be aspirated percutaneously at the same time as the procedure.

The incidence of perforation of the arterial wall has been reported at 3.7% in a large series by Hayes[39] comprising 1409 patients and 1532 limbs. Patients who had perforation were more likely to be older (median age 74.8 years vs 69.6 years) and/or diabetic. However, the perforation itself does not influence the ultimate outcome of the case.

Acute limb ischaemia can occur as a complication after attempted angioplasty, the incidence of which is <1.5%. In the past, this situation would have required an urgent bypass operation, but nowadays, fortunately, the majority of cases can be retrieved using a long self-expandable stent to counter the elastic recoil of the vessel, which causes acute shutdown to the flow acutely.

THROMBOLYSIS

Acute limb ischaemia occurs when a previously stenotic lesion progresses to an occlusion acutely, without adequate collateralisation around the stenotic lesion. This would most commonly occur in the femoro-popliteal segment. Symptoms include pain, pallor, decreased sensation and a cold foot.

There are two strategies for the management of this acute situation. If the limb is viable and not too threatened, it may be managed conservatively for 3 months and beyond, until the occlusion matures. There is usually symptomatic improvement during this interval through development of collateral circulation. It can then be dealt with by PTA or subintimal angioplasty, when the thrombus will be sufficiently hardened and therefore be amenable to balloon dilatation.

If the limb warrants treatment sooner rather than later, then thrombolysis can be started, using the lytic agent recombinant tissue plasminogen activator (rtPA). A suitable catheter is embedded into the thrombus and the lytic agent infused over several hours, with check angiograms performed at intervals to assess progress. The underlying stenosis will be revealed and balloon dilated, to achieve a satisfactory haemodynamic result. Thrombolysis can be used in conjunction with percutaneous aspiration thrombectomy (PAT) using a large-bore catheter. Thrombolysis is most effective when the thrombus load is not too large. Haemorrhagic complications are not uncommon, with a 1–3% stroke and up to 5% death risk.

CONCLUSION

PVD causes ulceration and gangrene in a substantial proportion of diabetic patients. In view of the aging population and increasing incidence of diabetes, it is likely to present as a substantial problem for vascular surgery/radiology departments. Fortunately, with the availability of refined and varied guidewires, low-profile coated balloons and the availability of newer and minimally invasive techniques such as subintimal angioplasty, it is possible to treat the majority of patients. In our unit the proportion of patients with critical limb ischaemia treated by angioplasty was 23% between 1988 and 1991,[29] 46% in 1994[40] and 64% in 1997.[32] Indeed, angioplasty has become the first-line treatment for the management of critical limb ischaemia, and with increasing experience, we believe that more than 75% of the patients with critical limb ischaemia can be treated in this minimally invasive fashion.

REFERENCES

1. NHS Centre for Reviews and Dissemination. Complications of diabetes. *Eff Health Care* 1999; 5:1–12.
2. Edmonds M, Boulton A, Buckenham T, *et al.* Report of the diabetic foot and amputation group. *Diabet Med* 1996;13:S27–S42.
3. World Health Organization. *Diabetes Care and Research in Europe: The St Vincent Declaration Action Programme* (implementation document). Copenhagen: World Health Organisation; 1995.
4. Edmunds ME. Progress in care of the diabetic foot. *Lancet* 1999;354:270–272.
5. McNeely MJ, Boyko EJ, Ahroni JH, *et al.* The independent contributions of diabetic neuropathy and vasculopathy in foot ulceration. How great are the risks? *Diabetes Care* 1995;18:216–219.
6. Alder AI, Boyko EJ Ahroni JH, Smith DG. Lower-extremity amputation in diabetes. The independent effects of peripheral vascular disease, sensory neuropathy and foot ulcers. *Diabetes Care* 1999;22:1029–1035.
7. Haimovici H. Patterns of arteriosclerotic lesions of the lower extremity. *Arch Surg* 1967;95:918–933.
8. Conrad MC. Large and small artery occlusion in diabetics and nondiabetics with severe vascular disease. *Diabetes* 1964;13:366–372.
9. London NJM, Cleveland TJ. Assessment of chronic lower limb ischaemia. In: Beard JD, Gaines PA, eds. *Vascular and Endovascular Surgery*. 2nd edn. Philadelphia: WB Saunders; 2001:27–54.
10. Jagger K, Phillips T, Martin RL, *et al.* Non invasive mapping of lower limb arterial lesions. *Ultrasound Med Biol* 1985;11:515–521.
11. Van Etter GI, Jaegar RA, Antonovic R, *et al.* Accuracy of lower extremity arterial duplex mapping. *J Vasc Surg* 1992;15:275–284.
12. Sensier Y, Hartshorne T, Thrush A, *et al.* A prospective comparison of lower limb colour coded duplex scanning with arteriography. *Eur J Vasc Endovasc Surg* 1996;11:170–176.
13. Sensier Y, Fishwick G, Owen M, *et al.* A comparison between colour duplex ultrasonography and arteriography for imaging infrapopliteal arterial lesions. *Eur J Vasc Endovasc Surg* 1998;15:44–51.
14. Pemberton M, London NJM. Colour flow duplex imaging of occlusive arterial disease of the lower limb. *Br J Surg* 1997;84:912–919.
15. Hertz SM, Baum RA, Owen RS, *et al.* Comparison of magnetic resonance angiography and contrast arteriography in peripheral arterial stenosis. *Am J Surg* 1993;166:112–116.
16. Owen RS, Carpenter JP, Baum RA, *et al.* Magnetic resonance imaging of angiographically occult run-off vessels in peripheral arterial occlusive disease. *N Engl J Med* 1992;326:77–81.
17. Bolia A, Brennan J, Bell PR. Recanalisation of femoro-popliteal occlusions: improving success rate by subintimal recanalisation. *Clin Radiol* 1989;40:325.
18. Bolia A, Miles KA, Brennan J, Bell PRF. Percutaneous transluminal angioplasty of occlusion of the femoral and popliteal arteries by subintimal dissection. *Cardiovasc Intervent Radiol* 1990;13:357–363.
19. Reekers JA, Kromhout JG, Jacobs MJ. Percutaneous intentional extraluminal recanalisation of the femoropopliteal artery. *Eur J Vasc Surg* 1994;8:723–728.
20. Reekers JA, Bolia A. Percutaneous intentional extraluminal (subintimal) recanalization: how to do it yourself. *Eur J Radiol* 1998;28:192–198.
21. Bolia A. Percutaneous intentional extraluminal (subintimal) recanalization of crural arteries. *Eur J Radiol* 1998;28:199–204.

22. Bolia A, Bell PRF. Femoropopliteal and crural artery recanalization using subintimal angioplasty. *Semin Vasc Surg* Sep 1995;8:253–264.

23. Bolia A, Sayers RD, Thompson MM, Bell PR. Subintimal and intraluminal recanalisation of occluded crural arteries by percutaneous balloon angioplasty. *Eur J Vasc Surg* 1994;8:214–219.

24. Bergqvist D, Karacagil S, Lofberg AM. Is balloon angioplasty below knee joint wise? In: Greenhalgh R, ed. *Indications in Vascular and Endovascular Surgery*. Philadephia: WB Saunders; 1988:353–365.

25. Matsi PJ, Manninen H, Laakso M, Jaakkola P. Impact of risk factors on limb salvage after angioplasty in chronic critical lower limb ischaemia. A prospective trial. *Angiology* 1994;45:797–804.

26. Parsons RE, Suggs WD, Lee JJ, *et al*. Percutaneous transluminal angioplasty for the treatment of limb threatening ischaemia. Do the results justify an attempt before bypass grafting? *J Vasc Surg* 1998;28:1066–1071.

27. Gutteridge W, Torrie EP, Galland RB. Cumulative risk of bypass, amputation or death following percutaneous transluminal angioplasty. *Eur J Vasc Endovasc Surg* 1997;14:134–139.

28. Danielsson G, Albrechtsson U, Norgren L, *et al*. Percutaneous transluminal angioplasty of crural arteries: diabetics and the factors influencing outcome. *Eur J Vasc Endovasc Surg* 2001;21:432–436.

29. London NJM, Varty K, Sayers RD, Thompson MM, Bell PRF, Bolia A. Percutaneous transluminal angioplasty for lower limb critical ischaemia. *Br J Surg* 1995;82:1232–1235.

30. Tisi PV, Mirnezami A, Baker S, Tawn J, Parvin SD, Darke SG. Role of subintimal angioplasty in the treatment of chronic lower limb ischaemia. *Eur J Vasc Endovasc Surg* 2002;24:417–422.

31. Lipsitz EC, Ohki T, Veith FJ, *et al*. Does subintimal angioplasty have a role in the treatment of severe lower extremity ischaemia? *J Vasc Surg* 2003;37:386–391.

32. Molloy KJ, Nasim A, London NJM, *et al*. Percutaneous transluminal angioplasty in the treatment of critical limb ischaemia. *J Endovasc Ther* 2003;10:298–303.

33. Florenes T, Bay D, Sandback G, *et al*. Subintimal angioplasty in the treatment of patients with intermittent claudication: long term results. *Eur J Vasc Endovasc Surg* 2004;28:645–650.

34. Lazaris AM, Tsiamis AC, Fishwick G, Bolia A, Bell PRF. Clinical outcomes of primary infrainguinal subintimal angioplasty in diabetic patients with critical lower limb ischaemia. *J Endovasc Ther* 2005;11:447–453.

35. Nydahl S, Hartshorne T, Bell PRF, Bolia A, London NJM. Subintimal angioplasty of infrapopliteal occlusions in critically ischaemic limbs. *Eur J Vasc Endovasc Surg* 1997;14:212–216.

36. Vraux H, Hammer F, Verhelst R. Subintimal angioplasty of tibial vessel occlusions in the treatment of critical limb ischaemia: mid-term results. *Eur J Vasc Endovasc Surg* 2000;20:441–446.

37. Ingle H, Nasim A, Bolia A, *et al*. Subintimal angioplasty of isolated infragenicular vessels in lower limb ischaemia: long-term results. *J Endovasc Ther* 2002;9:414–416.

38. Axisa B, Fishwick G, Bolia A, *et al*. Complications following peripheral angioplasty. *Ann R Coll Surg Engl* 2002;84:39–42.

39. Hayes PD, Chokkalingam A, Jones R, *et al*. Arterial perforation during infrainguinal lower limb angioplasty does not worsen outcome: results from 1409 patients. *J Endovasc Ther* 2002;9:422–427.

40. Varty K, Nydahl S, Nasim A, Bolia A, Bell PRF, London NJM. Results of surgery and angioplasty for the treatment of chronic severe lower limb ischaemia. *Eur J Vasc Endovasc Surg* 1998;16:159–163.

21 Peripheral Vascular Disease and Reconstruction

Malcolm Simms

THE PROBLEM

In Western society, the prevalence of symptomatic peripheral arterial occlusive disease (PAOD) producing intermittent claudication (IC) in men and women aged 55–74 years is 4.5%,[1] with people with diabetes being twice as susceptible as non-diabetics. In non-diabetic claudicants, the natural history of PAOD usually pursues a benign course with only 25% deteriorating over a 5-year period, 5% requiring vascular reconstruction and only 2% progressing to amputation. Continued smoking trebles the risk of disease progression.[2] Rather than suffering limb-related problems, the major hazard to which claudicants are subjected is mediated by the associated systemic atherosclerosis, with its attendant risk of heart attack and stroke, producing an increase in 5-year mortality from 5 to 30%. Risk factors other than smoking and diabetes include hypertension,[3] hyperlipidaemia[4] and hyperhomocysteinaemia.[5] The onset of symptomatic atherosclerosis tends to arise a decade later in women than in men.

In the diabetic population, the onset of PAOD is particularly sinister, since the risk of progression to amputation increases tenfold, to 20%. In the United Kingdom, 40% of all patients undergoing major limb amputation are people with diabetes, of an annual total of 15 000 operations performed.[6] Five years after amputation, only 50% of people with diabetes will be alive and only 20% will retain one intact leg.

The anatomical distribution of occlusion in the peripheral vasculature varies according to the risk factors implicated in its causation; thus smoking, hyperlipidaemia and male sex all favour iliac artery involvement,[7,8] smoking in both sexes is associated with femoro-popliteal disease [9,10] and in people with diabetes the infrapopliteal arteries are the most affected.[11–15]

The systemic complications of diabetes that concern interventionists are addressed elsewhere in this book. However, the pernicious trilogy of neuropathy, impaired tissue regeneration and increased infectivity that threatens the feet of people with diabetes supports the generalisation that '*every diabetic foot needs a pulse*'.

PRESENTATION AND EVALUATION OF PAOD IN DIABETES

Although palpation of ankle pulses should ideally be incorporated into diabetic clinic routine, the exercise is accurate and reliable in experienced hands only. Such hands, by definition,

The Foot in Diabetes, 4th Edition. Editors Andrew J.M. Boulton, Peter R. Cavanagh and Gerry Rayman.
© 2006 John Wiley & Sons, Ltd.

belong to trained clinicians who usually have other demands on their time. Consequently the development of PAOD in people with diabetes may be overlooked until the onset of symptoms prompts its detection.

In contrast to the generality of PAOD sufferers, IC is an uncommon presenting symptom in people with diabetes. The calf muscles that are most active during walking derive their blood supply from geniculate arteries that arise proximal to the popliteal trifurcation, and these are often spared in diabetic-pattern PAOD. Occlusion of the tibio-peroneal trunk and crural arteries is more likely to cause ischaemia at ankle and foot level. Although foot claudication is sometimes complained of by PAOD sufferers with a distal pattern of occlusion, in people with diabetes this symptom is likely to be obscured by peripheral neuropathy. As a result, the initial detection of PAOD in people with diabetes is often prompted by the onset of cutaneous trophic changes such as corns, calluses, blisters, ulcers or frank digital gangrene. Podiatrists and diabetic nurses are trained to investigate early phenomena, but uninformed patients may ignore what they see as minor problems until they become incapacitated, by which time the limb may be unsalvageable. Loss of skin integrity can be followed by rapid bacterial colonisation, particularly in the presence of interstitial oedema, and localised cellulitis can quickly progress to pyonecrosis.

Clinical Evaluation

In the majority of vascular patients, prognosis and therapeutic strategy can be determined clinically. Experience has shown that IC points to disease arising from a single anatomical level, whilst chronic critical limb ischaemia (CLI), characterised by rest pain or trophic change, requires disease to affect two or more levels. Proximally these levels comprise the aortic, iliac and femoral bifurcations and the superficial femoral artery (SFA) at the adductor hiatus. Below the knee, the relevant levels are the popliteal trifurcation, the malleolar anastomosis and the pedal arch. Reversal of symptoms requires restoration of flow across the appropriate number of levels. Thus, with a symptomatic history and careful mapping of pulses, it is possible to predict the urgency and likely extent of any revascularisation, as follows.

Femoral pulse palpation provides a reasonably accurate assessment of the adequacy of aorto-iliac inflow. The detection of obvious calcified plaque in the femoral artery by pressing firmly and rocking the fingertips from side to side is a reliable pointer to the presence of further calcification in the distal arterial tree.

Palpation of the popliteal pulse has considerable clinical significance; a strong pulse in the presence of CLI in the foot implies that there must be occlusion at trifurcation and malleolar levels, and so curative intervention will have to extend to the foot. Clinical accuracy in popliteal artery assessment is impaired by oedema and vascular calcification. When an absent popliteal pulse coincides with ischaemic trophic change in the foot, the popliteal trifurcation is probably diseased but the calf arteries are likely to be spared. If CLI is observed in the presence of a palpable ankle pulse, it is likely that the arteries of the foot are too extensively diseased for revascularisation to be profitable and that conservative treatment should be preferred.

Unfortunately, CLI is a concept that resists measurement, particularly in people with diabetes. The 2000 TransAtlantic Inter-Society Vascular Consensus Document defines it as rest pain, ulceration or gangrene attributable to objectively proven PAOD, predicting the need for major amputation within 6 months in the absence of successful intervention; ankle pressures should be below 50 mm Hg and toe pressures below 30 mm Hg.[16] Despite this apparently simple concept, publications describing vascular interventions for purported CLI do not routinely include data that would validate their categorisation and merely refer to the presence of rest pain or trophic change. This has contributed to misconceptions over the differing roles of angioplasty and surgical reconstruction. Factors that confound assessment include the effects of neuropathy and arthropathy on pain levels and of trauma, sepsis, neuropathy and venous disease in causing trophic change, particularly ulceration.

Ankle pressure measurement is fraught with the difficulties of interpreting sphygmomano-metric data in the presence of calcification of the leg arteries. Sometimes, observation of the height that induces the reproducible disappearance of the pedal Doppler signal whilst slowly elevating the leg from the supine position may provide a more accurate measure (in cm H_2O) of perfusion pressure (provided this is below 50 mm Hg, otherwise the leg cannot be elevated sufficiently high to lose the signal).[17]

In future, it may be helpful to define a subgroup of patients with subcritical ischaemia in whom rest pain or trophic change is not associated with the expected two anatomical levels of arterial occlusion on imaging, or in whom toe pressure measurement exceeds 30 mm Hg. In these patients, progression to limb loss in the absence of treatment is unlikely but vascular intervention, in combination with adjunctive measures, will improve symptoms and the prospects of healing.

Inspection of the affected limb should take into account swelling and pigmentation. Sym-metrical woody swelling and pigmentation of both calves point to longstanding congestive heart failure, whereas when occurring unilaterally, deep venous incompetence should be sus-pected. Uncomplicated superficial venous incompetence due to junctional or perforator reflux will give rise, on standing, to varicose veins (VVs) and purple telangiectases around the ankle. Calf swelling and ankle ulceration seldom develop as a result of primary VVs and if present they warrant a search for additional contributing factors such as post-phlebitic incompetence of deep veins.

Buerger's sign (ruddy hyperaemia of the foot in dependency, compared to deathly pallor and venous guttering on elevation) is a reliable pointer to the presence of CLI in non-diabetic patients. It indicates loss of the normal sympathetically mediated vasomotor tone in an extrem-ity that has suffered prolonged hypoperfusion. In people with diabetes, the onset of autonomic neuropathy may precede that of PAOD and this 'autosympathectomy' may mimic Buerger's sign. Similarly, combined motor and sensory neuropathy can predispose to the development of frictional, thermal or compression ulcers in feet that may not be suffering from ischaemia.

Portable (Continuous Wave) Doppler Ultrasound

The usefulness of portable Doppler devices is not confined to sphygmomanometric measure-ment of ankle systolic pressures and the calculation of the ankle–brachial pressure index (ABPI). Portable Doppler insonation of the ankle arteries with the patient seated upright and the legs dependent affords useful information on the distal vasculature, which, unlike pressure measurement, is not affected by arterial calcification. Patency of the anterior tibial, posterior tibial and peroneal arteries can be estimated, and the subjective quality of the signal (damped, staccato or vigorous) in systole and diastole can be interpreted to provide a crude estimate of inflow and outflow. If the deep plantar artery signal can be insonated (at the base of the first metatarsal space on the dorsum of the foot) then the effect on this plantar signal of manually occluding each of the ankle arteries in turn can be observed (peroneal artery compression is achieved by digital pressure postero-medial to the fibula, 5–10 cm above the lateral malleolus).

The artery providing dominant perfusion to the foot is the one that, when occluded, produces disappearance or weakening of the plantar signal.[18] Sometimes, failure to obliterate the plantar signal is observed whichever artery is compressed. This may reflect good bidirectional perfusion, or possibly heavy arterial wall calcification making the arteries incompressible.

For all the above reasons, evaluating and weighing the contribution of PAOD when assessing trophic changes in the diabetic foot requires experience and judgement. Therapeutic decision making will usually necessitate some form of arterial imaging. However, if it has been established previously by non-invasive means that endovascular intervention is not practicable, or if circumstances demand urgent intervention, direct surgical exploration and reconstruction can be undertaken on the basis of clinical and Doppler assessment only, with recourse to intra-operative on-table arteriography (OTA) as required.[19]

Duplex Ultrasonography

Duplex ultrasound merges greyscale imaging and Doppler velocity analysis into a single probe, so that both anatomical images and haemodynamic information can be provided at whichever site is chosen, at low cost and with no hazard to the patient. The only drawbacks are the expense and portability of the machines, both of which show steady improvement, and the training and expertise of the ultrasonographer, which are necessary to produce reliable and reproducible results.

In expert hands, duplex ultrasonography can provide comprehensive imaging and flow data throughout the peripheral vascular tree. Vessel diameter, wall thickness, consistency and compliance can be assessed, as can the presence of luminal plaque, thrombus and venous valves. In conjunction with this anatomical information, analysis of the Doppler spectrum enables calculation of the severity of stenoses and of the velocity and volume of blood flow. Limitations on the quality of information obtained are imposed by intervening tissues or gas or the presence of heavy vascular calcification, and because the resolution of the equipment is insufficient for vessels less than 2-mm diameter. However, in patients of normal build, it is possible to obtain diagnostic imaging and flow data from the aorta to the plantar arteries. This should be sufficient for the planning of therapeutic interventions such as angioplasty or bypass reconstruction, so that this exercise can take place routinely in the outpatient clinic. The need for contrast arteriography as a diagnostic tool has reduced further as a result of developments in computerised tomography and magnetic resonance imaging, and its main role now resides in therapeutic intervention.

Arteriography

This topic is covered in the preceding chapter but mention should be made of the place of intra-operative OTA.[20] In its simplest form, this consists of direct intra-arterial injection of contrast below a vascular clamp, with a sterile-wrapped X-ray plate placed under the site of interest. Because of the temporary circulatory arrest produced by clamping, it is possible to flood the outflow bed with contrast so that good images can be obtained reliably, using simple portable equipment rather than image intensifiers. A standard technique is to inject rapidly 50 ml of contrast into the proximally clamped common femoral artery (CFA) via a 19-gauge needle, and then wait for 5 s before making the X-ray exposure. This technique almost invariably yields perfect detailed images, the exception being the acutely ischaemic white leg, when flow in the affected part of the limb may be too slow to admit sufficient contrast.

The use of an image intensifier and a radiolucent remote-adjusting table in the operating theatre enables complex interventional manoeuvres such as stent deployment to be carried out through exposed arteries in a sterile environment, either alone or in combination with surgical reconstructive procedures.

SURGICAL RECONSTRUCTION

When contemplating reconstructive arterial surgery, the mantra should be

1. patient;

2. inflow;

3. graft;

4. outflow;

5. technique.

Patient

All vascular interventions must be preceded by a risk–benefit analysis that is shared with the patient and his/her family, taking into account the patient's expectations and overall prognosis, the difficulty, hazard and predicted success of the procedure and the long-term prospects. The analysis should cover all treatment options, whether conservative or palliative, endovascular or ablative.

Prior to any intervention, all available means should be implemented to optimise the condition of both patient and limb. Cardiorespiratory, nutritional and renal assessment should be undertaken and any deficits corrected as far as possible. Oedema, dermatitis, superficial ulceration and deep sepsis all impair tissue viability and prejudice outcome. As far as is practicable, these factors should be corrected prior to intervention. Bacterial culture and sensitivity testing is essential, and any deep collections of pus should undergo preliminary drainage. Adjunctive minor amputations should usually be postponed until after revascularisation is achieved, since incisions into ischaemic tissue always induce some degree of trauma-related local necrosis.

When surgical reconstruction is required, consideration must be given to the mode of anaesthesia, whether local, regional, neuraxial or general. This choice will normally be made with the advice of an experienced anaesthetic colleague, but it is worth remembering that all infrainguinal arterial bypass procedures can, if necessary, be performed using local anaesthesia only.[21] Prilocaine 0.5% is a useful agent, because of its rapidity of action and its low toxicity. The femoral exposure can be undertaken using local infiltration only, using a 25-gauge needle. When distal anaesthesia is required, blockade of the femoral nerve should be included, performed percutaneously or by direct infiltration of the nerve through the femoral wound. Usually additional local infiltration is needed to numb the medial thigh above the knee in order to enter the popliteal fossa. It is then a simple matter to locate the sciatic nerve, lying between the vascular bundle medially and the belly of biceps femoris muscle laterally. About 15 ml of 0.5% prilocaine is injected directly into the sciatic nerve, which can be felt bulging as it lies between finger and thumb. Within 1 min of this manoeuvre the onset of sciatic blockade should achieve complete anaesthesia of the remainder of the limb for at least 6 h. The author has encountered no complications from this technique in well over 100 applications. Adjunctive sedation can be employed to alleviate anxiety or positional discomfort but may produce disinhibition and confusion, and so should be used selectively.

Inflow

Success with infrainguinal bypass depends on adequate inflow to the CFAs and profunda femoris arteries (PFAs). Whenever there is doubt over the adequacy of the femoral pulse, angiographic or ultrasonic aorto-iliac assessment is required so that any stenoses can be corrected, preferably by endovascular means. Questionable stenoses can be evaluated by biplanar imaging or intra-operatively by papaverine testing.[22]

CFA disease is common in diabetes, and so extended open endarterectomy from the external iliac to the PFAs is needed in 30–50% of cases. Plaque in the profunda is best removed by retrograde squeezing using finger and thumb, since this is less likely to leave loose flaps.

Iliac angioplasty, endarterectomy or bypass can be performed synchronously with infrainguinal bypass. Extensive iliac atheroma with sparing of the aorta is not uncommon; if angioplasty fails or is contraindicated, this problem can usually be corrected by pulsion iliac endarterectomy. This entails exposing the iliac arteries from the aortic bifurcation through a small iliac extraperitoneal incision, then cracking and dissecting the plaque within the intact artery, beginning distally, by vigorous squeezing using finger and thumb. Once loosened in this way, the core of atheroma can be extruded distally in sections through the CFA arteriotomy. The resulting endarterectomised iliac segment makes a reliable autogenous conduit which appears resistant to infection and re-stenosis. Heavily calcified iliac arteries are unsuitable for this manoeuvre and aorto-femoral or ilio-femoral bypass will be required. In special circumstances (need for local or regional anaesthesia; hostile abdomen), extra-anatomical inflow procedures, such as axillo-femoral or cross-femoral bypass, may be considered.

When inflow enhancement is required, distal disease is likely to be less extensive, and so sequential distal bypass should not need to extend below popliteal level.

Graft

Autogenous vein remains the best conduit for infrainguinal bypass reconstruction, exhibiting low thrombogenicity and infectivity, with optimal properties of flexibility and compliance. It is a living graft, capable of repair and even, as shown when implanted in children, of growth. The ipsilateral long saphenous vein (LSV) is the first choice when available, because it is conveniently located in the leg and offers more options of length and calibre. It can be used in various configurations, either *in situ* (ISV), when valves and tributaries require extirpation,[23] or as a fully mobilised conduit, when it can be implanted reversed (RV) or non-reversed (NRV).[24] Randomised studies have shown no advantage for any particular configuration for vein grafts,[25] and the technique with which the surgeon is most familiar should be selected. When the LSV is partly or completely unavailable because of phlebitis, varicosity or previous excision, grafts can be constructed (in order of preference) from arm veins (cephalic, basilic, ulnar or linked configurations),[26] the contralateral LSV or from the short saphenous veins (SSV) of either leg. Conjoined lengths of vein make acceptable grafts and splicing together two or three lengths of good-quality vein is preferable to compromising by using narrow (<3 mm) or fibrosed phlebitic segments.

Venous valve extirpation is essential when using ISV or NRV configurations and is best performed after completion of the proximal arterial anastomosis. The valvulotome (developed by Hall and by Cartier but now available in various disposable forms) is passed retrogradely through the free open end of the graft up to the proximal anastomosis and then slowly withdrawn, so that after the pulsatile column of blood has shut each valve in turn, the valvulotome can engage and tear each pair of cusps sequentially as it progresses distally.

One advantage of not reversing the LSV is that since the proximal to distal taper of the vein is more compatible with arterial anatomy, veins with diameters as small as 2.5 mm can be considered for grafting. Consequently, vein utilisation is optimised. Other advantages are that the graft can be tunnelled when pulsating, minimising the risk of kinking, and finally, should the graft undergo thrombosis at any stage, the absence of valves facilitates embolectomy. Routing vein grafts through deep tunnels alongside the native arteries has the advantage of separating the grafts from skin wounds that, especially in diabetic patients, are susceptible to infection and breakdown. Wound dehiscence can leave subcutaneous grafts exposed to the air, with disastrous consequences.

When the length of LSV required for bypass is less than the full length of the leg, it is preferable to harvest the proximal section, from groin down, in order both to take advantage of what is usually the largest and most healthy section of vein and also to minimise dissection in the distal part of the leg, where tissue viability is usually poor.

A careful search for vein, assisted in obese patients by duplex ultrasound scanning, will invariably reveal sufficient for infrainguinal bypass in patients presenting with limb ischaemia for the first time. However, in some patients requiring secondary grafting, insufficient vein remains and alternative sources of graft must be considered if amputation is to be avoided. In this situation, up-to-date and clear arterial imaging is important in strategic planning. Combined endovascular and surgical options may still be feasible, and occasionally, total SFA endarterectomy may restore a useful conduit. Unlike iliac endarterectomy, special instrumentation is required and late re-stenosis is problematic.[27]

Prosthetic grafts should be regarded as a last resort in infrainguinal bypass for limb salvage in the diabetic population. When grafted to diseased arteries in the calf, the late results in term of patency and limb salvage are inferior[28] and the addition of distal anastomotic cuffs[29] or fistulae[30] confers little or no benefit. However, when used as the proximal component in a composite sequential femoral to popliteal to crural graft, in which the distal component is made of vein, prosthetic materials can yield satisfactory results.[31]

Outflow

Optimal tissue viability is sustained by normotensive pulsatile arterial flow and unimpeded venous drainage. Vascular reconstruction in diabetic PAOD should aim to restore this status. This can be achieved only if the arteries perfusing the arteriolar bed of the foot remain patent and accessible. When the obliterative process extends beyond the dorsalis pedis and plantar arteries into the pedal arch and the metatarsal and digital arteries, reconstruction is futile and healing of foot necrosis will not proceed, irrespective of the patency or otherwise of proximal bypass grafts. The development of ischaemic necrosis in a diabetic foot despite the presence of a palpable ankle pulse should deter thoughts of reconstruction; treatment should be conservative or ablative.

Arterial calcification on plain X-rays is commonly seen in diabetic patients and does not necessarily denote occlusion. Preliminary treatment planning, informing the choice of endovascular or surgical revascularisation, can often be based on clinical examination supported by duplex ultrasound scanning. When surgery is selected, the optimal siting of graft outflow requires good-quality arteriography, whether departmental or OTA. The purpose of outflow imaging is to demonstrate the most proximal arterial site that provides unimpeded perfusion of the distal vasculature through disease-free channels.

When arteriograms show that the occlusive process is confined to the distal vascular bed, commencing beyond the popliteal trifurcation, then it is highly likely to involve the pedal arch and its branches, in which case distal bypass is impracticable (Figure 21.1).

A common pattern of treatable occlusion in people with diabetes comprises a diffusely diseased SFA terminating in an occluded popliteal artery, with refilling of crural arteries in mid-calf (Figure 21.2). In skilled hands, angioplasty can recanalise about 80% of these cases and clinical success, though not necessarily patency, is reported in 69% at 1 year.[32] Surgical

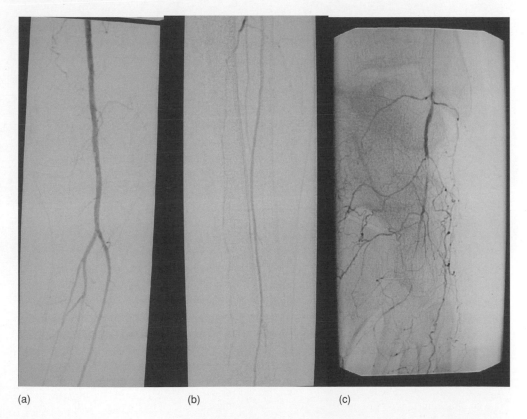

(a)   (b)   (c)

Figure 21.1   The unreconstructable leg; in the presence of distal ischaemic necrosis, a palpable popliteal pulse with arteriographic evidence of an open trifurcation points to occlusion of the pedal arch: (a) the arteriogram demonstrates a patent femoro-popliteal segment in continuity with an open trifurcation; (b) the posterior tibial artery is patent to ankle level; (c) both plantar arteries and the pedal arch are occluded. Bypass reconstruction is not feasible.

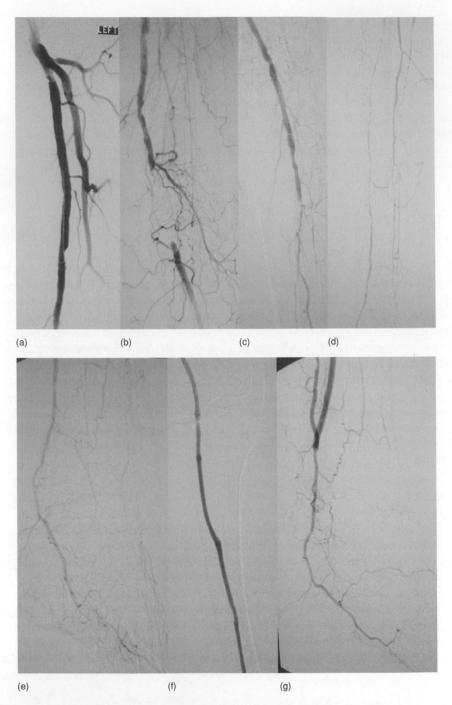

Figure 21.2 Collaboration between surgeons and radiologists; this arteriographic sequence demonstrates multi-segmental occlusion suitable for either angioplasty or bypass: (a) femoral bifurcation and outflow; (b) SFA occlusion at adductor level; (c) diseased but patent popliteal artery and trifurcation; (d) posterior tibial artery reconstitution; (e) posterior tibial and plantar continuity; (f) 6 months after failed angioplasty followed by common femoral to posterior tibial bypass using non-reversed long saphenous vein; duplex scan had suggested outflow stenosis; (g) a focal stenosis is shown in the posterior tibial artery at malleolar level. This was successfully dilated with a 4-mm balloon.

bypass using vein grafts offers durable patency with an acceptable complication rate.[33] Graft inflow should be sited above the commencement of the occlusive process but does not have to be from the CFA. Use of the SFA or the popliteal arteries for the proximal graft anastomosis has been found compatible with long-term graft patency, particularly in the diabetic population.[34]

Whichever disease-free crural artery is seen to be in continuity with the pedal arch (through collaterals in the case of the peroneal) can be considered a candidate for graft outflow. Vascular grafts should be as short and direct as possible, and the ankle joint should be crossed only if necessary; so the surgeon must be familiar with the approaches to all three arteries in the calf as well as to the pedal arteries.

Technique

Systemic anticoagulation is not essential for peripheral vascular reconstruction; neither is it a contraindication. Prophylaxis against venous thrombosis is advisable, commencing an agent such as enoxaparin 20 mg s.c. daily on admission to hospital. During the operation, local intra-arterial flushing with a 10 units/ml solution of heparin in Hartmann's solution delivered through a blunt cannula is sufficient to prevent local intra-arterial thrombosis during vascular clamping. Longstanding warfarinisation need not be reversed, provided pre-operative international normalised ratio (INR) levels do not exceed 3 and fresh frozen plasma is available, although neuraxial anaesthesia must be avoided in patients with anticoagulation. Excessive operative bleeding is likely in patients taking both aspirin and clopidogrel and one of these (usually the clopidogrel) should be withdrawn 7 days before surgery.

Following any successful revascularisation for CLI, a degree of post-operative soft tissue swelling is normal, partly due to tissue trauma and disturbance of venous and lymphatic drainage but largely through interstitial fluid accumulation, reflecting temporarily increased vascular permeability. This results from established circulatory adaptation to chronic underperfusion and is self-correcting over a period of weeks or months.

When revascularisation follows a period of severe ischaemia sufficient to produce muscle paralysis, pain or tenderness, then some degree of post-operative muscle swelling is inevitable, risking the development of compartment pressure syndrome (CPS). It is preferable to anticipate this and perform prophylactic fasciotomy, hopefully with the minimum of additional incisions, before wound closure. Grafts should not be left exposed to the air, but cover with viable muscle rather than skin is sufficient.

If post-operative CPS develops unexpectedly, then full compartmental decompression can be achieved with a single lateral calf incision along the line of the fibula, deepened to the bone, followed by splitting of all the attached fascial septa, both anterior and posterior. Fibular excision confers no additional benefit. With this technique, it is helpful to insert a loose-running monofilament subcuticular suture, with no initial attempt at skin closure. This manoeuvre controls retraction of the skin edges and permits delayed skin closure when the swelling subsides, simply by traction on the subcuticular suture, under sedation.

ADJUNCTIVE MEASURES AND MANAGING COMPLICATIONS

Intravenous antibiotic therapy should be administered prophylactically to all patients undergoing peripheral vascular reconstruction. The choice of agent should take into account the results of swab cultures from any ulcerated or necrotic areas of skin. Even when the skin is intact, patients should be routinely screened for methicillin-resistant *Staphylococcus aureus* (MRSA) colonisation prior to admission to hospital. A standard regimen might comprise flucloxacillin 1 g i.v. and gentamicin 120 mg i.v. on induction of anaesthesia, with a second dose on the first post-operative day. Prolonged antibiotic courses should not be administered prophylactically; they should be reserved for specific complications and modified according to the results of bacterial culture.

Once graft flow is established at operation, an intra-graft bolus dose of a vasodilator drug such as one of the prostacycline analogues[35] or papaverine 30 mg should abolish any tendency to vasospasm. There is also some support for giving an infusion of Dextran 40, 500 ml over 4 h, once daily for the first day or two, since this reduces platelet aggregation. None of the above will compensate for technical shortcomings.

Whenever possible skin wounds should be covered with waterproof occlusive dressings for 48–72 h, by which time they should have become sealed with a fibrin film and can be left uncovered. Haematomas and fluid collections should be drained promptly, with full sterile precautions, in theatre if necessary.

Graft patency can be checked by regular foot inspection and pulse palpation, but in case of doubt duplex ultrasound imaging is definitive and can also be used to diagnose deep vein thrombosis when swelling seems excessive. Graft occlusion should be tackled promptly and aggressively by operative re-exploration. It is vital to seek and rectify the cause of failure, so in addition to thrombectomy (by balloon catheter extraction and graft flushing), methodical checks of inflow, graft and outflow, with the possible assistance of OTA, are essential.

In the interests of minimising pain and reactive swelling, it is advisable to keep patients on bedrest with the leg elevated for the first 48 h. Care must be taken to protect pressure areas, particularly the heel of the operated leg or the sacrum in patients remaining on epidural analgesia. Thereafter, supervised mobilisation is desirable, tailored to the patient's abilities.

When soft tissue necrosis of the calf or foot is extensive, distal bypass and debridement can be combined with tissue reconstruction, using microvascular free grafts, comprising muscle, skin or both. Such grafts are fragile and insensate, and so they are unsuitable for weight-bearing surfaces. Initial enthusiasm for this approach in the United Kingdom has been tempered by poor long-term results, but encouraging reports continue to appear.[36]

RESULTS OF RECONSTRUCTION

These are usually presented in life-table format, quoting primary graft patency, primary assisted patency (including successful thrombectomy cases), secondary patency (including cases of successful re-grafting) and limb salvage (amputation avoided, irrespective of graft patency). When grafts occlude within the first 6 months of operation, before wound healing and collateral development are consolidated, it is likely that critical ischaemia will return and that, in the absence of successful re-grafting, amputation will prove necessary. After 6 months, graft failure is less likely to precipitate symptoms of recurrent critical ischaemia.

Somewhat surprisingly, the results of infrainguinal bypass procedures in diabetic patients have not been found inferior in terms of patency to those in non-diabetics, irrespective of anatomical level.[37] However, the diabetic population is more susceptible to neuroseptic and trophic complications that can precipitate limb loss despite graft flow being maintained. At 5 years, secondary graft patency rates of 80% and limb salvage rates of 95% have been reported

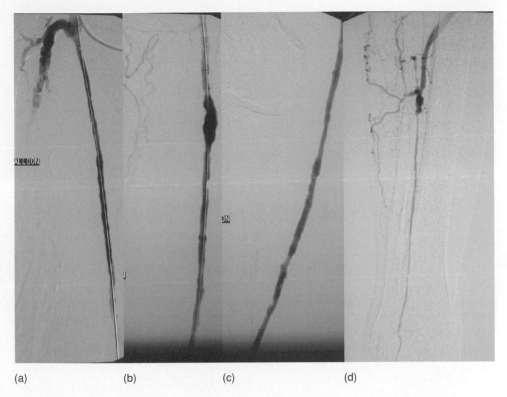

(a)   (b)   (c)   (d)

Figure 21.3   Arterialisation of vein grafts; a femoro-tibial vein graft in an insulin-dependent diabetic patient imaged 12 years after reconstruction, when angioplasty for stenosis was required for the third time: (a) proximal anastomosis to the common femoral artery; (b) aneurysmal dilatation and diffuse irregularity at mid-thigh level; (c) the atherosclerotic vein graft crosses the knee in a subcutaneous tunnel; (d) distal anastomosis to the atherosclerotic upper anterior tibial artery.

from centres with an interest in distal bypass, irrespective of inflow source or outflow vessel.[38] Beyond this time, survival declines more rapidly than graft failure. Good-quality vein grafts are capable of indefinite survival, as is seen when they have to be constructed in children. However, arterialised vein grafts in atherosclerotic hosts are eventually susceptible to the same degenerative processes as arteries (Figure 21.3).

ANGIOPLASTY OR BYPASS?

With increasing experience, these treatment options are coming to be regarded as complementary, rather than as competing alternatives. Attempts at conducting randomised prospective comparisons have been limited by the difficulty of recruiting cases in whom the choice of one or other method is not dictated by clinical or angiographic imperatives.

When the endovascular option is available, it will usually be preferred on grounds of safety, low morbidity and economy. Most vascular surgical units have seen at least a 50% reduction in the annual number of infrainguinal bypass operations performed since the introduction of endovascular interventions for CLI. The relative lack of durability of angioplasty is offset by its repeatability and the limited life expectancy of the subjects. These trends have meant that the rump of patients being considered for surgical bypass are likely to present complex challenges. The criteria influencing the choice of angioplasty or bypass are summarised below.

Surgical bypass	Angioplasty
Relative considerations	
SFA occlusion: flush origin or >20cm	Short stenoses, occlusions <20 cm
Advanced ischaemic necrosis	Venous or neuropathic ulceration
ABPI <0.5	ABPI >0.5
Life expectancy > 2 years	Life expectancy <2 years
Combined inflow and CFA disease	Aorto-iliacs dilatable, CFA clear
Inframalleolar occlusion	
Absolute indications for surgery	
Failed angioplasty	
Acute ischaemia	
Aneurysmal disease	
Heavy calcification	

CONCLUSIONS

Although developments in endovascular technique have reduced the volume of patients requiring bypass reconstruction for CLI, those that are ineligible or unsuitable for angioplasty, many of whom have diabetes, present complex challenges to vascular surgeons. In order to achieve optimal limb salvage with minimal morbidity, the surgical team requires multidisciplinary support and must have access to a wide range of skills and techniques. When revascularisation proves impossible, an equally positive approach to palliation, amputation and rehabilitation is necessary.

REFERENCES

1. Fowkes FGR, Housley E, Cawood EH, Macintyre CC, Ruckley CV, Prescott RJ. Edinburgh Artery Study: prevalence of asymptomatic and symptomatic peripheral arterial disease in the general population. *Int J Epidemiol* 1991;20:384–392.
2. Cronenwett JL, Warner KG, Zelenock GB, *et al*. Intermittent claudication. Current results of non-operative management. *Arch Surg* 1984;119:430–436.
3. Kannel WB, McGee DL. Update on some epidemiological features of intermittent claudication. *J Am Geriatr Soc* 1985;33:13–18.
4. Kannel WB, Skinner JJ Jr, Schwartz MJ, Shurtleff D, *et al*. Intermittent claudication: incidence in the Framingham Study. *Circulation* 1970;41:875–883.
5. Clarke R, Daly L, Robinson K, *et al*. Hyperhomocystinaemia: an independent risk factor for vascular disease. *N Engl J Med* 1991;324:1149–1155.
6. Dormandy J, Ray S. The natural history of peripheral arterial disease. In: Tooke JE, Lowe GD, eds. *A Textbook of Vascular Medicine*. London: Arnold; 1996:162–175.

7. Haltmayer M, Mueller T, Horvath W, Luft C, Poelz W, Haidinger D. Impact of atherosclerotic risk factors on the anatomical distribution of peripheral arterial disease. *Int Angiol* 2001;20:200–207.

8. Smith FB, Lee AJ, Fowkes FG, Lowe GD, Rumley A. Variation in cardiovascular risk factors by angiographic site of lower limb atherosclerosis. *Eur J Vasc Endovasc Surg* 1996;11:340–346.

9. Kannel WB, Shurtleff D. The Framingham Study. Cigarettes and the development of intermittent claudication. *Geriatrics* 1973;28:61–68.

10. Menzoian JO, LaMorte WW, Paniszyn CC, *et al.* Symptomatology and anatomic patterns of peripheral vascular disease: differing impact of smoking and diabetes. *Ann Vasc Surg* 1989;3:224–228.

11. Gensler SW, Haimovici H, Hoffert P, Steinman C, Beneventano TC. Study of vascular lesions in diabetic, nondiabetic patients. Clinical, arteriographic and surgical considerations. *Arch Surg* 1965;91:617–622.

12. van der Feen C, Neijens FS, Kanters SD, Mali WP, Stolk RP, Banga JD. Angiographic distribution of lower extremity atherosclerosis in patients with and without diabetes. *Diabet Med* 2002;19:366–370.

13. Strandness DE Jr, Priest RE, Gibbons GE. Combined clinical and pathologic study of diabetic and nondiabetic peripheral arterial disease. *Diabetes* 1964;13:366–372.

14. Conrad MC. Large and small artery occlusion in diabetics and non-diabetics with severe vascular disease. *Circulation* 1967;36:83–91.

15. Jude EB, Oyibo SO, Chalmers N, Boulton AJ. Peripheral arterial disease in diabetic and nondiabetic patients: a comparison of severity and outcome. *Diabetes Care* 2001;24:1433–1437.

16. TASC Working Group. Definition and nomenclature for chronic critical limb ischemia. *J Vasc Surg* 2000;31:Recommendations 73–74.

17. Smith FCT, Shearman CP, Simms MH, Gwynn BR. Falsely elevated ankle pressures in severe limb ischaemia: the Pole test – an alternative approach. *Eur J Vasc Surg* 1994;8:408–412.

18. Roedersheimer LR, Feins R, Green RM. Doppler evaluation of the pedal arch. *Am J Surg* 1981;142:601–604.

19. Shearman CP, Gwynn BR, Curran F, Gannon MX, Simms MH. Non-invasive femoropopliteal assessment. Is that angiogram really necessary? *Br Med J* 1987;293:1086–1089.

20. Flanigan DP, Wiliams LR, Keifer J, Schwartz JA, Gray B, Schuler JJ. Prebypass operative arteriography. *Surgery* 1982;92:627–633.

21. McKay C, Razik WA, Simms MH. Local anaesthetic for lower limb revascularisation in high-risk patients. *Br J Surg* 1997;84:1096–1098.

22. Flanigan DP, Ryan TJ, Williams LR, Schwartz JA, Gray B, Schuler JJ. Aortofemoral or femoropopliteal revascularisation? A prospective evaluation of the papaverine test. *J Vasc Surg* 1984;1(1);215–223.

23. Shearman CP, Gannon MX, Gwynn BR, Simms MH. A clinical method for the detection of arteriovenous fistulas during in situ great saphenous vein bypass. *J Vasc Surg* 1986;4:578–581.

24. Belkin M, Knox J, Donaldson MC, Mannick JA, Whittemore AD. Infrainguinal arterial reconstruction with nonreversed greater saphenous vein. *J Vasc Surg* 1996;24:957–962.

25. Harris PL, Veith FJ, Shanik GD, Nott D, Wengerter KR, Moore DJ. Prospective randomised comparison of in situ and reversed infrapopliteal vein grafts. *Br J Surg* 1993;80:173–176.

26. Holzenbein TJ, Pomposelli FB, Miller A, *et al.* Results of a policy with arm veins used as the first alternative to an available ipsilateral greater saphenous vein for infrainguinal bypass. *J Vasc Surg* 1996;23:130–140.

27. Smeets L, Ho GH, Haenaars T, van den Berg JC, Teijink JA, Moll FL. Remote endarterectomy: first choice in surgical treatment of long segmental SFA occlusive disease? *Eur J Vasc Endovasc Surg* 2003;25:583–589.

28. Veith FJ, Gupta SK, Ascer E, *et al.* Six year prospective multicentre randomised comparison of autologous saphenous vein and expanded poltetrafluorethylene grafts in infrainguinal arterial reconstructions. *J Vasc Surg* 1986;3:104–114.

29. Stonebridge PA, Prescott RJ, Ruckley CV. Randomised trial comparing infrainguinal polytetrafluorethylene bypass grafting with and without vein interposition cuff at the distal anastomosis. *J Vasc Surg* 1997;26:543–550.

30. Laurila K, Lepantalo M, Teittinen K, *et al.* Does an adjuvant fistula improve the patency of a femorocrural PTFE bypass with distal cuff in critical leg ischaemia? – a prospective randomised multicentre trial. *Eur J Vasc Endovasc Surg* 2004;27:180–185.

31. Mahmood A, Garnham A, Sintler M, Smith SRG, Vohra RK, Simms MH. Composite sequential grafts for femorocrural bypass reconstruction: experience with a modified technique. *J Vasc Surg* 2002;36:772–778.

32. Lazaris AM, Tsiamis AC, Fishwick G, Bolia A, Bell PRF. Clinical outcome of primary infrainguinal subintimal angioplasty in diabetic patients with critical lower limb ischaemia. *J Endovasc Ther* 2004;11:447–453.

33. Pomposelli FB, Kansal N, Hamdan AD, *et al.* A decade of experience with dorsalis pedis artery bypass: analysis of outcome in more than 1000 cases. *J Vasc Surg* 2003;37:307–315.

34. Reed AB, Conte MS, Belkin M, Mannick JA, Whittemore AD, Donaldson MC. Usefulness of autogenous bypass grafts originating distal to the groin. *J Vasc Surg* 2002;35:48–54.

35. Hickey NC, Shearman CP, Crowson MC, Simms MH, Watson H. Iloprost improves femoro-distal graft flow after a single bolus injection. *Eur J Vasc Surg* 1991;5:19–22.

36. Czerny M, Trubel W, Zimpfer D, *et al.* Limb salvage by femoro-distal bypass and free muscle flap transfer. *Eur J Vasc Endovasc Surg* 2004;27:635–639.

37. Wolfle KB. Bruijnen H, Loeprecht H, *et al.* Graft patency and clinical outcome of femorodistal arterial reconstruction in diabetic and non-diabetic patients: results of a multicentre comparative analysis. *Eur J Vasc Endovasc Surg* 2003;25:229–234.

38. Shah DM, Darling RC III, Chang BB, Fitzgerald KM, Paty PS, Leather RP. Long term results of in situ saphenous vein bypass. Analysis of 2058 cases. *Ann Surg* 1995;222:438–446.

22 Charcot Foot: What's New in Pathogenesis and Medical Management?

Edward B. Jude

INTRODUCTION

Charcot neuroarthropathy (CN) is a progressive condition affecting the bones and joints of the foot and is characterised by joint dislocation, subluxation and pathologic fractures of the foot of neuropathic patients, often resulting in a debilitating deformity. In developed countries, the condition is most commonly encountered in diabetic individuals.[1,2] The development of CN results in a foot that is 'at risk' for ulceration and amputation (Figure 22.1).

EPIDEMIOLOGY

The incidence of CN in diabetes is reported to be around 0.1–0.5%.[3–5] Bilateral involvement has been reported in up to 30% of patients with Charcot feet.[1] There is no sex predilection, and both type 1 and type 2 diabetic patients are at risk. It is commonly seen in the fourth or fifth decades of life and in patients with a long duration of diabetes.[3,6] The majority of lesions occur in the midfoot, but any bone or joint in the foot or ankle can be affected.[6,7]

PATHOGENESIS

The association between joint changes and neurological disease was observed as early as 1831 by Mitchell, who described a patient with 'rheumatism of the lower extremities' and 'caries of the spine'.[8] He noted the importance of 'that part of the spine, which supplies with nerves the parts in a state of active inflammation'. In 1868, Jean-Martin Charcot, a French neurologist, gave a detailed description of the arthropathy occurring in tabes dorsalis and this condition bears his name.[9] The association with diabetes was put forward by Jordan when he described a case of Charcot arthropathy in a diabetic patient.[10]

The aetiopathogenesis of diabetic CN is still unclear. Two theories have been put forward for the development of this joint condition. The first theory, known as the French theory, was

The Foot in Diabetes, 4th Edition. Editors Andrew J.M. Boulton, Peter R. Cavanagh and Gerry Rayman.
© 2006 John Wiley & Sons, Ltd.

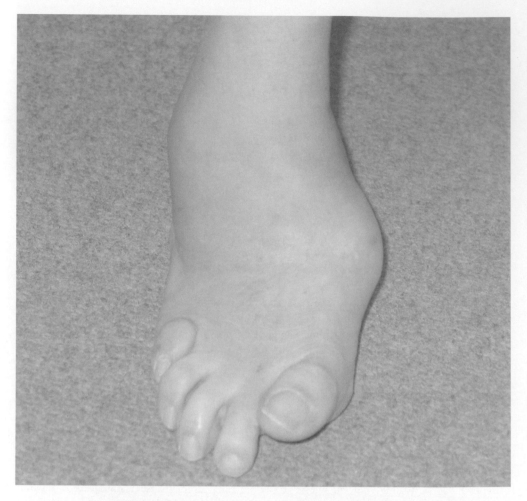

Figure 22.1   Acute Charcot foot with foot and ankle oedema

initially proposed by Charcot himself.[9] He suggested that arthritic changes were the result of damage to the central nervous system within the centres that control bone and joint nutrition. Therefore, neurological damage preceded the development of, and was in some way directly responsible for, the changes occurring in CN. The second theory, known as the German theory, was popularised by Volkman and Virchow.[11,12] This concept suggests that the changes in the bone were a result of a multiplicity of subclinical traumata, which went unperceived because of the insensitivity of the affected joint.

   Peripheral neuropathy and autonomic neuropathy are thought to be the pre-requisites for the initiation and progression of the Charcot process. Trauma may be an important precipitating factor in its development, although around two thirds of patients do not remember having injured the foot.[1,13] Continued weight bearing on the foot can result in a progression of the Charcot changes.[14] In a case series of 101 patients with CN, all patients had distal symmetrical sensory neuropathy,[3] and this was similarly observed in two other series.[6,15] Patients may also have motor nerve involvement, which may be the reason for the ligament stretching and spontaneous dislocations seen commonly in this condition.[16,17] However, it is thought that autonomic dysfunction leads to some of the circulatory changes that result in the gradual destruction of the foot. Sympathetic denervation results in increased blood flow to the foot, which has been demonstrated by plethysmography[18] and by increased uptake of isotope in patients with CN.[19]

Changes in the bones of the feet as a result of the peripheral nerve abnormality have been studied using bone turnover markers and bone density studies. Bone metabolism is characterised by two opposite activities: the formation of new bone by osteoblasts, and the degradation (resorption) of old bone by the osteoclasts. The rate of bone formation or resorption can be assessed either by measuring a prominent enzymatic activity, such as alkaline and acid phosphatase activity, of the bone-forming or resorbing cells, or by measuring bone matrix components released into the circulation during formation or resorption. Bone turnover markers have been shown to be increased in acute CN, indirectly indicating increased bone metabolism. Gough *et al.* measured pyridinoline cross-linked carboxy-terminal telopeptide domain of type 1 collagen (1CTP) and carboxy-terminal propeptide of type 1 collagen (PICP) as possible markers of bone resorption and bone formation, respectively, in diabetic patients with acute Charcot, chronic Charcot and in control subjects, in the systemic circulation (from a forearm vein) and in the foot.[20] They found an increase in the bone turnover marker 1CTP in patients with acute CN but no difference in the bone formation markers. In a similar study, Selby *et al.* measured urinary deoxypyridinoline (bone resorption marker) and bone-specific alkaline phosphatase (bone formation marker) in patients with acute CN and non-Charcot diabetic patients and found an increase in both these markers thus indicating an ongoing remodelling process, bone resorption and formation.[21] Edelson and colleagues employing a different urinary marker of bone resorption, cross-linked N-telopeptides of type I collagen (NTx), demonstrated increased levels of collagen breakdown in subjects with CN.[22] Therefore, a possible logical step in the treatment would be to dampen down this enhanced bone remodelling and hence retard the progression of the Charcot process.

In addition, studies have shown that there is reduced bone density in the foot in patients with diabetic CN.[23] Only one study has demonstrated, in a small group of patients presenting with a hot swollen foot, that reduced bone mineral density (using bone densitometry) in the lower limb led to subsequent development of CN, compared to patients with higher bone mineral density at baseline.[24] Broadband ultrasound attenuation studies have shown a reduction in bone density in the calcaneus in patients with CN.[25,26] The latter study by Jirkovska *et al.* also demonstrated an increase in 1CTP in patients with acute CN and a direct correlation between plasma 1CTP and bone density in the calcaneus.[26]

CLINICAL FEATURES AND DIAGNOSIS

Acute CN can be misdiagnosed as cellulitis, osteomyelitis or inflammatory arthropathy, and therefore a high index of suspicion is necessary so that appropriate treatment can be instituted immediately to prevent the severe deformities seen in this condition. The earliest manifestation of CN is swelling of the affected foot with pain or discomfort. On examination, the foot is generally warm, may be inflamed and swollen. There is a temperature differential of $>2°C$ when compared with the contralateral foot. Although patients have severe peripheral neuropathy, pain is the most common feature followed by discomfort in the foot.[6,27] In the acute state, the Charcot foot may be mistaken for gout, cellulits and osteomyelitis.[3] Sometimes, CN can be a diagnosis of exclusion, as most investigations in the early stages can be normal (see below).

Once the acute phase has subsided, which can take months, the foot then progresses into a chronic stage. The chronic Charcot foot is painless, without a temperature differential in a deformed foot. It can frequently become reactivated if there is further trauma to the foot, in which case differentiating it from osteomyelitis can be challenging. Therefore, long-term follow-up is necessary, as these patients are at high risk for reactivation of the Charcot process, foot ulceration as well as amputation.[28]

Investigations

CN can be diagnosed in the majority by plain X-rays, but at times specialised investigations may be required. Plain X-rays of the involved foot will reveal bone and joint destruction, fragmentation and remodelling in the advanced cases, but early changes may be subtle or undetectable.[29] The joints commonly involved are those of the phalanges and metatarsals and tarsal bones, but ankles can occasionally also be affected. Three-phase ^{99m}Tc bisphosphonate bone scans demonstrate an early increase in bone uptake, which is due to the increase in blood flow through the bone that accompanies the active Charcot process. Although a radiological diagnosis can be made with some confidence, it may be difficult to rule out osteomyelitis, especially in the presence of a foot ulcer. To exclude incidental osteomyelitis, [111] In-labelled leucocyte scans and magnetic resonance imaging may be required.[29,30]

TREATMENT

Management of CN is difficult and there is no specific treatment that can reduce or reverse the destructive changes. An increased awareness of this condition may help in enabling an earlier diagnosis, instituting earlier treatment and possibly preventing progression of the foot deformity and disability. The treatment offered to patients is usually long-term immobilisation in a total contact cast (TCC; made of plaster of Paris or fibreglass), Charcot restraint orthotic walker (CROW) or a Scotchcast boot (SCB; made of Deltalite plaster).[6,29,31] Two studies have shown that immobilisation may be necessary for between 14 and 18 weeks, but occasionally immobilisation for up to a year may be necessary. More recently, pneumatic walking braces have also been used and have been shown to reduce pressures similarly as plaster casting.[32] Surgical treatment has no role in the acute Charcot foot, but in the later stages, when the foot has achieved a stable shape, surgery may be necessary to remove bony deformities, and more extensive reconstructive surgery has, in some centres, led to excellent clinical results. Techniques include arthrodesis, exostectomies, reconstruction and Achilles tendon lengthening[33] (Chapter 23).

Immobilisation

Two studies have examined the use of TCC in the treatment of the Charcot foot. In one study, Armstrong and colleagues assessed the efficacy of serial TCC in 55 patients with acute CN until quiescence.[6] Following casting, patients were put into unprotected weight bearing via a removable cast walker, and then transferred to prescription footwear. Patients were transferred to cast walker when their temperature differential was less than 1°C for two consecutive weeks at the affected site compared with the corresponding site, contralaterally, and then to prescription footwear when temperature differential equilibrated for 1 month ($\pm 1°C$). All patients' feet became quiescent around 4 months (range 4–56 weeks) and progression to permanent footwear took just over 6 months. Therefore, the mean duration of immobilisation prior to return to permanent footwear was approximately 6 months, but some patients required this treatment for up to 12 months. In a separate study, McCrory et al. similarly examined the role of casting and foot temperature in active Charcot arthropathy.[34] In this study, they observed that skin temperature was possibly not a useful indicator of Charcot healing or progression. However, they found that radiographic healing usually began by 3–6 months and this roughly correlated around the time when 'foot cooling' began. Therefore, from these two studies, one can conclude that casting is necessary for a prolonged period, and clinical indicators are required to definitely ascertain the total duration of immobilisation. However, there have been no published studies on the use of the SCB in the acute Charcot foot.

Radiotherapy and Ultrasound

In the first randomised clinical trial in the CN, Chantelau et al. examined the use of radiotherapy in the acute Charcot foot.[35] In this study, they randomised 14 patients to receive radiotherapy or sham radiotherapy. All patients received standard treatment, which was offloading and bedrest. The end points of the study were clinical and radiological healing of the Charcot foot. There was no difference in healing of the Charcot foot in patients who received active treatment (radiotherapy) or sham radiotherapy (5.5 months vs 7 months; $p > 0.05$). This could have been a type 2 error resulting from the small number of patients in the study. However, patients who complied with offloading did much better than patients who were non-compliant. From this small study, it is difficult to rule out radiotherapy as a possible treatment of CN, and further studies are required to ascertain the usefulness of this modality of treatment in this condition. Low-intensity ultrasound has also been investigated in conjunction with offloading and was found to be useful.[36] However, both the above studies were done in small groups of patients and should be investigated in more robust trials.

Pharmacological Treatment – Bisphosphonates

Currently, treatments that are being used for the Charcot foot are unsatisfactory and do not modify the natural history of the condition or arrest the underlying bone resorption. There is no pharmacological treatment licensed for the treatment of CN. Although treatment with offloading has some clinical benefit, there is a need for pharmacological treatment.

In 1994, Selby and colleagues conducted a pilot study in the treatment of CN using a bisphosphonate, pamidronate.[37] This open-label study was designed to study the effect of bisphosphonates on the disease activity in CN and also on bone turnover markers. The effect of pamidronate on foot temperature and alkaline phosphatase was studied in a small number of patients ($n = 6$). All patients received infusions of pamidronate every 2 weeks (60 mg first dose and subsequently 30 mg fortnightly over 12 weeks), and foot temperature and alkaline phosphatase were measured at each visit. The treatment was associated with improvement in the patients' symptoms as well as a reduction in foot temperatures. A significant reduction was also seen in alkaline phosphatase over the 12 weeks of follow-up, which fell by about 25% at the end of the study.

Bisphosphonates are synthetic analogues of inorganic pyrophosphate that inhibit bone turnover by decreasing the resorption of bone. They do this directly, by inhibiting the recruitment and function of osteoclasts (the bone-resorbing cells), and indirectly, by stimulating osteoblasts (bone-forming cells).[38] Bisphosphonates may also shorten the lifespan of osteoclasts. Increased bone resorption is a prominent feature of many bone diseases, including CN. These characteristics make bisphosphonates the logical treatment for this condition. Pain is a major feature in CN, and it has been suggested that processes that affect the structure of bone are not necessarily those responsible for rapid pain relief, which is seen in CN patients.[39] Pain relief is thought to result from the effects of the bisphosphonate on prostaglandin E2 and other nociceptive substances.[40] Bisphosphonates may also affect the release of neuropeptides and neuromodulators from afferent nerve endings, the cytokines that could be responsible for producing vasodilatory and inflammatory changes seen in various bone conditions.[41,42]

Following on from the above pilot study, we proceeded to a randomised double-blind clinical trial using intravenous pamidronate in diabetic patients with CN. In this trial, we recruited 39 patients with active CN who were randomised to receive either placebo (normal saline) or pamidronate (90 mg) as a single intravenous infusion at baseline.[27] Disease activity (temperature differential), patients' symptoms and bone turnover markers were assessed at baseline and at each subsequent visit over the next 12 months. All patients received standard treatment of the affected foot, including immobilisation and bedrest. Reduction in temperature was seen in all patients and also symptoms score improved during follow-up.[27] There was a significant reduction in temperature in the placebo and active groups at 2 weeks when compared to baseline. There was a further reduction in temperature in the pamidronate group 4 weeks after the infusion, but this did not reach statistical significance when compared to the placebo group. All patients were asked about their symptoms related to the Charcot foot, which was scored using a visual analogue scale. Severe neuropathic pain was a major feature in the majority of patients, with discomfort being the next most common symptom. This has also been noted in other series.[6] Patients were asked to score the symptoms on a scale of 1–10 and this was measured quarterly. The patients' symptoms were significantly reduced in the pamidronate group when compared to the placebo group and this remained so until the end of the study.

Bone markers were measured to assess Charcot activity. We measured a bone resorption marker, deoxypyridinoline (in a second-void, early-morning sample and reported as a ratio with respect to urinary creatinine), and a bone formation marker, bone-specific alkaline phosphatase (in plasma in the fasting state). Both markers were measured at each visit. There was a marked reduction in urinary deoxypyridinoline and bone-specific alkaline phosphatase. A difference in these markers was seen around 4 weeks and remained until 12–24 weeks. This effect of pamidronate was limited and the bone markers returned towards baseline levels in 6–12 months after the infusion. The overall effect of pamidronate is thought to be due to a reduction in cytokines,[43] hence possibly reducing the inflammation within the bones and soft tissues of the foot. Whether this is the case in CN is interesting and needs further study. In this study, we did not do repeat X-rays or bone scans to assess the activity within the joints and bones of the foot.[44]

Although we found a reduction in the temperature (disease activity), the difference between placebo and pamidronate groups did not achieve statistical significance. To assess the number of patients required in the study, we performed power calculations that gave us a total of 38 patients to be recruited into the study in spite of which we did not find any difference in the temperature between the active and placebo groups. This may be because we did not take into account the simultaneous reduction in foot temperatures with simple offloading.[44] Therefore, we now feel that a larger clinical trial would be required to assess if bisphosphonates affect disease activity in CN and to determine the appropriate dose, duration and frequency of treatment. Further trials will also be needed to study other possible routes of administration, since in recent years potent oral bisphosphonates have become available.

There have been two further trials to study the benefit of bisphosphonates in CN. In a separate study, Anderson *et al.* treated 23 patients with acute CN with intravenous pamidronate (variable dose) or with standard care only.[45] Patients were followed up at 2 days and 2 weeks. Patients in the pamidronate group had a greater reduction in temperature than the standard care group. Patients also had a significant reduction in alkaline phosphatase. This however was not a randomised study, and there was a bias in the treatment strategy.

In a study from Italy, patients with acute CN were randomised to the oral bisphosphonate alendronate (70 mg once a week) or placebo.[46] Patients in both groups had reduction in temperature at the end of 6 months, which was not different; but patients in the active arm had a significant reduction in symptoms as well as a reduction in ICTP and hydroxyproline. Patients who received alendronate also showed an improvement in bone density in the foot.

From the above studies, it has been demonstrated that bisphosphonates do have some beneficial effects on the underlying Charcot process. However, all the studies had a small number of patients and larger randomised trials are urgently needed.

CONCLUSION

CN is a debilitating condition that requires prompt diagnosis and treatment. One can conclude from previous studies that immobilisation is an effective treatment for the active Charcot foot. The underlying pathogenesis is thought to be enhanced bone resorption, and there have been three trials using bisphosphonates as possible pharmacological treatment. Although some studies showed improvement in symptoms and bone turnover, a systematic improvement in disease activity has not been demonstrated. However, all the studies were underpowered and more robust trials are indicated. Irrespective of the treatment instituted, it must be started early in the disease process because once the bony changes and deformity have occurred they cannot be reversed. Therefore, immobilisation, bedrest, offloading and possibly pamidronate should be initiated as soon as possible and immediately after the diagnosis has been made, if one is to reduce the Charcot joint deformity and morbidity in diabetic patients with peripheral neuropathy.

REFERENCES

1. Shaw JE, Boulton AJM. The Charcot foot. *Foot* 1995;5:65–70.
2. Sanders LJ, Frykberg RG. Diabetic neuropathic osteoarthropathy: the Charcot foot. In: Frykberg RG, ed. *The High Risk Foot in Diabetes Mellitus.* New York: Churchill Livingstone; 1991:297–338.
3. Sinha S, Munichoodappa C, Kozak GP. Neuroarthropathy (Charcot's joints) in diabetes mellitus: a clinical study of 101 cases. *Medicine (Baltimore)* 1972;51:191–210.
4. Fabrin J, Larsen K, Holstein PE. Long-term follow-up in diabetic Charcot feet with spontaneous onset.*Diabetes Care* 2000;23:796–800.

5. Klenerman L. The Charcot neuroarthropathy joint in diabetes mellitus. *Diabet Med* 1996;13:S52–S54.

6. Armstrong DG, Tood WF, Lavery LA, Harkless LB, Bushman TR. The natural history of acute Charcot's arthropathy in a diabetic foot speciality clinic. *Diabet Med* 1997;14:357–363.

7. Codfield RH, Morrisson MJ, Beaubout JW. Diabetic neuroarthropathy in the foot: patient characteristics and patterns of radiographic change. *Foot Ankle* 1983;4:15–22.

8. Mitchell JK. On a new practice in acute and chronic rheumatism. *Am J Med Sci* 1831;8:55.

9. Charcot JM. Sur quelques arthropathies qui paraissent dependre d'une lesion du cerveau ou de la moelle epiniere. *Arch Physiol Norm et Pathol* 1868;1:161–178.

10. Jordan WR. Neuritic manifestations in diabetes mellitus. *Arch Intern Med* 1936;57:307–366.

11. Eloesser L. On the nature of neuropathic affections of the joint. *Ann Surg* 1917;66:201–206.

12. Brower AC, Allman RM. Pathogenesis of the neuropathic joint: neurotraumatic vs neurovascular. *Radiology* 1981;139:349–354.

13. Jeffocate W, Lima J, Norbrega L. The Charcot foot. *Diabet Med* 2000;17:253–258.

14. Sinha J, Thomas EM, Foster A, Edmonds M. Fractures in the neuropathic diabetic foot. *Foot* 1994;4:28–30.

15. Clouse ME, Gramm HF, Legg M, Flood T. Diabetic osteoarthropathy: clinical and roentgenographic observations in 90 cases. *Am J Roentgenol* 1974;121:22–23.

16. Newman JH. Spontaneous dislocation in diabetic neuroarthropathy: a report of six cases. *J Bone Joint Surg* 1979;61B:484–488.

17. El-Khoury GY, Kathol MH. Neuropathic fractures in patients with diabetic mellitus. *Radiology* 1980;134:313–316.

18. Archer AG, Roberts VC, Watkins PJ. Blood flow patterns in diabetic neuropathy. *Diabetologia* 1984;27:141–147.

19. Edmonds ME, Clarke MB, Newton S, Barrett J, Watkins PJ. Increased uptake of bone radiopharmaceutical in diabetic neuropathy. *Q J Med* 1985;57:843–855.

20. Gough A, Abraha H, Purewal TS, *et al.* Measurement of markers of osteoclast and osteoblastic activity in patients with acute and chronic diabetic Charcot neuroarthropathy. *Diabet Med* 1997;14:527–531.

21. Selby PL, Jude EB, Burgess J, *et al.* Bone turnover markers in acute Charcot neuroarthropathy. *Diabetologia* 1998;41:A275.

22. Edelson GW, Jensen JL, Kaczynski R. Identifying acute Charcot arthropathy through urinary cross-linked N-telopeptides. *Diabetes* 1996;45:108A.

23. Young MJ, Marshall A, Adams JE, Selby PL, Boulton AJM. Osteopenia, neurological dysfunction, and the development of Charcot neuroarthropathy. *Diabetes Care* 1995;18:34–38.

24. Rawesh A, Foster A, Barrett J, Buxton-Thomas M, Edmonds ME. A fall in bone mineral density of the foot predicts the development of Charcot foot (abstract). *Diabet Med* 1994;11:P26.

25. Jude EB, Hodgkinson M, Selby PL, Adams JE, Boulton AJM. Bone mineral density of the calcaneus in diabetic neuropathy. *Diabetologia* 1997;40:P2285.

26. Jirkovska A, Kasalicky P, Boucek P, Hosova J, Skibova J. Calcaneal ultrasonometry in patients with Charcot osteoarthropathy and its relationship with densitometry in the lumbar spine and femoral neck and with markers of bone turnover. *Diabet Med* Jun 2001;18:495–500.

27. Jude EB, Selby PL, Mawer B, *et al.* Pamidronate in diabetic Charcot neuroarthropathy: a randomised placebo controlled trial. *Diabetologia* 2001;44:2032–2037.

28. Fabrin J, Larsen K, Holstein PE. Long-term follow-up in diabetic Charcot feet with spontaneous onset. *Diabetes Care* 2000;23:796–800.

29. Jude EB, Boulton AJM. End stage complications of diabetic neuropathy. *Diabetes Rev* 1999;7:395–410.

30. Mayfield J, Reiber GE, Sanders LJ. American Diabetes Association technical review on preventative foot care in patients with diabetes mellitus. *Diabetes Care* 1998;21:2161–2177.

31. Morgan JM, Biehl WC, Wagner FW. Management of neuropathic arthropathy with the Charcot restraint orthotic walker. *Clin Orthop* 1993;296:58–63.
32. Baumbauer JF, Wervey R, McWilliams J, Harris GF, Shereff MJ. A comparison study of plantar foot pressures in a standardised shoe, total contact cast and prefabricated pneumatic walking braces. *Foot Ankle Int* 1997;18:26–33.
33. Rajbhandari SM, Jenkins RC, Davies C, Tesfaye S. Charcot neuroarthropathy in diabetes mellitus. *Diabetologia* 2002;45:1085–1096.
34. McCrory JL, Morag E, Norkitis AJ, *et al.* Healing of Charcot fractures: skin temperature and radiographic correlates. *Foot* 1998;8:158–165.
35. Chantelau E, Schnable T. Palliative radiotherapy for acute osteoarthropathy of diabetic feet: a preliminary study. *Pract Diabetes* 1997;14:154–157.
36. Strauss C, Gonya G. Adjunct low intensity ultrasound in Charcot neuroarthropathy. *Clin Orthop Relat Res* 1998;349:132–138.
37. Selby PL, Young MJ, Adams JE, Boulton AJM. Bisphosphonate: a new treatment for diabetic Charcot neuroarthropathy. *Diabet Med* 1994;11:14–20.
38. Fleisch H, Reszka A, Rodan G, Rogers M. Bisphosphonates: mechanism of action. In: Bilezikan JP, Raisz LG, Rodan GA, eds. *Principles of Bone Biology.* 2nd edn. San Deigo, CA: Academic Press; 2002:1361–1385.
39. Schott GD. Bisphosphonates for pain relief in reflex sympathetic dystrophy? *Lancet* 1997;350:1117.
40. Strang P. Analgesic effect of bisphosphonates on bone pain in breast cancer patients. *Acta Oncol Suppl* 1996;35:50–54.
41. Schott GD. An unsympathetic view of pain. *Lancet* 1995;345:34–636.
42. Dray A. Neurogenic mechanisms and neuropeptides in chronic pain. *Prog Brain Res* 1996;110:85–94.
43. Haworth CD, Selby PL, Webb AK, Mawer EB, Adams JE, Freemont AJ. Severe bone pain after intravenous pamidronate in adult patients with cystic fibrosis. *Lancet* 1998;352:1753–1754.
44. McGill M, Molyneaux L, Bolton T, Ionnou K, Uren R, Yue DK. Response of Charcot's arthropathy to contact casting: assessment by quantitative techniques. *Diabetologia* 2000;43:481–484.
45. Anderson JJ, Woelffer KE, Holtzman JJ, Jacobs AM. Bisphosphonates for the treatment of Charcot neuroarthropathy. *J Foot Ankle Surg* 2004;43:285–289.
46. Pitocco D, Ruotolo V, Caputo S, *et al.* Six-month treatment with alendronate in acute Charcot neuroarthropathy: a randomised controlled trial. *Diabetes Care* 2005;28:1214–1215.

23 The Operative Treatment of Charcot Neuroarthropathy of the Foot and Ankle

Michael L. Salamon and Charles L. Saltzman

Charcot neuroarthropathy of the foot and ankle (a Charcot foot) is characterised by destruction of bone and joints secondary to a neuropathic process. In developed nations, this neuropathy is most commonly a sequela of diabetes mellitus, and Charcot neuroarthropathy is strongly associated with the presence of sensory peripheral neuropathy. The presentation of a patient with Charcot neuroarthropathy is often difficult to distinguish from infection, and its symptoms include warmth, oedema, erythema and sometimes pain. Deep infection usually occurs by direct bacterial inoculation via skin ulceration. If there is no history of an ulcer, the acute symptoms of warmth, oedema and erythema are usually the result of a Charcot process.

Traditionally, the management of patients with Charcot neuroarthropathy has been non-operative. This management approach is founded on stabilising or immobilising the foot and ankle until the Charcot process consolidates into a solid, shoeable or braceable mass. Non-operative treatment includes either non-weight-bearing or weight bearing in a variety of immobilisation devices, and this treatment period usually lasts at least several months.[1] However, there are particular situations when surgery is warranted and is necessary in order to prevent instabilities and deformities that may lead to ulceration and possibly eventual amputation. The indications for, and timing of, surgery are controversial, since the surgical management of Charcot deformities of the foot and ankle continues to evolve.[2] In general, practitioners treating patients with neuroarthropathy of the foot and ankle should be experienced and should have the ability to hopefully recognise situations where conservative treatment may predictably fail.

The locations affected by Charcot neuroarthropathy in the foot and ankle are fairly consistent; they include the forefoot, midfoot and peri-talar region, the ankle and avulsion fractures of the posterior tuberosity of the calcaneus. In each of these general locations, a variety of recognisable deformity patterns may occur. We have found a clear relationship between bone mineral density of the unaffected limb and both the type of deformity that occurs (i.e. fracture vs dislocation) and the location. In general, fracture patterns occur in association with low bone mineral density and typically are located in the ankle or forefoot. Charcot patients who have higher bone mineral densities tend to develop midfoot deformities that occur via clean dislocations as opposed to fractures.[3]

The Foot in Diabetes, 4th Edition. Editors Andrew J.M. Boulton, Peter R. Cavanagh and Gerry Rayman.
© 2006 John Wiley & Sons, Ltd.

The overall goals of treating Charcot neuroarthropathy of the foot and ankle are the same for operative and non-operative treatments. These goals include providing the patient with a stable, well-aligned plantigrade foot that is free of infection and is shoeable or braceable. If this cannot be achieved non-operatively, surgery is indicated.[4] Surgery also is indicated in the presence of deep infection. In these cases, the infected bone and deep tissues must be debrided and then the foot or ankle stabilised in a plantigrade position using either internal fixation or external fixation, or a combination of the two. It is usually advisable not to place internal fixation devices into or through the chronically infected bone.

The other relative indication for operative management of Charcot neuroarthropathy is a deformity or instability pattern that is not yet ulcerated or infected but is not easily braceable or shoeable. These types of deformities create areas of pressure that put the local soft tissues at risk of ulceration with possible subsequent development of infection and need for amputation. According to the Seattle Diabetic Foot Study, having a Charcot foot was associated with the greatest relative risk for developing a foot ulcer and ultimate amputation.[5] Similarly, in a study of consecutive patients treated intensively for Charcot neuroarthropathy of the feet, survivorship of limbs with prior ulcerations or recurrent ulcerations was much poorer than survivorship of non-ulcerated feet.[6] The surgeon's goal in these situations is to operatively create a plantigrade limb via arthrodesis and/or osteotomies. If a particular fracture dislocation pattern is plantigrade but unstable after consolidation, it is at risk for further collapse and progression to an at-risk, non-plantigrade deformity. In these cases, stabilisation of the unstable segments via arthrodesis using fixation is indicated.

As a general rule, post-operative immobilisation and protected weight bearing is employed approximately twice as long as in cases where arthrodesis is attempted in non-neuropathic patients. This can be as long as 9 months and is guided by radiographic evidence of consolidation or fusion (both plain X-ray and computerised tomography).

MIDFOOT CHARCOT DEFORMITY

The most common anatomical site for diabetic Charcot foot is the tarso-metatarsal region. There are a variety of patterns that occur with Charcot neuroarthropathy of the midtarsus, depending on the anatomical location of the pathological process.[7] Recognising which patterns are at greatest risk of progressing to significant deformity and subsequent ulceration is important. Charcot foot deformities in the midfoot may progress to some variation of a rocker bottom pattern that may lead to increased areas of pressure and subsequent ulceration and osteomyelitis (Figures 23.1(a) and 23.1(b)). Non-operative treatment is indicated in cases where the foot is stable and has a longitudinal arch that is relatively preserved and devoid of deep infection. Again, the foot must also be braceable or shoeable with risk of ulceration minimised.

The simplest operative intervention involves exostectomy of a bony plantar prominence that has created an area of increased pressure on the underlying skin. This procedure should be performed only for well-consolidated, 'stable' midfoot problems. Situations where a plantigrade Charcot midfoot is present with an unstable yet relatively mild deformity may require *in situ* anatomical arthrodesis with internal fixation to prevent the progression of deformity.[8] If a significant rocker bottom deformity exists, the need for, and type of, surgery depends on the presence of deep infection. If the infection is chronic, widespread and involves the central portion of the foot, the patient may be best served by a well-performed partial foot or transtibial amputation. On the other hand, if the foot is severely deformed and ulcerated

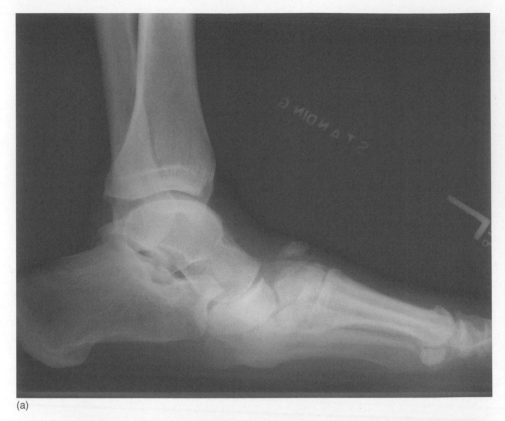

(a)

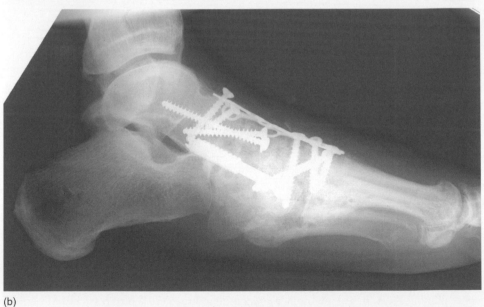

(b)

Figure 23.1 Pre-operative and post-operative lateral radiographs of a patient with Charcot midfoot deformity and subsequent surgical correction and arthrodesis. (a) The pre-operative image demonstrates collapse of the midfoot with resultant loss of the longitudinal arch; (b) post-operative image after reduction and reconstruction of the midfoot deformity, using screws and plates to achieve stability via arthrodesis

but not deeply infected, the basic longitudinal arch architecture of the foot may be re-built. This can be done via wedge resection of protruding bone and correction of deformity with external-fixation-enhanced fusion. With these surgeries, other conditions such as associated hindfoot and ankle contractures should be simultaneously treated with posterior soft tissue releases such as a tendoachilles lengthening. The reason for this is that the inability of the foot to achieve neutral ankle dorsiflexion can create areas of abnormally high plantar pressure that can later lead to re-ulceration.

HINDFOOT

The second most common anatomical site for diabetic Charcot foot destruction is the hindfoot, including the transverse tarsal joints (talo-navicular and calcaneocuboid) and the subtalar joint. Charcot deformities in this region may involve dislocation and fragmentation of all three joints, leading to a wide range of unstable rocker bottom patterns. Instability and progression tend to occur more often than early consolidation into fixed deformities. The progressive loss of hindfoot stability is often associated with substantial and clinically significant varus/valgus malposition.

Cases with minimal initial deformity and clear bony fracture are managed non-operatively with total contact casting or bracing until fully consolidated. However, cases with minimal fractures or greater deformity generally lead to unstable progressive rocker bottom deformity, increasing the likelihood of eventual ulceration and infection. In these situations, realignment/arthrodesis procedures are more appropriately indicated.

ANKLE

The ankle is affected by Charcot neuroarthropathy much less commonly than the midfoot and hindfoot. However, the destructive processes at the ankle often progress much more rapidly once the deformity is initiated, leading to coronal plane instability and ulceration over the malleoli. This is often associated with extremely low bone mineral density. The highly unstable cases, both varus and valgus, are generally unbraceable and coronal plane instability in the ankle is poorly tolerated. With fracture of the medial malleolus, the foot may invert, driving the distal tip of the fibula into the floor (or brace). Ulceration around the now prominent fibula often ensues and is very difficult to treat with casting or bracing. Conversely, ulcers on the medial border of the foot often develop with uncontrolled fibular fractures where the foot collapses into a valgus position.

Rotational ankle fractures in diabetic patients with other major identifiable end-stage diabetic co-morbidities are at much higher risk of initial treatment complications or the development of florid Charcot destructive changes, when compared to matched controls. Co-morbidities include insulin-requiring diabetes mellitus, previous history of Charcot neuroarthropathy and end-organ disease. These co-morbidities can be readily identified while conducting an intake history and physical examination. Ankle fractures in this challenging patient population are best treated with open reduction and internal fixation; however, complication rates regardless of treatment method approach 50%. The usual fixation techniques used in non-neuropathic ankle fractures are probably inadequate and must be supplemented with more robust internal fixation constructs, as the rates of catastrophic failure are high.[9]

The surgical management of complex Charcot ankle deformities follows the same principles of Charcot deformities in other regions of the foot. This frequently involves realignment of the hindfoot under the leg, combined with arthrodesis. The arthrodesis frequently includes the subtalar joint in addition to the ankle joint (tibio-talo-calcaneal fusion). A variety of fixation devices may be used, depending on the quality of the bone, presence of infection, condition of the soft tissues and whether or not significant systemic co-morbidities exist. Fixation devices include blade plates and other fixed-angle plating systems, tibio-talo-calcaneal nails and external fixation systems (Figures 23.2(a)–23.2(c)). The risks of surgical reconstruction, and the challenges of post-operative convalescence, can be considerable and should not be underestimated. The typical duration of post-operative recovery is long, often lasting up to 9 months. Sometimes, a transtibial amputation is a better treatment than complete reconstruction.

FOREFOOT

The typical location of bone and joint destruction in the forefoot is at the metatarso-phalangeal joint or metatarsal neck level. The pattern of Charcot changes is usually one of fracture, and pathologies at these sites are associated with low systemic bone density (Figure 23.3). The metatarso-phalangeal joints may dislocate without significant bony destruction but they will more likely demonstrate fragmented destructive changes. Plantar ulceration may accompany the Charcot changes in the forefoot potentially leading to infection and osteomyelitis.

Successful non-operative management includes initial total contact casting or bracing and then accommodation of forefoot deformity with wide toe box shoes and custom inserts. Resection arthroplasty and fusion are alternatives in situations where non-operative management fails or when recurrent ulceration occurs.

POSTERIOR CALCANEUS

The Charcot calcaneal deformity consists of an avulsion fracture of the posterior tuberosity of the calcaneus (Figure 23.4). This uncommon type of Charcot deformity may result in collapse of the longitudinal arch of the foot.[10] These fractures are usually adequately treated non-operatively with casting, bracing and limited weight bearing until consolidation occurs. Residual deformity can usually be accommodated by custom insoles or extra-depth shoes.[11] Occasionally, reduction and fixation may be necessary if the displaced fragment of the tuberosity creates an area of pressure on the overlying skin, which leads to ulceration. The bone is generally very soft and fixation may fail unless combined with an Achilles tendon or gastrocnemius muscle lengthening.

In conclusion, Charcot neuroarthropathy of the foot and ankle is traditionally treated non-operatively with total contact casting and bracing. This is done until consolidation occurs and the Charcot process solidifies into a stable mass. However, when a stable plantigrade foot cannot be achieved with non-surgical techniques, operative intervention may be warranted. This is essential so that ulceration and subsequent deep infection can be avoided and the goal of limb salvage can be achieved. The indications and techniques for operative intervention in Charcot neuroarthropathy cases are certain to evolve in the coming years.

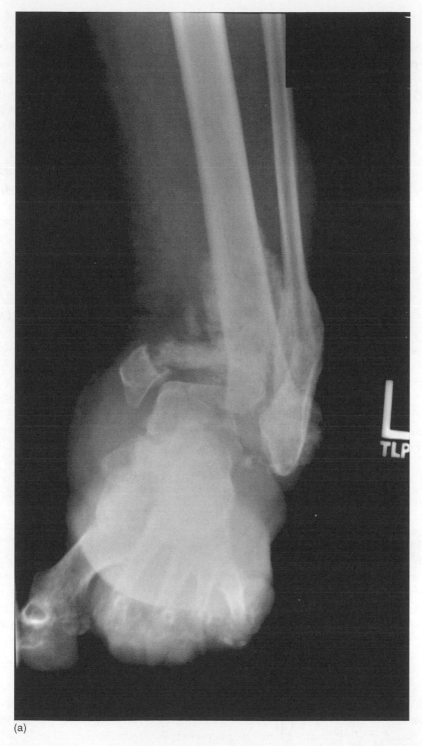

(a)

Figure 23.2 Example of patient with Charcot ankle deformity. (a) Charcot destruction of ankle joint with collapse into varus mal-alignment; (b) reconstruction of ankle with blade plate and supplemental fixation, using thin wire external fixation system; (c) healed ankle fusion after removal of external fixator. The distal end of the plate has been placed into the talus sparing the subtalar joint

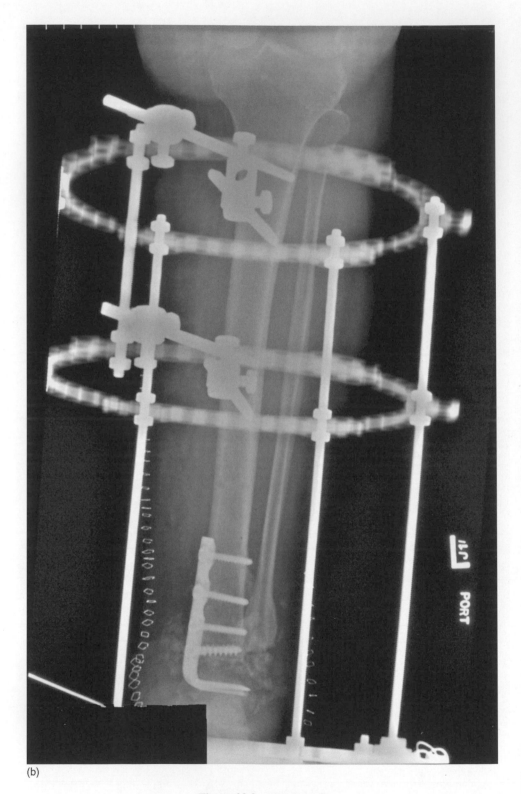

(b)

Figure 23.2 *(Continued)*

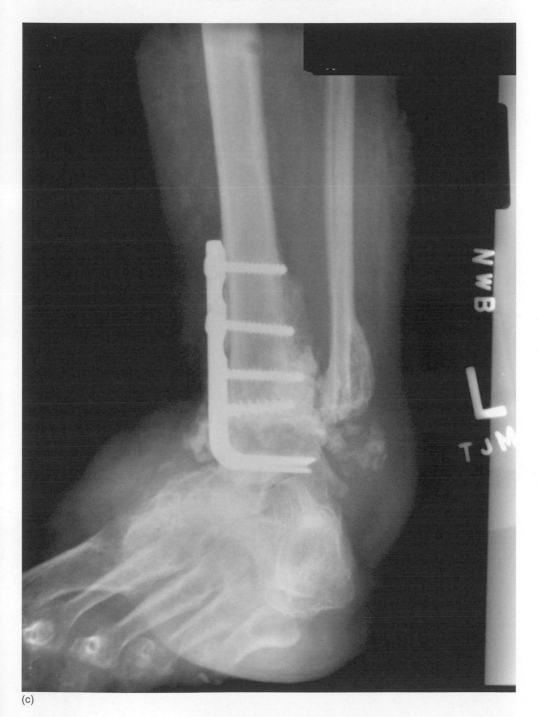

(c)

Figure 23.2   (*Continued*)

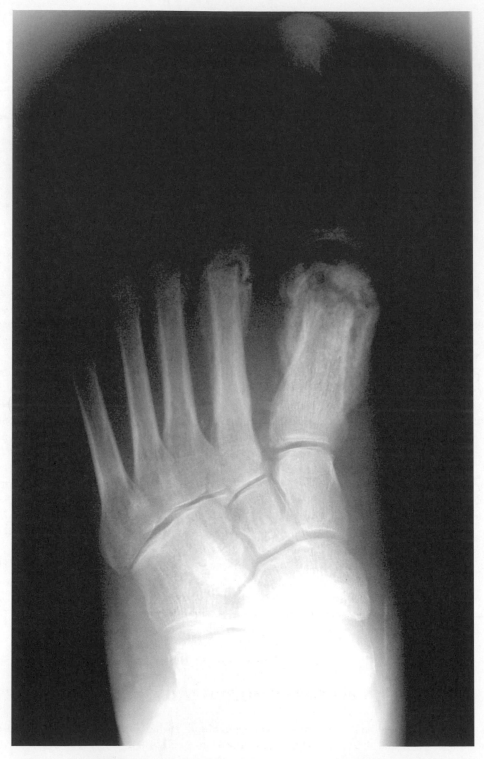

Figure 23.3 Anteroposterior (AP) radiograph of foot with osteopaenia secondary to diabetes and destructive changes consistent with Charcot forefoot destruction. Infection is unlikely, as this patient had no history of plantar ulceration

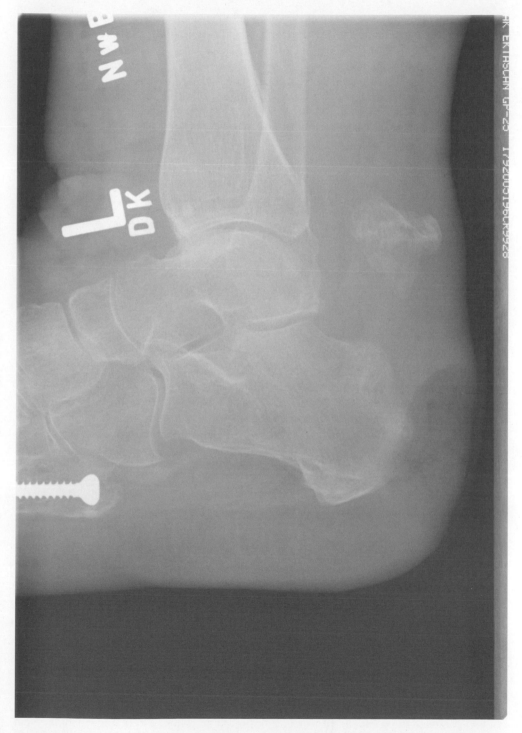

Figure 23.4 Lateral radiograph of the hindfoot, demonstrating avulsion of the posterior tuberosity of the calcaneus. An intramedullary screw is present within the fifth metatarsal after previous treatment of a fracture

REFERENCES

1. Pinzur MS, Shields N, Trepman E, Dawson P, Evans A. current practice patterns in the treatment of Charcot foot. *Foot Ankle Int* Nov 2000;21:916–920.
2. Simon SR, Tejwani SG, Wilson DL, Santner TJ, Denniston NL. Arthrodesis as an early alternative to nonoperative management of Charcot arthropathy of the diabetic foot. *J Bone Joint Surg* 2000;82A:939–950.
3. Herbst SA, Jones KB, Saltzman CL. Pattern of diabetic neuropathic arthropathy associated with the peripheral bone mineral density. *J Bone Joint Surg Br* Apr 2004;86:378–383.
4. Sammarco GJ, Conti SF. Surgical treatment of neuroarthropathic foot deformity. *Foot Ankle Int* 1998;19:102–109.
5. Boyko EJ, Ahroni JH, Stensel V, Forsberg RC, Davignon DR, Smith DJ. A prospective study of risk factors for diabetic foot ulcer. The Seattle Diabetic Foot Study. *Diabetes Care* 1999;22:1036–1042.
6. Saltzman CL, Hagy ML, Zimmerman B, Estin M, Cooper R. How effective is intensive nonoperative initial treatment of patients with diabetes and Charcot arthropathy of the feet? *Clin Orthop* Jun 2005;435:185–190.
7. Schon LC, Weinfeld SB, Horton GA, Resch S. Radiographic and clinical classification of acquired midtarsus deformities. *Foot Ankle Int* Jun 1998;19:394–404.
8. Pinzur MS, Sage R, Stuck R, Kaminsky S, Zmuda A. A treatment algorithm for neuropathic (Charcot) midfoot deformity. *Foot Ankle Int* May 1993;14:189–197.
9. Jones KB, Marsh JL, Estin M, Maiers-Yelden KA, Zimmerman MB, Saltzman CL. Ankle fractures in patients with diabetes mellitus. *J Bone Joint Surg Br* Apr 2005;87:489–495.
10. Brodsky JW. The diabetic foot. In: MJ Coughlin, RA Mann, eds. *Surgery of the Foot and Ankle*. 7th edn. St. Louis, MO: Mosby; 1999:895–969.
11. Schon LC, Easley ME, Weinfeld SB. Charcot neuroarthropathy of the foot and ankle. *Clin Orthop* 1998;349:116–131.

24 Surgery for Ulceration and Infection in the Diabetic Foot

James W. Brodsky

INTRODUCTION

Surgery of the diabetic foot is most often indicated for deep infection or for the treatment of recurrent and recalcitrant ulceration. Techniques for maximum tissue preservation and for salvage of the foot require conservative indications, clearly defined goals and definitive debridement methods. The overarching goal is complete healing of the soft tissues and maximum preservation of functional anatomy of the foot. The specific goals are to (1) achieve and maintain the foot plantigrade, i.e. functional for weight bearing; (2) restore and maintain an intact soft tissue envelope; (3) reduce the risks that *imminently* threaten either of these.[1] If a problem of ulceration or infection threatens the viability of the foot, or has proven recalcitrant to conservative measures, then the surgical goals are prevention of the spread of infection within the foot or proximal to the foot and salvage of the foot to prevent or minimise amputation.

While surgery of the diabetic foot has been advocated by some as 'prophylaxis', it is actually indicated to fulfil the goals defined above. By this definition, surgery for the diabetic foot should be practised as treatment of a pathologic condition rather than a form of prophylaxis of disease. In this sense, the concept of surgery as prophylaxis in the diabetic foot is not supported; rather, surgery should always be considered a form of treatment. While the difference may appear to be semantic at first glance, the concept reflects a fundamentally conservative surgical approach to diabetic foot problems.

SURGICAL INDICATIONS

Based on the goals noted above, common orthopaedic surgical indications include debridement of recalcitrant or infected ulcers; drainage and debridement of soft tissue infection; bone resection for relief of pressure and/or for osteomyelitis; closure techniques; Achilles lengthening surgery; and reconstruction of forefoot deformities.

With a few notable exceptions, recalcitrant or recurrent ulcerations are usually related to persistent or recurring pressure usually over a bony prominence. Once the soft tissue envelope has been breached, the risk for the development of deep infection or proximal extension of infection is the criterion for intervention. The failure of external, non-operative pressure relief

The Foot in Diabetes, 4th Edition. Editors Andrew J.M. Boulton, Peter R. Cavanagh and Gerry Rayman.
© 2006 John Wiley & Sons, Ltd.

interventions is the indication for surgical intervention. Ulcers that often require surgery are those classified as grade 2 on the Meggit–Wagner scale, i.e. with exposed tendon or joint, or those grade 3 ulcers in which there is exposure of the bone, osteomyelitis, abscess or soft tissue necrosis.[1,2]

Emphasis in pre-operative assessment of the patient must be given to adequate vascularisation or revascularisation of the foot. This is necessary for tissue healing, and is best done prior to reconstruction and preferably prior to any surgical procedure. However, in the presence of acute infection, emergent debridement often must precede the revascularisation, which in turn should precede definitive reconstruction and wound closure.

The anatomic location of the ulceration is important. The majority of recalcitrant ulcerations occur on the plantar forefoot area, i.e. distal to the tarsometatarsal joints. These, and midfoot ulcerations almost always associated with Charcot arthropathy, require evaluation and treatment of the bony prominence that underlies the ulceration.

The exceptions to the rule of underlying bone pressure can include ulcerations in the area of the heel and some plantar ulcerations due to soft tissue infection or soft tissue mass. Such lesions are more likely to be related to tissue ischaemia or infection alone.

DRAINAGE/DEBRIDEMENT OF SOFT TISSUE INFECTION

Drainage and debridement of soft tissue infection consists primarily of the treatment of abscesses that can occur either in the subcutaneous tissue or in any of the deep spaces of the foot. These most commonly occur in the forefoot and midfoot areas. It is important to note that not all abscesses are characterised by free-flowing purulence. Some consist strictly of necrotic tissue. Magnetic resonance imaging can be very helpful although not always essential in guiding the debridement.

The guiding surgical principle is to achieve adequate drainage and debridement. It is more conservative and more effective to create wide exposures and aggressive debridements than to attempt to minimise the surgical site over a deep infection. The infection frequently extends further into the deep spaces along tissue planes or along flexor and extensor tendons than is apparent from careful physical examination, from imaging studies or even at first inspection in surgery. An understanding of the surgical anatomy guides the debridement along the tissue planes and muscle compartments within the foot and the leg.

Incisions should be initiated over the area of greatest purulence, which is typically at or adjacent to the original breach of the skin. It is frequently necessary to create incisions in more than one area. The best example of this would be the patient with a plantar ulceration who demonstrates directly overlying dorsal erythema and swelling. This typically signifies a deep abscess formation. In this case, debridement of the plantar ulcer and drainage of the dorsal abscess are both required. This may be best achieved by a web-splitting incision that creates a U-shaped exposure from the dorsal intermetatarsal space to the plantar surfaces.

In physical assessment of deep space infection, localising signs are important to find, although the intensity of inflammatory signs can be blunted, especially in people with diabetes with advanced distal ischaemia. In contrast to an acute abscess, diffuse erythema and swelling of the entire region of the foot with mild inflammation may be a sign of an acute Charcot neuroarthropathy. In the very early stages, this can mimic infection. Initial radiographs may appear negative. Non-operative therapy and repetition of the radiographs at 1 or 2 weeks will usually reveal the neuroarthropathy. But the pace of modern medicine usually leads to early imaging with technetium-99 bone scans or magnetic resonance imaging, which will reveal early changes within the bone. In the case of plantar abscess formation, particular concern is required for extension of the infection into the leg compartments along the course of the flexor tendons.

BONE RESECTION FOR TREATMENT OF CHRONIC PRESSURE ULCERATION AND/OR OSTEOMYELITIS

Many surgical procedures for ulceration and infection involve the reduction of localised pressure due to bony deformity, and this category of operative procedures probably comprises the majority of all surgical interventions for the diabetic foot. There are three basic methods to relieve pressure of the bony prominence which underlies a neuropathic ulcer. These are (1) correction of a proximal deformity that increases weight-bearing pressure on the forefoot or midfoot; (2) realignment of the deformity; and (3) resection of the prominent bone. The first will be exemplified in the section on Achilles Tendon Lengthening. The latter of the three is the most common. It is the most straightforward, most effective and generally associated with lowest morbidity.

Together with adequate debridement of non-viable and infected tissues, reduction of local pressure is the key to healing of the soft tissue envelope. Perhaps as a function of the severity of neuropathy in the most distal regions, the greatest number of ulcerations in diabetic patients occur in the forefoot region. Hallux ulcerations frequently occur over the interphalangeal (IP) joint. Over the dorsum of the joint, these are usually caused by pressure of shoewear, and once the ulceration is healed, shoe modification must be undertaken. When ulcerations occur on the plantar surface, they are attributable to the combination of neuropathy and increased plantar pressure of weight bearing.[3] At the hallux IP joint, this most commonly occurs at the junction of the plantar and medial surfaces.

The three principles of surgical reconstruction can be applied to the hallux IP joint. First is simple resection, either of the IP joint itself or of the medial condyles on both sides of the joint. The second choice is realignment and arthrodesis, and the third choice is correction of proximal deformity if that is overloading the IP joint. Arthrodesis of the IP or even of the metatarsophalangeal joint (MTPJ) can be performed. One disadvantage in a neuropathic patient is the risk of non-union or secondary Charcot changes at the surgical site. Proximal intervention can be achieved through resection arthroplasty of the first MTPJ, i.e. a modification of the Keller bunion procedure, which has been reported to have excellent results.[4,5] This procedure leads to a reduction of toe plantar pressure through reduction of weight bearing (and reduced function) of the hallux.

Ulcerations are common in the area of the first MTPJ. These are typically troublesome, difficult to heal and associated with a considerable risk of partial foot amputation.[6] The extension of the ulceration into the sesamoid complex and then into the MTPJ of the great toe, as well as the difficulty in creating soft tissue coverage, warrants early surgical intervention. Surgical wound debridement is augmented by pressure reduction, frequently including medial sesamoidectomy (Plate 2). Resection of both sesamoids, as in non-neuropathic patients, is usually contraindicated because of the great likelihood of dorsal dislocation of the great toe. The elevated hallux will increase metatarsal plantar flexion and the subsequent pressure will exacerbate rather than resolve the problem. Basilar dorsiflexion osteotomy of the first

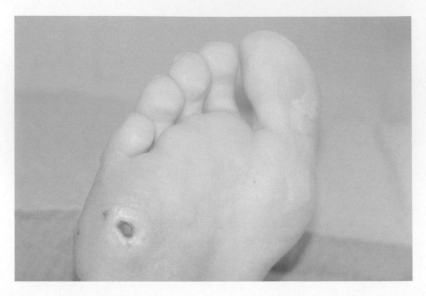

Figure 24.1   Chronic plantar fifth metatarsal ulceration, unresponsive to non-operative measures.

metatarsal has also been reported as a treatment for persistent first MTP ulcerations, and may be combined with sesamoidectomy.[7]

For discrete, recurrent plantar ulceration beneath a single metatarsal head, resection of the single distal metatarsal is frequently an efficacious method for resolving the ulcer that has failed the range of conservative measures, including total contact casting and bracing (Plate 3, Figure 24.1). The most common complication is transfer of increased pressure to an adjacent metatarsal, leading to a new ulceration. In cases such as this, resection of all the metatarsal heads has been described to create resolution of the otherwise intractable plantar forefoot ulceration.[8] There are reports suggesting that this can still result in increased plantar pressures, by pedobarographic measurement, but as yet, this has not been demonstrated to correspond to clinical outcomes.[9]

There is certainly an intermediate or grey zone between surgical treatment of infection by debridement of soft tissue and resection or realignment of selected portions of the osseous structure of the foot, and the often necessary and definitive procedures of partial foot amputation. The latter is the subject of a separate chapter within this book (Chapter 26). Suffice it to say that debridement, resection and amputation are different points along the same continuum. The goals of each are largely the same, namely to achieve a plantigrade foot with a stable and completely healed soft tissue envelope.

Posterior heel ulceration is a particularly troublesome problem. The normal soft tissue over the posterior calcaneus is thin. The options for soft tissue reconstruction are limited because of the paucity of adjacent tissue for rotation or translation. The relatively poor vascularisation of this tissue can retard both primary closure and healing by secondary intention. Exposure of the calcaneus or osteomyelitis of the calcaneal tuberosity must be resolved if the foot is to be salvaged. If the calcaneal wound cannot be healed or closed, then the foot cannot function, it is no longer possible for the patient to ambulate or wear a shoe and a below-knee amputation is the necessary next surgical intervention. Thus, resolution of these heel lesions is essential.

The methods for treating posterior calcaneal lesions include bony resection and free tissue transfer. The former has several variations that consist primarily of partial resection of the calcaneal tuberosity[10–12] and even complete resection of the calcaneus.[13] The principle of partial calcaneal resection is that removal of the calcaneal tuberosity removes the infected bone and at the same time reduces the amount of soft tissue required to close the wound. Of course, resection of the infected portions of the soft tissue and the non-viable edges of the flaps created by this procedure is necessary, and may even allow for primary or delayed primary closure of the wound. Provided that there is adequate perfusion of these tissues, this is the most direct and most successful method for a durable outcome to salvage the foot with a recalcitrant heel ulcer. This treatment is indicated primarily in patients who are able to walk pre-operatively. This requires the use of a custom ankle–foot orthosis. This usually will be a posterior shell polypropylene device lined with soft inner foam and moulded on its interior surface to accommodate the loss of the calcaneal tuberosity, while shaped on its external surface to mimic the contour of the heel in order to facilitate shoe fitting. The latter is necessary so that the foot and leg within the orthosis will stay securely within the shoe. Even in a non-ambulatory patient, this is a reasonable procedure for foot salvage. The salvaged foot can still be valuable for transfers and the lower limb for balance in a wheelchair.

The preferred surgical approach is a longitudinal incision. This can split the Achilles tendon or deviate to one side. The incision should be modified as necessary to incorporate resection of the ulceration. The entire zone of infected and even questionable tissue should be resected in full thickness from skin to periosteum. While less desirable, if the initial wound itself is oriented in such a way that a transverse incision is unavoidable, this can still be successful.

WOUND DEBRIDEMENT AND CLOSURE TECHNIQUES

Free tissue transfer can be indicated in the diabetic foot for foot salvage when local techniques are unsuccessful. The associated morbidity and success rate are functions of the surgical technique, the severity and location of the wound and the underlying health tissue status and vascularity of the patient's limb.

However, in the majority of cases, wound closure techniques are utilised through local tissue. The most common question is whether a wound should be allowed to close by secondary intention with gradual epithelialisation, followed by delayed skin grafting, or by primary or delayed primary closure. In general, primary or delayed primary closure is advocated as more effective, much more cost-efficient and successful.[14] Closure by secondary intention produces debilitation of the patient for the long period of healing. This has been reduced with innovations such as vacuum wound management. This innovation has provided a welcome and significant new tool for wound closure. Low pressure or vacuum-assisted closure is particularly valuable when there is insufficient soft tissue surplus to allow for primary closure of the wound edges.

The basis of the surgical technique dictates that there should be two criteria for primary or delayed primary closure. The first is that the wound is non-infected. This can be achieved by resection of the infected tissue, combined with antibiotics and local wound care. In this case, a return to surgery at an interval from several days to approximately 2 weeks can be used for repeat wound irrigation and debridement and then delayed primary closure. The second requirement is that there should be appropriate balance between bone and soft tissue (Plate 2(c)). Once stable, non-infected, soft tissue has been achieved, the level of bone resection must accommodate the degree of soft tissue translation and the adequacy of the soft tissue for coverage. Thus, the primary determinant of primary or delayed primary closure is the size and viability of the healthy soft tissue flaps.

These considerations for soft tissue closure after wound debridement and bone resection are the same principles used for achieving a stable, functional, healed foot in partial foot amputation.[1,14]

ACHILLES TENDON LENGTHENING

Achilles tendon lengthening has been shown to reduce forefoot and midfoot plantar pressure, and to aid plantar ulcer healing.[15–17] The indications for this procedure continue to evolve. The best results are in patients with forefoot plantar neuropathic ulcerations and limited ankle dorsiflexion of less than 5°. Achilles tendon lengthening is not used as an isolated treatment modality, rather as an adjunct to total contact casting in order to increase the duration and lower the risk of recurrence of ulceration, when compared to total contact casting alone. The triple hemisection technique uses a pointed scalpel with three separate, small incisions. Tendon elongation is then completed by pressure against the plantar surface of the foot to produce lengthening of the tendon along the weakened lines between the three hemisection points.

RECONSTRUCTION OF FOREFOOT DEFORMITIES

Reconstruction of forefoot deformities follows the general principles outlined above. The most common method is resection of a bony prominence. In the lesser toes, this can take the form of resection of the proximal interphalangeal (PIP) joint or resection of the distal phalanx for ulcerations at the tip. The two, not infrequently, must be combined to resolve distal osteomyelitis in the toe while preserving toe length and realigning the digit.

Realignment procedures of the toes together with resection of the infected tissue are indicated when the ulcer is caused by varus, valgus deformity or flexion deformities at the PIP joint. Flexion is the most common.

Fifth toe dorsal PIP joint ulcerations are most common because of the tapering of shoewear over the area. Shoe modifications can relieve dorsal pressure, and are indicated as a first intervention.

Surgical techniques include open flexor tenotomy in addition to resection of the joint to retard recurrent flexion deformities including those at the distal IP joint. Realignment of the toes is accompanied by temporary pin fixation for 4–5 weeks. Recurrent deformity is a risk in the first 6 weeks after pin removal. Careful attention to shoewear is necessary. Open-toed surgical shoes or appropriately designed sandals or wide-toed athletic shoes are generally recommended.

Reconstruction of hallux valgus deformities in the diabetic foot should be defined in terms of the same indications that would apply to neuropathic and non-neuropathic patients. If the diabetic patient does not have significant peripheral neuropathy, and has no history of prior ulceration and does not have increased risk factors for ulceration, it may be plausible that this patient has ordinary symptomatic, painful bunions equivalent to a non-diabetic, non-neuropathic patient. In non-neuropathic patients, bunion reconstruction should be indicated for pain rather than cosmesis. The majority of patients, both diabetic and non-diabetic, are best treated non-operatively with surgical interventions reserved for those patients with clear failure of the conservative measures of shoe and activity modification.

In the neuropathic diabetic patients, the indications revert to those of pressure relief surgery noted above. In these cases, failure to resolve recurrent or recalcitrant ulceration of the soft tissue is the primary indication. The surgeon must question the indication of pain for correction of hallux valgus deformities in a patient who has neuropathic ulceration. The risk is that the pain, while potentially severe, is most likely related to the dysesthesias of neuropathy rather than the deformity itself. This is frequently the case because an advanced measure of sensory neuropathy is required for most patients to develop ulceration. In this case, surgical technique may employ a combination of the principles of resection and/or realignment. Realignment or reconstructive procedures have a higher risk of failure in neuropathic patients, based upon reconstruction by soft tissue methods or by bony procedures. The patient should be warned that bony procedures of osteotomy or arthrodesis have a higher risk of non union. These complications should be thoughtfully considered by the surgeon and the patient. In the majority of cases, non-operative management of hallux valgus and hammer toe deformities in the neuropathic, diabetic patient is advised and is successful.

SURGERY OF THE TOENAILS

Surgery of the nails is indicated in diabetic patients for a deformity that results in breaks or threats to the soft tissue envelope, which could lead to deep infection. These would primarily be severely deformed onychomycotic nails or recurrent ingrown toenails leading to cellulitis or paronychia.

The essential first step is evaluation and documentation of the vascular status of the patient's forefoot. Pain in the toes, which can be attributed to the nail abnormalities, may be caused by the painful dysesthesias of neuropathy. Thus, as in other forefoot reconstructions, the primary indication in the neuropathic, diabetic patient is preservation or restoration of the intact and non-infected soft tissue envelope, rather than pain. Techniques can employ surgical resection of the bony matrix or chemical ablation of the nail.

In conclusion, surgery for ulceration and infection of the diabetic foot is indicated in the neuropathic, diabetic patient for maintenance or restoration of a functional, non-infected foot. When external offloading methods and antimicrobial therapies are unsuccessful, then surgical intervention is essential to treat or prevent deep infection. Salvage of a functional foot is the goal, and the indications appear to be rather durable while the techniques to achieve them will undoubtedly continue to evolve in the future.

REFERENCES

1. Brodsky JW. The diabetic foot. In: Coughlin, Mann, eds. *Surgery of the Foot and Ankle*. St. Louis, MO: Mosby; 1999:895–969.
2. Lavery LA, Armstrong DG, Harkless LB. Classification of diabetic foot wounds. *J Foot Ankle Surg* 1996;35:528–531.
3. Boulton AJ, Betts R, Franks CI, Newrick PG, Ward JD, Duckworth T. Abnormalities of foot pressure in early diabetic neuropathy. *Diabet Med* 1987;4:225–228.

4. Armstrong DG, Lavery LA, Vazquez JR, *et al.* Clinical efficacy of the first metatarsophalangeal joint arthroplasty as a curative procedure for hallux interphalangeal joint wounds in patients with diabetes. *Diabetes Care* 2003;26:3284–3287.
5. Downs DM, Jacobs RL. Treatment of resistant ulcers on the plantar surface of the great toe in diabetics. *J Bone Joint Surg Am* 1982;64:930–933.
6. Hong T, Brodsky J. Surgical treatment of neuropathic ulcerations under the first metatarsal head. *Foot and Ankle Clin* 1997;2:57–75.
7. Fleischli JE, Anderson RB, Davis WH. Dorsiflexion metatarsal osteotomy for treatment of recalcitrant diabetic neuropathic ulcers. *Foot Ankle Int* 1999;20:80–85.
8. Jacobs RL. Hoffman procedure in the ulcerated diabetic neuropathic foot. *Foot Ankle* 1982;3:142–149.
9. Cavanagh PR, Ulbrecht JS, Caputo GM. Elevated plantar pressure and ulceration in diabetic patients after panmetatarsal head resection: two case reports. *Foot Ankle Int* 1999;20:521–526.
10. Crandall RC, Wagner FW Jr. Partial and total calcanectomy. *J Bone Joint Surg Am* 1981;63:152–155.
11. Isenberg JS, Costigan WM, Thordarson DB. Subtotal calcanectomy for osteomyelitis of the os calcis: a reasonable alternative to free tissue transfer. *Ann Plast Surg* 1995;35:660–663.
12. Smith DG, Stuck RM, Ketner L, Sage RM, Pinzur MS. Partial calcanectomy for the treatment of large ulcerations of the heel and calcaneal osteomyelitis. An amputation of the back of the foot. *J Bone Joint Surg Am* 1992;74:571–576.
13. Baumhauer JF, Fraga CJ, Gould JS, Johnson JE. Total calcanectomy for the treatment of chronic calcaneal osteomyelitis. *Foot Ankle Int* 1998;19:849–855.
14. Brodsky JW. Amputations of the foot. In: Coughlin MD, Mann RA, eds. *Surgery of the Foot and Ankle.* St. Louis, MO: Mosby; 1999:970–1006.
15. Armstrong DG, Stacpoole-Shea S, Nguyen H, Harkless LB. Lengthening of the Achilles tendon in diabetic patients who are at high risk for ulceration of the foot. *J Bone Joint Surg Am* 1999;81:535–538.
16. Holstein P, Lohmann M, Bitsch M, Jorgensen B. Achilles tendon lengthening, the panacea for plantar forefoot ulceration? *Diabetes Metab Res Rev* 2004;20:S37–S40.
17. Mueller MJ, Sinacore DR, Hastings MK, Strube MJ, Johnson JE. Effect of Achilles tendon lengthening on neuropathic plantar ulcers. A randomized clinical trial. *J Bone Joint Surg Am* 2003;85A:1436–1445.

25 Conventional Offloading and Activity Monitoring

Lawrence A. Lavery and Douglas P. Murdoch

Ulcers in persons with diabetes and neuropathy often develop as a result of a moderate or high level of mechanical stress on the sole of the foot. The magnitude, duration, rate and direction of mechanical stress are pivotal factors in repetitive injuries. The number of times a day the foot is exposed to these forces or the number of steps the patient takes on a daily basis is the other part of the equation. Until recently, pressure at the site of foot ulceration has been the principal focus of much of the clinical and laboratory research, because there were tools readily available to measure foot pressures. Activity evaluation has only recently received attention in the literature, while other factors such as shear still do not have adequate clinical equipment for routine assessment.

Reduction of pressure and shear forces on the foot may be the single most important and most neglected aspect of neuropathic ulceration treatment. Offloading therapy is a pivotal part of the treatment plan for diabetic foot ulcers. The goal is to reduce or eliminate pressure at the ulcer while keeping the patient walking.[1,2] There are a variety of methods available to protect the foot from abnormal pressures. The selection of an offloading treatment must be tailored to the strength, activity, postural stability and co-morbidities of the patient. However, in most cases, the more restrictive the offloading strategy, the better the healing environment.[3] The patient and clinician must appreciate that foot ulcers are usually the result of repetitive injury and that every unprotected step is literally tearing the wound apart. Without addressing this important component of the causal pathway, the wound will continue to be re-injured, and in many instances, it will remain open. Obviously, patients prefer something that is light and easy to walk with, but in reality, the most effective treatment strategy requires a device that will severely disrupt normal activity for 6–8 weeks. Who would think of allowing a patient with a tibia or ankle fracture to walk without proper immobilisation? Yet, we often provide ineffective but convenient forms of offloading therapies in patients at risk of amputation.

The total contact cast (TCC) is considered the 'ideal' gold standard to heal diabetic foot ulcers.[4–10] The strength of this technique is that the extremity is protected every minute of the day. It is one of the techniques most often reported in the medical literature to facilitate wound healing in the insensate extremity (Table 25.1). Across centres, in descriptive cohort studies and randomised clinical trials, TCCs heal about 90% of foot ulcers. The average healing time ranges from 6 to 8 weeks. The consistency and high rate of wound healing with TCCs is much

The Foot in Diabetes, 4th Edition. Editors Andrew J.M. Boulton, Peter R. Cavanagh and Gerry Rayman.
© 2006 John Wiley & Sons, Ltd.

Table 25.1   Healing times with total contact casts

Offloading modality	Mean healing time	Type of study	% Healed	Type of wound	References
TCC	Forefoot ulcers: 30 days Rearfoot–midfoot ulcers: 63 days	Retrospective cohort[‡]	90	Wagner 1, 2	Myerson et al.[11]
TCC	Forefoot ulcers: 31 days Rearfoot–midfoot ulcers: 42 days	Retrospective cohort[‡]	Not reported	Wagner 1, 2, 3	Walker et al.[4]
TCC	40 days	Retrospective cohort[‡]	94	Wagner 1, 2	Birke[5]
TCC	38 days	Retrospective cohort[‡]	73	Wagner 1, 2, 3	Helm et al.[6]
TCC	44 days	Retrospective cohort[‡]	82	Wagner 1, 2	Sinacore et al.[7]
TCC	Midfoot ulcers: 28 days	Retrospective cohort[‡]	100	Wagner 1, 2	Lavery et al.[8]
TCC	34 days	RCT[†]	90	UT 1A	Armstrong et al.[9]
RCW	50 days		65		
Half shoe	61 days		58		
TCC	85 days	RCT[†]	90	Wagner 1, 2	Mueller et al.[10]
Shoe insole	65 days		32		
RCW	42 days	RCT	83	UT 1A– 2A	Armstrong and Lavery[12]
ITCC	58 days		52		

TCC, total contact cast; RCT, randomised clinical trial; UT, University of Texas; RCW, removable cast walker; ITCC, instant total contact cast.
[‡]Percentage healed no specified time.
[*]Percentage healed in 30 days.
[†]Percentage healed in 12 weeks.
[‡]Percentage healed in 10 weeks.

better than what has been reported in randomised clinical trials with 'advanced technologies' such as bioengineered tissue, growth factors and electrical stimulation. These types of advanced technologies report ulcer healing in 30–65% of patients in 12- to 20-week studies.[13–18] One of the most criticised design elements of 'advanced wound therapies' studies is their lack of a rigorous form of offloading as part of standard therapy. Most studies use a therapeutic shoe or healing sandal as the standard offloading technique, ensuring that their 'control group' will have suboptimal healing rates. There is no published work that compares an advanced wound therapy product with aggressive offloading with a TCC.

TCCs contrast with traditional fracture casts in several important ways. TCCs usually have very little cast padding. Felt padding is applied to the anterior crest of the tibia and over the medial and lateral prominences of the ankle bones (Figure 25.1). These are often sites of pressure, friction and iatrogenic ulceration, even when a well-moulded TCC is expertly applied. The toes are padded with foam and covered with cast material in order to protect them from injury. Well-moulded plaster cast material is the first layer used over the cast padding. It is applied to conform to the contour of the foot and ankle, then actively massaged and moulded

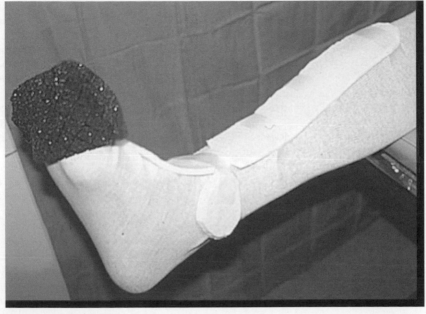

(a)

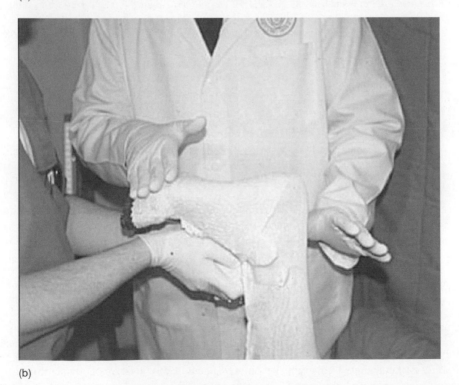

(b)

Figure 25.1   (a,b,c) Total contact cast application demonstrating padding over the toes and prominences of the ankle bones. The first layer of plaster is well moulded to conform to the foot and ankle

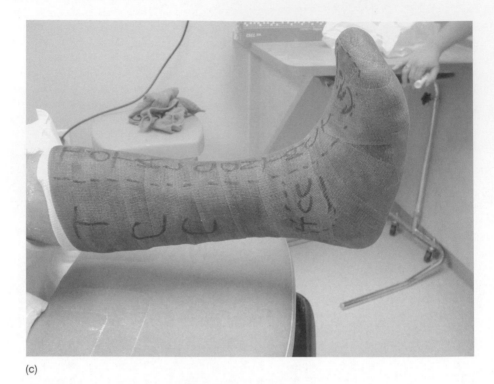

(c)

Figure 25.1   (*Continued*)

to achieve total contact with the surfaces of the lower extremity. This reduces motion as the cast dries and cast padding compresses. Fibreglass cast material is then applied as an outer layer, so that the patient can walk on the cast within 30 min. Classically, a 3-mm-thick board is incorporated into the fibreglass and a cast heel is positioned in the plantar central aspect of foot. This helps to further reduce pressure on the foot during ambulation.

TCCs are usually changed every week or two. Ideally, they are initially applied and scheduled to be changed in the morning, to reduce the severity of lower extremity swelling. If an extremity is severely swollen, a compression dressing should be applied for 2–5 days before a cast is applied. Walkers, canes or crutches should be used especially in older and obese patients or in patients with postural instability.

TCCs are often thought to be contraindicated in patients with infection and severe peripheral vascular disease (PVD). In fact, most published clinical studies of wound-healing therapies systematically eliminated these patients from consideration. It is therefore difficult to extrapolate much of the existing data to patients with neuroischaemic wounds or wounds with infection. Nabuurs-Franssen and colleagues reported clinical outcomes of TCC therapy in a prospective cohort of 98 patients with neuropathy (100%), PVD (44%) and infection (29%). As in other studies, 90% of patients without infection or ischaemia healed, and 87% of infected ulcers healed. In patients with vascular impairment, 69% healed. However, in patients with PVD and infection, only 36% healed.[19]

TCCs are advantageous for several reasons. They allow complete rest of the foot, even though the patient can be mobile and active during the therapy. They help control oedema that can impede healing and protect the foot from trauma and infection.[20] Perhaps, most importantly, because casts cannot be removed by patients, there is a strong element of forced compliance with this therapy. Patients have no choice but to keep pressure off their ulcer during every step they take during the day. It has been theorised that the total contact nature of the cast disperses forces to the lower tibia; however, there is little evidence to support this notion. TCCs probably reduce shear forces on the sole of the foot because they limit joint motion of the foot and ankle, force an apropulsive gait pattern and reduce stride length and cadence. TCCs have been shown to reduce pressure at the site of ulceration by 84–92%.[21,22] This is far superior to most other commercially available products.

TCCs have a significant impact on patients' level of activity. Because a TCC is confining and heavy, patients simply walk less. For instance, in a randomised clinical trial that compared TCCs, removable cast walkers (RCW) and healing sandals, patient treated with TCCs had a higher proportion of wounds that healed (90%) compared to either the RCW (65%) or the healing sandal (58%) group.[9] In addition, patients in TCCs took 58% fewer steps than subjects treated with healing sandals and 22% fewer steps than subjects treated with RCWs.[9,23]

BARRIERS TO USING TOTAL CONTACT CASTS

The TCC was a concept that was developed and popularised by Dr Paul Brand as a tool to heal neuropathic foot wounds in people with leprosy (Hansen's disease) in India. It was ideal for this rural setting because it was inexpensive and the materials were readily available even in an impoverished area with few medical resources. Dr Brand subsequently taught this technique at workshops on the insensate limb at the Gillis W. Long Hansen's Disease Centre in Carville, Louisiana. It is ironic that despite a large body of clinical and laboratory evidence in post-industrialised countries with advanced therapies and abundant resources, TCCs are not widely used.

There are several practical barriers that limit their adoption by the general medical community. TCCs are difficult to apply. TCCs require a physician, therapist or cast technician who is skilled at using this technique. In an insensate patient, tight or incorrectly applied casts can cause iatrogenic wounds. Total contact casting can require a significant amount of human resources, materials and space in a busy clinic. In addition, TCCs must be removed and then fully reapplied every 7 to 14 days. In settings with a low volume of foot wounds, dedicating the resources and training to safely and effectively apply TCCs may not be practical.

However, even when TCCs are applied correctly, patients often complain that the cast is hot and heavy. It is difficult to bathe and sleep with a TCC, especially in the elderly, obese patients. Many patients will refuse this type of therapy without a dedicated clinician to explain the risks and benefits of this form of TCCs.

REMOVABLE CAST WALKERS

There are a number of removable cast walkers (RCWs) that have been designed to help protect and heal foot wounds in people with diabetes. RCWs offer several advantages compared to TCCs. RCWs are relatively inexpensive, and the protective inner sole can be easily replaced if it shows signs of wear. The DH pressure relief walker (Royce Medical, Camarillo, CA, USA) has been shown to be almost identical to TCCs in pressure reduction at the site of ulcerations on the sole of the foot (Figure 25.2).[21,22] It does not require special training to correctly and

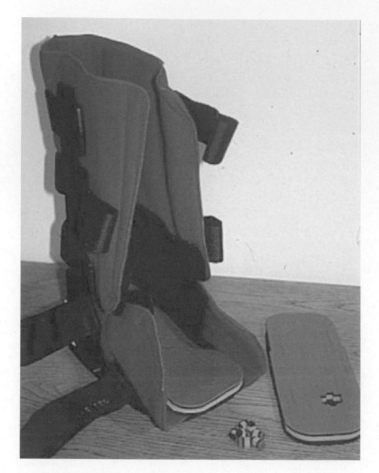

Figure 25.2   Removable cast walker. Active offloading walker, Royce Medical, Camarillo, CA, USA

safely apply these devices. In addition, they can be easily removed to assess and debride the wound, to bathe or to sleep. And they can be used in patients with infection or severe PVD.

Standard RCWs have been demonstrated to reduce peak pressures as effectively as TCCs,[21,22] but in both descriptive studies and randomised clinical trials, TCC have higher rates of healing.[9,12,24] A logical explanation for RCWs' less effective clinical performance is non-compliance to treatment: these devices are being removed by the patients who use them.[23] Armstrong and colleagues measured the number of steps taken with and without a removable cast boot in 20 patients with neuropathic foot ulcerations. Activity was measured from a waist-worn computerised accelerometer and correlated to activity recorded on an accelerometer mounted on the RCW, which was not readily accessible to the patient. Surprisingly, patients removed the RCW for 72% of their daily activity on average. Although a total of 30% of the patients in the study recorded more daily activity while wearing the device, this subgroup wore the RCW only for 60% of their total daily activity.[23]

It would be ideal to be able to take the clinical efficacy of the TCC and combine it with the relative ease of application of the RCW.[25,26] In an effort to achieve this, Armstrong and Katz modified the RCWs by merely wrapping them with a layer of cohesive tape or plaster bandage. This technique has been termed the 'instant' total contact cast (ITCC).[24–26]

In two randomised clinical trials, this technique has demonstrated clinical efficacy and safety. Armstrong et al.[26] compared a commercially available cast boot (Royce Medical, Camarillo, CA, USA) and the same RCW but making it 'irremovable'. A significantly higher proportion of patients healed at 12 weeks in the ITCC group when compared with the RCW (86.4% vs 58.3%). Of the patients that healed, persons treated with the ITCC healed significantly faster (41.6 ± 18.7 days vs 58.0 ± 15 days). Katz and colleagues[24] then compared the ITCC concept to a traditional TCC and found no difference in clinical outcomes or complications. The mean healing time was 5.4 weeks in the TCC group and 5.1 weeks in the ITCC group. We conclude that the ITCC is equally efficacious in healing diabetic foot ulcers, when compared to the TCC. However, it was quicker, easier and more cost-effective than the TCC.

The concept of an ITCC allows physicians, nurses and technicians to significantly improve the effectiveness of offloading with no additional training or expertise. The cost of many RCWs is similar to the cost of materials required to apply a TCC. Initial studies demonstrate the same proportion and rate of wound healing compared to TCCs. This is a very straightforward approach that can be adopted by most physicians that care for the diabetic foot.

CHARCOT RESTRAINT ORTHOTIC WALKER

The Charcot restraint orthotic walker (CROW) is a custom-made lower extremity clamshell foot and ankle orthosis that is designed to protect the neuropathic foot and aids in controlling lower extremity oedema. The CROW is a rigid polypropylene shell with a rocker bottom sole (Figure 25.3). The primary drawback to this type of device is that it is custom made and often takes several weeks to manufacture. It is very expensive, and if the structure or size of the lower extremity changes because of oedema or muscle atrophy, the custom device will no longer fit properly, and it cannot be used. Unfortunately, there is very little evidence in the medical literature that supports the effectiveness of this offloading technique.[27]

HEALING SANDALS AND HALF SHOES

There are growing numbers of healing sandals, half shoes and wedged shoes designed to reduce pressure on the forefoot. Half shoes such as the OrthoWedge or Darco products were originally designed to protect the forefoot after elective surgery (Figure 25.4). Half shoes are not very well accepted by patients. They are difficult to walk in. They often cause pain of the contralateral extremity, and patients with postural instability cannot safely use the device. As a result, compliance with these modalities is generally poor, and this is reflected in the clinical outcomes reported in the medical literature.[9,22,28,29]

Healing sandals can be custom made and moulded to the contour of the foot (Figure 25.5). Surgical shoes can be quickly modified by adding a pressure-reducing insole. In addition, there are a number of commercially available products designed specifically for the diabetic foot. These are easy to use and ideal for patients with impaired balance. They are tolerated well, but offer a significant compromise in pressure reduction and healing potential.

There are a number of reports that give us insight into the effectiveness of various healing sandals to treat foot ulcers in persons with diabetes. Veves and colleagues[18] used a

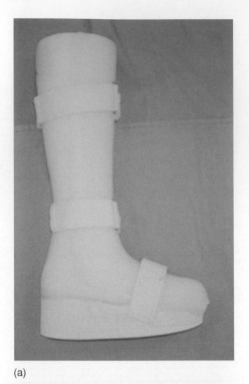

(a)

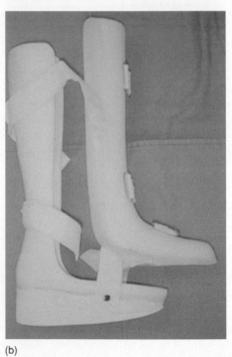

(b)

Figure 25.3   (a,b) Charcot restraint orthotic walker (CROW)

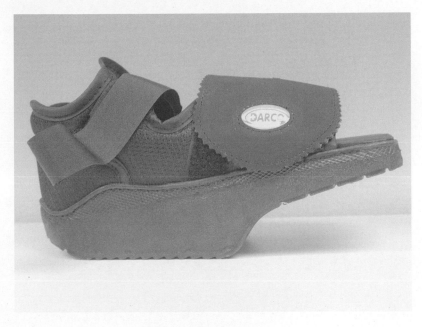

Figure 25.4 Darco half shoe

custom-healing sandal as the standard offloading modality in the pivotal, randomised clinical trail of Graftskin. Only 38% of subjects healed in the control arms, with an average healing time of 90 days. Likewise, Armstrong and colleagues[9] evaluated a half shoe (Darco, Huntington, WV, USA) compared to a removable cast boot and TCC, in a 12-week randomised clinical trial. Subjects treated with the half shoe had the lowest proportion of healed wounds (58%) and slowest rates of healing, with an average healing time of 61 days, compared to 33.5 days in the TCC group and 50.4 days in the RCW group.

Likewise, Ha Van and colleagues[28] reported that more patients with neuropathic ulcers healed faster when immobilised with a fibreglass cast (81%) compared to healing sandals (70%). Cast therapy was also protective against deep infection. In addition, very poor compliance was observed with the healing sandal. Only 10% of patients were compliant with the healing sandal compared to 98% of patients treated with fibreglass casts.

FELTED FOAM PADDED DRESSINGS

Padding techniques that use glue or tape to secure a pad around or over an ulcer on the sole of the foot have also been reported in the medical literature with success. This type of technique can be used in the patients' shoes if they have a deep toe box, with healing sandals or in removable cast boots (Plate 4). This is an easy technique to use and can be mastered by many members of the health care team. This technique involves two basic materials, adhesive felt and adhesive foam. The non-ulcerated skin is usually prepared with a standard skin adherent for protection and to assist in keeping the felt in place. The felt, which can be of different

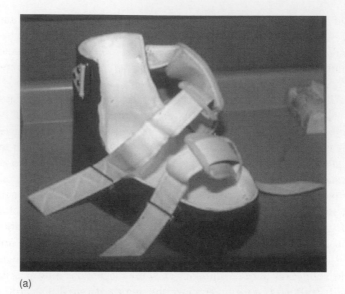

(a)

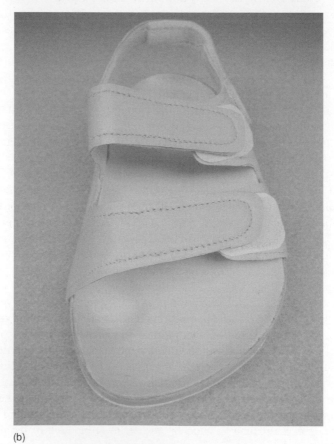

(b)

Figure 25.5   (a,b) Custom healing sandal

thicknesses (typically 0.125 in., 0.25 in.), is cut to support the areas around the ulcer site, taking into account specific anatomical variations. Additional pieces of felt can be added as needed to effect a flat plantar surface (much like the TCC concept). The ulcer is treated with the topical and primary dressing to fill the apertured part of the felt. The foam is then cut to cover the entire dressing including the felt and ulcer site. Tape is then utilised to seal the edges. It is a quick and inexpensive technique. However, patients must leave it in place for a week at a time. It is often malodorous and surrounding soft tissue is easily macerated.

Healing with this offloading approach is usually less successful than with more aggressive immobilisation. Zimny *et al.*[29] compared felted foam padded dressings to conventional wound therapy and found that healing times were almost identical. The padded dressing group healed in 79.6 days (range 75–84 days) compared to 83.2 days (range 77–90 days) using conventional therapy. In contrast, Birke and colleagues[30] reported an average healing time of 36 days with 93% complete wound closure, using felted foam in a retrospective cohort of diabetic foot wounds. Special load-relieving dressings are also available (Chapter 30).

THERAPEUTIC SHOES AND INSOLES

Therapeutic shoes and insoles are often the easiest choice for the busy clinician. They are always a choice of compromise for patients that cannot tolerate other offloading strategies. They are widely available, but manufactured with considerable variability in quality, customisation and effectiveness. Therapeutic shoes and insoles offer only a fraction of the pressure reduction at the site of ulceration provided by casts, removable cast boots or even padded dressings and healing sandals (Table 25.2).[22] The magnitude of pressure reduction is variable and depends on the location of the ulceration. In a gait lab study, therapeutic shoes with insoles reduced pressure at the site of ulceration in a wide range, from 3.4 to 48.4% (Table 25.3).[31]

Data regarding the effectiveness of therapeutic shoes and insoles are sparse. Most often, therapeutic shoes and insoles have been used as a control group in clinical trials of advanced

Table 25.2 Pressure reduction with removable cast walkers, half shoes, felted foam and surgical shoes

	% Change[a]	
Modalities	Great toe ulcer group	Forefoot ulcer group
Royce walker	79	85
Total cotact cast	85	76
Half shoe	64	66
Felted foam dressing	34	48
Post-operative shoe	7	36

[a]Percent change from the baseline measurements in canvas Oxford shoes.

Table 25.3 Percent pressure reduction from baseline among diabetic patients with foot ulcers treated with off-the-shelf footwear with and without accommodative insoles

	Xtra Depth		Cross Trainer		San Antonio shoes	
Insole	Yes	No	Yes	No	Yes	No
First metatarsal	42.9	28.5	42.6	34.7	45.0	41.3
Second to fifth metatarsal	47.2	38.8	45.5	41.4	48.4	45.4
Great toe	18.3	8.8	3.2	−12.2	16.8	6.2

wound therapies (Table 25.4).[15,17] In randomised clinical trials of Dermagraft, only 18% of patients healed in 12 weeks in the control group that was offloaded with extra-depth shoes with custom insoles. In a 12-week randomised clinical trial by Mueller and colleagues,[10] therapeutic shoes and insoles were evaluated against TCCs. Only 32% of subjects treated with therapeutic shoes and insoles healed, compared to 90% of subjects treated with TCCs.

Table 25.4 Healing times with shoes, healing sandals, half shoes and felted foam dressings

Offloading modality	Mean healing time	Type of study	% Healed	Type of wound	References
Fibreglass cast shoe	34	Retrospective cohort[†]	91	Wagner 1	Hissink et al.[32]
Fibreglass cast, shoe and insole	Not reported	RCT*	50 21	Wagner 1	Caravaggi et al.[33]
Scotchcast boot	130 days	Retrospective cohort[‡]	80	Wagner 1, 2, 3	Knowles et al.[34]
Fibreglass cast	69 days	Prospective	81	UT 2A	Ha Van et al.[28]
Half shoe	134 days	cohort[‡]	70	UT 1A	
Custom splint	300 days	Retrospective cohort[‡]	Not reported	Not stated	Boninger and Leonard[27]
Felted foam dressing	80 days	RCT	Not reported	Wagner 1, 2	Zimny et al.[29]
Half shoe	83 days				
TCC	48 days	Retrospective	92	Wagner	Birke et al.[30]
Felted foam dressing	36 days	cohort[†]	93	1, 2, 3	
Healing shoe	42 days		81		
Walking splint	51 days		83		

RCT, randomised clinical trial.
[‡]Percentage healed no specified time.
[*]Percentage healed in 30 days.
[†]Percentage healed in 12 weeks.
[‡]Percentage healed in 10 weeks.

ACTIVITY AS A TREATMENT TOOL

The patient's activity is an important component of developing and healing foot wounds. The most effective offloading devices limit activity because they restrict joint motion and make it difficult to walk. Until recently, measurements of patients' activity have been missing from our evaluation of cumulative stress on the diabetic foot. With the availability of inexpensive computerised activity monitors, the ability of patients and physicians to accurately evaluate activity as a clinical tool is at hand.[35,36] In many cases, persons with diabetes and foot ulcers are less active than non-diabetic and diabetic controls. Armstrong *et al.*[37] and Maluf and Mueller[38] have reported that the variability in activity is more significant than the total numbers of steps per day. Smoothing out the peaks and troughs may help with prevention and treatment of foot wounds. Using embedded monitoring instruments in removable offloading devices may improve patients' understanding of the treatment process and enhance the abysmal compliance with healing sandals and RCWs.[23,28] We may be able to dose activity to facilitate healing and prevent ulceration just as we would a drug. Or, we could simply make the offloading device in a way so it cannot be removed by the patient.

CONCLUSION

Attention to offloading should be a basic element of every treatment plan for diabetic foot ulcers. It is often neglected entirely or provided half-heartedly. Offloading is not an easy part of the treatment plan for either the patient or the physician, but it is one of the most critical aspects of care.

REFERENCES

1. Lavery LA, Vela S, Quebedeaux T, Lavery LA. Total contact casts: pressure reduction at ulcer sites and the effected on the contralateral foot. *Arch Phys Med Rehabil* 1997;78:1268–1271.
2. Armstrong DG, Lavery LA, Nixon BP, Boulton AJM. It is not what you put on, but what you take off: techniques for debriding and offloading the diabetic foot wound. *Clin Infect Dis* Aug 2004;39:S92–S99.
3. American Diabetes Association. Consensus Development Conference on Diabetic Foot Wound Care. *Diabetes Care* 1999;22:1354–1360.
4. Walker SC, Helm PA, Pullium G. Total contact casting and chronic diabetic neuropathic foot ulcerations: healing rates by wound location. *Arch Phys Med Rehabil* 1987;68:217–221.
5. Birke JA. Healing rates of plantar ulcers in leprosy and diabetes. *Lepr Rev* 1992;63:365–374.
6. Helm PA, Walker SC, Pullium G. Total contact casting in diabetic patients with neuropathic foot ulcerations. *Arch Phys Med Rehabil* 1984;65:691–693.
7. Sinacore DR, Mueller MJ, Diamond JE, *et al.* Diabetic plantar ulcers treated by total contact casting. A clinical report. *Phys Ther* 1987;67:1543–1549.
8. Lavery LA, Armstrong DG, Walker SC. Healing rates of diabetic foot ulcers associated with midfoot fracture due to Charcot's arthropathy. *Diabet Med* 1997;14:46–49.
9. Armstrong DG, Nguyen HC, Lavery LA, van Schie CH, Boulton AJ, Harkless LB. Offloading the diabetic foot wound: a randomized clinical trial. *Diabetes Care* 2001;24:1019–1022.
10. Mueller MJ, Diamond JE, Sinacore DR, *et al.* Total contact casting in treatment of diabetic plantar ulcers. Controlled clinical trial. *Diabetes Care* 1989;12:384–388.

11. Myerson M, Papa J, Eaton K, Wilson K. The total-contact cast for management of neuropathic plantar ulceration of the foot. *J Bone Joint Surg Am* 1992;74A:261–269.
12. Armstrong DG, Lavery LA. Evaluation of removable and irremovable cast walkers in the healing of diabetic foot wounds: a randomized controlled trial. *Diabetes Care* 2005;28:551–554.
13. Steed DL, Donohoe D, Webster MW, Lindsley L, for the Diabetic Ulcer Study Group. Effect of extensive debridement and treatment on the healing of diabetic foot ulcers. *J Am Coll Surg* 1996;183: 61–64.
14. Wieman TJ, Smiell JM, Su Y. Efficacy and safety of a topical gel formulation of recombinant human platelet-derived growth factor-BB (becaplemin) in patients with chronic neuropathic diabetic ulcers. A phase III randomized placebo-controlled double-blind study. *Diabetes Care* 1998;21:822–827.
15. Hanft J. Healing of chronic foot wounds in diabetic patients treated with human fibroblast derived dermis. *J Foot Ankle Surg* 2002;41:291–299.
16. Peters EJ, Lavery LA, Armstrong DG, Fleischli JG. Electric stimulation as an adjunct to heal diabetic foot ulcers: a randomized clinical trial. *Arch Phys Med Rehabil* 2001;82:721–725.
17. Marston WA, Hanft J, Norwood P, Pollak R. The efficacy and safety of Dermagraft in improving the healing of chronic diabetic foot ulcers: results of a prospective randomized trial. *Diabetes Care* 2003;26:1701–1705.
18. Veves A, Falanga V, Armstrong DG, Sabolinski ML. Graftskin, a human skin equivalent, is effective in the management of noninfected neuropathic diabetic foot ulcers: a prospective randomized multicenter clinical trial. *Diabetes Care* 2001;24:290–295.
19. Nabuurs-Franssen M, Sleegers R, Huijberts MSP. Total contact casting of the diabetic foot in daily practice. *Diabetes Care* 2005;28:243–247.
20. Coleman WC, Brand PW, Birke JA. The total contact cast. A therapy for plantar ulceration on insensitive feet. *J Am Podiatry Assoc* 1984;74:548–552.
21. Lavery LA, *et al.* Reducing dynamic foot pressures in high risk diabetics with foot ulcerations: a comparison of treatments. *Diabetes Care* 1996;19:818–821.
22. Fleischli JG, Vela S, Lavery LA. Comparison of strategies for reducing pressure at the site of neuropathic ulcers. *J Am Podiatr Med Assoc* 1997;87:466–447.
23. Armstrong DG, Lavery LA, Kimbriel HR, Nixon BP, Boulton AJ. Activity patterns of patients with diabetic foot ulceration: patients with active ulceration may not adhere to a standard pressure off-loading regimen. *Diabetes Care* 2003;26:2595–2597.
24. Katz IA, Harlan A, Miranda-Palma B, Armstrong DG, Boulton AJ. A randomized trial of two irremovable offloading devices in the management of neuropathic diabetic foot ulcers. *Diabetes Care* 2005;28:555–558.
25. Armstrong DG, Short B, Espensen EH, Abu-Rumman PL, Nixon BP, Boulton AJ. Technique for fabrication of an 'instant total contact cast for treatment of neuropathic diabetic foot ulcers. *J Am Podiatr Med Assoc* 2002;92:405–408.
26. Armstrong DG, Lavery LA, Wu S, Boulton AJM. Evaluation of removable and irremovable cast walkers in the healing of diabetic foot wounds: a randomized controlled trial. *Diabetes Care* 2005;28:551–554.
27. Boninger ML, Leonard JA Jr. Use of bivalved ankle–foot orthosis in neuropathic foot and ankle lesions. *J Rehabil Res Dev* 1996;33:16–22.
28. Ha Van G, Siney H, Hartmann-Heurtier A, Jacqueminet S, Greau F, Grimaldi A. Nonremovable, windowed, fiberglass cast boot in the treatment of diabetic plantar ulcers: efficacy, safety, and compliance. *Diabetes Care* 2003;26:2848–2852.
29. Zimny S, Meyer MF, Schatz H, Pfohl M. Applied felted foam for plantar pressure relief is an efficient therapy in neuropathic diabetic foot ulcers. *Exp Clin Endocrinol Diabetes* 2002;110:325–328.
30. Birke JA, Pavich MA, Patout CA Jr, Horswell R. Comparison of forefoot ulcer healing using alternative off-loading methods in patients with diabetes mellitus. *Adv Skin Wound Care* 2002;15:210–215.

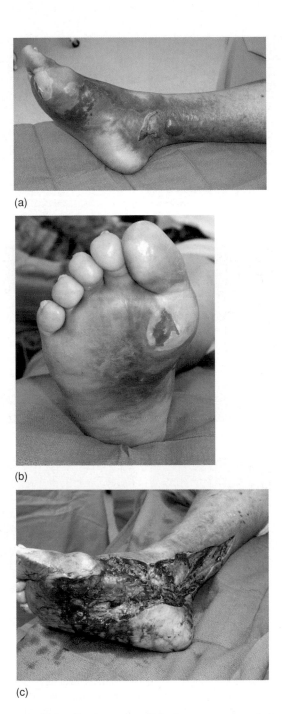

(a)

(b)

(c)

Plate 5 (a,b) This 61-year old insulin-dependent diabetic woman was admitted to the hospital with clinical signs of sepsis. Her condition continued to worsen in spite of parenteral broad-spectrum antibiotic therapy and medical management. (c) Following thorough debridement of necrotising fasciitis, her clinical condition rapidly improved. She was treated with culture-specific antibiotic therapy and vacuum-assisted wound healing. Split-thickness skin grafting and therapeutic footwear allowed her to resume her independent ambulatory status

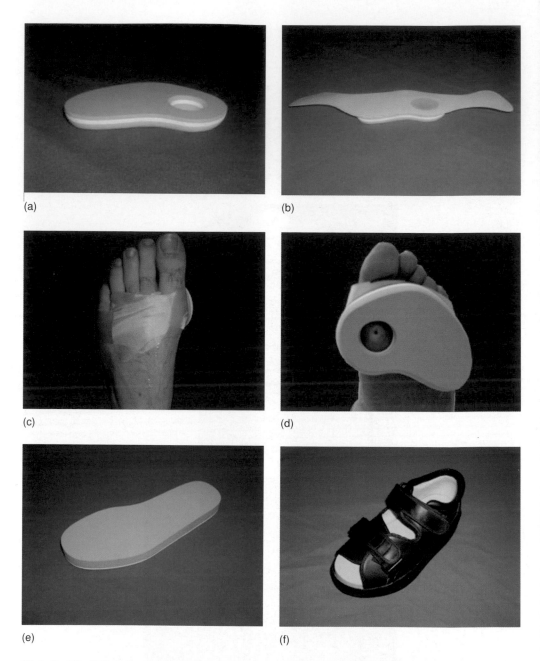

Plate 6 The DIApedia pressure-relieving dressing (PRD) ulcer-healing prototype system. (a) The PRD has three primary layers, from top (patient side) down: shear reducing, offloading and conforming (the adhesive and dorsal anchor straps are *not* shown in this view); note the profiled edges and pressure-relieving aperture. (b) The adhesive dorsal anchor straps provide (c) a continuous adhesive system. (d) Here, the PRD is shown in place with the pressure-relieving aperture over the ulcer; the aperture would usually be 'filled' with a product that controls the wound environment (e.g. product for exudate absorption). (e) For ambulation, the PRD is accommodated by a viscoelastic footbed (f) in a healing shoe (here a Darco product)

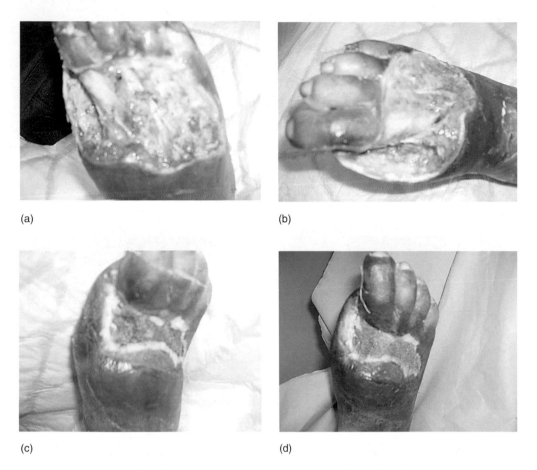

(a)

(b)

(c)

(d)

Plate 7 (a,b,c,d) Post-operative wound before NPWT

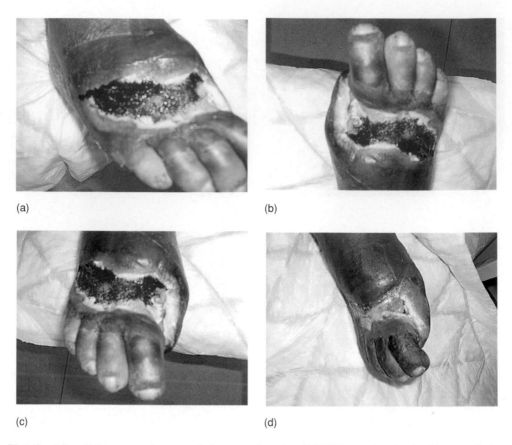

(a)

(b)

(c)

(d)

Plate 8 (a,b,c,d) Post-operative wound after several weeks of NPWT, now showing healthy granulation tissue

31. Lavery LA, Vela S, Quebedeaux T, Lavery DC. Reducing plantar pressure in the neuropathic foot: a comparison of footwear. *Diabetes Care* 1997;20:1706–1710.

32. Hissink RJ, Manning HA, van Baal JG. The MABAL shoe, an alternative method in contact casting for the treatment of neuropathic diabetic foot ulcers. *Foot Ankle Int* 2000;21:320–323.

33. Caravaggi C, Faglia E, De Giglio R, *et al*. Effectiveness and safety of a nonremovable fiberglass off-bearing cast versus a therapeutic shoe in the treatment of neuropathic foot ulcers: a randomized study. *Diabetes Care* 2000;23:1746–1751.

34. Knowles EA, Armstrong DG, Hayat SA, Khawaja KI, Malik RA, Boulton AJ. Offloading diabetic foot wounds using the scotchcast boot: a retrospective study. *Ostomy Wound Manage* 2002;48:50–53.

35. Armstrong DG, Boulton AJ. Activity monitors: should we begin dosing activity as we dose a drug? *J Am Podiatr Med Assoc* 2001;91:152–153.

36. Armstrong DG, Abu-Rumman PL, Nixon BP, Boulton AJ. Continuous activity monitoring in persons at high risk for diabetes-related lower extremity amputation. *J Am Podiatr Med Assoc* 2001;91:451–455.

37. Armstrong DG, Lavery LA, Holtz-Neiderer K, *et al*. Variability in activity may precede diabetic foot ulceration. *Diabetes Care* 2004;27:1980–1984.

38. Maluf KS, Mueller MJ. Comparison of physicial activity and cumulative plantar tissue stress among subjects with and without diabetes mellitus and a history of recurrent plantar ulcers. *Clin Biomech* 2003;18:567–575.

26 Amputations in the Diabetic Foot

Michael S. Pinzur

Partial or whole foot amputation requires special consideration in the diabetic population. Virtually all of the patients have peripheral neuropathy with loss of protective sensation, and accompanying deficits in walking balance. Many have peripheral vascular disease. By the time these patients require an amputation, they will likely have the associated co-morbidities of ischaemic cardiovascular disease, renal failure, protein-losing malnutrition and vision deficits. Salvage of a functional terminal organ of weight bearing allows these individuals to remain more mobile and independent, as compared with patients who have undergone transtibial or proximal level amputations.[1-5]

LIMB SALVAGE VERSUS AMPUTATION

Individuals with diabetes generally face lower extremity amputation as a consequence of foot infection and/or gangrene. The first step in the decision-making process is determination of whether the intervention has the potential to maintain a viable and functional limb. If the patient does not use the foot for walking or transferring from bed to chair, then heroic measures should not be undertaken. If treatment offers the potential for maintaining a functional organ of weight bearing, four issues need to be addressed:

1. Will limb salvage outperform amputation and prosthetic limb fitting? If all transpires as one could reasonably predict, will the functional independence of the patient following limb salvage or reconstruction be greater, or less, than that after amputation and prosthetic limb fitting? This will vary greatly with age, vocational ability, medical health, lifestyle, education and social status.

2. What is a realistic expectation of functional capacities at the completion of treatment? A realistic appreciation of functional end results should be made with respect to both limb salvage and amputation. Consultation with physical medicine and rehabilitation, social work and physical therapy can assist in determining reasonable outcome expectations.

3. What is the cost to the patient? One should consider both the financial and time allocation costs to the patient, and the time and resources required of the health care system. Both

The Foot in Diabetes, 4th Edition. Editors Andrew J.M. Boulton, Peter R. Cavanagh and Gerry Rayman.
© 2006 John Wiley & Sons, Ltd.

the physician and patient must have a reasonable understanding of the resource and time commitments that will be necessary to either maintain the limb, or undergo amputation and rehabilitation.

4. What are the risks associated with each option? One must consider the treatment-specific potential morbidities. For example, when a distal vascular bypass graft gets infected, the limbs of many patients cannot be salvaged at the transtibial level, and often require transfemoral amputation.[6]

WOUND-HEALING PARAMETERS

Healing of surgical wounds in individuals with diabetes poses several special concerns due to the metabolic deficiencies associated with the disease, the disease-specific deficiencies in the patients' immune system, the oft-associated relative malnutrition and the ever-present micro- and macroscopic central and peripheral vascular disease. Specifically, healing of an amputation wound requires a combination of arterial blood supply, tissue nutrition and immunocompetence. The development of peripheral vascular disease is a slow process, allowing patients to develop collateral blood flow during the period of time when the major vessels are slowly occluding. Unlike the vascular surgeon or interventional radiologist who is looking for a 'pressure head' or a reconstituted vessel, surgical wound healing simply requires a threshold level of oxygenated blood. Both Yao and Wagner have shown that one needs approximately one-half the normal blood flow to support wound healing in the dysvascular limb.[4,5,7]

The most common method of measuring arterial inflow is accomplished by measuring ultrasound Doppler arterial pressures. In the normal arterial waveform, the area under the waveform curve represents blood flow. The ankle–brachial index (ABI) is the ratio of the ultrasound Doppler pressure, taken at the level of the dorsalis pedis or posterior tibial artery, to the brachial pressure. Wagner described the 'ischaemic index' as the ratio of the ultrasound Doppler pressure at the level of interest, i.e. popliteal for healing of a transtibial amputation, to the brachial pressure. The threshold measure of arterial inflow sufficient to support wound healing in a dysvascular limb is an ischaemic index of approximately 0.5.[4,5,7] Unfortunately, calcification of the leg arteries makes the measured ultrasound Doppler falsely elevated in at least 15% of patients with longstanding diabetes.[8,9] This has prompted many to use transcutaneous oximetry as a measure of the oxygen-delivering capacity of the cardiovascular system to the area in question.[8,10] When transcutaneous oxygen measurement is not locally available, the vascular laboratory can measure toe pressure as an indicator of arterial inflow to the foot. This is due to the observation that arteries of the hallux do not seem to be calcified, as do the vessels of the leg.[11–13] The accepted threshold toe pressure is 30 mm Hg.

There is a significant impairment to wound healing in diabetic individuals for several reasons, in addition to the presence of peripheral vascular disease. Diabetic patients with foot infection tend to exhibit parameters of malnutrition due to a combination of their inherent metabolic disease and the co-morbidity contribution of impaired renal function.[14,15] While the nutrition literature has accepted a standard serum albumin of 3.5 g/dl as the lower limits of normal, it is currently accepted that the threshold serum albumin necessary to support wound healing in the diabetic dysvascular limb is 3.0 g/dl.[2,14,15]

In addition to these factors, individuals with diabetes have a multifactorial impairment in their immune system. This may explain why the offending organisms seen in diabetic foot infection are so unusual, and seemingly non-'pathogenic'. Immunoglobulin production and competence are impaired, as well as leucocyte function. Affected individuals are often incapable of mounting a white blood cell response, demonstrating low or 'normal' white blood cell counts in the face of life-threatening infection. The accepted threshold marker for lymphocyte function is a total (absolute) lymphocyte count of 1500.

SURGERY FOR INFECTION AND/OR GANGRENE

When patients present with clinical signs of sepsis and wound-healing thresholds below the accepted wound-healing parameters, surgery should involve debridement (removal) of all infected or gangrenous tissue, combined with open wound management. Broad-spectrum parenteral antibiotic therapy can be initiated until culture-specific antibiotic therapy is instituted (Chapters 13 and 14). The overall metabolic and medical condition of the patient can be optimised, and nutritional support should be initiated.[2,14] When both the systemic medical condition and the nutritional environment have been clinically optimised, a definitive amputation or wound closure can be performed (Plate 5).

Osteomyelitis, diabetic foot abscess and gangrene are surgical diseases. All dead and infected tissue must be removed. Resolution of these disease processes cannot be accomplished with antibiotic therapy alone. Antibiotic therapy augments wound management, following removal of all infected and non-viable tissue. Swab cultures are inadequate. The adjunctive antibiotic therapy should be determined by surgically obtained tissue cultures. Following removal of infected and gangrenous tissue, and clinical resolution of the infection, a terminal end organ of weight bearing must be created from the remaining tissue. The optimal goal is to provide an ulcer-free plantar grade foot that will allow the patient to bear weight and maintain walking independence with commercially available therapeutic footwear[3,16] (Plate 5).

AMPUTATION LEVEL SELECTION

The first step in determination of specific surgical amputation level is to establish reasonable goals for the patient. In patients with severe peripheral vascular disease, the vascular surgeon can advise on the probability of providing improved vascular inflow. Consultation with physical medicine and rehabilitation can help determine the patient's ambulatory potential.[17,18] Distal bypass surgery, endovascular surgery and foot and ankle amputation should generally be performed only in patients with the potential to ambulate. When the reasonable goal is chair sitting and wheelchair ambulation, more proximal amputation at the transtibial or knee disarticulation level should be performed. The questionable benefit of partial limb retention to assist in wheelchair transfer does not justify the surgically associated morbidity.

The second step is an assessment of wound-healing capacity. The patient must possess an adequate bony platform and soft tissue envelope sufficient to create a functional terminal organ of weight bearing. The roles of plastic surgical soft tissue transfer and free tissue transfer and the use of vacuum-assisted wound healing provide interesting potential to expand the surgeon's capacity for function-sparing limb salvage. Their roles will be better defined with more experience. Wound-healing parameters should be above threshold to predict acceptable wound failure rates. When patients have adequate vascular inflow, serum albumin above 2.5–3.0 g/dl and a total lymphocyte count greater than 1500, one can expect a wound-healing rate of greater than 90%. When one of the parameters is below threshold values, the wound-healing rate drops to 60%.[2,8,14,15]

The clinical examination of the patient and an assessment of the wound-healing parameters provide the surgeon with a biological amputation level. A realistic assessment of the patient's rehabilitation potential will then provide guidance for the surgeon on the appropriate rehabilitation amputation level.

THE END ORGAN OF WEIGHT BEARING

The human foot is uniquely adapted for its role as a terminal end organ of weight bearing. The engineer refers to this interaction as load transfer, and quantifies that load with a measure of the vertical ground reaction force (GRF). During the period of time that the GRF is applied, the multiple joints of the foot allow optimum positioning of the foot to maximise the surface area and the ability to distribute the load. The plantar skin and underlying connective tissue are uniquely evolved to manage the load without breaking down. One must understand both these concerns, and the availability of specialised therapeutic footwear to distribute forces and reduce plantar pressure.[16]

The residual limb needs to be positioned in a plantar grade orientation to optimise its capacity as a platform. There should be no bony prominences, as the insensate foot ulcerates when shear forces are applied over a bony prominence with an adherent or poorly cushioned soft tissue envelope. The soft tissue envelope needs to be sufficiently cushioned and covered with durable skin to tolerate the loads associated with daily living. Split-thickness skin graft and bioengineered skin substitutes are rarely sufficiently durable to achieve these tasks.[3,19]

FUNCTIONAL AMPUTATION LEVELS

Toe Amputation

The hallux (great toe) acts as the stabiliser of the medial column of the foot during the terminal stance phase. If possible, the proximal metaphysis of the proximal phalanx should be preserved in order to maintain the insertion of the flexor hallucis brevis. If this insertion cannot be maintained, important stability during the terminal stance phase will be lost and such patients will become relatively apropulsive. Some (a minority of) authors suggest that these patients would be better served with midfoot amputation (Figures 26.1 and 26.2).

The lesser toes serve very little function. Preservation of some proximal phalanx of the second toe will prevent lateral migration of the hallux, preventing a severe 'bunion' deformity that may be prone to ulceration (Figure 26.3). A smooth contour of remaining toes will avoid potential pressure concentration (Figure 26.4).

Ray Resection

Longitudinal amputation of a toe and its corresponding metatarsal is generally performed only for infection. One would not expect healing following resection of longitudinal gangrene, as peripheral vascular disease worsens with distance from the core. As a primary procedure,

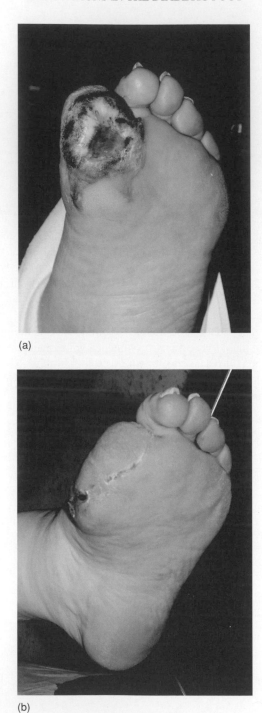

(a)

(b)

Figure 26.1   (a) A 51-year old overweight insulin-dependant diabetic male had a persistent plantar ulcer that continued to return after several episodes of treatment. (b) A dorsal skin flap was used to obtain successful healing at hallux amputation level

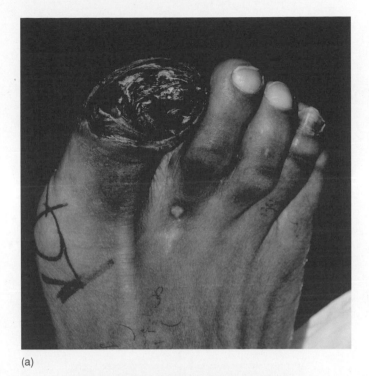

(a)

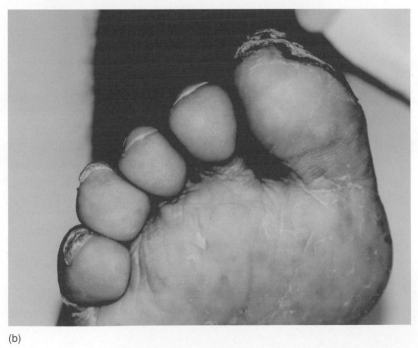

(b)

Figure 26.2 (a,b) The 53-year old diabetic patient developed this ischaemic ulcer. (c) A plantar-based flap was successful in providing a stable amputation through the proximal phalanx of the hallux

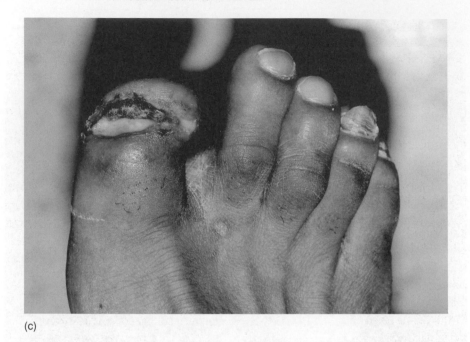

(c)

Figure 26.2   (*Continued*)

the best results are achieved following resection of a lateral (first or fifth) metatarsal. Central metatarsal resection requires sufficient bony resection to allow secondary wound closure. When more than one metatarsal needs to be removed, the residual forefoot becomes very narrow and tends to develop an equinus (plantar flexion) deformity, which is difficult to accommodate with therapeutic footwear. To ensure the most favourable outcome, these individuals are best treated with midfoot amputation.[20]

Midfoot Amputation

Amputation at the middle level of the foot can be performed at the transmetatarsal or tarsal–metatarsal (Lisfranc) levels. Both provide an excellent weight-bearing platform for walking. Late equinus deformity can be avoided by performing a percutaneous Achilles tendon lengthening at the time of surgery, and managing the patient in a below-knee total contact walking cast for 4 weeks following the surgery.[14] Amputation through the distal metatarsal shafts minimises the loss in walking propulsion at the cost of an appreciable rate of re-ulceration under one or all of the residual metatarsal ends. This can be avoided by performing the surgery through the proximal metaphyses, at the cost of a decreased lever arm to assist propulsion.[21,22]

Hindfoot Amputation

Except for special circumstances, hindfoot amputation should be avoided due to the high risk for the late development of non-correctable ankle equinus due to the overpowering effect of the ankle plantar flexors (Figure 26.5). There is recent interest in performing this amputation level

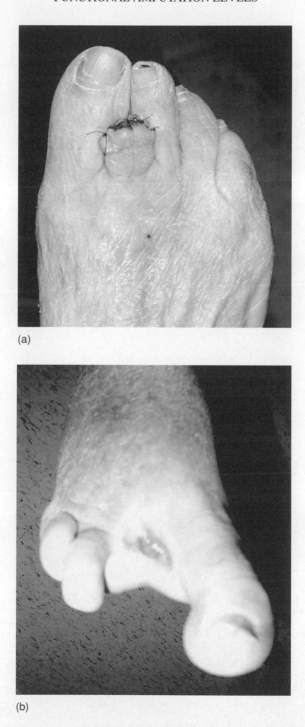

(a)

(b)

Figure 26.3 (a) Preservation of the proximal metaphysis of the second toe prevented the hallux from migrating laterally. (b) This foot had a complete amputation of the second toe. The foot is at high risk for the development of a severe hallux valgus deformity with a bony prominence prone to ulcerate

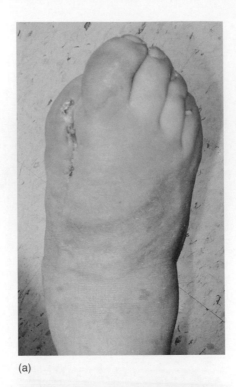

(a)

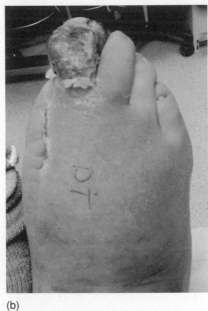

(b)

Figure 26.4   (a) A partial first ray resection allowed the second toe to be prominent. (b) Pressure in the early post-operative period produced a transfer pressure lesion in the second toe. (c,d) Multiple toe resections created a smooth border. The absence of prominent toes allowed successful therapeutic shoe fitting

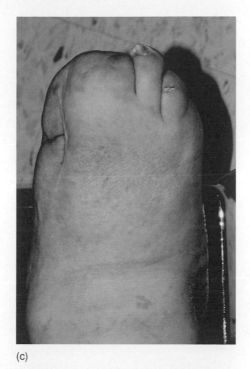

(c)

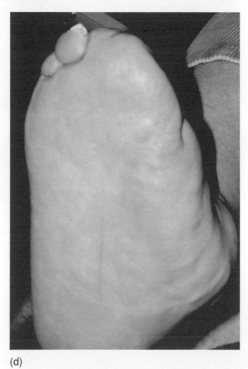

(d)

Figure 26.4 (*Continued*)

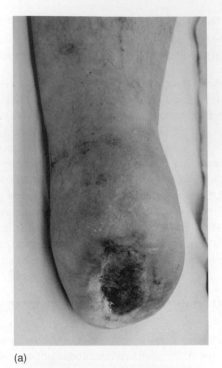

(a)

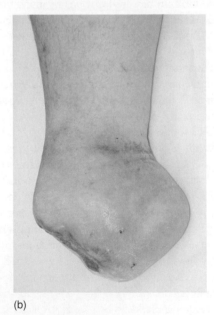

(b)

Figure 26.5   (a,b,c,d) This insulin-dependent diabetic male underwent open hindfoot amputation as treatment for infection. In spite of immobilisation in a below-the-knee cast, the patient has developed a severe equinovarus deformity that precluded weight bearing. Note the significant bony prominence underlying the anterior aspect of the calcaneus. This deformity cannot be accommodated with therapeutic footwear. The patient will require an ankle disarticulation (Syme's)

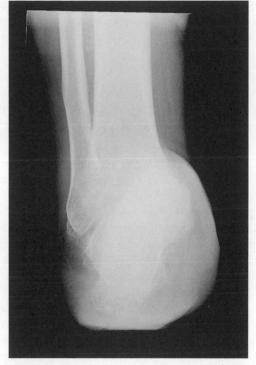

(c)

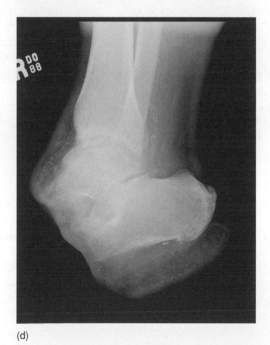

(d)

Figure 26.5   (*Continued*)

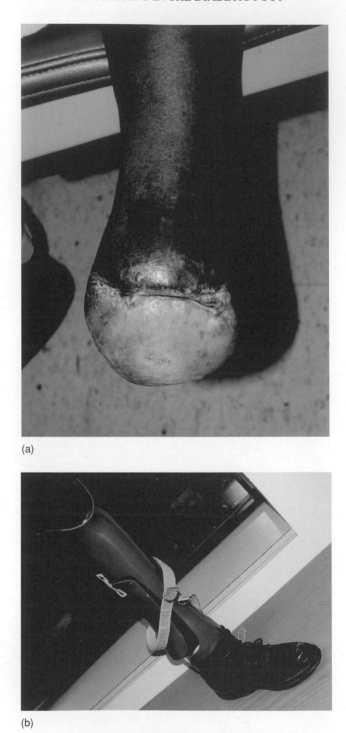

(a)

(b)

Figure 26.6 (a) Residual limb following one-stage Syme's ankle disarticulation. (b) This patient was able to quickly become a successful walker with a 'Canadian' Syme's prosthesis

in conjunction with ankle fusion only in individuals who do not, or will not be able to, obtain a prosthesis (Syme's ankle disarticulation) due to entitlement or financial reasons. Combining ankle fusion with hindfoot amputation allows apropulsive ambulation with a modified high-topped shoe.

Syme's Ankle Disarticulation

Syme's ankle disarticulation allows end bearing within a prosthetic socket, using the normal weight-bearing tissue of the heel. When the surgery is successful, these individuals resume normal walking with a prosthesis and rarely have late complications (Figure 26.6).[2] The two critical factors necessary to achieve a successful Syme's ankle disarticulation are preservation of the posterior tibial artery and securing the heel pad to the tibia with non-absorbable sutures.[2,23]

REFERENCES

1. Pinzur MS, Gottschalk F, Smith D, *et al*. Functional outcome of below-knee amputation in peripheral vascular insufficiency. *Clin Orthop* 1993;286:247–249.
2. Pinzur MS, Stuck R, Sage R, Hunt N, Rabinovich Z. Syme's ankle disarticulation in patients with diabetes. *J Bone Joint Surg* 2003;85A:1667–1672.
3. *International Consensus on the Diabetic Foot*. Amsterdam: The International Working Group on the Diabetic Foot; 1999.
4. Wagner FW Jr. Amputations of the foot and ankle. Current status. *Clin Orthop* 1977;122:62–69.
5. Wagner FW Jr. Management of the diabetic neurotrophic foot, Part II: a classification and treatment program for diabetic, neuropathic, and dysvascular foot problems. *Instr Course Lect* 1979;28:143–165.
6. Pinzur MS, Guedes de souza pinto M, Schon LG, Smith DG. Controversies in lower extremity amputation. *Instr Course Lect* 2003;52:445–454.
7. Yao ST, Hobbs JT, Irvine WT. Ankle systolic pressure measurements in arterial disease affecting the lower extremities. *Br J Surg* 1969;56:676–679.
8. Pinzur MS, Sage R, Stuck R, Ketner L, Osterman H. Transcutaneous oxygen as a predictor of wound healing in amputations of the foot and ankle. *Foot Ankle* 1992;13:271–272.
9. Emanuele MA, Buchanan BJ, Abraira C. Elevated leg systolic pressures and arterial calcification in diabetic occlusive vascular disease. *Diabetes Care* 1981;4:289–292.
10. Wyss CR, Harrington RM, Burgess EM, Matsen FA. Transcutaneous oxygen tension as a predictor of success after an amputation. *J Bone Joint Surg* 1988;70A:203–207.
11. Pahlsson HI, Wahlberg E, Olofsson P, Swedenborg J. The toe pole test for evaluation of arterial insufficiency in diabetic patients. *Eur J Endovasc Surg* 1999;18:133–137.
12. Carter SA, Tate RB. The value of toe pulse waves in determination of risks for limb amputation and death in patients with peripheral arterial disease and skin ulcers or gangrene. *J Vasc Surg* 2001;33:708–714.
13. Ubbink DT, Tulevski II, de Graaff JC, Legemate DA, Jacobs JHM. Optimisation of the non-invasive assessment of critical limb ischaemia requiring invasive treatment. *Eur J Endovasc Surg* 2000;19:131–137.
14. Pinzur MS, Kaminsky M, Sage R, Cronin R, Osterman H. Amputations at the middle level of the foot. *J. Bone Joint Surg* 1986;68A:1061–1064.
15. Dickhaut SC, DeLee JC, Page CP. Nutritional status: importance in predicting wound healing after amputation. *J Bone Joint Surg* 1984;66A:71–75.

16. Pinzur MS, Dart H. Pedorthic management of the diabetic foot. *Foot Ankle Clin* 2001;6:205–214.
17. Keenen MA, Perry J, Jordan C. Factors affecting balance and ambulation following stroke. *Clin Orthop* 1984;182:165–171.
18. Pinzur MS, Graham G, Osterman H. Psychological testing in amputation rehabilitation. *Clin Orthop* 1988;229:236–240.
19. Pinzur MS. Current concepts: amputation surgery in peripheral vascular disease. *Instr Course Lect* 1997;46:501–509.
20. Pinzur MS, Sage R, Schwaegler P. Ray resection in the dysvascular foot. *Clin Orthop* 1984;191:232–234.
21. Pinzur MS, Gold J, Schwartz D, Gross N. Energy demands for walking in dysvascular amputees as related to the level of amputation. *Orthopaedics* 1992;15:1033–1037.
22. Pinzur MS, Wolf B, Havey RM. Walking pattern of midfoot and ankle disarticulation amputees. *Foot Ankle Int* 1997;18:635–638.
23. Smith DG, Sangeorzan BJ, Hansen ST, Burgess EM. Achilles tendon tenodesis to prevent heel pad migration in the Syme's amputation. *Foot Ankle* 1994;15:14–17.

27 Rehabilitation of the Amputee with Diabetes

E.R.E. Van Ross and T. Carlsson

INTRODUCTION

In previous editions of this book, this chapter was entitled 'Rehabilitation After Amputation'. However, the authors recognise this title to be misleading. The term 'diabetic foot' implies a chronic impairment with irreversible pathology. The preceding chapters written by physicians, podiatrist, nurses and surgeons really do come within the definition of 'rehabilitation'. Amputation is but an episode within a diabetes management process that began many years previously. Also, amputee rehabilitation begins prior to amputation and not, as is traditionally viewed, after the completion of surgical limb ablation. Rehabilitation is the process of obtaining optimal function despite residual disability.[1] Physical, sensory and mental capacities are restored or developed in people with disabling conditions, and so rehabilitation may be viewed as an enabling process.

Comprehensive rehabilitation should address all of the following issues[2]:

- the damaged system or part (the amputation stump);
- other body systems (cardiovascular, respiratory system, also the contralateral limb);
- psychological attitudes;
- immediate factors affecting the material environment, e.g. clothes, prosthesis, etc.;
- the near environment, e.g. housing, stairs;
- distant environment, e.g. access to shops, social outlets, etc.;
- social support networks.

Much too often, we hear patients say 'I wish they had done the amputation earlier'. This simple admission by the patient should provoke all professionals to review their clinical practice and decision making. When it is advised, amputation should be a positive treatment offered at the appropriate time. This is by no means an argument for increased or hasty amputation surgery but rather a statement that treatment is directed towards the interests of the patient,

The Foot in Diabetes, 4th Edition. Editors Andrew J.M. Boulton, Peter R. Cavanagh and Gerry Rayman.
© 2006 John Wiley & Sons, Ltd.

rather than the foot lesion alone. Extended attempts to save the foot, whether successful or not, may be at the expense of general deconditioning, joint contractures, loss of motivation and severely reduced mobility. Clinical decision making is enhanced by excellent communication and even crossover between the team caring for the foot lesion and the amputee rehabilitation team. Professionals should provide complete information to patients, allowing them to face potentially unpalatable situations with calmness and dignity, knowing they have made the best decision for themselves.

THE AMPUTEE POPULATION

About 1 in 15 foot ulcers result in amputation.[3] It is estimated that only 50% of all people undergoing lower extremity amputation are referred to the amputee rehabilitation team for fitting of a prosthesis or appliance. Those not referred to the amputee rehabilitation team either have a 'minor' amputation of a toe, or part of a toe, and continue to be managed by the foot team, or are considered to be so severely impaired that they would not benefit from rehabilitation.

Patients referred to the amputee rehabilitation team have usually undergone a 'major' amputation at the transmetatarsal level or at a more proximal site. Figures for the United Kingdom show a 35% increase in new dysvascular amputees referred to artificial limb centres over the last 8 years[4] with the majority of amputations performed at the transtibial or the transfemoral level.

Surgical teams are aware that the more distal the amputation the better the outcome for the amputee. Some recent studies indicate that an increasing percentage of partial foot amputations are now being performed.[5]

APPROACHING AMPUTATION

Rehabilitation must be perceived as a continuum, with a seamless transition from the team providing foot care to the amputee rehabilitation team. The multidisciplinary amputee rehabilitation team is now accepted as the best working model for the delivery of care.[6] At the centre of the team is the patient, his/her carers and family. The other members of the team include a rehabilitation physician, prosthetist, nurse, physiotherapist and occupational therapist, clinical psychologist/counsellor and, importantly, a podiatrist who links in with the foot care team. This close-knit team must have access to clinicians from other disciplines in the medical and surgical specialities besides primary care, community rehabilitation, vocational rehabilitation, benefits agencies, etc.

The Pre-amputation Phase

The pre-amputation phase begins as soon as amputation is contemplated. It includes a full medical, psychological, environmental and social evaluation of the patients and their home circumstances. Time must be spent to explain the reasons for amputation together with the potential advantages and disadvantages and the likely functional outcome. In our practice, whenever possible, the patient is invited to the artificial limb centre to meet the rehabilitation team, see the range of available prosthetic hardware and get a clear idea of the planned rehabilitation process. Counselling the patient and the family and introducing them to an amputee who has already been through the experience can be an invaluable preparation.

The psychologist should assess the person's own psychological perceptions of his/her medical condition and personal health beliefs. The assessment can highlight the patient's hopes, motivation and dissatisfaction and indeed direct extra attention to vulnerable personalities requiring additional support in the post-surgical phase.

The key to pre-amputation planning is to choose the correct level of amputation to be performed at the most propitious time, on a well-informed patient.

The Surgical Phase

The aim of amputation surgery is to produce a residual limb (stump) that is functional and will control a prosthesis. Amputation surgery is a positive treatment and should not be viewed by surgeons as a failure of surgical practice, to be performed as the unsterile last case on the operating list by the most junior surgeon. Surgeons should be proficient with modern techniques and knowledgeable of available prosthetic hardware.

GENERAL PRINCIPLES APPLICABLE TO AMPUTATION SURGERY

Skin

The scar should be healed and not adherent to underlying bone. Scar placement is almost immaterial – modern socket materials can cope with fragile scars in any position. Full-thickness and partial-thickness skin grafts should be used only when absolutely essential and not located over bony prominences. Skin flaps must be sutured at the correct tension if they are to remain healthy and pressure tolerant. Skin clips used for closure inhibit early mobilisation on a pre-prosthetic device. Instead, nylon sutures supplemented with adhesive skin strips work well.

Muscle

Muscle flaps should be stabilised by reattachment to bone (myodesis) or attached to their opposing muscle (agonist to antagonist myoplasty). Bulky myocutaneous flaps are undesirable, and the more vulnerable ischaemic muscle should be excised.

Nerves

Neuroma formation is inevitable after amputation. Large and obvious nerves should be placed under gentle traction and cleanly divided in order to allow the ends to retract into underlying muscle. Coagulation, diathermy and cold blocks of nerves are not routinely used.

Blood Vessels

It is a fallacy to believe that the absence of bleeding is an indication for higher level of amputation.[7] Wound healing is more subtle and depends on the microcirculation. Arteries should be suture ligated separately and away from veins in order to avoid fistula formation.

Bones

Preparation of the bone end is of the greatest importance. The bone must be cut to the correct length and the distal edges bevelled and then smoothed, in order to avoid prominent sharp bony edges under the skin.

Dressings

A wool bandage followed by a crepe over bandage is the commonest method of dressing following surgery and, in general, these dressings work well. For the below-knee amputation in particular, stump bandaging is generally unsatisfactory and there is often evidence of iatrogenic oedema caused through the bandage acting as a tourniquet. A removable rigid plaster of Paris cast dressing[8] is advocated for control of oedema and protection of the wound or, if impractical, a commercial stump shrinker is used.

Post-surgical Care

The immediate post-surgical management following amputation is the responsibility of the anaesthetist and the surgical team. Routine care involves correcting metabolic and electrolyte imbalances. Most patients will have stump pain and phantom sensation and/or phantom pain.[9] In the immediate aftermath of surgery, opiates are usually essential. Following recovery of full consciousness, it is important to monitor the patient's response to surgery. High levels of phantom pain are an indication to start on anti-epileptic-type medication such as gabapentin, pregablin, carbamazepine, etc. This should be supplemented by simple analgesics. Recalcitrant pain is treated by stage 2 analgesics such as tramadol. Additionally, amitriptyline may be added at night to provide sedation and pain relief, but doses used may not be sufficient to act as an antidepressant. (Textbooks on pain relief should be consulted for further details.)

As soon as the patient's general health and cognition have stabilised, the physiotherapist should begin a programme of joint mobilisation in order to prevent contractures, maintain fitness and reduce stump oedema. Patients should be instructed on stump elevation and avoidance of injury. During the time of surgery, the remaining foot is often neglected. Attention must be paid to caring for the foot and avoiding heel ulcers.

When medically stable, the patient should be transferred to a rehabilitation ward, where the ethos should be to promote function and independence. The ward should run at a slower pace, with greater access to clinical psychologists and therapists. Medical staff have a responsibility to ensure that the patient is haematologically and biochemically stable. Anaemia should be corrected and diabetes well controlled. Appropriate analgesia should be instituted and can often be given on an 'as-needed' basis. It is unnecessary for the patient to have unreasonable levels of pain; yet at the same time, they should not be over-sedated and, thus, unable to work with the therapist.

Care of the amputation stump wound should be supervised by specialist nurses. Appropriate dressings should be used. For the transtibial (below-knee) amputee, a rigid plaster of Paris cast is advocated. If this is not feasible, an 'off-the-shelf' stump shrinker should be used. The pneumatic post-amputation mobility aid (PPAM aid)[10] may be used from day 7 to mobilise the transtibial and transfemoral amputee. The device is easily applied and gets the patient standing upright and weight bearing. If used appropriately, it helps stump shrinkage, reduces pain, initiates aerobic exercise and gives an immense morale boost to the patient through the sheer joy of standing and walking.

About 40% of amputation stumps[11] do not heal by primary intention. Some of these heal by secondary intention often after a prolonged period of time. In our practice, patients with unhealed stumps are dressed using the hospital dressing protocol and then mobilised on the PPAM aid. Stump shrinkage and exercise are most beneficial for healing. Stump shrinkage reduces oedema thereby reducing wound tension. Reduction in oedema immediately increases the measured tissue partial pressure of oxygen $(TcpO_2)$.[12] In addition, exercise improves peripheral circulation, which boosts the $TcpO_2$. Infected stumps require debridement, drainage and sometimes antibiotics. Occasionally surgical debridement under anaesthetic is required. Hasty conversion to a higher level of amputation should be avoided, particularly if it results in the loss of the knee joint.

PSYCHOLOGICAL ASSESSMENT

Ablating a limb produces an obvious and visible defect which is often painful and distressing. There is a high incidence of anxiety and depression following amputation, particularly in younger patients who may have lost their limbs through an element of neglect. The Hospital Anxiety and Depression Scale[13] and Beck Inventory[14] are standardised scales that are easily administered.

Various psychological treatments are available. Cognitive behavioural therapy helps patients to realise that feelings interact with thoughts, fears and behaviour and that all of these are under their own control. Antidepressant medication may be used to supplement this therapy. The psychologist should observe the relationship between the amputee and the rehabilitation ward staff. Over-protective ward staff can create a state of helplessness and dependency. The clinical psychologist should work with the staff to encourage the patient to gain as much functional independence as is safely possible. The locus of control[15] measures the patients' views of their own sense of control of their environment. Amputees generally have an external locus of control soon after surgery and feel they are unable to make progress, unless help is provided. They accept that their future is controlled by other staff, social services, etc. On the other hand, patients with an internal locus of control have a firm belief that the outcome of their rehabilitation depends on their motivation and actions. They take charge of their future and work with the team in planning their discharge. A good rehabilitation team will foster an internal locus of control among its patients.

Some patients are unrealistic in their abilities, their achievements and the outcome following amputation. This group may display mild dementia, or memory impairment, as assessed by the Mini Mental Score[16] and they may require counselling and guidance. (Care should be taken if the patient is on opiates, or other drugs likely to impair cognition.) The rehabilitation team must work with the patients and their family and carers.

The role of family and carers is important in the outcome (generally single people do less well than those with a family). A sudden change in the person's function following amputation may compel his/her partner to change from being a friend or sexual partner into adopting the role of nurse. This role change can cause the partner to react with denial, anxiety, disgust, guilt and depression, and to become obsessed with a need for information and a desire to protect the patient. Psychologist should be aware of this change and work with the team to provide appropriate support, counselling and information. Sexual dysfunction is unfortunately a common consequence of diabetes. The burden of amputation causes additional psychological difficulties and physical problems. If requested, referral should be made to a specialist sexual dysfunction team.

The occupational therapist should begin very early the process of teaching the patient to become independent in activities of daily living: sitting balance to allow hand function, independent transfers, dressing, washing, toileting, etc. The therapist should also be involved in choosing an appropriate wheelchair and cushion. Amputees have formed support groups (Limbless Association in the United Kingdom, Amputee Coalition in the United States) that play an invaluable role in providing 'buddy schemes', information, support and visiting services, besides collecting money for ongoing research and welfare.

LEVELS OF AMPUTATION

This chapter allows only a brief description of management for different levels of amputation. See also the discussion of amputation in Chapter 26.

Toes

It is traditional that 'minor amputations' are not often referred to the 'amputee rehabilitation centre'. Excision of a toe, part of a toe or a ray of the foot alters the biomechanics to a limited extent. The patient, however, is still burdened by having a neuropathic foot that requires continued vigilance, podiatry and orthotics. Orthotics should be limited to pressure-relief insoles and surgical shoes and should not attempt to provide material that fills in the space left by the missing digit. This can expose a foot with neuropathy to the risk of developing pressure ulcers over the neighbouring toes.

Transmetatarsal Amputations

Excision of all the toes is usually performed through the necks of the metatarsals. The surgeon should endeavour to provide a long full-thickness plantar flap with the suture line placed anteriorly and not adherent to the bone. Foot amputations through the tarsometatarsal joint (Lisfranc amputation) or the more proximal amputations through the talo-navicular joint (Chopart amputation) require more care. The dorsiflexors should be reattached in order to avoid development of an equinus contracture.

Partial foot amputations are appropriate for the less active patient where the expectation is of limited mobility over flat terrain. These amputations are generally associated with lower mortality, but with a higher chance of non-healing. About 40% of these procedures eventually require more proximal surgery.[11] The main functional consequence of partial foot amputation is the shortening of the toe lever. This results in some loss of postural stability as well as loss of the terminal stance support during gait. This is observed as increased postural sway, shortening of the stride and loss of forward propelling power.

A prosthetic replacement is not always necessary. Depending on the functional length that has been lost and the anticipated level of activity, it may be addressed by provision of a combination of shoe filler orthosis and footwear. The orthosis protects and supports the foot remnant. The footwear, designed to minimise stress on vulnerable skin, has a rigid sole to compensate for the loss of toe lever and a rocker base to allow rollover at the metatarsal joints.

Alternatively, partial foot prostheses can be used, especially when higher levels of mobility are predicted. Biomechanically, a full-length toe lever is restored. This is connected to the anterior aspect of the leg, which counteracts the force generated by the toe lever during gait. A higher anterior support will reduce the direct pressures and shear forces generated over the amputation site hence reducing the stress on the skin. There is no need to enclose the posterior aspect of the leg, as this serves no mechanical purpose (Figure 27.1).

Syme's Amputation/Ankle Amputation

Syme's amputation is classically performed just proximal to the ankle joint, using the strong heel pad to cover the distal end of the tibia. The advantage is a very strong end-bearing stump, where the person may even take a few steps without the aid of a prosthesis (such as for walking from bed to the toilet at night). The major disadvantage is the poor cosmesis caused through the bulbous distal end of the stump. The Wagner modification[17] where the malleoli are excised has improved the appearance.

An ankle amputation generally creates a good strong lever below the knee that can be utilised to power prosthetic ambulation. The limb segment shortening caused by an ankle amputation is often less than 50 mm, which restricts the prosthetic hardware that can be used. Consequently, only a small selection of commercially available prosthetic foot components can be fitted into the available space below the stump. The circumference at the level of the malleoli is typically greater than the lower third of the shin. Not only does this make it impossible to match the contralateral ankle dimensions for cosmetic purposes, but any prosthetic socket must allow this large distal circumference to enter through a narrower section of the socket. This can be achieved in different ways. An 'access trap' (a removable section of the socket that is repositioned once the residual limb is *in situ*) can be used (Figure 27.2). Alternatively, an open cross section can be used where the posterior aspect is left open, since it serves no mechanical purpose. The socket above the level of the malleoli effectively consists of an anterior support ending slightly below the patella. This support resists the floor reaction force during terminal stance, hence providing forward propulsion. Other variations exist and the choice of socket is dictated by individual factors.

Transtibial (Below-Knee) Amputation

This is an important amputation where the knee joint is preserved. The ideal stump length should be approximately 15 cm as measured from the medial tibial plateau to the end of the tibia. Even very short stumps, barely 7 cm long, can be fitted with a prosthesis and produce a result functionally superior to the transfemoral (above-knee) amputation. The advantages of preserving the knee joint are

1. lower energy requirement for walking;

2. a vastly improved gait, particularly when walking outdoors over rough terrain;

3. ease of donning and doffing the prosthesis;

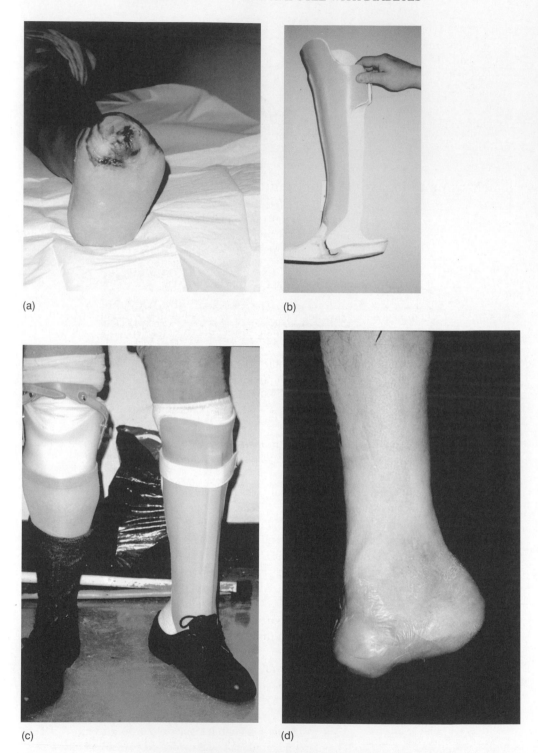

(a)   (b)

(c)   (d)

Figure 27.1   A 54-year-old man with diabetes, who is a blind double amputee: (a) transmetatarsal ulcer; (b) partial foot appliance with anterior extension; (c) in use; (d) after 6 weeks

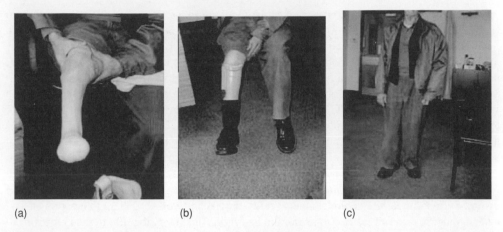

(a)   (b)   (c)

Figure 27.2   Syme's amputation: (a) well-healed stump with tough end-bearing heel pad; (b) a plunge fit socket is applied by the patient, despite cheiroarthropathy of hands; (c) functions as a community ambulator

4. lighter weight;

5. improved functional ability and lower dependency;

6. shorter rehabilitation period;

7. cheaper prosthesis as compared to the above-knee prosthesis.

Modern transtibial prostheses are built from modular components. There is a multitude of components available along with numerous socket concepts that can be applied to this common level of amputation. Choices are based on the individual user's presentation. Specific to the diabetic person is that sensation as well as healing capacity may be impaired in the residual limb. Neuropathy in the contralateral leg may reduce proprioception, affecting balance and increasing risk. Hand function and vision may be impaired.

These factors need to be considered when determining the prosthetic specification. Good suspension is important in order to maximise proprioception and minimise ground impact on the residual limb during ambulation. The suspension is a function of the interface (socket design) that connects the prosthesis to the residual limb. Materials such as silicones and polyurethanes that combine good suspension and pressure-distributing properties are used in either prefabricated or bespoke interface stump sleeves. A lightweight modular system (Figure 27.3) and a reasonably responsive composite foot help to minimise the energy loss associated with prosthetic use.

Knee Disarticulation (Through-Knee) Amputation

This is considered to be an atraumatic surgical procedure that involves no disturbance to the bone. It is especially indicated when the patient's general condition is poor and a decision has been made that the patient will not (for other medical reasons) be a suitable candidate for mobilisation with a prosthesis. Functioning hamstrings allow controlled hip extension, thereby

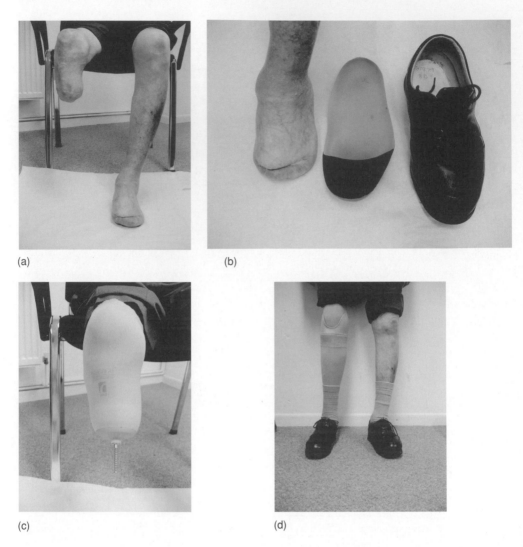

Figure 27.3 (a,b) A 79-year-old man with type 2 diabetes; (c) fitted with appropriate appliances; (d) functions as community ambulator

improving sitting balance, as compared to the transfemoral amputation. Knee disarticulation produces a very strong, functional level of amputation because of the long skeletal lever and the natural ability of the femoral condyles to carry weight. Nevertheless, it is not very commonly done, perhaps due to the restricted prosthetic solutions, which makes it cosmetically and biomechanically mismatched when compared to the contralateral knee.

As in the case of ankle amputation, the shape of the residuum may be bulbous distally due to the presence of the femoral condyles. When designing the prosthetic socket, access traps and differential liners allow a wider circumference to enter through a narrower section of the socket. Differential liners are flexible inner sockets, which have been built up on the outside of the narrower sections to form an almost uniform external circumference, enough to allow the bulbous portion of the residuum to pass through the narrower section during donning. Consequently, the rigid outer socket with marginal undercut will help to maintain good suspension of the prosthesis.

As the femur retains its full length, the prosthetic knee joint will inevitably be placed below the level of the anatomical knee joint of the contralateral side. This causes a thigh segment length discrepancy that is particularly noticeable whilst sitting. The effect can be minimised by the use of polycentric knee joints. These knee joints have a complex centre of rotation, typically involving four axes. As a result, they protrude less than single axis knees when flexed, making the prosthesis cosmetically more acceptable. The restricted space for knee components also limits the functionality of the knee. The choice of foot component is dependent on the type of knee in use.

Transfemoral (Above-Knee) Amputation

Transfemoral amputations should only rarely be performed on people with diabetes. At surgery, about 12–15 cm of distal femur should be removed and the thigh muscles should be reattached to the femoral end in order to avoid muscle retraction. Secure attachment of the hip adductors as advocated by Gotschalk[18] allows better control of the stump within the prosthetic socket.

When amputation takes place at this level because of diabetes, the patient's general health is likely to be poor and the functional deficit is likely to be considerable. The loss of the knee joint and shortening of the femur limits propulsive power and control of the prosthesis. The increase in energy expenditure when walking is significant. Consequently, the weight of the prosthesis needs to be kept to a minimum.

Critical for safe ambulation is the user's ability to control the prosthetic knee joint. Many different knees are available, featuring varying degrees of functionality and safety. In general terms, increased functionality results in increased weight of the component. In practice, this often restricts the choice of knee joints for diabetic patients. For the lowest functional levels, a locked knee joint can be used to achieve safe low-level ambulation with a stiff knee. The knee is manually unlocked when the user wants to sit down and locks automatically when the knee is fully extended for standing. The prosthetic foot choice is dependent on the type of knee in use. Such components are light and safe but result in an uncosmetic, asymmetric, high-energy gait. For the more able person, sophisticated hydraulic and microprocessor swing/stance control are available.

Suspension is important as it contributes to the control of the prosthesis. The stump is often cylindrical in cross section. Therefore, rotational stability of the prosthesis may be difficult to achieve and there will occasionally be a requirement to add auxiliary suspension such as a belt around the waist.

Second Limb (Bilateral Amputations)

For people with diabetes, there is a significant chance of loosing the second limb. Before undertaking surgery, it is important to assess the patient's medical condition. Should there be a good chance of walking and prosthetic rehabilitation is to be considered, only the most distal amputation possible should be performed. On the other hand, if the person is too ill and unlikely to walk, the amputation should be designed to allow good sitting balance and ease of transfers.

PROBLEMS PARTICULAR TO THE PERSON WITH DIABETES

Fluctuating stump volume is associated with the occurrence of cardiac failure and nephropathy. This makes fitting an accurate prosthetic socket extremely difficult. Such patients require regular prosthetic adjustment and review. Using two or more stump socks when measuring for the prosthetic socket allows flexibility in coping with the fluctuating stump volume. Impaired vision makes accurate donning and doffing of the prosthesis extremely difficult. Walking, particularly over uneven surfaces, can be hazardous. Many of these patients restrict walking to indoors, or when outdoors link arms with a companion. Peripheral neuropathy is generally associated with poor balance,[19] and increases the risk of falling.

Cheiroarthropathy (limited joint mobility) and muscle wasting are common in people with diabetes. When determining the prosthetic specification, consideration needs to be given to any loss of hand function and/or vision impairment, as the complexity of the donning and doffing process can vary. If at all possible, the goal should be for an individual to be able to don and doff the prosthesis independently.

CONCLUDING REMARKS

Diabetes is a medical condition that affects multiple systems. Limb amputation is only one part of the picture. Simply replacing the lost limb with a prosthesis will produce an unsatisfactory result. The coordinated efforts of a multidisciplinary team are crucial in providing physical, psychological, social and environmental support. The rehabilitation team has an extended duty to help the amputees in their return to society. Lord Holderness, politician, soldier, campaigner for the disabled and double above-knee amputee, summed it up when he said, 'Rehabilitation converts a patient back into a person'.

REFERENCES

1. DeLisa JA. *Rehabilitation Medicine: Principles and Practice*. 2nd edn. Philadelphia: JB Lippincott; 1993.
2. British Geriatric Society. *Rehabilitation of Older People*. BGS Compendium document (revised), 2004.
3. Defronzo RA, Ferrannini E, Keen H, Zimmet P, eds. *International Textbook of Diabetes*. 3rd edn. Wiley; 2004:Chap 73.
4. *The Amputee Statistical Database for the United Kingdom 2003/2004*. Gyle Square, Edinburgh: ISD Publications; 2005.
5. Dupre JC, Dechamps E, Pillu M, Despyroux L. The fitting of amputated and non-amputated diabetic feet: a French experience at the Villiers–Saint–Denis Hospital. *J Am Podiatry Med Assoc* 2003;93:221–228.
6. Ham R, Regan JM, Roberts VC. Evaluation of introducing the team approach to the care of the amputee: the Dulwich Study. *Prosthet Orthot Int* 1987;11:25–30.
7. Kendrick RR. Below knee amputation in arteriosclerotic gangrene. *Br J Surg* 1956;44:13–17.
8. Wu Y. Post operative and pre-prosthetic management of lower extremity amputations. *Capabilities* 1996;5:2.
9. Sherman RA, Arena JG. Phantom limb pain mechanisms. Incidence and treatment. *Clin Rev Phys Rehabil Med* 1992;4:1–26.

10. Redhead RG. The early mobilisation of lower limb amputees using a pneumatic walking aid. *Prosthet Orthot Int* 1983;7:88–90.
11. Dillingham TR, Liliana M, Pezzin E, Shore AD. Reamputation, mortality and health care costs among persons with dysvascular lower limb amputations. *Arch Phys Med Rehabil* Mar 2005;86:480–486.
12. Kolari PJ, Pekanmaki K, Pohjola RT. Transcutaneous oxygen tension in patients with post thrombotic leg ulcers: treatment with intermittent pneumatic compression. *Cardiovasc Res* Feb 1988;22:138–141.
13. Zigmond AS, Snaith RP. The Hospital Anxiety and Depression Scale. *Acta Psychiatr Scand* 1983;67:361–370.
14. Beck AT, Ward C, Mendelson M, Mendelson M, Mock J, Erbaugh J. An inventory for measuring depression. *Arch Gen Psychiatry* 1961;4:561–571.
15. Partridge L, Johnson M. Perceived control of recovery from physical disability: measurement and prediction. *Br J Clin Psychol* 1989;28:53–60.
16. Hodkinson HM. Evaluation of a mental test score for assessment of mental impairment in the elderly. *Age Ageing* 1972;1:233–238.
17. Wagner FW. Amputation of the foot and ankle: current status. *Clin Orthop* 1977;122:62–69.
18. Gotschalk FA, Jaegers HJ. Transfemoral amputation. In: Murdoch G, Bennett-Wilson A, eds. *Amputation: Surgical Practice and Patient Management.* Butterworth-Heinemann; 1996.
19. Richardson JK, Ashton-Miller JA, Lee SG, Jacobs K. Moderate peripheral neuropathy impairs weight transfer and unipedal balance in the elderly. *Arch Phys Med Rehabil* Nov 1996;77:1152–1156.

28 Footwear for People with Diabetes

Peter R. Cavanagh and Jan S. Ulbrecht

INTRODUCTION

One afternoon, almost 20 years ago, during a visit to our laboratory, the late Dr Paul Brand – who was still engaged in an active clinical practice of hand and foot surgery – was musing about his potential activities after retirement. Only partly in jest, he declared that he thought he might become a shoemaker, because he had the impression that more diabetic patients had congratulated him on the shoes he had prescribed for them than on the foot surgery he had performed.

Dr Brand actually 'retired' to an active lecture schedule, but the anecdote reflects the importance that this eminent scholar and teacher of neuropathic foot pathology placed on therapeutic footwear. Despite his own pioneering experimental work more than 40 years ago,[1,2] the state of the art in footwear prescription for patients with diabetes is still rudimentary. Studies have shown that different practitioners faced with the same patient devise very different solutions, which can differ greatly in their efficacy.[3] (Some of the prescribed interventions even increased pressure at a region of interest, something that would certainly be categorised as a negative outcome.) The authors of the above study have urged the development of 'unambiguous guidelines that enable improved education and consequently less variation between therapists'.[3]

Unfortunately, such guidelines have been slow to emerge from the research laboratories. As we shall discuss, there have been important technical developments – notably, good in-shoe pressure measurement techniques and computer-aided design–computer-aided manufacture (CAD-CAM) systems to make insoles. Scientists have embraced these tools to show that technology can produce improved products or at least evaluate the effectiveness of footwear prescriptions. However, these tools have been slow to flow to the practitioner. Trends in footwear prescription have also been influenced by cost constraints – such as those in the United Kingdom that require at least 75% of items dispensed to be 'off-the-shelf', or the Medicare guidelines in the United States that reimburse for one pair of custom-made shoes plus two pairs of insoles (or one pair of extra-depth shoes and three pairs of insoles) per calendar year to qualified patients.

In this chapter, we shall examine the evidence that guides the prescription of therapeutic footwear, discuss the mechanisms whereby therapeutic footwear is believed to exert its effect and make recommendations for best practice in the absence of clear, evidence-based guidelines. The physician seeing a patient for diabetes-related medical issues should understand which

The Foot in Diabetes, 4th Edition. Editors Andrew J.M. Boulton, Peter R. Cavanagh and Gerry Rayman.
© 2006 John Wiley & Sons, Ltd.

patients will need footwear, what can safely be dispensed to a given patient and what conditions require a referral to a local provider of therapeutic footwear.

WHAT DOES THE LITERATURE SAY?

Three subsets of the literature are relevant to therapeutic footwear for people with diabetes: retrospective studies, in which the role of footwear in injury is inferred from charts or self-report; clinical trials and controlled studies, in which patients have been prescribed footwear, and the outcomes, usually ulcer prevention, have been examined; and biomechanical studies, in which different interventions have been tried, and some component of the foot–shoe interface has been measured. All of these approaches are potentially instructive, and all have shed some light on the role of therapeutic footwear in people with diabetes.

Retrospective Studies

Footwear is widely believed to cause many foot injuries, ulcers and even amputations in persons with diabetes. Various authors have retrospectively identified 'narrow shoes',[4] 'pressure from footwear',[5] 'inadequate footwear',[6] 'trauma from footwear'[7] and footwear in general[8] as being responsible for between 21 and 89% of ulcers. The 'pivotal event' in a series of 80 consecutive patients with amputations was reported to be 'shoe related' in 42% of cases.[9] To prevent injury from simple mis-sizing, it is essential for diabetic patients that shoe length and width be carefully determined by measurement, since a neuropathic patient will not be able to give adequate feedback regarding shoe fit. One study showed that in 66% of cases, the foot width of neuropathic patients was much broader than that of conventional shoes.[10] This suggests that shoes with additional width and/or depth should often be prescribed.

Clinical Trials and Controlled Studies

Very few randomised controlled studies have tested the effectiveness of therapeutic footwear in preventing foot ulceration or re-ulceration.[11,12] One study, which showed no effect in a large number of patients,[13] was probably influenced by study design issues, including the fact that a break in the skin that lasted less than 30 days was not defined as an ulcer.[14] Those studies that have shown a benefit to wearing prescription footwear are generally smaller and less well controlled. Three studies in which a control group of patients used their own footwear after healing an ulcer have shown, not surprisingly, that a therapeutic intervention reduces the risk of re-ulceration.[15–17] The reductions observed were substantial (28% vs 50% at 12 months,[16] 15% vs 60% at 12 months,[15] and 4% vs 33% at 9 months[17] for therapeutic vs own shoes, respectively). A significant problem in designing a study of therapeutic shoes is determining, preferably *a priori*, whether or not the footwear prescription used is effective for every patient in the trial – that is, does it reduce plantar pressure at the regions of interest (see below). The doctor who recommends prescription footwear also faces this problem, as will be discussed further below.

Biomechanical Studies

Studies in this category do not use a clinical outcome to judge the effectiveness of shoes. Most frequently, they use the measurement of pressure exerted between the bottom surface of the

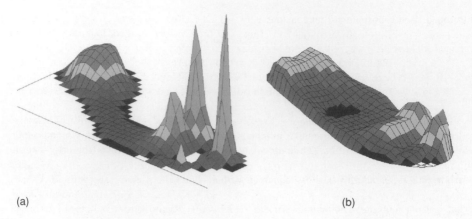

(a)   (b)

Figure 28.1 Peak plantar pressure during walking, measured in the same subject, (a) under the foot during barefoot walking and (b) inside a shoe which provides pressure relief at areas of elevated pressure under the metatarsal heads and hallux. Both data sets are to approximately the same scale. Peak pressure in barefoot walking > 1 MPa

foot as it meets the insole of the shoe (plantar pressure) usually during walking, as shown in Figure 28.1.[18] Early studies were done with individual pressure sensors,[2] but these tended to cause a concentration of pressure at the site being measured. Today, there are a variety of products that comprise a matrix of flat sensors embedded in a thin insole, and the patient walks for 20–30 steps while data are captured on a computer. It is also now possible to monitor for longer periods of up to 8 h. Although the results from sensors made by different manufacturers are not comparable (because of different surface areas and other issues), comparative studies are possible with a given insole: e.g., is shoe condition A better than shoe condition B? Using this methodology, strategies for the reduction of plantar pressure have been tested. It can reasonably be assumed that if plantar pressure at a site of importance (such as a prominent metatarsal head (MTH)) is reduced in a given condition, and the prescription shoe is worn consistently by the patient (see below), then the clinical outcome may be improved.

A variety of interventions, including custom insoles,[19] metatarsal pads,[20,21] metatarsal bars[22] and rigid or semi-rigid shoes[23] (see below), have been studied.[24] The results have led to insight into the placement and design of the various interventions. Making the sole of the shoe rigid and contoured (rather like a Dutch clog, see below), together with the provision of an appropriate insole, has been shown to be the most successful intervention, reducing plantar pressures by up to 50%.[23,25]

HOW DOES THERAPEUTIC FOOTWEAR WORK?

The designer of therapeutic footwear attempts to do a number of things, depending on the needs of the diabetic patient. Some of the most frequently used strategies are (1) providing room to accommodate deformity (most often prominent dorsal surfaces of toes and medial and lateral prominences); (2) providing adequate depth to allow thick insoles, thick socks and special features of the insoles – such as metatarsal pad and bars and arch supports – without putting pressure on the dorsum of the foot; (3) reducing load at critical areas of focal pressure, such as MTHs, the tips of clawed toes or midfoot prominences secondary to Charcot fractures;

(4) transferring load from regions thought to be at risk, to regions – such as the mid-metatarsal shaft area or the arch – that are able to accommodate more load; and (5) changing the patient's gait and the motion of the foot during walking by making the shoe rigid. All of the above changes must be accomplished in a way that does not compromise the stability of the patient during gait and, most importantly, in a manner that is acceptable to the patient from an aesthetic standpoint (see below for a discussion on patient compliance). Comfort, usually a dominant factor in everyday footwear, can often not be perceived by the neuropathic patient.

The terms 'insole' and 'orthosis' are often used interchangeably, although an orthosis usually implies that some custom attempt to alter the load distribution has been implemented. As we have discussed elsewhere,[26] insoles for patients with loss of sensation should usually be 'accommodative' rather than 'corrective'. The 'functional orthotics' that are often used to correct foot alignment – in sports medicine, for example – are typically not appropriate for neuropathic patients, because they tend to increase loading in order to change foot function.

Cushioning

'Cushioning' is a rather vague term that has both static and dynamic connotations.[18] The most useful visualisation of cushioning in footwear is to contrast the interface conditions of the foot of a patient standing on a rigid flat surface with those of the same patient standing on a soft foam mat. The foam mat 'cushions' the foot by providing a surface that accommodates to the contours of the bony prominences, applying load to surfaces that were not previously loaded. The 'stock' insoles delivered with most therapeutic shoes are meant only as fillers and usually need to be replaced before footwear is provided to the patient. Significant cushioning can be derived from flat insoles, often up to 10 mm (3/8 in.) thick, if there is room in the shoe. A completely custom-moulded insole is the extreme of this approach to reduction in plantar pressure. Such an insole is typically made based on an impression of the foot (either a plaster cast, a foam box or, more recently, a digital scan; see below). Although a custom-moulded insole can be effective in reducing pressure, it will usually require some of the load-relief and load-redistribution functions described below to achieve optimal efficacy.

It is easy to underestimate the pressure that can exist underneath the foot during walking, as well as the consequent compression of soft insole materials that essentially 'bottom-out' such that they no longer offer significant cushioning. This implies that both thickness and stiffness are important in insoles designed to provide cushioning. If the insole can be significantly compressed (by more than 50%) by pinching it between the thumb and finger, then it is probably too soft for effective cushioning of the foot. Insoles also lose the ability to provide cushioning with repeated use.[27,28] The practitioner should examine insoles at every visit to see if replacement is required. Telltale deep impressions under bony prominences where the material may be extremely thin are signs that the insole should be replaced. Dispensing several pairs of insoles with a pair of new shoes is recommended if it is economically feasible.

Load Relief

An alternative strategy to address high pressure at bony prominences is to provide load relief. Load reduction has traditionally been accomplished by using metatarsal pads and bars (Figure 28.2), which are intended to elevate one or more MTHs. Such pads have an asymmetrical

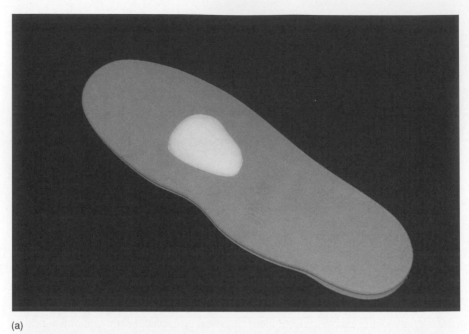

(a)

(b)

Figure 28.2   Interventions to relieve high pressures under metatarsal heads by transferring load to other regions. (a) Metatarsal pad; (b) customised metatarsal bar; (c) schematic diagram of rigid rocker shoe with a plug under a metatarsal head region and metatarsal pad.

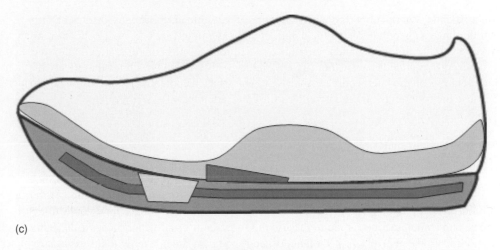

(c)

Figure 28.2 (*Continued*)

section in the sagittal plane and the exact location of the apex in relation to the MTH is critical to their effectiveness. Studies have shown, for example, that a 5-mm difference in positioning can markedly affect the load relief provided[20] and that one standard position is not best for all feet. Some placements have been shown to result in minimal reduction in pressure[29] or even to increase in pressure at the target site.[30] This variation in response makes effective prescription difficult, especially since determining the exact location of the plantar prominence on an insole can be problematic. In general, the closer the apex is placed to the MTH, without being underneath it, the more effective it is likely to be. Pads are available in different heights (typically between 1/4 and 3/8 in. (6 and 10 mm)), and the higher the pad that can be accommodated in a given shoe, the better. They usually have an adhesive to allow attachment atop an existing insole.

Load relief can also be achieved at a plantar prominence by altering the material properties or configuration of the insole directly under the prominence. Historically, some concern has been expressed regarding annular pads that remove pressure on one area and redistribute it to the immediate surrounding areas.[31] However, our own experiments have shown that a pad appropriately contoured across all the MTHs with an annular aperture under one MTH can relieve load without causing unacceptable local increases in pressures. Another possibility is to excavate a 'well' in the insole (and sometimes also in the midsole) directly under the prominence. This well is then filled with a soft compressible material that will reduce pressure at the MTH. The edges of the well must be designed such that they do not cause a local increase in pressure, and the best way to do this is to extend and taper the posterior border.[32] It is also important not to fill the well with incompressible material (such as silicone) because this may result in an increase in plantar pressure.

Load Redistribution

This strategy involves changing the interface between the foot and the shoe so that load is transferred away from areas at risk for ulceration or tissue damage. The medial longitudinal arch of the foot is the preferred region to receive transferred load because of its broad area;

thus, so-called 'arch supports' or 'scaphoid pads' are a feature of many insoles or orthoses. Studies have shown that raising the height of an insole in the arch area can relieve areas such as the heel, the first MTH and the hallux.[19] The premise of this intervention is that the arch can accept the added load without risk of injury. Little is known about the effects of such interventions on the lateral border of the foot, which has the potential to be additionally loaded because the foot tends to roll outward off the elevated arch.

Rigid Outsoles (Rocker and Roller Shoes)

All of the above interventions are designed to be placed between the foot and the shoe, but important reductions in forefoot pressure can be obtained by making the shoes rigid and contouring the outsole. The patients walk somewhat differently than they would in flexible shoes, and some practice is required to use the shoes comfortably and successfully. This type of modification can be performed on almost any shoe by a shoemaker who inserts a rigid plate (often of carbon fibre) into the midsole. The two basic designs are the 'rocker' – where there is an abrupt transition between front and back of the sole – and the roller – where the transition is made by a smooth curve (Figure 28.2(c)).

Some shoe manufacturers offer 'off-the-shelf' rocker shoes. As discussed above, rigid shoes can be remarkably effective, reducing peak plantar pressure in the forefoot by 20–50%. Studies have shown that their effectiveness depends on specification of appropriate design parameters for rocker height and for position of the rocker axis (and probably the orientation of the axis)[23,25] and that different individuals respond to the same shoe design in different ways. A rule of thumb from these studies is to place the axis of the rocker at approximately 55–60% of shoe length forward from the heel and to give the platform on which the foot rests a minimum amount of toe spring ('turn-up' at toe). Even though such a configuration will not be optimal for all subjects, it will almost certainly result in reduced plantar pressure at the MTHs.

Rigid shoes appear to reduce pressure because they allow the patient to ambulate without extending the toes (at the metatarso-phalangeal joints). This change probably prevents prolonged load bearing on the fragile tissues underlying the MTHs. Patients should be encouraged to walk more slowly and to take shorter strides than normal in rocker shoes, since this will prevent load bearing on the flattened surface of the rocker.

CHOOSING THE APPROPRIATE FOOTWEAR FOR THE PATIENT

In this section we will give guidance to the practitioner who needs to make decisions regarding footwear for patients who may range from those who are recently diagnosed with diabetes and are concerned about their feet to those who have experienced recurrent ulcers in the past and are at high risk for amputation.

Ideally, decisions regarding the complexity (and, therefore, the expense) of footwear that a patient should receive would be based on a detailed biomechanical examination using the tools described above to measure pressure distribution. However, such equipment is still beyond the financial reach of all but a few specialised centres, and footwear prescription decisions must be based on surrogate measures of risk. Two such indicators are the extent of deformity and the presence of callus on the patient's foot; the assumption is that more of either factor will lead to (or reflect) higher pressures and greater risk. Risk of ulcer recurrence is high; thus, patients with prior ulcers are also at higher risk. In addition, it seems to be intuitively obvious that a

Table 28.1 A general guide to footwear prescription based on risk status

Prior plantar ulcer/deformity/callus/ high plantar pressure	Activity		
	Low	Moderate	High
No	Sports shoe with a soft insole	Sports shoe or extra-depth shoe with a thick insole	Sports shoe or extra-depth shoe with a thick insole; consider rocker bottom
Yes/moderate	Sports shoe or extra-depth shoe with a thick insole	Sports shoe or extra-depth shoe with a thick insole, metatarsal pads or bar; consider rocker bottom	Sports shoe or extra-depth shoe with a thick insole, metatarsal pads or bar, rocker bottom; consider custom insole
Yes/severe	Customised upper or custom shoe, thick insole; consider custom insole	Customised upper or custom shoe, thick custom insole with reliefs, rocker bottom	Customised upper or custom shoe, thick custom insole with complex reliefs, rocker bottom

Adapted from Ref. 26.

patient who is habitually more active will require greater protection, although the few studies that are available are equivocal on this issue.[33–35] All of these factors can be put together in the risk matrix shown in Table 28.1, which guides the prescriber towards an appropriate level of footwear intervention.

The Newly Diagnosed Diabetic Patient

Many patients who are newly diagnosed with diabetes will visit a foot specialist for a 'foot check-up' because they know that diabetes carries an increased risk for foot complications. Invariably, these patients will have good pulses, good sensation and no significant foot deformity and will not, therefore, have special requirements in footwear. The provider should take the opportunity to explain why they are not 'at risk' for immediate foot problems and to suggest that they return for an annual examination to reassess their risk. It is not too early for these individuals to begin adopting good footwear habits, and they should be educated at every visit to their physician about the need for shoes that do not apply excessive loads to the foot, on either the dorsal or the plantar surfaces. Patients should shake out their shoes before putting them on, carefully wash and thoroughly dry their feet daily (including the web spaces) and begin to inspect their feet regularly.

The Patient Who Is at Risk for an Ulcer

How to perform a foot examination to help determine the risk for ulceration or other foot injury is described elsewhere in this volume (Chapter 6). The most important sign is loss of protective sensation (LOPS), implying that the patient cannot feel the stimuli that would otherwise be interpreted as leading to foot injury. LOPS alone is sufficient to result in ulceration, e.g. if the patient were to wear shoes that apply pressure along the lateral border of the foot. However, when LOPS is combined with foot deformity, the risk is likely to be even greater. Special prescription footwear should always be provided in such cases. The deformity may be obvious (a large bunion, for example) or more subtle (a mildly prominent MTH). There may be indications of the at-risk areas such as redness, warmth or callus (which has been shown to be a risk factor for ulceration).[36]

A first line of defense for at-risk patients, as shown in Table 28.1, is a quality sports shoe, as long as any deformity can be accommodated. Sport shoes can reduce plantar pressures compared to conventional shoes[37] and can also reduce the accumulation of callus.[38] There will, however, be some patients who cannot safely wear sports shoes because of their need for more cushioning in certain locations under the foot or their significant foot deformity. For example, toes that are dorsally prominent because of clawing or hammering will need more room in what is called the 'toe box' – the front part of the shoe. In such cases, the patient will need an extra-depth shoe or a super-extra-depth shoe,[39] which have, respectively, approximately 1/4 and 1/2 in. (6 and 13 mm) of additional space in the toe box. This space can accommodate prominent toes when a normal insole is used, or, in patients without dorsal deformity but with plantar prominences, allow the use of a thick insole or orthosis with features that distribute pressure or unload regions of focal pressure. Certain deformities will need to be accommodated by stretching a specific region of the shoe upper, using special tools. Some shoes are designed to stretch easily when heated. In many instances, a thick 'off-the-shelf' insole without customisation or modification will suffice, but in a patient who is at least moderately active or has at least moderate foot deformity, customisation of the insole will be required. Cost is usually an issue in the prescription because (as short sighted as such a policy is) many health services will not pay for primary prevention.

The Diabetic Patient with an Ulcer

With rare exceptions, shoes should not be worn at all by diabetic patients with active ulcers, except special prescription shoes (sometimes called 'half shoes'[40]), which isolate regions of the foot completely from weight bearing. Patients who walk into an examination room wearing the very shoes in which their foot became ulcerated should not walk out wearing those same shoes. Some form of offloading such as a cast or other device (Chapters 25 and 30) must be immediately employed until the ulcer is healed. However, while an ulcer is healing, the practitioner should be making plans for the footwear that the patient will need after the ulcer has healed; any delay in providing definitive footwear to the patient, after the treated ulcer has healed, can result in rapid re-ulceration in the same or an associated area. Any impressions that need to be taken of the foot (for custom-made insoles, for example) can be made even on the healing ulcer if it is fully covered with a clear film dressing.

The Diabetic Patient with a Recently Healed Ulcer

The first few weeks following return to normal ambulation after ulcer healing is a period of very high risk, and it may be preferable to transition the patient into new therapeutic footwear by providing a very well-cushioned walking splint or orthopaedic walker to enable the fragile new tissue to consolidate. Recurrence of foot ulcers is a significant clinical problem.[41] Estimates of recurrence range from 28% at 12 months[42] to 100% at 40 months.[16] It has been suggested that ulcer-free survival should be used as an indicator of the effectiveness of foot ulcer management in different centres.[43]

Once a patient's ulcer has healed, the clinician needs to mount a major initiative, first, to get the patient into appropriate therapeutic shoes, and second, to convince the patient that wearing the shoes may be critical to preventing another ulcer and a possible amputation (see below). Since there is a high likelihood that the original ulcer was footwear related, the patient's previous footwear is often not a good starting point for the new footwear prescription. It can, however, be an extremely useful piece of evidence of what did not work and can guide the next iteration of footwear. Depending on the patient's level of activity and extent of foot deformity (Table 28.1), the practitioner will need to be prepared to take extraordinary steps to provide a protective shoe. This will likely involve a footwear professional who can implement necessary modifications to the foot–shoe interface and convert the shoe into one with a rocker sole, if needed. Sizing the shoe to accommodate thick socks and insoles provides another means of reducing the pressure on the foot,[44] but care must be taken to ensure that this does not result in excessive pressure on the dorsum of prominent toes. As with all new footwear, the patients should wear their new shoes in a graduated manner, starting with a few hours per day, after which they, or a companion, should inspect their feet carefully. Any excessive redness or damage to the skin should be the trigger for an immediate return visit to the footwear provider for modifications. Unfortunately, the prescription and dispensing of therapeutic shoes is still very much a trial-and-error process, and it is not unusual for a new pair of shoes to require several such modifications before they are satisfactory.

In addition to a pair of shoes for use outside the home, several centres also provide custom-moulded sandals or slippers to patients with healed ulcers for use in the home. This implicitly acknowledges that patients are unlikely to wear their therapeutic shoes consistently at home and provides an interface that is better than that during barefoot walking. Since many diabetic patients wake during the night to urinate, footwear that can be easily slipped on may make the difference between staying healed and creating new ulcers resulting from barefoot walking.

Occasionally, the practitioner will recognise that the patient's most dangerous activities from a foot injury standpoint occur during an activity for which the prescribed shoes cannot be worn. One example was a factory worker for whom it was necessary to make extra-depth shoes with steel toecaps, and another was a special pair of shoes for horse riding. In such cases, an effort should be made to provide a footwear solution that facilitates the activity and prevents injury.

The Charcot Patient

Conservative treatment of patients with plantar deformities secondary to Charcot neuroarthropathy is a challenging and time-consuming process.[45] The typical midfoot collapse can leave a 'rocker bottom foot' with a midfoot prominence that becomes the only weight-bearing surface on the plantar aspect of the foot, resulting in extremely high plantar pressures. Surgery may be required to provide a plantigrade foot that can function without ulceration.[46] The deformity will often mandate a custom-made shoe, requiring the skills of an orthopaedic shoemaker who will make measurements and a cast of the entire foot to produce a shoe that will fit the Charcot foot. A custom-moulded interface between the foot and the shoe, including special load relief from plantar prominences, is often built directly into the midsole of such shoes, and a custom-made orthosis is then placed inside the shoe. Traditionally, Charcot patients have often been provided with a brace – such as a patellar-tendon-bearing brace (PTB)[47] – to transfer some of the load to the leg. However, patients often dislike PTBs,[47] and it is not clear that load bearing is always reduced on the braced foot.[48]

COMPLIANCE IN WEARING THERAPEUTIC FOOTWEAR

The most advanced and well-designed prescription shoe can be effective only if it is worn by the patient on a continuing basis. However, a number of studies have shown that consistent use of such footwear is rarely the case and that poor compliance with wearing therapeutic footwear is associated with increased risk of re-ulceration.[49,50] It has been suggested that to be effective, shoes must be worn for at least 60% of the time,[51] but this number would seem to be low. One study reported that only 22% of the sample 'regularly wore' prescribed footwear, and only 38% of the subjects wore slippers indoors.[52] Another study found that only 12% of patients wore their shoes at home more than 80% of the time. Patients can often be compliant for the majority of the time, only to fail, and ulcerate, after a holiday or special event such as a wedding at which they felt the need to wear attractive (but unsafe) footwear.[53]

No research has yet established the optimal approach to maximize patient compliance with footwear. Many authorities feel strongly that when patients are given shoes that they perceive to be 'ugly', compliance will be poor.[54] However, others believe that the key is in the patient's perceived value of the shoe, and not in a previous history of foot complications or the aesthetics of footwear. The role of education in compliance with footwear is not yet known. In the absence of better evidence, it seems reasonable to attempt (1) to produce attractive therapeutic shoes; (2) to make sure that the patients know the cost of their shoes; (3) to carefully explain the reason for the shoes and the role that footwear can play in ulcer and amputation prevention; and (4) to remind the patients and their family members as frequently as possible about the need to wear the shoes at all times.

FUTURE TRENDS

The design of therapeutic footwear remains an art that is only just beginning to be influenced by science. The early progress that Dr Brand and his colleagues made[1,2] did not herald the revolutionary change that they hoped for. Yet, the digital world is knocking at the door, and an array of tools such as contact foot digitisers, in-shoe pressure mapping, finite element method simulations and CAD-CAM[55] are beginning to make contributions that will eventually change the face of footwear design and prescription. These developments will not filter through to practice until the value of therapeutic footwear in reducing morbidity can be demonstrated and shown to be cost-effective.

NOTE

The authors own stock in DIApedia LLC.

REFERENCES

1. Bauman J, Girling E, Brand PW. Plantar pressures and trophic ulceration. An evaluation of footwear. *J Bone Joint Surg Br* 1963;45B:652–673.
2. Bauman JH, Brand PW. Measurement of pressure between foot and shoe. *Lancet* 1963;1:629–632.
3. Guldemond NA, Leffers P, Schaper N. Clinical proficiency of Dutch podiatrists, pedorthists, and orthotists regarding plantar pressure reduction. In: *Biomechanics of the Lower Limb in Health and Disease*. University of Salford, UK; 2005:210–211.
4. Edmonds ME, Blundell MP, Morris ME, Thomas EM, Cotton LT, Watkins PJ. Improved survival of the diabetic foot: the role of a specialised foot clinic. *Q J Med* 1986;60:763–771.
5. Macfarlane RM, Jeffcoate WJ. Factors contributing to the presentation of diabetic foot ulcers. *Diabet Med* 1997;14:867–870.
6. Benotmane A, Mohammedi F, Ayad F, Kadi K, Azzouz A. Diabetic foot lesions: etiologic and prognostic factors. *Diabetes Metab* 2000;26:113–117.
7. McGill M, Molyneaux L, Yue DK. Which diabetic patients should receive podiatry care? An objective analysis. *Intern Med J* 2005;35:451–456.
8. Apelqvist J, Larsson J, Agardh CD. The influence of external precipitating factors and peripheral neuropathy on the development and outcome of diabetic foot ulcers. *J Diabetes Complications* 1990;4:21–25.
9. Reiber GE. Who is at risk of limb loss and what to do about it? *J Rehabil Res Dev* 1994;31:357–362.
10. Chantelau E, Gede A. Foot dimensions of elderly people with and without diabetes mellitus – a data basis for shoe design. *Gerontology* 2002;48:241–244.
11. Maciejewski ML, Reiber GE, Smith DG, Wallace C, Hayes S, Boyko EJ. Effectiveness of diabetic therapeutic footwear in preventing reulceration. *Diabetes Care* 2004;27:1774–1782.
12. Spencer S. Pressure relieving interventions for preventing and treating diabetic foot ulcers. *Cochrane Database Syst Rev* 2000;3:CD002302.
13. Reiber GE, Smith DG, Wallace C, *et al*. Effect of therapeutic footwear on foot reulceration in patients with diabetes: a randomized controlled trial. *JAMA* 2002;287:2552–2558.
14. Cavanagh PR, Boulton AJ, Sheehan P, Ulbrecht JS, Caputo GM, Armstrong DG. Therapeutic footwear in patients with diabetes. *JAMA* 2002;288:1231; author reply 1232–1233.
15. Busch K, Chantelau E. Effectiveness of a new brand of stock 'diabetic' shoes to protect against diabetic foot ulcer relapse. A prospective cohort study. *Diabet Med* 2003;20:665–669.
16. Uccioli L, Faglia E, Monticone G, *et al*. Manufactured shoes in the prevention of diabetic foot ulcers. *Diabetes Care* 1995;18:1376–1378.
17. Viswanathan V, Madhavan S, Gnanasundaram S, *et al*. Effectiveness of different types of footwear insoles for the diabetic neuropathic foot: a follow-up study. *Diabetes Care* 2004;27:474–477.
18. Cavanagh PR, Ulbrecht JS, Caputo GM. The biomechanics of the foot in diabetes mellitus. In: Bowker JH, Pfeifer MA, eds. *Levin and O'Neal's The Diabetic Foot*. 6th edn. St Louis, MO: Mosby; 2001.
19. Bus SA, Ulbrecht JS, Cavanagh PR. Pressure relief and load redistribution by custom-made insoles in diabetic patients with neuropathy and foot deformity. *Clin Biomech (Bristol, Avon)* 2004;19:629–638.
20. Hayda R, Tremaine MD, Tremaine K, Banco S, Teed K. Effect of metatarsal pads and their positioning: a quantitative assessment. *Foot Ankle Int* 1994;15:561–566.
21. Hsi WL, Kang JH, Lee XX. Optimum position of metatarsal pad in metatarsalgia for pressure relief. *Am J Phys Med Rehabil* 2005;84:514–520.
22. Jackson L, Binning J, Potter J. Plantar pressures in rheumatoid arthritis using prefabricated metatarsal padding. *J Am Podiatr Med Assoc* 2004;94:239–245.

23. van Schie C, Ulbrecht JS, Becker MB, Cavanagh PR. Design criteria for rigid rocker shoes. *Foot Ankle Int* 2000;21:833–844.

24. Ashry HR, Lavery LA, Murdoch DP, Frolich M, Lavery DC. Effectiveness of diabetic insoles to reduce foot pressures. *J Foot Ankle Surg* 1997;36:268–271; discussion 328–329.

25. Nawoczenski DA, Birke JA, Coleman WC. Effect of rocker sole design on plantar forefoot pressures. *J Am Podiatr Med Assoc* 1988;78:455–460.

26. Ulbrecht JS, Cavanagh PR. Shoes and insoles for at-risk people with diabetes. In: Armstrong DG, Lavery LA, eds. *Clinical Care of the Diabetic Foot*. Alexandria, VA: American Diabetes Association; 2005:36–44.

27. Brodsky JW, Kourosh S, Stills M, Mooney V. Objective evaluation of insert material for diabetic and athletic footwear. *Foot Ankle* 1988;9:111–116.

28. Foto JG, Birke JA. Evaluation of multidensity orthotic materials used in footwear for patients with diabetes. *Foot Ankle Int* 1998;19:836–841.

29. Chang AH, Abu-Faraj ZU, Harris GF, Nery J, Shereff MJ. Multistep measurement of plantar pressure alterations using metatarsal pads. *Foot Ankle Int* 1994;15:654–660.

30. Holmes GB Jr, Timmerman L. A quantitative assessment of the effect of metatarsal pads on plantar pressures. *Foot Ankle* 1990;11:141–145.

31. Armstrong DG, Liswood PJ, Todd WF. Potential risks of accommodative padding in the treatment of neuropathic ulcerations. *Ostomy Wound Manage* 1995;41:44–46, 48–49.

32. Erdemir A, Saucerman JJ, Lemmon D, *et al.* Local plantar pressure relief in therapeutic footwear: design guidelines from finite element models. *J Biomech* 2005;38:1798–1806.

33. Armstrong DG, Abu-Rumman PL, Nixon BP, Boulton AJ. Continuous activity monitoring in persons at high risk for diabetes-related lower-extremity amputation. *J Am Podiatr Med Assoc* 2001;91:451–455.

34. Lott DJ, Maluf KS, Sinacore DR, Mueller MJ. Relationship between changes in activity and plantar ulcer recurrence in a patient with diabetes mellitus. *Phys Ther* 2005;85:579–588.

35. Maluf KS, Mueller MJ. Novel Award 2002. Comparison of physical activity and cumulative plantar tissue stress among subjects with and without diabetes mellitus and a history of recurrent plantar ulcers. *Clin Biomech (Bristol, Avon)* 2003;18:567–575.

36. Murray HJ, Young MJ, Hollis S, Boulton AJ. The association between callus formation, high pressures and neuropathy in diabetic foot ulceration. *Diabet Med* 1996;13:979–982.

37. Perry JE, Ulbrecht JS, Derr JA, Cavanagh PR. The use of running shoes to reduce plantar pressures in patients who have diabetes. *J Bone Joint Surg Am* 1995;77:1819–1828.

38. Soulier SM. The use of running shoes in the prevention of plantar diabetic ulcers. *J Am Podiatr Med Assoc* 1986;76:395–400.

39. Kaye RA. The extra-depth toe box: a rational approach. *Foot Ankle Int* 1994;15:146–150.

40. Chantelau E, Breuer U, Leisch AC, Tanudjaja T, Reuter M. Outpatient treatment of unilateral diabetic foot ulcers with 'half shoes'. *Diabet Med* Apr 1993;10:267–270.

41. Mantey I, Foster AV, Spencer S, Edmonds ME. Why do foot ulcers recur in diabetic patients? *Diabet Med* 1999;16:245–249.

42. Chantelau E, Kushner T, Spraul M. How effective is cushioned therapeutic footwear in protecting diabetic feet? A clinical study. *Diabet Med* 1990;7:355–359.

43. Pound N, Chipchase S, Treece K, Game F, Jeffcoate W. Ulcer-free survival following management of foot ulcers in diabetes. *Diabet Med* 2005;22:1306–1309.

44. Garrow AP, van Schie CH, Boulton AJ. Efficacy of multilayered hosiery in reducing in-shoe plantar foot pressure in high-risk patients with diabetes. *Diabetes Care* 2005;28:2001–2006.

45. Saltzman CL, Hagy ML, Zimmerman B, Estin M, Cooper R. How effective is intensive nonoperative initial treatment of patients with diabetes and Charcot arthropathy of the feet? *Clin Orthop Relat Res* 2005;435:185–190.

46. Trepman E, Nihal A, Pinzur MS. Current topics review: Charcot neuroarthropathy of the foot and ankle. *Foot Ankle Int* 2005;26:46–63.

47. Trepman E, Donnelly P. Patellar tendon-bearing, patten-bottom caliper suspension orthosis in active Charcot arthropathy: crutch-free ambulation with no weight bearing in the foot. *Foot Ankle Int* 2002;23:335–339.

48. Saltzman CL, Johnson KA, Goldstein RH, Donnelly RE. The patellar tendon-bearing brace as treatment for neurotrophic arthropathy: a dynamic force monitoring study. *Foot Ankle* 1992;13: 14–21.

49. Chantelau E, Haage P. An audit of cushioned diabetic footwear: relation to patient compliance. *Diabet Med* 1994;11:114–116.

50. Connor H, Mahdi OZ. Repetitive ulceration in neuropathic patients. *Diabetes Metab Res Rev* 2004;20:S23–S28.

51. Macfarlane DJ, Jensen JL. Factors in diabetic footwear compliance. *J Am Podiatr Med Assoc* 2003;93:485–491.

52. Knowles EA, Boulton AJ. Do people with diabetes wear their prescribed footwear? *Diabet Med* 1996;13:1064–1068.

53. Armstrong DG, Dang C, Nixon BP, Boulton AJ. The hazards of the holiday foot: persons at high risk for diabetic foot ulceration may be more active on holiday. *Diabet Med* 2003;20:247–248.

54. Boulton AJ, Jude EB. Therapeutic footwear in diabetes: the good, the bad, and the ugly? *Diabetes Care* 2004;27:1832–1833.

55. Cavanagh PR. Therapeutic footwear for people with diabetes. *Diabetes Metab Res Rev* 2004;20:S51–S55.

29 New Casting Techniques: Introduction to the 'Instant Total Contact Cast'

David G. Armstrong, Stephanie C. Wu and Ryan C. Crews

Foot ulceration is one of the most common complications associated with diabetes and often plays a central role in the causal pathway to lower extremity amputation.[1] Amelioration of pressure, shear and repetitive injury to the sole of the foot are principal tenets of diabetic ulcer care.[2] Numerous offloading modalities are currently available to practitioners. Total contact casting is considered by many clinicians to be the gold standard in redistribution of pressure over the plantar aspect of the diabetic foot.[3–9] Total contact casts (TCCs) have been shown to reduce pressure at the site of ulceration by 84–92%,[10] and there is a large body of work that supports the clinical efficacy of TCC. In two randomised controlled trials comparing the proportion of healed ulcers treated with the TCC compared with other readily available and popular devices, such as removable cast walkers (RCWs), half shoes and therapeutic depth inlay shoes, TCC healed a higher proportion of wounds compared to other modalities.[9,11] This was an interesting finding because certain types of RCWs, including the one used in one of the above-mentioned trials, often reduce pressure on the plantar aspect of the foot as well as TCCs.[11] If patients do not heal as well in the RCWs, and yet they offloads pressure almost likewise, then a logical explanation for their less effective clinical performance is that the patients are simply not wearing these devices.[12] As easy as it was for the clinicians to apply these devices, the patients can remove them just as easily.

The question of compliance with removable devices has been studied by the authors in a recent study where the activity of patients with diabetic foot ulcers and their offloading regime were assessed. In this study it was postulated that although the RCW and TCC may offload (more or less) equally well, patients, because of their dense neuropathy, might not strictly adhere to a standard pressure-offloading regimen. In the study, accelerometers were worn on the patients' waist and hidden in the RCW. It revealed that patients wore their offloading device for less than 30% of their total daily activity.[12] This disappointing result has prompted us to search for simple solutions.

Understanding that most centres do not have the infrastructure, expertise or personnel to apply TCCs, in light of the previous data, we have suggested that a potential alternative might be to make the RCW less easily removable. This simple concept, termed an 'instant total

The Foot in Diabetes, 4th Edition. Editors Andrew J.M. Boulton, Peter R. Cavanagh and Gerry Rayman.
© 2006 John Wiley & Sons, Ltd.

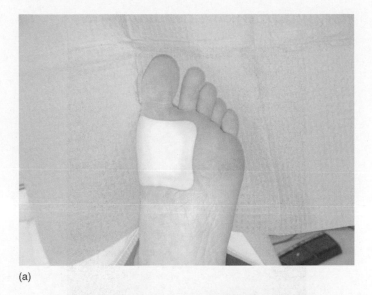

(a)

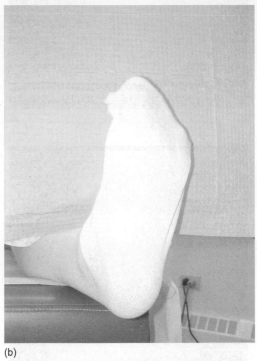

(b)

Figure 29.1 Application of the instant total contact cast (iTCC). (a) Preparation of the foot: (i) Debride ulcer as necessary. Apply dressing to ulcer. The dressing may be held in place with paper tape or, as is the case in the figure, may be self-adherent. No circumferential dressing is generally applied, as this could pose a risk of irritation to the skin. (ii) If the iTCC is being applied for persons with Charcot and no ulcer, then no special dressing is required. (iii) Be sure that all toenails are debrided and the skin is well hydrated, using an emollient of choice. (iv) Cotton or lamb's wool may be placed between the toes to reduce maceration if this is a concern in the specific patient being treated. (b) Cotton stockinette is applied to the foot and leg: (i) Stockinette should be snug and form fitting. (ii) Fold stocking over the toes dorsally and tape it in place. (iii) Make a cut in the stockinette at anterior ankle and tape in place to reduce wrinkles, as required. The goal is to provide minimal wrinkling over areas of potential pressure.

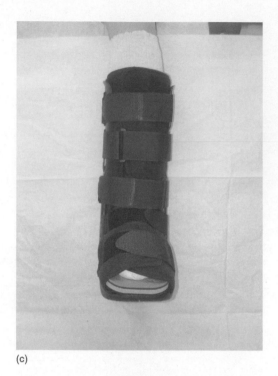

(c)

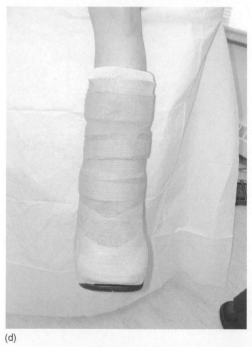

(d)

Figure 29.1 (*Continued*) (c) A robust removable cast walker is then applied to the foot. One should use a device that has been shown to reduce pressure to a similar extent as a total contact cast. (d) The device is then wrapped with a single layer of cohesive bandage or plaster of Paris. The device may be initially changed at 2–3 days to ensure no irritation. If irritation is noted, that site may be accommodated with cotton padding or other similar modalities. Following re-examination, the device may be changed as is typical by the treating clinic.

contact cast' (iTCC),[13] involves simply wrapping the RCW with either a layer of cohesive bandage or a plaster/fibreglass (Figure 29.1), thereby making it more difficult for patients to remove. The iTCC then may have the benefit of adequate offloading (on par with the TCC) as well as adequate adherence to the prescribed course of pressure reduction.

Two recent randomised controlled trials seemed to support the above-mentioned postulate. In the first study, subjects given an iTCC appeared to heal as readily at 12 weeks as patients given a standard TCC (80% iTCC vs 74% TCC).[14] A second study performed in parallel with this project compared the iTCC with a standard RCW. This study suggested substantial differences in healing at 12 weeks between the irremovable and removable devices (83 vs 52%).[15]

While wound healing is clearly a complex process, the act of offloading (a relatively simple concept) is rarely addressed appropriately and even more rarely adhered to. It may be argued that the results realised in the data presented above represent highly specialised conditions in highly specialised centres dedicated to diabetic foot wound healing. Some would argue that it is a moot point to try to compare trials performed at one or two so-called 'centres of excellence' with a multitude of industry-sponsored trials conducted at centres, worldwide. We, however, would not propose a comparison. We would, rather, propose a compromise.

We propose marrying wound-healing agents that do not require frequent dressing changes with robust pressure offloading modalities that are, by design, less easily removable. In a clinical trial sense, this would (by virtue of higher healing rates in both experimental and control groups) require greater numbers to show superiority. However, this same higher healing rate might also lead to more consistent results in more centres around the world and (commensurately) fewer lower extremity amputations.

REFERENCES

1. Singh N, Armstrong DG, Lipsky BA. Preventing foot ulcers in patients with diabetes. *JAMA* Jan 12, 2005;293:217–228.
2. Brand PW. The diabetic foot. In: Ellenberg M, Rifkin H, eds. *Diabetes Mellitus, Theory and Practice*. 3rd edn. New York: Medical Examination Publishing; 1983:803–828.
3. American Diabetes Association. Consensus Development Conference on Diabetic Foot Wound Care. *Diabetes Care* 1999;22:1354–1360.
4. Coleman W, Brand PW, Birke JA. The total contact cast, a therapy for plantar ulceration on insensitive feet. *J Am Podiatr Med Assoc* 1984;74:548–552.
5. Helm PA, Walker SC, Pulliam G. Total contact casting in diabetic patients with neuropathic foot ulcerations. *Arch Phys Med Rehabil* 1984;65:691–693.
6. Walker SC, Helm PA, Pulliam G. Total contact casting and chronic diabetic neuropathic foot ulcerations: healing rates by wound location. *Arch Phys Med Rehabil* 1987;68:217–221.
7. Walker SC, Helm PA, Pulliam G. Chronic diabetic neuropathic foot ulcerations and total contact casting: healing effectiveness and outcome probability (abstract). *Arch Phys Med Rehabil* 1985;66:574.
8. Sinacore DR, Mueller MJ, Diamond JE. Diabetic plantar ulcers treated by total contact casting. *Phys Ther* 1987;67:1543–1547.
9. Mueller MJ, Diamond JE, Sinacore DR, *et al.* Total contact casting in treatment of diabetic plantar ulcers. Controlled clinical trial (see comments). *Diabetes Care* 1989;12:384–388.
10. Lavery LA, Vela SA, Lavery DC, Quebedeaux TL. Reducing dynamic foot pressures in high-risk diabetic subjects with foot ulcerations. A comparison of treatments. *Diabetes Care* 1996;19:818–821.
11. Armstrong DG, Nguyen HC, Lavery LA, van Schie CH, Boulton AJM, Harkless LB. Offloading the diabetic foot wound: a randomized clinical trial. *Diabetes Care* 2001;24:1019–1022.

12. Armstrong DG, Lavery LA, Kimbriel HR, Nixon BP, Boulton AJ. Activity patterns of patients with diabetic foot ulceration: patients with active ulceration may not adhere to a standard pressure off-loading regimen. *Diabetes Care.* Sep 2003;26:2595–2597.
13. Armstrong DG, Short B, Nixon BP, Boulton AJM. Technique for fabrication of an 'instant' total contact cast for treatment of neuropathic diabetic foot ulcers. *J Am Podiatr Med Assoc* 2002;92:405–408.
14. Katz IA, Harlan A, Miranda-Palma B, *et al.* A randomized trial of two irremovable offloading devices in the management of neuropathic diabetic foot ulcers. *Diabetes Care* 2005;28:555–559.
15. Armstrong DG, Lavery LA, Wu SC, Boulton AJM. Evaluation of removable and irremovable cast walkers in the healing of diabetic foot wounds: a randomized controlled trial. *Diabetes Care* 2005;28:551–554.

30 New Technologies in Wound Healing: Pressure-Relieving Dressings

Carine van Schie and Jan Ulbrecht

OFFLOADING DIABETIC FOOT ULCERS

Wound healing is prolonged or prevented if the wound is subjected to ongoing trauma,[1] which explains why pressure relief or offloading is considered a key factor in healing diabetic foot ulcers.[2] Effective offloading techniques include off-the-shelf and custom-made removable and irremovable casts, walkers and 'half shoes', as reviewed in Chapter 25. However, removable devices may not be efficacious if patients do not appreciate and comply with the need for 100% mechanical protection. Thus, unfortunately in many patients the majority of their walking involves steps that are not adequately protected by offloading.[3] This, together with the fact that many practitioners fail to prescribe devices with proven offloading efficacy, has lead to relatively poor healing rates of diabetic neuropathic ulcers being the norm.[4]

The strongest evidence that offloading is key in healing diabetic foot ulcers comes from studies of total contact casting, where healing of well-perfused plantar neuropathic ulcers is almost 100% in 6 weeks (Chapter 25), because of the almost complete mechanical protection offered by total contact casts (TCCs).[5] However, TCCs are not as frequently utilised as would be expected, for two principal reasons: fear of enclosing a wound in a cast, lest unrecognised infection should develop; and because TCCs are labour intensive. Furthermore, patients also do not like TCCs, because they are awkward, limit mobility and affect personal hygiene.

Offloading options that have efficacy similar to that of the TCC but are more acceptable to practitioners and patients are therefore needed. As discussed previously, one such option is the irremovable cast walker. The simplest measures in wound care are often the most effective, or have the most impact,[6] and this may well be true of the attempts to transfer load from the ulcer to the healthy skin around the ulcer, using a load-relieving dressing. The following section describes such measures and considers their potential benefits and drawbacks.

The Foot in Diabetes, 4th Edition. Editors Andrew J.M. Boulton, Peter R. Cavanagh and Gerry Rayman.
© 2006 John Wiley & Sons, Ltd.

THE FELTED FOAM DRESSING METHOD

The concept of transferring load away from the ulcer to the skin around the ulcer is simple and has been put into practice using the method referred to as felted foam dressing (FFD) for well over 20 years, with descriptions in the literature for over 10 years.[7–10] Although many have raised concerns about the likelihood of transfer lesions and edge effect lesions,[11] these are in fact not reported in the FFD literature. FFDs have been shown to be effective in pressure reduction in diabetic patients with neuropathic foot ulcers,[10, 12] with pressure reduced in the initial 3 days, but followed by an increase in pressure if the FFD is used beyond 3 days.[12] In a recent randomised controlled trial, Zimny et al.,[7] using the protocol of changing the FFD every 3 days, noted that the healing of neuropathic plantar ulcers achieved was somewhat better than that achieved using a 'half shoe' (average 75 (95% CI, 67–84) vs 85 (95% CI, 79–92) days; $p = 0.03$). It should be noted, however, that these healing times are considerably longer than those achieved with the TCC, where 42 days is the typical average.[13] To our knowledge, a direct comparison of the TCC and FFD methods have not been performed.

Unfortunately, there are a variety of variables involved in the preparation and use of FFD, which may explain the less-than-ideal healing rates. An important variable is the variety of different ways of making FFDs. Thus, the FFD usually includes a number of layers of a product that already combines felt and foam, some employing just one layer, while others use multiple layers.[7–10, 12] The mechanical properties of these layers are usually not defined and are presumably variable among different investigators. In addition, the area of the FFD can also vary from covering all or most of the plantar surface to being much smaller and localised to the lesion. Methods of adhesion can also vary, the traditional method being to attach the FFD to the foot by rubber cement. This is not accepted by all. Some additional wrap, such as an Unna boot bandage, is also often employed. In addition, the footgear utilised varies widely from putting the patient back into his/her own shoes, to using a removable cast walker.

Thus, at least two companies are in the process of developing commercial products based on the FFD method.

PROTOTYPE PRESSURE-RELIEVING DRESSINGS FOR DIABETIC FOOT ULCERS

One prototype pressure-relieving dressing (PRD) specifically designed to offload pressure under individual plantar metatarsal head (MTH) areas was recently developed and investigated (Coloplast A/S, Denmark). The PRD was tested in the laboratory of one of the authors (van Schie),[14] and was a prototype of a sterile dressing especially designed for diabetic foot ulcers. Besides exhibiting normal qualities of dressing, such as absorption and retention, it also has a built-in pressure-relieving cushion in order to relieve pressure at the active MTH site only (Figure 30.1). The dressing is designed and indicated for plantar foot ulcers of grade 1 or 2 (according to Wagner scale)[15] without infection. The absorbing part of the non-adhesive dressing, which is capable of absorbing exudate from the wound, is designed to cover the MTH wound area. The pressure-relieving part of the dressing (silicone), which is 4 mm thick on average and slightly adhesive, is placed on the intact skin. It has a built-in 'woven tread' to maintain shape and thickness. This is an important feature of the prototype PRD, which is especially designed to keep the structure and pressure-relieving properties of the pressure-relieving material

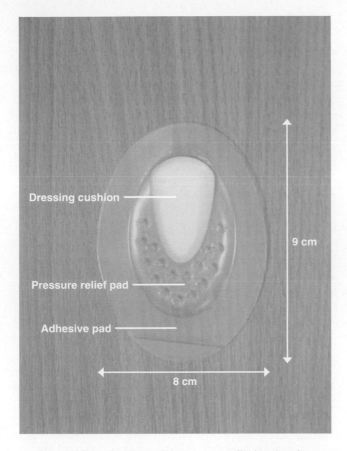

Figure 30.1   Example of the pressure-relieving dressing

throughout its wear time. The material and design used will not collapse as, for example, felt does.

A mean pressure reduction of 30% was observed at the PRD MTH site of interest (817.2 $\pm$ 139.3 barefoot vs 573.2 $\pm$ 166.1 kPa; $p < 0.0001$; mean $\pm$ SD; optical pedobarograph (Department of Medical Physics and Clinical Engineering, Royal Hallamshire Hospital, Sheffield, UK)) as was assessed in 18 patients with diabetic peripheral neuropathy without prior ulceration. A mean pressure reduction of 30% compares well with other protective shoes or offloading techniques,[16–21] and the offloading effect was sustained for at least 3 days. However, 30% offloading is much less than usually seen in devices with proven healing efficacy such as the TCC,[5] FFD[10, 12] and various walkers.[22] Therefore, this PRD cannot be used on its own as an alternative to other offloading modalities for ulcer healing. However, its goal would be to offer a supplement to the existing offloading modalities in order to improve wound healing. It may be sufficient to allow a few 'barefoot' steps to be taken when a patient is not wearing the removable device but chooses to ambulate without it. This PRD may also have a role in prevention, where the patient does not accept special shoes or insoles, but might be willing to utilise the PRD with his or her own shoes. In this circumstance, when the shoe is removed, excessive pressure during 'barefoot' walking would also be mitigated.

Importantly, the prototype dressing was shown to be effective at reducing pressures not only at the MTH of interest, but also at both neighbouring MTHs. The medial and lateral MTH showed a 16% pressure reduction and there was no edge effect or transfer effect pressure increases.

Another prototype PRD is under development by DIApedia, LLC (United States) (J. Ulbrecht *et al.*, in preparation) (Plate 6). This device is much thicker (13 mm) and because of that its offloading is similar to that of a TCC (J. Ulbrecht *et al.*, in preparation). For instance, in one study of ten healthy volunteers with high forefoot pressure, a mean pressure reduction of 85% was observed at the MTH site of interest (610 ± 80 barefoot vs 98 ± 62 kPa; $p < 0.0001$; mean $\pm$ SD; Pliance (Novel GMBH, Munich, Germany)). In addition, the well of the PRD can be 'loaded' with a dressing product that can have a positive impact on wound healing – for instance, for exudate absorption or growth factor release. Because of its thickness, this PRD would be difficult to accommodate in a regular shoe, but rather is best used with another footgear device, such as a healing shoe and a specific footbed that can be provided as part of a system.

Thus, offloading by this PRD prototype is similar to that seen in a TCC and is reproducible, offloading is independent of patient compliance (as long as the patient does not remove the PRD adhered to the foot), the wound can be examined at will and the wound can be exposed to active agents – all attributes that make this potentially a very useful product that now must go through clinical testing.

SUMMARY

The concept of offloading plantar neuropathic ulcers locally, using a PRD, as embodied in the FFD method, is not new. Progress is now being made to enhance this method with reliable products with proven efficacy. The two PRD 'off-the-shelf' prototype products appear effective in reducing plantar pressure at individual MTHs. While one may be easier to use, the other offers offloading similar to that of the TCC, with the potential for similar healing success, but without the problems of the TCC. While the developments are promising, these novel devices now need to be further evaluated in patients with active foot ulceration.

REFERENCES

1. Piagessi A, Viacava P, Rizzo L, *et al.* Semiquantitative analysis of the histopathological features of the neuropathic foot ulcer: effects of pressure relief. *Diabetes Care* 2003;26:3123–3128.
2. Cavanagh PR, Ulbrecht JS, Caputo GM. The non healing diabetic foot wound: fact or fiction? *Ostomy Wound Manage* 1998;44:6S–13S.
3. Armstrong DG, Lavery LA, Kimbriel HR, Nixon BP, Boulton AJ. Activity patterns of patients with diabetic foot ulceration: patients with active ulceration may not adhere to a standard pressure off-loading regimen. *Diabetes Care* Sep 2003;26:2595–2597.
4. Margolis DJ, Allen-Taylor L, Hoffstad O, Berlin JA. Healing diabetic neuropathic foot ulcers: are we getting better? *Diabet Med* Feb 2005;22:172–176.
5. Petre M, Tokar P, Kostar D, Cavanagh PR. Revisiting the total contact cast: maximizing off-loading by wound isolation. *Diabetes Care* Apr 2005;28:929–930.
6. Calne S. Achieving innovation in wound care. *J Wound Care* Feb 1999;8:47.

7. Zimny S, Schatz H, Pfohl U. The effects of applied felted foam on wound healing and healing times in the therapy of neuropathic diabetic foot ulcers. *Diabet Med* Aug 2003;20:622–625.

8. Ritz G, Kushner D, Friedman S. A successful technique for the treatment of diabetic neurotrophic ulcers. *J Am Podiatr Med Assoc* Sep 1992;82:479–481.

9. Kiewied J. Felt therapy for leprosy patients with an ulcer in a pressure area (letter). *Lepr Rev* 1997;68:378–381.

10. Fleischli JG, Lavery LA, Vela SA, Ashry H, Lavery DC. Comparison of strategies for reducing pressure at the site of neuropathic ulcers. *J Am Podiatr Med Assoc* 1997;87:466–472.

11. Armstrong DG, Liswood PJ, Todd WF. Potential risks of accommodative padding in the treatment of neuropathic ulcerations. *Ostomy Wound Manage* 1995;41:44–48.

12. Zimny S, Reinsch B, Schatz H, Pfohl M. Effects of felted foam on plantar pressures in the treatment of neuropathic diabetic foot ulcers. *Diabetes Care* 2001;24:2153–2154.

13. Armstrong DG, Nguyen HC, Lavery LA, van Schie CH, Boulton AJ, Harkless LB. Off-loading the diabetic foot wound: a randomized clinical trial. *Diabetes Care* 2001;24:1019–1022.

14. van Schie CH, Rawat F, Boulton AJ. Reduction of plantar pressure using a prototype pressure-relieving dressing. *Diabetes Care* Sep 2005;28:2236–2237.

15. Wagner FW. The dysvascular foot: a system of diagnosis and treatment. *Foot Ankle* 1981;2:64–122.

16. Perry JE, Ulbrecht JS, Derr JA, Cavanagh PR. The use of running shoes to reduce plantar pressures in patients who have diabetes. *J Bone Joint Surg* 1995;77A:1819–1828.

17. van Schie C, Ulbrecht JS, Becker MB, Cavanagh PR. Design criteria for rigid rocker shoes. *Foot Ankle Int* 2000;21:833–844.

18. van Schie CHM, Whalley A, Vileikyte L, Wignall T, Hollis S, Boulton AJM. Efficacy of injected liquid silicone in the diabetic foot to reduce risk factors for ulceration: a randomized double-blind placebo-controlled trial. *Diabetes Care* 2000;23:634–638.

19. Lobmann R, Kayser R, Kasten G, *et al.* Effects of preventative footwear on foot pressure as determined by pedobarography in diabetic patients: a prospective study. *Diabet Med* 2001;18:314–319.

20. Lord M, Hosein R. Pressure redistribution by molded inserts in diabetic footwear: a pilot study. *J Rehabil Res Dev* 1994;31:214–221.

21. Veves A, Masson EA, Fernando DJS, Boulton AJM. Use of experimental padded hosiery to reduce abnormal foot pressures in diabetic neuropathy. *Diabetes Care* 1989;12:653–655.

22. Lavery LA, Vela SA, Lavery DC, Quebedeaux TL. Reducing dynamic foot pressures in high-risk diabetic subjects with foot ulcerations. *Diabetes Care* 1996;19:818–821.

31 Negative Pressure Wound (VAC) Therapy

David G. Armstrong and Andrew J.M. Boulton

Over the past several years, negative pressure wound therapy (NPWT) has emerged as a commonly employed option in the treatment of complex wounds. This therapy involves the delivery of intermittent or continuous subatmospheric pressure through a specialised pump connected to a resilient open-celled foam surface dressing covered with an adhesive drape to maintain a closed environment. This pump is connected to a canister, which serves to collect wound discharge and exudate.

Previous work has suggested that the application of negative pressure optimises blood flow, decreases local tissue oedema and removes excessive fluid and pro-inflammatory exudates from the wound bed.[1,2] These physiological changes promote a moist wound-healing environment and may facilitate the removal of bacteria from the wound. Additionally, the application of subatmospheric pressure may help increase the rate of cell division and subsequent formation of granulation tissue. Although the exact mechanism of action of NPWT on wound healing is not clear, some authors postulate that the application of these so-called microdeformational forces to wounds *in vivo* can promote wound healing by deforming or stretching individual cells in the wound-healing environment to stimulate proliferation and wound healing.[3]

While there has been much anecdotal 'evidence' bolstering the significant clinical enthusiasm for the use of this modality, higher level evidence had been largely absent in the medical literature. Two technical reviews on the subject, from the Cochrane Collaboration and the US Agency for Health Care Quality, could identify only a small handful of randomised studies supporting the use of NPWT delivered through vacuum-assisted closure (VAC). This cohort, totalling 135 patients, was from small, underpowered projects mainly from single centres.[4,5] These studies, in some cases, pooled various wound aetiologies and did not focus on safety issues. Therefore, the purpose of a recent study[6] was to determine, in a randomised clinical trial, the effect of NPWT relative to the standard of care in patients with complex wounds secondary to partial foot amputation in patients with diabetes.

In this study, 162 patients were enroled into a 16-week, 18-centre randomised clinical trial.[6] Inclusion criteria consisted of partial foot amputation wounds up to the transmetatarsal level and evidence of adequate perfusion. Patients randomised to NPWT ($n = 77$) received therapy with dressing changes every 2 days. Control patients ($n = 85$) received standard moist wound care according to consensus guidelines. NPWT was delivered through the vacuum-assisted closure

The Foot in Diabetes, 4th Edition. Editors Andrew J.M. Boulton, Peter R. Cavanagh and Gerry Rayman.
© 2006 John Wiley & Sons, Ltd.

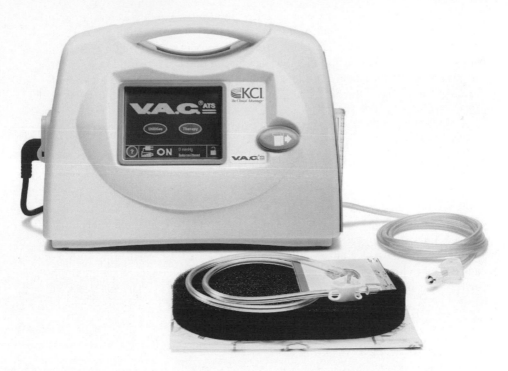

Figure 31.1 The VAC system, showing the vacuum pump, tubing and, in the foreground, the foam dressing.

(VAC®) therapy system (Figure 31.1). Wounds were treated until healing or completion of the 112-day active treatment period.

Significantly more subjects healed in the NPWT group (55.8% (95% CI, 44.1%–67.2%); $p = 0.040$) compared to the standard therapy group (38.8% (95% CI, 28.4%–50.0%)). Both the rate of wound healing, based on the time to complete closure ($p = 0.005$), and the rate of granulation tissue formation, based on the time to 76–100% formation in the wound bed ($p = 0.002$), were faster in the NPWT group. Finally, there was a strong trend towards fewer amputations in the NPWT group (2/11 vs 9/11, $p = 0.060$) compared to standard therapy.

The above-mentioned study supports the contention that NPWT delivered through the VAC therapy system yielded a higher proportion of healed wounds, faster time to wound closure, a more rapid and robust granulation tissue response and a trend towards reduced risk for a second amputation, compared to the control group. We believe this to be the first randomised clinical trial in the medical literature to evaluate these outcomes in wounds secondary to open amputation of the foot.

A rather important differentiating factor between the above-mentioned study and previous works is that the wounds in this study were larger and more complex than those in previous randomised trials. Many prior studies primarily evaluated superficial diabetic foot ranging in size from 2.4 to 2.97 cm^2 compared to 20·7 cm^2 in the NPWT-VAC study.[6–11] The fact that the prevalence and rate of healing was at least the same and in some cases superior in the NPWT-VAC study compared with previous studies of smaller, more superficial wounds may be important to consider and be worth further evaluation.

A frequent observation made by clinicians is that NPWT as delivered through the VAC therapy system appears to stimulate a rapid granulation tissue response compared to other available therapies (Plates 7 and 8): an observation strongly supported by the results of this recent study. While it has been difficult to measure in the past, the time to 100% granulation tissue may be an important clinical end point, as it is frequently the triggering event for further clinical decision making such as skin grafting, delayed closure or modification of dressing regime.

A number of questions pertaining to the clinical use of NPWT were posed at a recent consensus conference that focused entirely on diabetic foot wounds.[12] It was agreed that smaller wounds responding to debridement, appropriate offloading and standard care would not be suitable candidates for NPWT. Larger, deeper and, in view of more recent evidence,[6] post-surgical debridement or partial foot amputation wounds are most likely to benefit from NPWT. With respect to duration of NPWT treatment, this should generally be continued until there is a healthy granular bed. NPWT should not be applied to any wound prior to debridement, but can be applied after bypass surgery, provided there are no signs to suggest residual infection, necrotic tissue or active bleeding. Similarly, although NPWT is not a therapy for osteomyelitis, it can be used following surgical incision and drainage, provided that a period of observation (usually at least 24 h) occurs before the application of NPWT. Evidence also exists to support the use of NPWT on complex plantar wounds during outpatient management using removable offloading[13]: using a bridging technique to lead the tubing to the dorsum of the foot, NPWT did not result in any clinically significant increase in pressure while walking with the pressure-relief walker and the bridged NPWT *in situ*.

In conclusion, it appears that NPWT as delivered through the VAC therapy system may be an effective treatment for complex diabetic foot wounds. Treatment with this therapy seems to result in a higher proportion of wounds that heal, faster healing rates and potentially fewer re-amputations. Further randomised controlled trials using NPWT for other indications in the diabetic foot need to be planned with both primary and secondary end points. Secondary end points might include rates of healing, quality of life, pain reduction, cost of care, requirement for further procedures and the proportion of patients requiring further surgery/amputations.

REFERENCES

1. Banwell PE, Teot L. Topical negative pressure (TNP): the evolution of a novel wound therapy. *J Wound Care* 2003;12:22–28.
2. Armstrong DG, Boulton AJM, Banwell P. *Topical Negative Pressure: Management of Complex Diabetic Foot Wounds.* Oxford: Oxford Wound Healing Society; 2004.
3. Saxena V, Hwang CW, Huang S, Eichbaum Q, Ingber D, Orgill DP. Vacuum-assisted closure: microdeformations of wounds and cell proliferation. *Plast Reconstr Surg* 2004;114:1086–1096, discussion 1097–1098.
4. Evans D, Land L. Topical negative pressure for treating chronic wounds (Cochrane review). *Cochrane Database Syst Rev* 2001;1:CD001898.
5. Samson DJ, Lefevre F, Aronson N. Blue Cross and Blue Shield Association Technology Evaluation Center Evidence-Based Practice Center, under Contract No. 290-02-0026. Rockville, MD: Agency for Health Care Quality; 2004. (Publication No. 05-E005-2).
6. Armstrong DG, Lavery LA. Negative pressure wound after partial diabetic foot amputation: a multicentre, randomised controlled trial. *The Lancet* 2005;366:1704–1710.

7. Veves A, Sheehan P, Pham HT. A randomized, controlled trial of Promogran (a collagen/oxidized regenerated cellulose dressing) vs standard treatment in the management of diabetic foot ulcers. *Arch Surg* 2002;137:822–827.

8. Veves A, Falanga V, Armstrong DG, Sabolinski ML. Graftskin, a human skin equivalent, is effective in the management of noninfected neuropathic diabetic foot ulcers: a prospective randomized multicenter clinical trial. Apligraf Diabetic Foot Ulcer Study. *Diabetes Care* 2001;24:290–295.

9. Marston WA, Hanft J, Norwood P, Pollak R. The efficacy and safety of Dermagraft in improving the healing of chronic diabetic foot ulcers: results of a prospective randomized trial. *Diabetes Care* 2003;26:1701–1705.

10. Steed DL. Clinical evaluation of recombinant human platelet-derived growth factor for the treatment of lower extremity diabetic ulcers. Diabetic Ulcer Study Group. *J Vasc Surg* 1995;21:71–78.

11. Gentzkow GD, Iwasaki SD, Hershon KS. Use of Dermagraft, a cultured human dermis, to treat diabetic foot ulcers. *Diabetes Care* 1996;19:350–354.

12. Armstrong DG, Attinger CE, Boulton AJM, *et al.* Guidelines regarding negative pressure wound therapy in the diabetic foot: results of the Tucson Expert Consensus Conference. *Ostomy Wound Manage* 2004;50:3S–27S.

13. Armstrong DG, Kunze K, Martin BR, Kimbriel HR, Nixon BP, Boulton AJM. Plantar pressure changes using a novel negative pressure wound therapy technique. *J Am Podiatr Med Assoc* 2004;94:456–460.

32 The Diabetic Foot in Brazil

*Hermelinda Pedrosa, Andrew JM Boulton and
Maria Stela Oliveira Dias*

THE SITUATION OF DIABETES MELLITUS IN BRAZIL

The care of chronic diseases in Brazil had been restricted to cancer until the late 1980s, when the Ministry of Health decided to include the problems related to hypertension and diabetes mellitus (DM), besides aging, eye diseases and health promotion and prevention, in the National Division of Chronic Degenerative Disease. In 1988, as a first step to implement policies for DM, a national survey was conducted with the scientific support of the Brazilian Diabetes and Endocrinology societies, the National Council of Research (CNPq), the Pan-American Health Organization and the Juvenile Diabetes Association, to determine the prevalence of DM in the population between 30 and 69 years. As in many developing and newly industrialised countries, a high age-adjusted prevalence rate of 7.6% was found with the highest numbers in the most developed areas: São Paulo (9.7%) and Rio Grande do Sul (8.9%).[1] In line with other countries, the burden of DM is rising rapidly in Brazil: the current figure of nearly 5 million people with diabetes is expected to more than double by 2025 reaching nearly 12 million, when the country will be among the ten countries (Table 32.1) with the largest diabetic population in the world.

Following the National Diabetes Census, a programme for education and control of DM was then initiated by the Brazilian government, focusing on the organisation of diabetes care at university, public state and county hospitals with the main goal of linking them to the health centres. The establishment of diabetes teams at different skill levels (low, medium and high complex) aimed to cater for patients according to their type of diabetes, treatment and presence or absence of complications, with attention focused at retinopathy, nephropathy and neuropathy, in addition to cardiovascular disease.[3]

However, the late complications of neuropathy, including foot ulcers and amputations, received no emphasis, presumably as it was believed that such conditions were under surgical care (vascular and orthopaedic specialties). In Brasilia, the capital of Brazil, in the early 1990s, however, the first outpatient foot clinic was established, linked to the hospital diabetes staff according to approaches reported from the United States and the United Kingdom. The strategies were adapted to the reality of scarce resources and inaccessibility to health care, which are the main causes of amputations in developing countries, and even to poor knowledge of foot problems among health professionals at that time, who were mainly ignorant as to the correct management of ulcers.[4,5]

The Foot in Diabetes, 4th Edition. Editors Andrew J.M. Boulton, Peter R. Cavanagh and Gerry Rayman.
© 2006 John Wiley & Sons, Ltd.

Table 32.1 Diabetic population: current figures and estimates to 2025

Country	Estimates (2003) (in millions)	Country	Estimates (2025) (in millions)
India	31.5	India	79.4
China	20.8	China	42.3
United States	17.7	United States	30.3
Indonesia	8.4	Indonesia	21.3
Japan	6.8	Pakistan	21.1
Pakistan	5.2	*Brazil*	*11.3*
Russia	4.6	Bangladesh	11.1
Brazil	*4.6*	Japan	8.8
Italy	4.3	Phillipines	7.8
Bangladesh	3.2	Egypt	6.7

Note: Brazil has a high prevalence of diabetes mellitus, 7.6%, and current figures place it as the eighth largest diabetic population worldwide, but WHO has estimated it to double and reach the sixth position in 2025, as has been verified among other developing countries.[2] Copyright © 2004 American Diabetes Association. From Diabetes Care, Vol. 27, 2004; 11047–1053. Reprinted with permission from The American Diabetes Association.

Therefore, in order to circumvent this adverse situation, with the agreement of the local state health department and the coordination of the new national diabetes care programme, a project was designed based on the very well-known British experience of Manchester and London[6,7] and was named *Save the Diabetic Foot Project*, which received further support of both Brazilian Diabetes and Endocrinology scientific societies.[8]

SAVE THE DIABETIC FOOT PROJECT: INTRODUCING BRAZIL INTO THE FOOT CARE SCENE

The current lifetime incidence of foot ulcer, based on recent studies, may be as high as 25%,[9,10] and it has been well recognised that a multidisciplinary team, preventative policies and education of professionals, patients and carers can succeed in the reduction of foot problems, with a great impact on the dramatic costs of this devastating diabetic complication.[11–14] In Brazil, the data collection performed by the National Health System (*DataSUS*) registers neither amputation by causes nor foot ulcers: the available data on foot problems come from isolated hospital studies.[8] A similar problem is faced regarding costs: they derive from total numbers of diabetic complications requiring hospital treatment and are under-estimated, although considered high, comparing to private services: *DataSUS* reported the costs to be US$15.5 million in 2000.[15] Another difficulty concerning the care of foot problems in Brazil is the lack of podiatrists to set up specialist teams or even to provide basic care at health centres. This would have been an important barrier to start running the project, considering the crucial role of these professionals in the care and prevention of the diabetic foot.[16] Therefore, the initial approaches to deal with these obstacles, initially in Brasilia and later elsewhere, included the following:

1. to persuade the policymakers to understand huge impact of the problem particularly relating to health economics;

2. to train professionals in foot examination techniques and diabetic foot care at the hospital and health centres;

3. to implement a specialist diabetic foot clinic;

4. to spread the project to other Brazilian states.

The project was initially established in 1991 when the nurses were invited to educate patients and perform basic podiatry care, and in 1992 a weekly foot clinic was opened at the general diabetic and endocrine outpatient clinic at the hospital.[17] There were no sophisticated procedures, with the key message being the mandatory removal of shoes/sandals and socks in order to detect those at risk of foot problems. The success of the clinic was such that it soon accounted for 13% of all the annual appointments,[8,17] and professionals from other health centres also started to be trained to implement a foot network in the health district of Taguatinga, near Brasilia. In 1993, a better podiatric training was provided with the support of British and North American podiatrists during the first national foot workshop held in Brasilia and São Paulo, mainly based on the Malvern National Foot Conference in the United Kingdom.[18] It was then agreed that a 2-day foot workshop was the way of motivating professionals, when theoretical and practical activities were organised (Table 32.2). An intense participation of patients, who were willing to relate their own experience of dealing with deformities, amputation, ulcers and even difficulties to health care access for financial reasons and lack of resources, had a great impact among professionals who left the training period with enthusiasm and anticipated what it has been nowknown to be shared with professionals: a better holistic and psychological approach to diabetic patients with foot problems.[12,17–21]

Table 32.2 Foot workshops: materials and methods applied

Methods	Materials
Themes	Neurological and vascular tests
Epidemiology, social and economic	10-g monofilament
aspects of foot problems	Tuning fork 128 Hz
Pathophysiology: neuropathy,	Cottonwool
peripheral arterial disease, roles of	Pins
biomechanics on ulcer development	Hammer
Ulcer management	Handheld Doppler
Screening techniques	Monofilament, biosthesiometer (at the hospital only)
Biomechanics	Harris mat, Pressure stat® Goniometer
Basic podiatry	
Callus removal, superficial ulcer	Snippers
debridement	Scalpel
Nail care, dressings, hydration	Files, vegetable oils
Prevention	
Proper shoe, daily inspection	Education flowchart (based on the daily
Family and patient education	foot clinic activity)
Organisation of basic foot care	Practical Guidelines – International Consensus (from 1999)

Note: The themes for theoretical and practical activities have been adapted from the very successful foot workshops that took place in Malvern National Diabetic Foot Conference (United Kingdom), involving crucial issues to be discussed among health professionals, which have been enriched by diabetic patients' participation.[8]

EDUCATION AND SCREENING PROCEDURES

Identification of foot complications is the main step towards prevention, and this is a message for specialist and general clinicians who deal with diabetic patients. There are many reports on what to inquire about risk factors, and those most frequent as based on robust studies include previous history of ulcer and amputation, long duration of DM, poor glycaemic control, impaired vision, lack of education and inaccessibility to health care.[21,22] Concerning the physical examination, as peripheral neuropathy is the main permissive factor among the several causes of ulceration in the limbs,[23-26] one should also search for insensitivity, deformities (clawed- and hammer toes, bone prominences) and signs of high plantar pressure (hyperkeratosis, callus) besides evaluation of footwear conditions.[22]

There are no barriers to identifying the at-risk diabetic foot, and this has been the main message to the professionals who have learned how to apply simple techniques, which include the assessment of plantar protective sensation employing the 10-g monofilament[27,28,29]: this was used for the very first clinical activities after the project received financial support from the Brasilia branch of the Brazilian Endocrine Society, importing the instruments from Carville, United States. Years later, the local government and the Ministry of Health itself provided the health professionals, after their training during the national foot workshop sessions, with tuning forks, education flowchart and the monofilaments used by the leprosy programme. The participation of those professionals followed established criteria: a nurse and a doctor selected by each state health department or university would attend the training, and after returning to their services they would start the process of setting up basic foot outpatient clinics in their services and a further referral system following the model in Brasilia.[8,30]

In the past 4 years, the workshops have been linked to the scientific programmes of national meetings of Brazilian Diabetes and Endocrine societies with an active participation of well-known international speakers promoting the aim of saving the foot in the country: the success can be judged by the number of participants attending such meetings (Table 32.3). Meanwhile, some teams have come to Brasilia for a week for training at the diabetic foot centre and some are currently attached to the orthotic and prosthetic department.[8]

The increase in the number of basic foot clinics has been impressive, although simple and mostly on an outpatient basis. The latest estimates after the training in the Brazilian capital show how the scenario has changed: in 1992 there was only one foot clinic linked to the general diabetes clinic, and in 2005 the number reached 62 plus the foot centre in Brasilia (Figure 32.1), which has become a regional and national reference for the Ministry of Health.

Table 32.3 Project demonstration and workshop attendance: 1992–2005

Workshops	38
Workshop participants (n)	4035
National congress/regional meetings and seminars	21
National congress/regional meetings and seminars participants	4950
Total estimate	8985

Note: The foot workshops were first held in Brasilia and São Paulo (1993) when the first podiatrists from the United Kingdom and the United States helped to teach basic podiatry. Since that time, the workshops have been either held in Brasilia or more recently linked to scientific meetings of both diabetes and endocrine Brazilian societies (mean attendance: 100 per workshop; 200 per meeting).

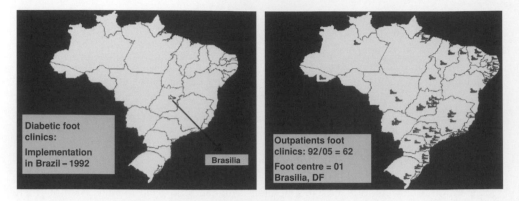

Figure 32.1　Brazilian foot clinics: spread from 1992 to 2005. The first basic foot clinic was set up in Brasília, in 1992, linked to the general diabetes outpatient clinic. Nowadays, there has been an impressive increase in the number of other outpatient foot clinics in the country, and the clinic in the Brazilian capital has become a foot centre and a national reference for training health professionals[8]

The north region (Amazonian), however, still represents a complex problem, which hopefully will be solved in the near future when those clinics will be re-evaluated by the Brazilian Diabetic Foot Task Force (BDFTF), a very important initiative of the National Coordination of Diabetes and Hypertension (Ministry of Health).

The project has been implementing the Practical Guidelines since the International Consensus was translated into Portuguese and distributed free of charge among all professionals trained on foot examination and care.[21] A pilot study was carried out involving the hospital and two health centres in Brasilia: of 82.3% of the 367 records analysed, 40.4% of the patients in hospital care and 26% of those in primary care were found to have loss of protective sensation.[31] Applying the International Consensus[21] risk category system, a remarkable finding was shown related to category 3 (previous amputation or ulcer): 57.7% at the hospital had had an ulcer in comparison with 9% at the health centres.[8,31] This demonstrated that the referral system is functioning, although the situation remains suboptimal for footwear, which is not provided either by the public or by the private health system. Individual analysis of all three centres verified that 35.8% of those attending the federal senate foot clinic, set up in 1999 to make the politicians more sensitive to DM problems, were found to have inadequate footwear, while it was verified that the patients from the hospital and health centre did not have appropriate footwear, 65.5% and 62.2% respectively, probably due to a lower socio-economic conditions.[32]

Another tool implemented by the project was a specially designed foot card (Figure 32.2) to be given to patients after being screened, which has proven to be useful at both hospital and health centres: the patients can keep it and show it at other services in a similar manner to what has been done with diabetes identification cards.[31,32]

ACHIEVEMENTS RELATED TO FOOT TEAM, AMPUTATION RATES AND INSOLE PROVISION

During the period 1992–2004, there have been encouraging developments in the Brasilia project, although many remain to be achieved: this relates to the development of a true interdisciplinary cooperation when compared to the basic team back in 1992. The vascular surgeons

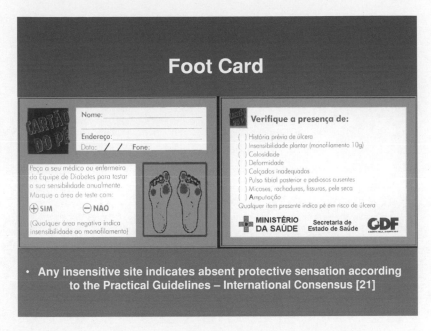

Figure 32.2 Foot card: a useful tool to identify patients screened for neuropathic ulcer risk. The foot card has been designed to be given to patients after being screened for foot problems, and it was based on the Practical Guidelines of the International Consensus.[21] The new original format[8] has been changed and the number of areas of tests for protective sensation is only three: hallux, first and fifth metatarsal heads

have become an integrated part and are now having daily clinics, as do the social workers. Other specialists regularly involved include dermatologists, infectious disease specialist, orthopaedists, orthotists, physiatrist, physiotherapists, plastic surgeons and psychiatrists.

An important link has been obtained with the extension of the project to the family health programme and other health districts, as there are six other outpatient foot clinics at those regional hospitals, which integrate the public health system of Brasilia.

A retrospective analysis performed at the hospital in Brasilia showed that 45% of the amputations in period 1989–1991 were registered among diabetic patients.[17] Evaluating data from 1992 to 2000, there was a trend towards reduction, with an overall decrease of 77.8%, with decrease particularly among female patients.[8] More recently, applying the Lower Extremity Amputation Study (LEAS) group protocol,[33] after the diabetic foot centre was inaugurated and linked to the orthotics and prosthetics department, a significant statistical difference between above-knee and below-knee amputations (Figure 32.3), with a trend towards reduction in the major procedures, has been found. The increase in the minor amputations was observed after the vascular team daily activities, which can be seen as good practice although increasing the overall number of amputations. The LEAS protocol is expected to be applied to other hospitals where surgical procedures have been carried out since the project implementation, to verify its overall impact among amputations.

The orthotists have joined the diabetic foot team in 1999 and have integrated well with the nurses on the team. The provision of free insoles in the early stages has increased significantly, as it is now not only involving hospital patients but encompassing all the other regional foot

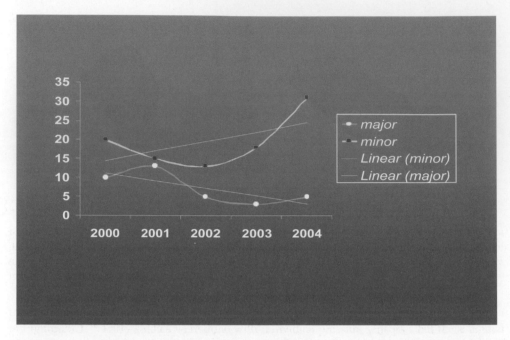

Figure 32.3   Amputation rate according to level of procedure
Note: Lower Extremity Amputation Study protocol and guidelines[33] on data collection were restricted to the reference hospital where the diabetic foot centre is based: a trend towards major amputation (above ankle) reduction and an increase in minor procedures (below ankle) has been verified

clinics of other health districts of Brasilia: from 198 (1999) it reached 1249 (2004), with a little decline to 1138 (2005) reaching a total of 6279 in the whole period (Figure 32.4).

PROBLEMS TO BE SOLVED

Despite many good achievements, many problems still exist. The project faces a low investigation and management of peripheral arterial disease: the more complex diagnosis or intervention that has been shown in recent studies in Rio de Janeiro[34] is difficult to achieve due to a lack of vascular surgeons and resources in many public hospitals. There is a need to re-evaluate the foot clinics in the country in order to provide them with a better structure and more qualified professionals, particularly concerning the implementation of casting clinics and including simple techniques to evaluate plantar pressures. An interesting study recently performed at the diabetic foot centre in the Brazilian capital compared Pressure stat® and Harris mat, showing the former to take significantly less time (1.70 min versus 2.61 min, $p < 0.05$) and to be able to evaluate the requirement of insoles with its pressure calibration card.[35] Extension of the links with the primary care and health family professionals in the rest of the country might be achieved with the inclusion of a foot workshop during the Diabetes and Hypertension National Training where nearly 4000 primary care health professionals are expected to be trained. The application of the International Consensus questionnaire might be a way to verify these issues and is expected to be in the agenda of the BDFTF with the support of the Ministry of Health

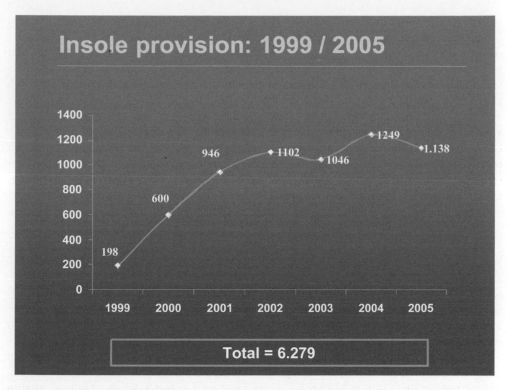

Figure 32.4 Free insole provision from the orthotic and prosthetic department. The insole provision was started in 1999 when the diabetic foot centre was inaugurated in Brasilia, linked to the orthotic and prosthetic department of the State Health Secretary. There has been an important increase in the number of free insoles given to the diabetic patients with either high plantar pressure or foot deformities[8]

in 2006. The provision of free insoles and prosthesis must be included in other state health departments as it has been done in Brasilia. Free customized footwear, at least for those with deformities, would represent a preventative approach, as it has been done in India,[36] and could be reached due to the abundance of leather in Brazil.

The links with the International Working Group on the Diabetic Foot since 1998 have represented a great opportunity to consolidate Brazil in the international scene, but throughout the period of its early steps the project has maintained an enriching scientific integration with the Manchester Diabetes Centre. Other academic links have been gathered with the Medical School and the Catholic University of Brasilia, which have both included medical and physiotherapy students[37] activities which may help future professionals to be more aware about the diabetic foot problems. The lack of podiatrists in the country is also an important issue to be resolved, and discussion has been conducted with well-known North American and British professionals for the possibility of a course in the near future.

The social deprivation and inaccessibility to health care does account for the difference between management in developed and underdeveloped countries.[8,37,38] During these 13 years of its activities, the Save the Diabetic Foot Project has made notable achievements that have contributed to change the concerning, perception and management of foot problems in the country.[8] No sophisticated plan was ever made, and the crucial approach for a country with scarce resources was education of health professionals involving general clinicians, specialists and nurses from distant Amazonian states, underdeveloped areas of north, northeast and centre-west to the more developed areas in the southeast and south of Brazil. It seems that the lesson of interdisciplinary management and prevention[6,7,12,13,39,40] has been learned by many of them, and this certainly will help to circumvent the difficulties still currently being faced. The scientific support of the Brazilian Diabetes and Endocrine societies plus the recent involvement in Clinical Guidelines Task Force of the International Diabetes Federation,[41] which is represented in the BTFDF, hopefully encouraged the diabetic foot not be seen as the Cinderella of all diabetic complications. The financial support of the Brazilian government through the Ministry of Health certainly will help the patients to be given the opportunity to receive a proper foot care.

REFERENCES

1. Malerbi D, Franco LJ, and the Brazilian Cooperative Group on the Study of Diabetes Prevalence. Multicentre study of the prevalence and impaired glucose tolerance in the urban population aged 30–69. *Diabetes Care* 1996;19:704–709.
2. Wild S, Roglic G, Green A, Sicree R, King H. Global prevalence of diabetes: estimates for the year 2000 and projections for 2030. *Diabetes Care* 2004;27:1047–1053.
3. *Manual de Diabetes*. Brasília: Ministério da Saúde; 1990. (ISBN 85-334-0031-4)
4. Gadsby R. The diabetic foot in primary care: a UK perspective. In: Boulton AJM, Connor H, Cavanagh PR, eds. *The Foot in Diabetes*. Chichester: Wiley; 2000:95–104.
5. Chaturvedi N, Stevens LK, Fuller JH, Lee ET, Lu M, and the WHO Multinational Study Group. Risk factors, ethnic differences and mortality associated with lower-extremity gangrene and amputation in diabetes. The WHO multinational study of vascular disease in diabetes. *Diabetologia* 2001; 44:S65–S71.
6. Thomson FJ, Veves A, Ashe H, *et al.* A team approach to diabetic foot care: the Manchester experience. *Foot* 1991;1:75–82.
7. Edmonds ME, Blundell MP, Morris ME, *et al.* Improved survival of the diabetic foot: the role of specialized foot clinic. *Q J Med* 1986;232:763–771.
8. Pedrosa HC, Leme LAP, Novaes C, *et al.* The diabetic foot in South America: progress with the Brazilian save the diabetic foot project. *Int Diabetes Monit* 2004;16:17–24.
9. Williams R, Airey M. The size of the problem: epidemiological and economic aspects of foot problems in diabetes. In: Boulton AJM, Connor H, Cavanagh PR, eds. *The Foot in Diabetes* 3rd edn. Chichester: Wiley; 2000:3–18.
10. International Working Group on the Diabetic Foot. Epidemiology of diabetic foot infections in a population based cohort. Paper presented at: International Consensus on the Diabetic Foot; May 22–24, 2003; Noordwijkerhout, the Netherlands.
11. Lavery LA, Armstrong DG, Wunderlich RP, Tredwell J, Boulton AJM. Diabetic foot syndrome: evaluating the prevalence and incidence of foot pathology in Mexican Americans and non-Hispanic whites from a diabetes disease management cohort. *Diabetes Care* 2003;26:1435–1438.
12. Boulton AJM. Why bother educating the multidisciplinary team and the patient – the example of prevention of lower extremity amputation in diabetes. *Patient Educ Couns* 1995;26:183–188.
13. Dargis V, Pantelejeva O, Jonushaite A, Vileikyte L, Boulton AJM. Benefits of a multidisciplinary approach in the management of recurrent diabetic foot ulceration in Lithuania. *Diabetes Care* 1999;22:1428–1431.
14. Pecoraro RE, Reiber GE, Burgess EM. Pathways to diabetic limb amputation: basis for prevention. *Diabetes Care* 1990;13:513–521.

15. *Campanha Nacional de Detecção de Suspeitos de Diabetes Mellitus – Março/Abril 2001*. Ministério da Saúde, Secretaria de Políticas de Saúde, Editora MS, Setembro; 2001.

16. Berry BL, Black JA. What is chiropody/podiatry? *Foot* 1992;2:59–60.

17. Pedrosa HC, Silva EM, Dias MSO, Farias LFCS, Miziara MDY. É possível salvar o Pé Diabético? (estudo-piloto do projeto Salvando o Pé Diabético). *Arq Bras Endocrinol Metabol* 1991;35:24.

18. Shaw J, Vileikyte L, Connor H, Boulton AJM. The diabetic foot 1994. *Diabet Med* 1995;12:88–90.

19. Vileikyte L. Psychological and behavioural issues in diabetic neuropathic foot ulceration. In: Boulton AJM, Connor H, Cavanagh PR, eds. *The Foot in Diabetes* 3rd edn. Chichester: Wiley; 2000:121–130.

20. Pedrosa HC, Lima LP. *Album Seriado Vamos Pegar no Pé*. Brasília: Ministério da Saúde; 1998. (ISBN 85-334-0158-2)

21. International Working Group on the Diabetic Foot. *International Consensus on the Diabetic Foot* (Brazilian version, translated by Pedrosa HC, Andrade AC). Brasilia: Secretaria de Estado de Saúde, Distrito Federal; 2001.

22. Singh N, Armstrong DG, Lipsky BC. Preventing foot ulcers in patients with diabetes. *JAMA* 2005;293:217–228.

23. Young MJ, Boulton AJM, Macleod AF, Williams DR, Sonksen PH. A multicentre study of the prevalence of diabetic peripheral neuropathy in the United Kingdom hospital population. *Diabetologia* 1993;36:150–154.

24. Reiber GE, Vileikyte L, Boyko ET, *et al.* Causal pathway for incident lower extremity ulcers in patients with diabetes from two settings. *Diabetes Care* 1999;22:157–162.

25. Young MJ, Breddy JL, Veves A, Boulton AJM. The prediction of diabetic neuropathic foot ulceration using vibration perception thresholds: a prospective study. *Diabetes Care* 1994;17:557–560.

26. Boulton AJM, Malik RA, Arezzo JC. Diabetic somatic neuropathies. *Diabetes Care* 2004;27:1458–1486.

27. Burden M. Providing a diabetes foot care service. In: Boulton AJM, Connor H, Cavanagh PR, eds. *The Foot in Diabetes* 3rd edn. Chichester: Wiley; 2000:73–80.

28. Gadsby R, McInnes A. The at risk foot: the role of the primary care team in achieving St Vincent targets for reducing amputation. *Diabet Med* 1998;15:S61–S64.

29. Kumar S, Fernando DJS, Veves A, Knowles EA, Young MJ, Boulton AJM. Semmes–Weinstein monofilaments: a simple, effective and inexpensive screening device for identifying diabetic patients at risk of foot ulceration. *Diabetes Res Clin Pract* 1991;13:63–68.

30. Pedrosa HC, Alves FS, Nery ES, *et al.* Current status of foot care: preliminary clinical audit – based on the International Consensus on the Diabetic Foot. Paper presented at: the DFSG Meeting (Diabetic Foot Study Group) of the European Association for the Study of Diabetes; 2001; Crieff, Scotland.

31. Pedrosa HC, Novaes C, Mendes V, *et al.* A ten year sensibilization saga on the diabetic foot: time to turn into a national (official) programme in Brazil. Paper presented at: the Joint Meeting of the Neurodiab (Diabetic Neuropathy Study Group of the EASD) and the DFSG (Diabetic Foot Study Group of the EASD), Balantonfured, Hungary; 2002:A10, 115.

32. Mendes VB, Novaes C, Santos EG, *et al.* Screening of patients for the at risk foot at the Federal Senate: an approach to make politicians more sensitive? (abstract) *Arq Bras Endocrinol Metabol* 2001;45:143.

33. The LEA Study Group. Comparing the incidence of lower extremity amputations across the world: the global lower extremity amputation study. *Diabet Med* 1995;12:14–18.

34. Spiechler ERS, Spiechler D, Martins CSF, Franco LJ, Lessa I. Health Ministry, Rio de Janeiro, Brazil. Diabetic lower extremities amputation – Rio de Janeiro, BR, 90–96 (abstract). *Diabetologia* Aug 1998;41:279.

35. Pedrosa HC, Gomes EB, Assis MA, *et al.* Is a mat just a mat? Paper presented at: Proceedings of the Diabetic Foot Study Group; 2005; Chalkidiki, Greece.

36. Viswanathan V, Madhavan S, Rajasekar S, Chamukuttan S, Amabady R. Amputation prevention initiative in South India: positive impact of foot care education. *Diabetes Care* 2005;28:1019–1021.

37. Gomes E, Leme L, Saigg M, Sena F, Pedrosa H, Boulton AJM. The diabetic foot as a physiotherapy training academic activity (abstract). *Diabetes* 2003;52:A507.
38. Ward J. Introduction: the diabetic foot – the good news, the bad news. In: Boulton AJM, Connor H, Cavanagh PR, eds. *The Foot in Diabetes* 3rd edn. Chichester: Wiley; 2000;01–02.
39. Boulton AJM. Lowering the risk of neuropathy, foot ulcers and amputations. *Diabet Med* 1998; 15:S57–S59.
40. Boulton AJM. The diabetic foot: from art to science. *Diabetologia* 2004;47:1343–1353.
41. International Diabetes Federation. *Global Guidelines for Type 2 Diabetes*. Clinical Guidelines Task Force, International Diabetes Federation; 2005.

33 Recent International Developments: India

V. Viswanathan

Diabetes mellitus is recognised to be common in Indians in the Asian subcontinent, and currently 25 million Indians have diabetes. The projections indicate that India will have the largest number of diabetic patients by the year 2025.

Epidemiological studies among migrant Asian Indians in many countries showed a higher prevalence of type 2 diabetes compared with the host populations and other migrant ethnic groups.[1] Studies conducted in India in the last decade have highlighted that not only the prevalence of type 2 diabetes is high, but also it is increasing rapidly in the urban population.[2,3] Diabetes develops at a younger age in Indians, i.e. at least a decade or two earlier than in the Western population.[4,5]

An urban–rural difference in the prevalence rate was found, indicating that the environmental factors related to urbanisation had a significant role in increasing the prevalence of diabetes.[6] The prevalence of diabetes in the urbanising rural population was found to be midway between the rural and urban populations.[7]

EPIDEMIOLOGY OF DIABETIC FOOT INFECTION IN INDIA

In India, the prevalence of diabetic foot ulcers in clinic population was estimated to be 3.6%.[8] Socio-cultural practices such as barefoot walking and certain religious practices, use of improper footwear and lack of knowledge regarding foot care contributes towards increase in the prevalence of foot complications in India.[9]

Costs are substantially higher for those who develop foot ulcers. In a study from southern India, it was found that patients without foot problems spent 9.3% of the total income, while patients with foot problem had to spend 32.3% of the total income towards treatment.[10] This huge challenge imposed by diabetic foot problem calls for prevention and effective management at initial stages of the complication.

PATHOPHYSIOLOGY OF FOOT INFECTION IN INDIA

A retrospective study[11] to evaluate the clinical profile of diabetic foot infection showed that the recurrence of foot infections was common among south Indian type 2 diabetic patients.

The Foot in Diabetes, 4th Edition. Editors Andrew J.M. Boulton, Peter R. Cavanagh and Gerry Rayman.
© 2006 John Wiley & Sons, Ltd.

Of 374 patients, 198 (53%) patients had recurrence of foot infection (relapsers) and had to be hospitalised again. The relapsers had a higher prevalence of peripheral vascular disease (PVD) and neuropathy than the non-relapsers.

A multicentric and multinational study[12] among 613 type 2 diabetic patients from Tanzania, Germany and India was conducted to determine the differences in underlying risk factors and clinical presentation of foot problems. It was found that PVD was frequent in Germany, while in Tanzania and India it was far less common. The lower prevalence in India was probably due to younger age of the patients, shorter diabetes duration, lower proportion of smokers and ethnicity-related factors. A lesser prevalence of PVD but a higher prevalence of amputation was noted among Indians when compared with those in Western countries, which was related to progressive infection.

It has been reported that smoking is associated with higher prevalence of foot problems in diabetic subjects.[13] Patients who wore footwear both inside and outside their homes developed lesser foot problems than those who wore footwear only when they went outside.

Limited joint mobility (LJM) and foot pressure were measured in 345 subjects, of whom 295 had diabetes and the remaining 50 were non-diabetic controls.[14] It was observed that the joint mobility at the ankle and at the big toe was significantly reduced in the diabetic patients when compared with controls. Among the diabetic patients, those with neuropathy and those with a history of foot ulcer had significantly lower joint mobility. LJM and increased foot pressure appear to be important determinants of foot ulcerations in south Indian diabetic subjects.

INITIATIVES TO MANAGE THE BURDEN OF DIABETIC FOOT IN INDIA

Considering the high rate of diabetic foot infections and the economic burden imposed by the same, there is an urgent need for preventive foot care in India. It was found necessary to form an apex body to formulate strategies to address the following deficiencies:

- no concept of diabetes foot care;

- no trained personnel;

- no standards for podiatry care;

- no structured curriculum and educational inputs to develop a cadre of podiatrists.

In order to improve the awareness about diabetic foot among health care professionals, podiatry workshops were conducted in seven cities of India, between April 2000 to December 2001.

The Diabetic Foot Society of India (DFSI) was formed in March 2002. The formation of the DFSI was an important step in improving diabetic foot care in India. It is a forum where surgeons, diabetologists and nurses come together for a common cause of tackling the problem of diabetic foot amputations in India.

In an Amputation Prevention Initiative[15] in south India, it was shown that strategies like intensive management and foot care education were helpful in preventing recurrent problems and surgery. Type 2 diabetic patients with high-risk foot were selected for the study. Ulcers present during the recruitment had healed in 81% subjects who followed the advice, whereas among the non-adherent subjects, complete healing occurred only in 49%. A significantly larger proportion of subjects who did not follow the advice developed newer problems (26%) and required surgical procedures (13%), when compared with those who followed the advice (7 and 3%, respectively).

DEVELOPMENT OF DIAGNOSTIC AND WOUND MANAGEMENT TOOLS

In India, vibration perception threshold (VPT) measurement is seldom done due to higher cost of the imported biothesiometer. An indigenous biothesiometer was developed in India, which has a good specificity and sensitivity.[16] The cost of the equipment is low.

FOOTWEAR

Until recently, the footwear made of microcellular rubber (MCR) prescribed for patients with leprosy was provided to diabetic patients. These MCR footwears were not liked by many patients due to the stigma attached with leprosy. In a prospective study,[17] patients were randomly assigned to wear either their own footwear or therapeutic footwear made of some indigenously available insole materials. After 9 months, re-ulceration occurred only in 4% of the therapeutic footwear group versus 32% in the control group. Acceptance of this footwear is better, compared to the MCR footwear, and the cost of each pair is also affordable to most patients ($12).

CONCLUSION

The staggering human and economic costs of diabetes foot disease may be reduced significantly by several simple preventive measures designed to prevent foot ulcers and lower extremity amputations in developing countries. The key elements of preventive care practised in India include: annual examination of the feet by health care providers to determine risk factors for ulceration, subsequent examination of high-risk feet at each patient visit, patient education about daily self-care of the feet and careful diabetes management.

REFERENCES

1. Zimmet PZ. Diabetes epidemiology as a tool to trigger diabetes research and care. *Diabetologia* 1999;42:499–518.
2. Mohan V, Shanthirani S, Deepa R, Premalatha G, Sastry NG, Saroja R. Intra-urban differences in the prevalence of the metabolic syndrome in southern India – the Chennai Urban Population Study (CUPS No. 4). *Diabet Med* 2001;18:280–287.
3. Verma NPS, Madhu SV. Prevalence of known diabetes in urban east Delhi. 17th International Diabetes Federation Congress, Mexico City. *Diabetes Res Clin Pract* 2000;50:515.
4. Ramachandran A, Snehalatha C, Kapur A, *et al.* High prevalence of diabetes and impaired glucose tolerance in India – National Urban Diabetes Survey (NUDS). *Diabetologia* 2001;44:1094–1101.

5. UK Prospective Diabetes Study Group. UK Prospective Diabetes Study XII: differences between Asian, Afro-Caribbean and white Caucasian type 2 diabetic patients at diagnosis of diabetes. *Diabet Med* 1994;11:670–677.
6. Ramachandran A, Snehalatha C, Daisy D, Viswanathan M. Prevalence of glucose intolerance in Asian Indians. Urban–rural difference and significance of upper body adiposity. *Diabetes Care* 1992;15:1348–1355.
7. Ramachandran A, Snehalatha C, Latha E, Manoharan M, Vijay V. Impacts of urbanization on the life style and on the prevalence of diabetes in native Asian Indian population. *Diabetes Res Clin Pract* 1999;44:207–213.
8. Pendsey SP. Epidemiological aspects of diabetic foot. *Int J Diabetes Dev Countries* 1994;14:37–38.
9. Vijay V, Snehalatha C, Ramachandran A. Socio-cultural practices that may affect the development of the diabetic foot. *IDF Bull* 1997;42:10–12.
10. Shobhana R, Rama Rao P, Lavanya A, Vijay V, Ramachandran A. Cost burden to diabetic patients with foot complications – a study from Southern India. *J Assoc Physicians India* 2000;48:1147–1150.
11. Vijay V, Narasimham A, Seena R, Snehalatha C, Ramachandran A. Clinical profile of diabetic foot infections in South India – a retrospective study. *Diabet Med* 2000;17:215–218.
12. Morbach S, Lutale JK, Viswanathan V, *et al*. Regional differences in risk factors and clinical presentation of diabetic foot lesions. *Diabet Med* 2003;21:91–95.
13. Vijay V, Seena R, Snehalatha C, Ramachandran A. Routine foot examination: the first step towards prevention of diabetic foot amputation. *Pract Diabetes Int* 2000;17:112–114.
14. Vijay V, Snehalatha C, Sivagami M, Seena R, Ramachandran A. Association of limited joint mobility and high plantar pressure in diabetic foot ulceration in Asian Indians. *Diabetes Res Clin Pract* 2003;60:57–61.
15. Vijay V, Sivagami M, Seena R, Snehalatha C, Ramachandran A. Amputation prevention initiative in south India: a positive impact of foot care education. *Diabetes Care* 2005;28:1019–1021.
16. Vijay V, Sanjeev K, Kelkar DK, Seena R, Ramachandran A. Validation of indigenously made biothesiometer. *Asian J Diabetol* 2003;5:13–14.
17. Vijay V, Sivagami M, Saraswathy G, *et al*. Effectiveness of different types of footwear insoles for the diabetic neuropathic foot. *Diabetes Care* 2004;27:474–477.

34 Recent International Developments: Africa

Zulfiqarali G. Abbas and Lennox K. Archibald

The incidence of diabetes mellitus is increasing in populations across Africa; a parallel increase in the number of foot ulcers in these populations has been documented. Data from Tanzania suggest that these increases might partly be associated with urbanisation. Although most published reports from Africa suggest that foot ulcers generally are associated with underlying peripheral neuropathy, recent data from Tanzania established that peripheral vascular disease might be playing a more substantial role in ulcer causation than was previously thought. Other data from Tanzania indicate that ulcers due to both neuropathy and vascular disease (i.e. neuroischaemia) are increasingly being seen. Factors associated with poor outcomes include delays in seeking medical attention, neuroischaemia or ulcers that have progressed to gangrene at presentation. Key prevention measures include regular feet inspection, minimisation of barefoot walking, stopping the treatment of callosities at home with sharps and avoidance of delays in seeking medical attention for foot lesions, however minor.

INTRODUCTION

Diabetes mellitus has now become a major public health problem in underdeveloped countries: on the African continent the number of people with diabetes is projected to be more than double by 2025.[1] An association with urbanisation is suggested by data from Tanzania, where the prevalence of diabetes in urban areas is estimated at 12.2% versus 1% in rural areas.[1] Foot complications now constitute a major public health problem among diabetic patients: 40–60% of non-traumatic lower limb amputations are performed on patients with diabetes.[2–9] Most published reports confirm that foot lesions in African diabetic patients are associated with peripheral neuropathy, commonly have an infectious aetiology and result in prolonged hospital stays and substantial morbidity or mortality.[2–8, 10–12]

PATHOPHYSIOLOGY OF FOOT ULCERS

The pathophysiology of diabetic foot lesions is complex and multifactorial. Contributory factors include peripheral neuropathy, peripheral vascular disease, infection, biomechanics and local trauma. The pattern of foot ulcer occurrence depends on the varying degrees of contribution of each of these factors. For example, ulcers may be secondary to both ischaemia and neuropathy (so-called mixed types of neuroischaemic ulcers).

Peripheral Neuropathy

Peripheral neuropathy is one of the most common complications affecting diabetic patients in both developed and less-developed nations.[2] The resulting loss of sensation in the feet invariably leads to sequelae that include callosities, cracked soles, breakdown of skin or non-discernable injuries, such as burns or rat bites. These complications can result in foot ulcers, which can progress to infection, necrosis, gangrene, loss of the limb or death.

The prevalence of peripheral neuropathy in diabetic populations across Africa has been documented in several studies and range from 6 to 84% (Table 34.1).[13] In a major study performed in Tanzania, Abbas *et al.* found no differences in the rates of peripheral neuropathy among African (80%) and Asian (81%) diabetic patients with ulcers.[10] In another comparative study, Abbas and colleagues found no significant differences in the prevalence of neuropathy in patients with foot ulcers from Tanzania (82%), Germany (78%) and India (82%).[11]

Peripheral Vascular Disease

Although relatively common in industrialised countries, peripheral vascular disease is not a common cause of gangrene in the lower limb of diabetic patients in Africa. In the three-nation study cited above, Abbas *et al.* found that the occurrence of peripheral vascular disease in diabetic patients from Germany was significantly higher (48%) than comparable populations in India (13%) or Tanzania (12%).[11] Because communities across Africa are becoming more urbanised, the prevalence rates of peripheral vascular disease in diabetic populations are increasing in some of these regions, ranging from 1 to 79% (Table 34.2).[13]

Abbas *et al.* established that rates of peripheral vascular disease in Tanzania varied by ethnicity, with rates of 26 and 34% in African and Asian patients, respectively.[10] Moreover, they also showed that peripheral vascular disease might be playing a more substantial role in the causation of foot ulcers in African diabetic patients than was previously thought.[10] Likely reasons for this include increased urbanisation and adoption of behaviours and diets from the West.

Neuroischaemia

Neuroischaemia occurs in patients with both peripheral neuropathy and vascular disease and is characterised by pain at rest, ulceration on the margins of the foot resulting from localised pressure necrosis, or digital necrosis or gangrene. Infection often complicates ulceration in both the neuropathic and the neuroischaemic foot. Abbas *et al.* have documented a 17.5% prevalence rate of neuroischaemic lesions among diabetic patients in Tanzania.[4] Other published data confirm that despite a low prevalence rate of peripheral vascular disease in African diabetic patients with foot ulcers, amputation is a frequent outcome and is generally attributed to neuroischaemic lesions or progressive infection.[4]

Table 34.1 Literature review of peripheral neuropathy rates across the African continent

Publication year	Author	Country	No. of patients	Prevalence of peripheral neuropathy (%)
2003	Moulik *et al.*	Zambia	185	61
2000	Abbas *et al.*	Tanzania	200	25.5
2000	Benotmane *et al.*	Algeria	132	84.4
1999	Kadiki *et al.*	Libya	8922	45.7
1997	Wikbald *et al.*	Tanzania	153	28.1
1997	Levitt *et al.*	South Africa	300	27.6
1996	Nambuya *et al.*	Uganda	252	46.4
1995	Lester	Ethiopia	43	50
1995	Gill *et al.*	South Africa	64	42
1995	Elbagir *et al.*	Sudan	128	37.5
1993	Lester	Ethiopia	1386	10.5
1992	Lester	Ethiopia	431	8
1991	Lester	Ethiopia	121	36.4
1991	Friend *et al.*	Malawi	100	59
1991	Elmahdi *et al.*	Sudan	413	31.5
1990	Akanji *et al.*	Nigeria	50	68
1989	Elmahdi *et al.*	Sudan	448	28.1
1988	Rolfe	Zambia	600	31.2
1987	McCance *et al.*	South Africa	118	11.9
1984	Omar *et al.*	South Africa	133	21.7
1984	Lester	Ethiopia	847	9.4
1984	Gill *et al.*	South Africa	475	5.9
1983	Lester	Ethiopia	105	46.7
1980	Mhando *et al.*	Tanzania	139	32.4
1977	Morley *et al.*	South Africa	170	50
1976	Adetuyibi	Nigeria	52	69.6
1971	Osuntokum *et al.*	Nigeria	832	49.2
1970	Belcher	Ethiopia	94	47
1968	Greenwood *et al.*	Nigeria	240	58.3
1964	Haddock *et al.*	Tanzania	116	31
1964	Goodall *et al.*	Malawi	90	6
1963	Kinnear *et al.*	Nigeria	309	33.3
1963	Gelfand *et al.*	Zimbabwe	99	4
1961	Gelfand *et al.*	Zimbabwe	150	6

Table 34.1 was adapted from Ref. 13. Permission to use Table 34.1 was granted by International Scientific Literature, Inc., publishers of the *Medical Science Monitor*.

FOOT ULCERATION IN AFRICA

A recent outcomes study in Tanzania showed that 15% of diabetic patients admitted to the inpatient medical service of the largest hospital in the country have foot ulcers – 80% of these ulcers were first-time occurrences.[4] Moreover, the highest inpatient mortality rate has been documented in diabetic patients with severe foot ulcers, who do not undergo amputation of

Table 34.2   Literature review of peripheral vascular disease rates across the African continent

Publication year	Author	Country	No. of patients	Prevalence of peripheral vascular disease (%)
2003	Moulik et al.	Zambia	185	41
2002	Abbas et al.	Tanzania	92	21
2000	Benotmane et al.	Algeria	132	78.7
2000	Abbas et al.	Tanzania	200	12.5
1997	Wikbald et al.	Tanzania	153	12.5
1997	Levitt et al.	South Africa	300	8.2
1995	Lester	Ethiopia	43	11.6
1995	Elbagir et al.	Sudan	128	10
1991	Friend et al.	Malawi	100	15
1991	Elmahdi et al.	Sudan	413	3.4
1990	Akanji et al.	Nigeria	50	54
1989	Elmahdi et al.	Sudan	448	6.2
1988	Rolfe	Zambia	600	1.7
1987	McCance et al.	South Africa	118	10.2
1984	Lester	Ethiopia	847	0.9
1984	Gill et al.	South Africa	475	2.1
1980	Mhando et al.	Tanzania	139	2.9
1971	Osuntokun et al.	Nigeria	832	4.4
1970	Belcher	Ethiopia	94	1.1
1968	Greenwood et al.	Nigeria	240	1.7
1963	Gelfand et al.	Zimbabwe	99	0

Table 34.2 was adapted from Ref. 13. Permission to use Table 34.2 was granted by International Scientific Literature, Inc., publishers of the *Medical Science Monitor*.

the relevant limb.[4] Specific factors contributing to development of diabetic foot ulcers include walking barefoot or delays in seeking medical attention for seemingly innocuous foot lesions. Poverty and absence of access to health care certainly underscore foot ulceration in African diabetic populations. For diabetic patients living at or below the poverty level, the purchase of appropriate footwear might not be feasible or of high priority (barefoot walking, a common practice in rural communities in Africa, is commonly associated with low income but may be cultural as well).[2]

Abbas et al. have recorded some unusual examples of foot ulcerations among attendees at their outpatient clinic in Dar es Salaam – in particular, patients with peripheral neuropathy were found to be at risk of acquiring rodent bites on their feet; diabetic rather than non-diabetic patients appear to be singled out by rodents.[12] For diabetic patients with peripheral neuropathy, such trauma or injuries might go unnoticed until the patient finally becomes symptomatic and presents to the diabetes clinic with an ulcer or injury that has progressed to fulminating foot sepsis.

Although patients who neither take the time to take care of themselves and address foot care nor attend the diabetes outpatient clinic for follow-up or education are most at risk of developing infected foot ulcers, lack of sensation in the anaesthetic foot may cause ordinarily conscientious and responsible patients to be unaware of injuries sustained through inappropriate

Table 34.3 Non-ulcerative pathology leading to foot ulcers among patients attending the diabetes clinic, Muhimbili National Hospital, Dar es Salaam, Tanzania

Complications	Frequency ($n = 200$)	%
Dry skin	79	39.5
Callus	68	34.0
Fungal infection	66	33.0
Onycholysis	65	32.5
Cracked skin on sole	31	15.5
Corns	14	7.0
Scabies	4	2.0
Ingrowing toenail	1	0.5

or ill-fitting footwear, to walk barefoot on hot asphalt under the midday sun or to use keratolytic agents or razor blades to treat callosities.[2] Any foot lesion, however innocuous it may appear, should never be disregarded.[9] Ostensibly minor lesions can progress to an ulcer and provide an entry point for rapidly ascending infection. In a study of patients with symptomatic peripheral neuropathy in Tanzania, non-ulcerative sequelae included dry skin, callosities, fungal infection or onycholysis (Table 34.3).[2]

FOOT INFECTION

Diabetic foot infections usually begin in ulcers that are sequelae of existing neuropathy, macrovascular disease or certain metabolic disturbances.[14] Such infections have been shown to be the immediate cause of foot or leg amputation in 25–50% of diabetic patients and may result in death.[9] In Tanzania, Abbas *et al.* have described a population of diabetic patients with infected ulcers who have neither neuropathy nor vascular disease.[3,4] Typically, these patients are young adults with type 1 diabetes, who were diagnosed during their initial presentation to the outpatient clinic with infected feet. The pathogenesis of these infections usually starts with a non-specific injury, followed by breakdown of skin and spread of infection to deeper tissue layers.

Patients in African communities often present to hospital only after the onset of gangrene or during a stage of sepsis that might be intractable to conventional supportive treatment.[2–6,12] Because patients with infected ulcers often feel no pain because of neuropathy, or may have no systemic symptoms until late in the course of the condition, medical providers often presume (incorrectly) a degree of self-neglect among affected patients. Fungal infection of toenails or in the intertriginous areas may lead to cracked skin or fissures on the soles of the feet. This type of infection produces relatively slight discomfort, but its real importance lies in the fact that these lesions pave the way for the entry of microorganisms into the foot, leading to secondary bacterial infection.[2] It is not surprising, therefore, that foot infections are especially common where there are no available services for follow-up of the diabetic foot, or lesions are ignored or detected relatively late in the course of the infection after unsuccessful home therapy, such as soaking in hot water, or application of unproven herbal remedies prescribed by traditional healers. Foot infections of this nature culminate in the onset of gangrene or disseminated infection with ensuing amputation of the foot or entire limb, or death from overwhelming sepsis.

MORTALITY

Abbas and colleagues ascertained clinical correlates for mortality among diabetic patients with foot ulcers in Tanzania. They found that overall mortality rate among patients with foot ulcers was 27% and was significantly higher among patients who had peripheral vascular disease, neuroischaemia or non-healing ulcers.[4] In addition, patients with foot ulcers that had progressed to gangrene (Wagner score ≥4) were significantly more likely to die, compared with patients with ulcers of Wagner score <4. Patients with ulcers of Wagner score ≥4 were more likely to have delayed presentation to hospital from the time of onset of the foot ulcer.[4] In the same study, the highest mortality rate (54%) was observed among patients with ulcers of Wagner severity score ≥4, who did not undergo surgery.[4]

AMPUTATION

Gangrene and infection appear to be the most commonly cited indications for foot amputation in diabetic patients.[9] However, the true lower limb amputation rate resulting from foot infections in African diabetic patients remains underestimated.[3,4,9,14] The non-healing ulcer is not generally considered an indication for amputation except in certain instances where patients have developed chronic osteomyelitis.[14,15] In Tanzania, neither peripheral vascular disease nor microvascular disease appears to be an important factor for surgeons when making the decision to operate.[3,4] The importance of delayed presentation to hospital is underscored by the fact that 10% of patients who needed and had agreed to undergo surgery died from advanced sepsis before the planned surgical procedure was actually carried out.[3,4]

PREVENTION

The two most significant risk factors for foot complications are social deprivation and limited access to health care. Motivation, education and action by diabetic patients are essential for protecting the feet from complications. In industrialised countries, numerous clinical studies have demonstrated that special diabetic foot clinics reduce the incidence of serious foot problems and that patient education results in unequivocal reduction in the occurrence of ulcers and amputations among diabetic patients. In contrast, relatively little outcomes research has been performed to study the effectiveness of various primary and secondary interventions in the prevention of diabetic foot ulcers or infection in Africa.

The golden rules of prevention are maintenance of glycaemic control to prevent or delay the onset of peripheral neuropathy, podiatric care that includes regular feet inspection, making an effort not to walk barefooted or cut foot callosities with razors or knives at home and avoidance of delays in presenting to hospital when a foot lesion, however minor, has developed. These simple rules, if followed, will go a long way in reducing adverse events associated with the diabetic foot in Africa.

CONCLUSION

While it may be impossible to totally prevent foot ulceration, it is certainly feasible to prevent the progression of small ulcers to infection, sepsis, osteomyelitis or gangrene. Education remains the most important preventive tool in Africa and should be an integral part of preventive programmes: simple and repetitive, and targeted at both health care workers and patients alike. Diabetic patients must be educated on the importance of foot care and of consulting a doctor during the early stages of foot-related symptoms. Ultimately, success will depend on the ability of health care providers to inculcate the motivation and self-help that are essential for the well-being of diabetic patients.

REFERENCES

1. International Diabetes Federation. *Diabetes Atlas*. 2nd edn. Brussels, Belgium: International Diabetes Federation; 2003.
2. Abbas ZG, Archibald LK. Foot complications in diabetes patients with symptomatic peripheral neuropathy in Dar es Salaam, Tanzania. *Diabetes Int* 2000;10:52–56.
3. Abbas ZG, Gill GV, Archibald LK. The epidemiology of diabetic limb sepsis: an African perspective. *Diabet Med* 2002;19:895–899.
4. Abbas ZG, Lutale JK, Morbach S, Archibald LK. Clinical outcome of diabetes patients hospitalised with foot ulcers, Dar es Salaam, Tanzania. *Diabet Med* 2002;19:575–579.
5. Dagogo-Jack S. Pattern of diabetic foot ulcer in Port Harcourt, Nigeria. *Pract Diabetes Dig* 1991;2:75–78.
6. Akanji AO, Famuyiwa OO, Adetuyibi A. Factors influencing the outcome of treatment of foot lesions in Nigerian patients with diabetes mellitus. *Q J Med* 1989;73:1005–1014.
7. Rolfe M, Tanga CM, Walker RW, Bassey E, George M. Diabetes mellitus in the Gambia, West Africa. *Diabet Med* 1992;9:484–488.
8. McLarty DG, Pollitt C, Swai ABM. Diabetes in Africa. *Diabet Med* 1990;7: 670–684.
9. International Working Group on the Diabetic Foot. *International Consensus on the Diabetic Foot*. Amsterdam, The Netherlands; 1999. (ISBN 90-9012716-X). Available at: www.iwgdf.org. Accessed Mar 4, 2006.
10. Abbas ZG, Lutale JK, Archibald LK, and the Tanzania Diabetic Ulcer Surveillance System (TANDUSS). Epidemiology of foot ulcers in Tanzania: a contrast between African and Asian diabetes populations. *Diabetologia* 2002;45:1042.
11. Morbach S, Lutale J, Viswanathan V, *et al*. Regional variation of risk factors and clinical presentation of diabetic foot lesions. *Diabet Med* 2004;21:91–95.
12. Abbas ZG, Lutale J, Archibald LK. Rodent bites on the feet of diabetes patients in Tanzania. *Diabet Med* 2005;22:631–633.
13. Abbas ZG, Archibald LK. Epidemiology of the diabetic foot in Africa. *Med Sci Monit* 2005;11: RA262–RA270.
14. Larsson J, Apelqvist J. Towards less amputations in diabetic patients. *Acta Orthop Scand* 1995; 66:181–192.
15. Cavanagh P, Ulbrecht J, Gregory M. The non-healing diabetic foot wound: fact or fiction? *Ostomy Wound Manage* 1998;44:6–12.

35 The International Consensus on the Diabetic Foot

N.C. Schaper and K. Bakker

INTRODUCTION

More than 200 million people in the world have diabetes mellitus, and too many of these subjects suffer from diabetic foot ulcers, which may eventually lead to an amputation (Table 35.1).[1] Given the high costs associated with these ulcers, this disorder is a major burden not only to the patient but also to the health care system.[2,3] Although the pathways to ulceration and amputation do not differ throughout the world, the prevalence of ulcers and amputations varies markedly between different countries.[4–6] These differences probably reflect variations in population characteristics and wound management strategies across geographic regions.[5–7] Usually, several mechanisms are involved simultaneously, stressing the need for a patient-oriented, multidisciplinary, approach to reduce the number of ulcerations, amputations and associated health care costs.[8–10] Furthermore, a well-structured organisation with facilities for providing diabetic foot care should be present.[11] For such an approach to be useful, concerted action by all persons working with diabetic subjects is required, and specific guidelines are needed to realise uniformity in diabetic foot care.[4] Unfortunately, lack of awareness, knowledge and skills by both patients and health care providers still results in insufficient prevention and management in too many patients.[12]

THE INTERNATIONAL WORKING GROUP ON THE DIABETIC FOOT

In the last decade, guidelines on prevention and management of the diabetic foot have been formulated in several countries. However, differences in specialists involved, aims and target groups resulted in different documents. Furthermore, in several countries, the diabetic foot is not on the agenda of the policymakers in health care, and arguments are needed to reallocate resources. Clearly, there was a need for an international consensus, which could be the starting point for the formulation of guidelines in different countries or geographical areas. Also, from quite a different field, a need for consensus was expressed. The number of scientists involved in research in the diabetic foot is steadily increasing, but in several areas different definitions of items such as an ulcer, osteomyelitis, 'severe' or 'mild' ischaemia were used by different

The Foot in Diabetes, 4th Edition. Editors Andrew J.M. Boulton, Peter R. Cavanagh and Gerry Rayman.
© 2006 John Wiley & Sons, Ltd.

Table 35.1   Foot facts[12]

- One in every six people with diabetes will have a foot ulcer during his/her lifetime.
- Every year, 4 million people with diabetes will develop a foot ulcer.
- Every 30 seconds a leg is lost due to diabetes, somewhere in the world.
- Foot problems are the most common cause of admission to hospital, for people with diabetes.
- In developing countries, foot problems may account for up to 40% of health care resources.
- The direct cost of an amputation is estimated to be between US$30 000 and US$60 000.
- Ulcers can be prevented, and up to 85% of amputations can be avoided.

---

specialists involved.[13] Moreover, several ulcer classification systems have been promoted, but no system has found universal acceptance. This lack of common language and a common ulcer classification system hampers both the formulation of unambiguous guidelines for daily practice and the uniform reporting of scientific data. To fulfill these needs, the International Consensus on Guidelines of the Diabetic Foot has been developed by a group of independent experts, in close association with several international organisations involved in the care of subjects with diabetes mellitus.

The International Working Group on the Diabetic Foot (IWGDF) coordinates the production of consensus documents. This worldwide organisation was instituted in 1996 and is, since 2000, also the Consultative Section on the Diabetic Foot of the International Diabetes Federation (IDF). Currently, 82 countries from all continents are represented in this unique multidisciplinary team of experts on the diabetic foot, including general practitioners, diabetologists, podiatrists, diabetic nurses and general, vascular and orthopaedic surgeons. Since its creation, the IWGDF has produced 'The International Consensus on the Diabetic Foot' in 1999 and three supplements in 2003 on infection, classification and wound healing.[14-16] During the three meetings of the IWGDF, in 1997, 1998 and in 2003, the consensus process, the documents produced and the implementation of the guidelines were discussed. Moreover, several working groups on specific topics have met more frequently under the guidance of an editorial board. All materials produced by the IWGDF can be ordered at the IDF office in Brussels, Belgium.

THE INTERNATIONAL CONSENSUS ON THE DIABETIC FOOT (1999)

The aim of the 1999 consensus document was to provide guidelines for prevention and treatment that will reduce the impact of diabetic foot disease, with consideration of costs and using the principles of evidence-based medicine (Table 35.2).[4] In the document, the basic concepts

Table 35.2   Documents produced by the IWGDF

- The International Consensus on the Diabetic Foot (1999)
- Practical Guidelines on the Management and Prevention of the Diabetic Foot (1999)
- Interactive CD-ROM (2003) with
     International Consensus on Diagnosing and Treating the Infected Diabetic Foot
     Report on wound healing and treatments
     Report on classification of foot ulcers for research purposes

---

in diabetic foot care are addressed, with clear description of the various diagnostic, preventive or therapeutic strategies. Furthermore, the organisation of care and the implementation of the guidelines are described. The document consists of three different texts, written for policymakers in health care, general foot care specialists and health care professionals, respectively. The text for policymakers focuses on the socio-economic impact of the diabetic foot and the possibility to reduce this impact by well-targeted intervention strategies. The Practical Guidelines on the Management and Prevention of the Diabetic Foot describes the basic principles of prevention and treatment. All health care workers involved in the care of diabetic patients can use these guidelines. The International Consensus on the Management and Prevention of the Diabetic Foot serves as a reference to The Practical Guidelines. Furthermore, it summarises the strategies in management and prevention, gives a set of definitions of the essential topics in diabetic foot disease and can be used by the various specialists involved in diabetic foot care.

THE 2003 CONSENSUS DOCUMENT AND REPORTS

After the successful launching of the consensus documents at the Third International Symposium on the Diabetic Foot in 1999, the IWGDF decided in 2000 that additional documents were to be produced on the infected diabetic foot, wound healing and on an ulcer classification for research purposes. These topics were not covered in depth by the 1999 consensus document.

Infection

Infection is a frequent complication of diabetic foot ulcers and is, in many patients, the pivotal event leading to amputation. The IWGDF observed that there were worldwide large differences in the definition of infection, its diagnosis and its management. Therefore, a working group of experts in the field was instituted, with B.A. Lipsky (United States) as chairman. This group produced a state-of-the-art consensus document on diagnosis and treatment of the infected diabetic foot, and moreover, it provides practical guidelines for daily practice.[14] A summary of this consensus document and, in particular, of the practical guidelines is given below.

Wound Healing

The aims of the wound care document were to provide a state of the art on wound healing, on barriers to healing and on treatments for diabetic foot ulcers; a summary of this document is given below.[15] Unfortunately, it became clear to the working group, with K.G. Harding (United Kingdom) as chairman, that the evidence base to produce practical guidelines on wound care is lacking. The current document should therefore be seen as a progress report; however, the IWGDF hopes that within the next few years more solid data will become available. Given the great need for practical, evidence-based guidelines, the present consensus process will be continued, and hopefully within the next few years practical guidelines will be produced on this topic, in combination with a shorter version of the current document.

Classification

More than ten different systems have been developed to classify diabetic foot ulcers for daily clinical practice, and different centres of excellence use different classification systems;

reaching consensus on this topic was clearly a challenge for all experts involved.[13] In the earlier projects of the IWGDF, solid scientific data were the basis for consensus, but in the present project, much more arbitrary choices had to be made. Moreover, the design and content of a classification strongly depends on its aims, and the current system is to be used in research; a more simple system for daily clinical practice still needs to be developed. In addition to some members of the IWGDF, all researchers who had developed an ulcer classification scheme in the past were asked to participate in a working group, with N.C. Schaper (the Netherlands) as chairman. The newly designed classification system has been primarily developed to characterise patients participating at a certain time point in a research project, usually during the inclusion phase, and should be the basis for the inclusion and exclusion criteria.[16] The system, which is summarised below, aims to create a reproducible categorisation scheme; however, this assumption needs to be tested. Therefore, the classification system needs to be validated, and indeed the process of validation has recently been started.

CONSENSUS PROCESS

The international guidelines are produced by the IWGDF (Table 35.3) following a clear set of rules. An evidence-based approach is the aim of the development of the guidelines. The information used during this process is obtained from literature research, several Cochrane analyses and consensus statements from other documents. However, at present, solid scientific information on many relevant topics is lacking, and the documents should be regarded as the consensus reached by a group of independent well-known experts from the different fields involved in the care of diabetic patients with foot disease. The International Consensus was written by experts in the field, under the guidance of an editorial board. All members of the IWGDF agreed upon the final texts after several cycles of writing, commenting and editing by the editorial board. Subsequently, this document was endorsed by international organisations such as the World Health Organisation (WHO) and the IDF. The three supplements on infection, wound care and classification were written by three separate working groups. The chairman of each consensus group communicated with the editorial board of the IWGDF, which in turn was responsible for the communication with the members of the IWGDF. The members of each group were representatives of the IWGDF and/or well-known experts in the field. Each group was asked to produce a text that was in line with the consensus of 1999 and with other related consensus projects, such as the TransAtlantic InterSociety consensus group on peripheral arterial disease and the guidelines on diabetic foot infections of the Infectious Diseases Society of America.[17] After a cycle of writing, editing and commenting by all members of the IWGDF, the texts were discussed in depth and modified during a meeting of the IWGDF in the Netherlands in 2003. During this meeting, the three final documents were produced and subsequently agreed upon by all 62 IWGDF members, with their signatures.

Table 35.3 List of useful addresses

- Web site of the IWGDF: www.iwgdf.org
- Web site of the IDF: www.idf.org/bookshop (documents and CD-ROM)
- IWGDF e-mail address: karel.bakker@hetnet.nl

The consensus documents were, as stated earlier, developed by a group of independent experts, and the documents were created without any influence of pharmaceutical companies. However, the development of the consensus and the implementation programme were greatly facilitated by the financial support given by pharmaceutical companies. Until now, Johnson & Johnson and Dermagraft Joint Venture (Advanced Tissue Sciences/Smith & Nephew) generously supported the initiative. Furthermore, a donation was received from the Dutch EASD (European Association for the Study of Diabetes) Fund and from NovoNordisk. In several countries, the translation of the International Consensus was supported by local pharmaceutical companies, which facilitated the worldwide implementation of the consensus project, as described in the next paragraph.

IMPLEMENTATION

The International Consensus was originally produced as a booklet in 1999. An interactive CD-ROM was printed in 2003, containing the original International Consensus document (1999), and the newly approved documents on infection, classification and wound healing. Furthermore, the Spanish and French versions of the Practical Guidelines on the Management and Prevention of the Diabetic Foot were included in the CD-ROM, as well as a picture gallery and an interactive search system.

Depending upon local circumstances, the principles outlined in the documents have to be translated for local use, taking into account regional differences in socio-economics, accessibility to health care and cultural factors. In almost all regions and countries, contact was made with organisations or individuals involved in diabetes care. Local champions of the diabetic foot were recruited, resulting in a total of 82 persons (as per June 2005) as representatives of their country or region. The International Consensus document was created in such a way that it enabled the production of translated (and if necessary adapted) versions for local use, with relatively low costs. Moreover, in the relatively rich developing countries, national pharmaceutical companies sponsored some of these versions, and this money was used to support the production of guidelines in some lesser developed countries. Under guidance of the board of the IWGDF, the International Consensus was translated in 25 languages in 2005, including Russian, Chinese, Japanese and Arabic. These translated versions were endorsed by the local diabetic organisations and were subsequently presented in most countries at national meetings on the diabetic foot. Members of the IWGDF participated in several of these meetings and also helped to organise practical training sessions. Subsequently, the IWGDF developed the 'Step by Step' programme with the aim to improve diabetic foot care in developing countries. With the financial support of the World Diabetes Foundation, projects have been initiated in countries such as India, Sri Lanka, Bangladesh and Tanzania. Also, an IWGDF Web site was created to inform all health care workers in the field of the diabetic foot on the consensus projects and on the current status of diabetic foot management. In addition, more specific information is provided on future meetings, and also personal experiences of people in the field are displayed as 'Foot Notes'.

Finally, the IWGDF is, as a Consultative Section, involved in several IDF initiatives, such as the 2005 worldwide campaign on foot care. This campaign culminated in the World Diabetes Day on this topic, with press conferences in all the IDF regions, a travelling photographic exhibition and with special issues of well-known journals specifically dedicated to this topic

(*Lancet, Diabetes Voice*). Moreover, a 200-page book (an IDF *Time To Act* publication) has been published in English; later it will be followed by versions in Spanish and French if sufficient funding can be found.[12]

FUTURE PROJECTS

The IWGDF is currently involved in the following projects:

- The worldwide implementation of the current international guidelines on diabetic foot care will be continued, with support of local working group members in their activities.

- The current guidelines will be evaluated and adapted, if necessary.

- The IWGDF will soon initiate new consensus projects, which will be ready in 2007.

- The network of country representatives will continue to expand as part of the wider move towards the stimulation of local initiatives to collect data and launch prevention programmes.

CONCLUSIONS

The International Consensus on the Diabetic Foot is a unique project. It is characterised by the worldwide involvement and commitment of many different experts in the field, working in various areas of foot care and research. It is not only involved in guideline development and evaluation, but also has a strong emphasis on worldwide implementation. The consensus project has helped to create an active international network of diabetic foot experts and researchers. Perhaps more importantly, it has helped to put the diabetic foot on the agenda of policymakers, by raising awareness not only in the Western world but also particularly in developing countries (e.g., the Just Qatar International Diabetic Foot Conference, held in April, 2006). The International Consensus is a continuous process and new and/or updated documents will be presented during the Fifth International Symposium on the Diabetic Foot in May 2007, Noordwijkerhout, the Netherlands.

APPENDIX 1 – SUMMARY OF THE GUIDELINES ON DIAGNOSING AND TREATING THE INFECTED DIABETIC FOOT[14]

Diagnosis

An infected foot ulcer is diagnosed clinically, by the presence of purulent secretions or local evidence of inflammation, or occasionally systemic toxicity. Clinical signs, however, may be subtle as the inflammatory response may be mitigated by diabetic complications. Laboratory tests, including cultures, may suggest but do not establish the presence of infection, with the exception of reliably obtained deep bone cultures in suspected osteomyelitis. Classifying infections by their severity helps determine the site, type and urgency of treatment. The severity of the infection should be assessed by examining the wound, limb and the overall status of the patient, to determine the appropriate approach to treatment.

Microbiology

Obtaining proper specimens for culture is usually advisable, to help select an appropriate antibiotic regimen. Cultures may not be necessary in previously untreated, mild infections.

Wound cultures should be taken by obtaining tissue (by curettage or biopsy) of the debrided wound base or by aspirating pus, rather than by swabbing. If swabs are the only option, take them from the ulcer base after debridement, and process quickly. Consider obtaining blood cultures from patients with systemic toxicity, and consider bone cultures from patients with osteomyelitis.

Aerobic Gram-positive cocci (especially staphylococci) are usually the initial, often the only, and almost always the most frequently isolated pathogens in soft tissue and bone infections.

Gram-negative and anaerobic bacteria are commonly isolated, but usually as part of a polymicrobial, chronic or necrotic infection.

Treatment

Consult a diabetic foot care team or specialist, where available. Hospitalise patients with a severe infection, needing multiple or complex procedures; having critical foot ischaemia; needing intravenous therapy; or unlikely to comply with therapy. In case of severe infection, consult appropriate specialists promptly for any necessary invasive diagnostic or surgical procedures.

Prescribe antimicrobial therapy for all clinically infected wounds immediately, but not for uninfected wounds. Select the narrowest spectrum therapy possible for mild or moderate infections. Choose initial therapy based on the commonest pathogens and known local antibiotic sensitivity data. Adjust (broaden or constrain) empiric therapy, based on the culture results and clinical response to the initial regimen.

The prescription must cover staphylococci and streptococci in almost all cases. Broaden the spectrum, if necessary, based on the clinical picture, or on previous culture or current Gram-stained smear results. Topical therapy for mild superficial infections has not been adequately studied; oral therapy is effective for most mild to moderate infections; parenteral therapy (at least initially) is advisable for severe infections.

Choose agents that have demonstrated efficacy in treating complicated skin infections and soft tissue infections. These include semi-synthetic penicillins, cephalosporins, penicillin–lactamase inhibitors, clindamycin, fluoroquinolones, carbapenems and oxazolidinones. Treat soft tissue infections for 1–2 weeks if they are mild infections, and for about 2–4 weeks for most that are moderate and severe. When the clinical evidence of infection has resolved, antibiotic therapy can be stopped.

In case of osteomyelitis, consider surgically removing any infected and necrotic bone, if possible. Unless all infected bone is resected, provide antibiotic treatment (with parenteral therapy, at least initially) for at least 4 weeks; treating for several months with highly bioavailable oral agents (especially fluoroquinolones) without surgical resection may be effective in selected patients.

APPENDIX 2 – SUMMARY OF THE REPORT ON WOUND HEALING AND TREATMENTS[15]

Background

Diabetic foot ulcers readily become chronic, and chronic ulcers have biological properties that differ substantially from acute ones. Much of the available information on the biology of wound healing relates to acute and experimental wounds and may not be directly relevant. It follows that there is limited evidence currently available to underpin protocols for the management of diabetic foot ulcers, or to guide choice of applications and dressings. Nevertheless, it is possible to define certain principles, and whichever strategy is selected, wound management has to be integrated into an effective programme of multidisciplinary care.

Glycaemic Control

While chronic complications of diabetes such as peripheral vascular disease and neuropathy may be largely irreversible, aspects of structure and function of connective tissue and cells may be impaired by hyperglycaemia, and their function should be improved if normoglycaemia is achieved.

Promotion of Healing

Active promotion of wound healing can be attempted by (1) surgical revascularisation and (2) specific efforts to correct defined biological abnormalities thought to be hindering the healing process. These include the use of a variety of applications, dressings and technologies, which may stimulate healing by applying, or stimulating the release of, growth factors and cytokines. While this approach holds the greatest promise for the future, it will be dependent on defining defects that need correction in specific individuals, and having technologies available to address them. This field is in its infancy.

Wound Care

Management of the wound and its surrounding tissue in order to promote healing includes regular inspection, cleansing and removal of surface debris, elimination of pathogenic bacteria and creation of an appropriate environment to facilitate endogenous tissue regeneration. Debridement – in either the operating room or in the outpatient clinic – should be employed to remove surface debris and necrotic material. Wide excision of the ulcer and surrounding tissue has also been promoted by some authors as a means of replacing the biology of the chronic wound with that of an acute one. Autolytic debridement may be facilitated by the use of moisture-retentive dressings, to maintain an appropriately moist environment. A variety of enzymatic agents have been developed to debride necrotic and sloughy wounds without damaging healthy tissue. Enzymatic debridement is, however, expensive and requires a certain amount of skill to apply, and convincing evidence of effectiveness is still required. Larval therapy may also be suitable as biological debridement and helps minimise the risk of maceration. Data on efficacy are currently limited to that from small case series, but more robust studies are underway. Oedema predisposes to infection, and fluid from chronic wounds may block cellular proliferation and angiogenesis. Oedema may be reduced by compression or negative pressure and the accumulation of excess fluid may be limited, while maintaining sufficient hydration of the wound surface by more frequent dressing changes and/or the use of preparations with appropriate absorptive capacity.

Dressings

The term dressing applies to products chosen to cover the wound and to insulate it from the environment. Inevitably, however, dressing products have been developed which combine this function with other properties, such as debridement or regulation of wound moisture. It follows that the potential properties of dressings are many. There are a large number of dressings available, and although there are theoretical criteria that could be used to direct choice, there is little hard evidence to guide practice. Unfortunately, there have been no quality controlled trials of traditional therapies in diabetic foot ulcers. The evidence to support the use of some newer technologies is stronger, but is limited by studies having been undertaken almost exclusively in uninfected neuropathic diabetic foot ulcers. Conclusions drawn from these studies cannot be extrapolated to other ulcer types, which constitute the majority of those seen in clinical practice.

General Principles

In conclusion, wound care should be based on the following principles.

- Ulcers that remain contaminated by debris and surface slough after sharp debridement should be managed with an agent, treatment or application with debriding properties.

- Antiseptic agents may help clean the surface of the wound, but there is little justification for using an antiseptic on clean ulcers.

- The wound surface should be kept appropriately moist; hydrogels and hydrofibres may benefit drier wounds, while excessive exudate should be removed with absorbent preparations, for example alginates and foams.

- Some newer applications, dressings and technologies may influence the healing process, but their place in ulcer management has not been established to date.

- Ulcers should be covered to protect them from trauma and to maintain appropriate warmth and hydration of the wound bed. However, the inappropriate use of occlusive dressings and/or failure to change dressings and clean the wound surface with sufficient regularity may worsen prognosis by allowing the accumulation of excessive exudate and causing maceration of the surrounding skin.

APPENDIX 3 – SUMMARY OF THE REPORT ON CLASSIFICATION OF FOOT ULCERS FOR RESEARCH PURPOSES[16]

Background

The aim of the research classification is to enable the categorisation of different populations of diabetic patients with a foot ulcer for the purposes of research, at a certain time point, according to strict criteria and using the terms that are relevant, unambiguous and applicable worldwide. Such a classification system should facilitate communication and enable the comparison of the results of different research projects. It was not the aim to develop a classification system that can be used to predict the outcome of an individual patient or that can act as a guide for daily management. The consequence is that, as far as possible, objective, reproducible techniques should be used. However, in several categories a compromise had to be made between the ideal world and daily life, and a minimal set of criteria was given. Depending upon the aim of an individual research project, additional criteria can and, in some cases, should be added to the current system to improve correct categorisation. The current system is primarily developed to characterise patients participating at a certain time point in a research project, usually during the inclusion phase of a project, and it should be the basis for the inclusion and exclusion criteria. Therefore, temporal aspects are not included in the current system. However, wounds clearly change in time, and complications can develop. When, for instance, the chronobiology of wounds is studied, an extra category on wound characteristics can be added. Finally, the current system needs to be validated before it can be introduced formally as an international classification system.

The Classification System

Five categories were created: Perfusion, Extent/size, Depth/tissue loss, Infection and Sensation. For each category, a grading system is provided.

Perfusion

Grade 1: No symptoms or signs of peripheral arterial disease (PAD)[17] with

- Palpable dorsal pedal and posterior tibial artery or
- Ankle–brachial index between 0.9 and 1.10 or
- Toe–brachial index >0.6 or
- Transcutaneous oxygen pressure (TcpO$_2$) >60 mm Hg.

Grade 2: Symptoms or signs of PAD present, but not of critical limb ischaemia (CLI).

- Presence of intermittent claudication or
- Ankle–brachial index <0.9, but with ankle pressure >50 mm Hg or

- Toe–brachial index <0.6, but systolic toe blood pressure >30 mm Hg or

- $TcpO_2$ 30–60 mm Hg or

- Other abnormalities on non-invasive testing, compatible with PAD (but not with CLI).

Grade 3: Critical limb ischaemia, as defined by

- Systolic ankle blood pressure <50 mm Hg or

- Systolic toe blood pressure <30 mm Hg or

- $TcpO_2$ <30 mm Hg.

Extent size

Wound size (measured in square centimetres) should be determined after debridement, if possible.

Depth/tissue loss (evaluated after initial debridement)

Grade 1   Superficial full-thickness ulcer, not penetrating any structure deeper than the dermis.

Grade 2   Deep ulcer, penetrating below the dermis to subcutaneous structures, involving fascia, muscle or tendon.

Grade 3   All subsequent layers of the foot involved, including bone and/or joint (exposed bone, probing to bone).

Infection

Grade 1   No symptoms or signs of infection.

Grade 2   Infection involving the skin and the subcutaneous tissue only. At least two of the following items are present: local swelling or induration; erythema >0.5 to 2 cm around the ulcer; local tenderness or pain; local warmth; purulent discharge. No systemic signs, as described below.

Grade 3   Erythema >2 cm plus one of the items described above, or infection involving structures deeper than skin and subcutaneous tissues such as abscess, osteomyelitis, septic arthritis, fasciitis. No systemic signs.

Grade 4   Any foot infection with two or more of the following conditions: temperature >38 or <36°C; heart rate >90 beats/min; respiratory rate >20 breaths/min; $PaCO_2$ <32 mm Hg; white blood cell count >12 000 or <4000/mm^3; >10% immature (band) forms.

Sensation

Grade 1   No loss of protective sensation on the affected foot

Grade 2   Loss of protective sensation on the affected foot, defined as the absence of perception in the affected foot to pressure (10-g monofilament) or vibration (128-Hz tuning fork), or a vibration perception threshold >25 V.

REFERENCES

1. Wild S, Roglic G, Green A, Sicree R, King H. Global prevalence of diabetes: estimates for the year 2000 and projections for 2030. *Diabetes Care* 2004;27:1047–1053.
2. Vileikyte L. Diabetic foot ulcers: a quality of life issue. *Diabetes Metab Res Rev* Jul/Aug 2001;17:246–249.
3. Ragnarson Tennvall G, Apelqvist J. Prevention of diabetes-related foot ulcers and amputations: a cost-utility analysis based on Markov model simulations. *Diabetologia* 2001;44:2077–2087.
4. International Working Group on the Diabetic Foot. *International Consensus on the Diabetic Foot.* Apelqvist J, Bakker K, Van Houtum WH, Nabuurs-Franssen MH, Schaper NC, eds. Maastricht: Schaper NC, 1999.
5. Jeffcoate WJ, van Houtum WH. Amputation as a marker of the quality of foot care in diabetes. *Diabetologia* 2004;47:2051–2058.
6. Ramachandran A. Specific problems of the diabetic foot in developing countries. *Diabetes Metab Res Rev* 2004;20:S19–S22.
7. Boulton AJ. The diabetic foot: from art to science. The 18th Camillo Golgi lecture. *Diabetologia* Aug 2004;47:1343–1353.
8. Jeffcoate WJ, Harding KG. Diabetic foot ulcers. *Lancet* 2003;361:1545–1551.
9. Singh N, Armstrong DG, Lipsky B. Preventing foot ulcers in patients with diabetes. *JAMA* 2005;293:217–228.
10. Reiber GE, Vileikyte L, Boyko EJ, *et al.* Causal pathways for incident lower-extremity ulcers in patients with diabetes from two settings. *Diabetes Care* 1999;22:157–162.
11. Apelqvist J, Larsson J. What is the most effective way to reduce incidence of amputation in the diabetic foot? *Diabetes Metab Res Rev* 2000;16:S75–S83.
12. IDF. *Diabetes and Foot Care: Time to Act.* Brussels: IDF; 2005. Online at http://www.idf.org/webdata/T2A.Introduction.pdf.
13. Armstrong DG, Peters EJG. Classification of wounds of the diabetic foot. *Curr Diabetes Rep* 2001;1:233–238.
14. Lipsky BA. International consensus group on diagnosing and treating the infected diabetic foot. A report from the international consensus on diagnosing and treating the infected diabetic foot. *Diabetes Metab Res Rev* 2004;20:S68–S77.
15. Jeffcoate WJ, Price P, Harding KG, and the International Working Group on Wound Healing and Treatments for People with Diabetic Foot Ulcers. Wound healing and treatments for people with diabetic foot ulcers. *Diabetes Metab Res Rev* 2004;20:S78–S89.
16. Schaper NC. Diabetic foot ulcer classification system for research purposes: a progress report on criteria for including patients in research studies. *Diabetes Metab Res Rev* 2004;20:S90–S95.
17. Dormandy JA. Management of peripheral arterial disease (PAD). TASC Working Group. TransAtlantic Inter-Society Consensus (TASC). *J Vasc Surg* 2000;31:S1–S296.

36 The Organisation of Diabetic Foot Care: Evidence-Based Recommendations

Robert J. Young

WHY IS A STRUCTURE OR SYSTEM OF CARE NECESSARY?

Wherever there is good evidence about the beneficial nature of a particular sequence of health care interventions, it is necessary to put in place organisational arrangements that will maximise the chance that the interventions will be performed and that the arrangements are effective. Thus, it is not sufficient simply to train health care professionals to perform their technical and professional roles adequately. Nor can one reasonably expect that patients will inevitably turn up for a due intervention in the right place at the right time. Rather, there need to be structures or pathways of care capable of supporting professionals in ways that enable them to apply their knowledge and training consistently and efficiently. And there need to be signposts or self-enabling information for patients. This is just as true for the unpredictable and extended course of interventions that comprise care for long-term conditions as it is for the more predictable and short-term interventions associated with elective medicine.

In respect of the diabetic foot, there is appreciable evidence for the effectiveness of interventions that can minimise the onset of neuropathy and peripheral vascular disease (primary preventive care), that can detect and minimise the consequences of early peripheral neuropathy, peripheral vascular disease and other susceptibility factors (secondary preventive care) and that will minimise limb loss and maintain mobility if serious problems arise (tertiary preventive care or salvage therapy). It is the systems that underpin this approach to primary, secondary and tertiary prevention of diabetic foot disease that form the content of this chapter. The approach is consistent with presently accepted models of long-term condition management such as are advocated in the English National Service Framework for Diabetes: Standards,[1] and with the detailed evidence that led to the recommendations assembled in the formulation of the National Institute for Clinical Excellence (NICE) guidelines[2] (http://www.nice.org.uk/page.aspx?o=dg .endocrine).

The Foot in Diabetes, 4th Edition. Editors Andrew J.M. Boulton, Peter R. Cavanagh and Gerry Rayman.
© 2006 John Wiley & Sons, Ltd.

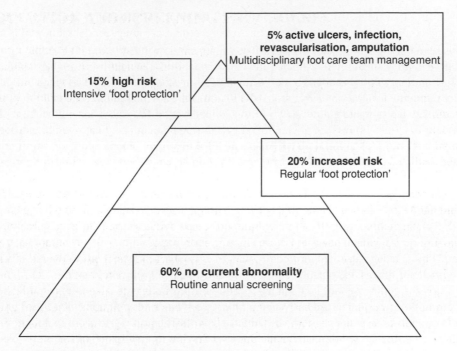

Figure 36.1 The 'Pyramid of Foot Care' for a population of people with diabetes

THE SCALE OF THE TASK

Foot complications are common in diabetes. Everyone with diabetes is potentially susceptible. Overall, about 30% of people with diabetes have neuropathy and 30% have peripheral vascular disease. These conditions and other vulnerabilities of the foot increase with advancing age. Around 5% of people with diabetes may develop a foot ulcer in any one year, and major amputation rates are currently around 0.5% per year. Given that the prevalence of diabetes is presently of the order of 3–4%, and likely to increase by 50–100% over the next 10 years, care structures need to be organised on a communitywide basis and resourced to a level commensurate with the volumes of patients that will require screening or intervention at each level (Figure 36.1).

CARE NEEDED BY EVERYONE WITH DIABETES

Registration, recall and regular review are at the heart of continuing care for people with diabetes. Continuing care encompasses reviews of glucose control and vascular risk factors. Optimisation of these factors is the means whereby the onset and progression of the cardinal risk factors for diabetic lower limb disease (peripheral neuropathy and peripheral vascular disease) can be attenuated. There is therefore a set of tasks that relates to reviewing the current management plan and agreeing on a future plan.

In addition, the review process offers a systematic opportunity to identify early evidence of emerging complications. For the eyes the process is retinal screening, for the kidneys it is testing the urine for microalbuminuria, but in the feet it requires examination for early evidence of peripheral neuropathy or peripheral vascular disease plus the evaluation of any supplementary risk factors that might intensify their effect (e.g. foot deformity, poor vision or balance problems). Pragmatically and for administrative convenience (this is a formidable administrative task for primary care providers) these routine reviews are usually organised annually.

CARE THAT SOME DIABETIC PATIENTS NEED

If, during the continuing care review process, significant risk factors for diabetic foot disease are discovered, then preventive care needs to be enhanced. The person who has intact sensation, palpable pulses and warm feet is at *low current risk* of a diabetic foot problem and can simply be rescheduled for repeat examination, usually in a year. However, a person with diabetes who has impaired sensation and/or absent pulses is at *increased risk* of diabetic foot ulceration.

This risk can be contained (secondary preventive care). Accordingly, there needs to be a system whereby the people with increased risk receive enhanced foot care education, particularly with regard to choice of footwear (minimally traumatic, maximally protective), more regular foot review (3–6 monthly) and, ideally, intensified efforts to optimise glucose control and cardiovascular risk factors. Sometimes, the identification of an early abnormality and an explanation of its attendant implications may facilitate greater ongoing engagement in the relevant aspects of preventive care, i.e. it creates a state of 'readiness to change'. Such explanation, discussion and shared decision making require significant amounts of time if they have to be effective.

Whereas in many models of care the primary care provider will carry out the routine foot examination, these enhanced services are usually organised by podiatrists as a service to primary care providers and constitute what is sometimes known as a 'foot care protection programme'. In respect of realising the opportunities to intensify glucose control and cardiovascular risk factor reduction, it is clearly essential that podiatric and primary care services communicate effectively.

CARE THAT A FEW DIABETIC PATIENTS NEED

Some people with diabetes are not just at increased risk but at *high risk* of foot ulceration. They not only have reduced sensation and/or absent pulses but also have a history of previous ulceration and/or foot deformity. More intensive 'foot care protection' reduces the risk that such people will progress to (re-)ulceration. Such patients require all the interventions offered to people with increased risk but in addition require more frequent (1–3 monthly) podiatric reviews that include foot care education, reassessment of the need for revascularisation, skin and nail care and, where necessary, the provision of specialist orthotics and footwear to offload vulnerable areas of intense pressure.

CARE FOR DIABETIC PATIENTS WITH ACTIVE FOOT PROBLEMS

People with new ulcers, swelling or skin discolouration should be referred to a multidisciplinary foot care team within 24 h. A multidisciplinary high-risk foot care team should comprise highly trained specialist podiatrists and orthotists, nurses with training in the dressing of diabetic foot wounds and diabetologists with expertise in lower limb complications; such a team requires unhindered access to suites for managing major wounds, inpatient facilities that are accessible urgently, multi-route antibiotic administration, community nursing, diagnostic and clinical advisory microbiology services, orthopaedic/podiatric surgery, vascular surgery, radiology and orthotics.

Organisationally, this means that such a team should be established in every health economy, and people with diabetes, primary care providers and emergency services must know of its existence and understand how to refer new problems without delay. By bringing together relevant expertise and deploying it without delay, both temporary and permanent disability can be minimised.

The evidence as to which interventions the multidisciplinary foot care teams should best deploy is patchy. But there is consensus or better support for wound monitoring, debridement and regularly changed dressings, intensive antibiotic therapy for invasive infection (cellulitis, osteomyelitis), offloading measures including total contact casting, revascularisation where appropriate, high-impact education and optimisation of metabolic and cardiovascular risk factors. Some of the patients referred acutely according to the above criteria will have Charcot neuroarthropathy. Immobilisation of the affected area plus other emerging interventions should also be a responsibility of the multidisciplinary team.

ALGORITHM OF CARE PATHWAYS

The NICE guideline contains an algorithm that describes on one page (Figure 36.2) the organisational arrangements outlined above.

LOCAL ORGANISATIONAL ARRANGEMENTS

An average local health care economy in the United Kingdom comprises approximately 250 000 people, of whom 8000–10 000 will presently have diagnosed diabetes. Local provider services will usually include about 120 primary care practitioners and their teams, community-based services (usually the prime working location for podiatrists and district nurses) and an acute hospital.

The workload implied by the above recommendations means that

- Primary care services need to perform up to 6000 foot examinations per year;

- Community podiatry services need to see and provide a foot care protection programme to 2000 people with increased risk (approximately 5000 contacts per year) and 1500 people with high risk (approximately 9000 contacts per year);

- A multidisciplinary foot care team needs to see and treat 500 people with new ulceration (approximately 10 000 contacts per year, including up to 50 minor and major amputations, up to 50 revascularisations, large numbers of casts, bespoke shoes, etc.).

This is clearly a formidable management task and will deliver the evidence-based benefits safely, efficiently, effectively, equitably and in a 'patient-centred' manner only if each of the

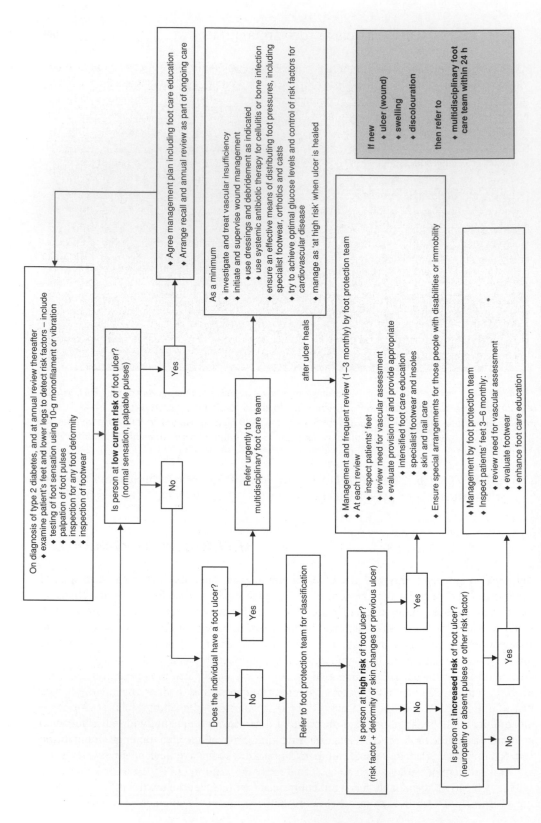

Figure 36.2 NICE Foot Care Guideline: algorithm[3]

components is integrated effectively with the others. Accordingly, there must be some form of local coordination (e.g. a multidisciplinary steering group) that keeps all members of the distributed diabetes care team up to date with local organisational arrangements, that maintains the competencies of all personnel, that creates a framework for good communication including shared record keeping and that, by means of continuous clinical audit, evaluates the service structures, processes and outcomes in order to prioritise, implement and re-evaluate incremental improvements as required.

REFERENCES

1. Department of Health (London, England). National Service Framework for Diabetes: Standards (14/12/2001; supplementary material published 15 March 2002). Crown copyright. Product code: 26192. Available online at http://www.dh.gov.uk/PublicationsAndStatistics/Publications/Publications PolicyAndGuidance/PublicationsPolicyAndGuidanceArticle/fs/en?CONTENT_ID=4002951&chk= 09Kkz1 [accessed 22 April 2006].
2. National Health Service (UK). National Institute for Health and Clinical Excellence (NICE). Endocrine, nutritional and metabolic. Copyright 2006. Available online at www.nice.org.uk/page .aspx?o=dg.endocrine [accessed 22 April 2006].
3. National Health Service (UK). National Institute for Health and Clinical Excellence (NICE). NICE Guideline: Type 2 diabetes, foot care: Appendix E. NICE Foot Care Guidelines (Revision): Algorithm. Available online at www.nice.org.uk/page.aspx?o=208094 [accessed 22 April 2006].

37 Primary Care: Delivery/Translation of Guidelines into Practice

Eva-Lisa Heinrichs and Michael Clark

INTRODUCTION

The management of diabetes is consuming an increasingly significant portion of an already restricted health care budget. As both the incidence and the prevalence of diabetes escalate, pressures to manage this pandemic cost-effectively will increase.[1] Managing the diabetic foot and its complications has been presented as the most costly part of managing diabetes.[2] To ensure that scarce resources achieve maximum health gain, health care policy strategies worldwide are shifting the main responsibility for prevention and treatment of chronic disease from secondary care to primary care.[3] Consequently, this has been a key area of change in the management of diabetes. The primary care sector is required to cope with increasing requirements of cost containment and efficiency whilst at the same time raising standards of care.

Clinical Practice Guidelines (CPGs) are by definition systematically developed recommendations to assist practitioner and patient decisions about appropriate health care for specific clinical circumstances.[4] They are widely viewed as a summary of the best available research evidence together with recommendations for practitioners.[5] It is universally acknowledged that evidence-based decision making and CPGs may serve as important tools to reduce variations in practice, contain costs and ultimately increase the effectiveness of clinical practice.[6,7] Over the past several decades, there has been not only a remarkable growth in the development of CPGs, but also a greater appreciation of their value.[5]

Whilst the development of clinical guidelines regionally, nationally and internationally has increased substantially in recent years, less attention has been paid to guideline dissemination and implementation, and it would be naïve to suggest that just because guidelines exist, their implementation automatically follows.[8] In fact, large gaps exist between best practice and evidence in the implementation of CPGs, and we still lack in-depth knowledge of which factors are decisive in achieving changes, in which target groups and in which settings.[9,10]

The process of implementing CPGs has been likened to the process required to bring about organisational change.[11,12] Many of the principles applicable to organisational change could

The Foot in Diabetes, 4th Edition. Editors Andrew J.M. Boulton, Peter R. Cavanagh and Gerry Rayman.
© 2006 John Wiley & Sons, Ltd.

therefore be applicable to CPGs implementation, and where relevant these principles have been applied in the discussion of the implementation process in this chapter.

CHOICE OF GUIDELINE

Because of the wide variation in the quality of CPGs, it is important that users critically appraise available guidelines before implementing these in their practice setting.[11,13] Not surprisingly, the quality of a CPG is an important variable that has been shown to affect its implementation.[5] Guideline implementation continues to be a major challenge for those working in the health service, due in large part to the great number of practice guidelines available, some being more 'evidence based' than others.[5,8,14] Thus, the first problem facing the primary care professional is the plethora of CPGs choices available, necessitating a suitable tool or means by which to make an optimal choice for the health care setting in question.

'AGREE': AN INSTRUMENT FOR APPRAISING GUIDELINES

In 1998, the requirement for a tool to assist in guideline assessment and selection was recognised by international researchers and policymakers in Europe. Subsequently, in 2001, an EU-funded collaboration resulted in the development of an instrument for appraising the quality and applicability of clinical guidelines – the so-called AGREE instrument.

'AGREE' stands for Appraisal of Guidelines Research and Evaluation. The ongoing project's aims are to improve medical knowledge and the health of the European population. The main specific objective was to develop an appraisal instrument to assess clinical guidelines in order to promote the transfer of research results into clinical practice. The AGREE instrument has subsequently become an internationally recognised generic tool for appraising the quality of CPGs. It is designed to assess guidelines developed locally, regionally, nationally and internationally, and it can be applied to new guidelines as well as existing guidelines and updates to guidelines.[15]

The AGREE instrument can be used by guideline developers to assess whether their guidelines are sound, by policymakers to help decide which guidelines could be recommended for use, by health care providers who wish to undertake an assessment before adopting the guideline recommendations and finally by educators and teachers to help enhance critical appraisal skills amongst health care professionals. Whilst the AGREE instrument assesses the likelihood that a guideline will achieve its intended result, it is important to note that it does not assess the impact on patient outcomes.[15]

The AGREE instrument consists of 23 items (criteria) organised into six sections or domains. Each domain is intended to capture a separate guideline quality. The six domains are as follows:

- Scope and purpose;

- Stakeholder involvement;

- Rigour of development;

- Clarity and presentation;

- Applicability;

- Editorial independence.

Table 37.1   An example of guidelines appraisal results using the AGREE instrument

Domain	Item
Scope and purpose	• The clarity of the overall objective • The expected health benefits to the specific clinical problem • Whether the target population is clearly described
Stakeholder involvement	• The information provided in the guidelines about the composition, discipline and relevant expertise of the guideline development group • The evidence that the patients' experiences and expectations of health care have been taken into consideration • Clear definition of target user(s) • Whether the guidelines have been pre-tested
Rigour of development	• The strategy used to search for evidence • The criteria for including/excluding evidence • The methods used to formulate the recommendations and how the final decisions were reached • The extent to which the guidelines consider health benefits, side effects and risks of the provided recommendations
Clarity and presentation	• Whether the recommendations are concrete and precise, as permitted by the evidence, or if the evidence is not clear-cut, whether this uncertainty is stated in the guidelines • Have the possible different options for screening, prevention, diagnosis or treatment of the clinical problem in question been covered? • Is it easy to find the most relevant recommendations? • Has additional material been provided to assist in the dissemination and implementation?
Applicability	• Issues such as potential changes to the current organisation of care • Requirement for possible additional resources • Implications for the budget • Review criteria derived from the key recommendations have been defined so that adherence to the guidelines can be measured in case of implementation of the guideline in question
Editorial independence	• Independence of financial support provided for guidelines development • Declaration of conflict of interest on individual development group member level.

Items in each domain, shown in Table 37.1, measure the extent to which that criterion has been fulfilled using a rating on a 4-point scale. The item scores are added to achieve a total score for the particular domain. It should be emphasised that the six domain scores are independent and therefore not aggregated into a single score. Although domain scores may be useful for comparing guidelines and for decision making, it is important to note that it is not possible to set thresholds for the domain score that would indicate a 'good' or a 'bad' guideline.[15] The instrument comes with detailed instructions, and it is recommended that a minimum of two or ideally four appraisers perform the guideline assessment.

APPRAISING GUIDELINES USING THE AGREE INSTRUMENT: A PRACTICAL EXAMPLE

The following is a practical example of an appraisal of a selection of guidelines using the AGREE instrument. Five well-known guidelines were chosen from a wide range available for the management of the diabetic foot.

- Type 2 Diabetes Prevention and Management of Foot Problems by the National Institute for Clinical Excellence in the United Kingdom (NICE).[16]

- Management of Diabetes by the Scottish Intercollegiate Guidelines Network (SIGN).[17]

- Clinical Guidelines and Evidence Review for Type 2 Diabetes: Prevention and Management of Foot Problems by the Royal College of General Practitioners in the United Kingdom (RCGP).[18,36]

- Management of Type 2 Diabetes by the New Zealand Guidelines Group (NZGG).[19]

- Practical Guidelines on the Management of the Diabetic Foot based upon the International Consensus on the Diabetic Foot (ICG).[20]

Following the AGREE instrument instructions for use, the above guidelines were evaluated by four appraisers – a professor in health care research science, a podiatrist and the two authors of this chapter. The results are shown in Table 37.2.

Results

Scope and purpose

All guidelines have scores that indicate that the appraisers found all the relevant information.

Stakeholder involvement

For all the guidelines, concern on pre-testing prior to issuing the guidelines is reflected in the scores. The lower scores for RCGP and ICG guidelines are due to lack of clarity on whether patients' experiences and expectations of health care had been taken into consideration.

Rigour of development

The appraisers gave the lowest scores in this domain to the NICE and the ICG guidelines. Separate analysis of the individual item scores for NICE showed a lack of clarity on the criteria for including/excluding evidence, on the method by which final decisions were made and whether health benefits, side effects and risks of the recommendations in the guidelines have been clearly presented. The results for the ICG guidelines reflect a lack of clarity of the criteria for including/excluding evidence and on the explicit link between the recommendations and the supporting evidence.

Table 37.2 An example of using the AGREE tool to evaluate five well-known practice guidelines for the management of the diabetic foot

Guideline	Year of publication	Scope and purpose	Stakeholder involvement	Rigour of development	Clarity and presentation	Applicability	Editorial independence
				AGREE domain scores (%)			
NICE	2004	100.0	72.9	55.9	81.2	72.2	33.3
SIGN	2001	80.5	68.7	83.3	81.2	25.0	54.2
RCGP	2000	97.2	56.2	83.3	66.7	33.3	41.7
NZGG	2003	97.2	75.0	84.5	83.3	33.3	100.0
ICG	1999	75.0	54.2	51.2	68.7	58.3	45.8

Clarity and presentation

All guidelines scored high on this item. The RCGP guidelines scored lower than the three national guidelines mainly because the guidelines are not supported by tools for application. The ICG guidelines have a lower score mainly due to a lower average score on most of the items in this domain compared to the other guidelines.

Applicability

The results for the SIGN, RCGP, NZGG and ICG guidelines express to varying degrees a level of doubt as to whether points such as potential organisational barriers, cost implications and criteria for monitoring and/or auditing purposes are clearly addressed.

Editorial independence

All but the NZGG received low scores in this particular domain.

The ultimate choice of guideline for implementation purposes, which would normally follow an appraisal process, should be based on the scores, taking into account the relative importance of the various domains and items to the health care setting in question.

IMPLEMENTING A CLINICAL PRACTICE GUIDELINE

A flowchart of the key components of the CPGs' implementation process is presented in Figure 37.1. These key components are discussed below.

Stakeholders

Management and organisational environment

Delivering an adopted guideline into current practice is likely to be a challenging process. It is important to realise that at least some change in behaviour and policy as well as in resource allocation will most probably be required. Implementing CPGs nearly always requires some organisational changes and substantial time and resources. These are important reasons for consulting senior management as a threshold step to gain their support at the outset, if the decision to implement the guideline does not originate from them. Effective managerial–clinical relations, where managers understand what clinicians value and where clinicians think like managers, have been shown to facilitate implementation of innovations requiring change in practice.[21]

The speed of adoption is influenced by the degree to which the new practice requires changes in the organisational culture.[22] Ensuring that the implementation project fits with the organisation's overall strategy and resource commitments will eliminate possible organisational issues that could act as barriers.[8] Compatibility with the existing organisational norms, values and ways of working is likely to be a determinant of successful assimilation.[23]

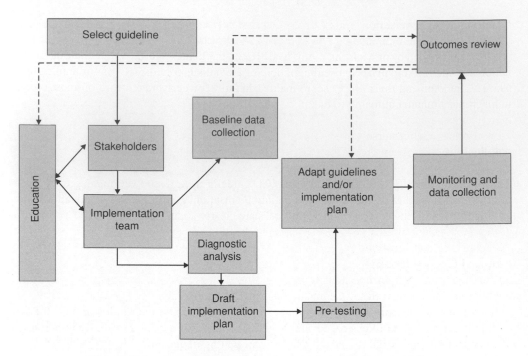

Figure 37.1   An overview of the implementation process for guidelines

Attempts should be made to identify key issues in the organisational culture and environment immediately at the outset of the process. This assessment is essential in order to fully comprehend the resources and changes essential for success. All possible implications on cost and resources need analysis and clarifying. Resources include materials, technologies, monies and networks as well as people required for a successful implementation. Lack of such resources and time are recognised barriers to change, and restraining forces that are likely to require resolution include increased workload, lack of time, poor communication, traditional working practices and resistance to change.[12,24] Therefore, identifying workload implications and discussing and addressing these at the onset have been shown to be important considerations for successful implementation.[11] A key element to success may be ensuring that relevant clinical and administrative systems are in place to facilitate adherence to the CPGs, and because it is likely that new administrative systems are required, administrative staff should be involved and invited to provide input.[25] Restructuring of medical records to provide either detailed care plans or at least prompts about actions required during the consultation has been recommended.[20] Systematic reviews indicate that prompts appear to be consistently effective in achieving change of practice. Their frequency and proximity to the point of clinical decision making may influence the size of their impact.[26]

The health care professionals

Preference should be given to considering professional group specific issues at the outset. Encouraging a feeling of ownership may create a more positive attitude to the guideline and facilitate the process for addressing possible barriers and necessary changes in behaviour required for implementation. It is worth noting that health care professionals as stakeholders include, in addition to the members of the multidisciplinary team, all groups of professionals who may be affected by or who may influence the new guidelines in practice.[12] These health care professionals are likely to play different roles at different times throughout the implementation process. Recognising their roles will allow members of the health care team to engage in a more focused manner at the relevant time, and therefore avoid imposing on their limited time more than necessary.

Whilst the practice nurse's role in the care of persons with diabetes has substantially grown, physicians remain a key group. They need to be involved early on, and a determination of the level of support of key physicians who influence clinical practice is essential.[11] Among the documented physician-related barriers are changes to standards of practice such as usual routines; opinion leaders not agreeing with the evidence; insufficient medical training; or obsolete knowledge.[27] If the new practice is compatible with the practitioners' individual or professional values, norms and perceived needs, it will be more readily adopted.[23]

Identifying and involving the key players acknowledges their importance and sets up a transparent process for identification of issues that need to be addressed to ensure success of the implementation.[11] Requiring others to change necessitates an understanding of the problems they face.[12] Innovations that are compatible with the intended adopters' values, norms and perceived needs are more readily adopted.[28] It is recognised that a person can play both a negative and a positive role in effecting change and implementing guidelines, and inviting them to provide input on their individual concerns about the recommendations and engaging in the adaptation process may have a positive influence on implementation.[8] Rather than being passive recipients, people tend to a greater or lesser extent to find (or fail to find) meaning in new recommendations, develop feelings (positive or negative) about them, challenge them, worry about them, complain about them, 'work around' them, gain experience with them, modify them to fit particular tasks and try to improve or redesign them – often through dialogue with other users.[23] Strategies for change should provide mechanisms that reinforce desired behaviour and as such, incentives for change may be required. Such incentives can include financial reward, resource reallocation, education and training, performance feedback and empowerment.[12] If the changes are likely to be widespread, securing support of a strong coalition of key players is essential for the implementation process to succeed.[12] Until this important step has been completed, it is not advisable to commence a project, which otherwise may only disrupt practice and fail, due to lack of necessary support, resources and time.

The patients

In chronic illness, day-to-day care responsibilities fall most heavily on patients and their families.[29] Patients' adherence to recommended treatment protocols is vital to successful disease management. Therefore, recognising that patients are key stakeholders will encourage their participation and ultimately serve to improve care.[10]

The referral practice

The particular collaboration between primary and secondary care should be carefully considered and taken into account and included at the outset, as this will inevitably be affected by the change. Success is much harder to achieve if the new recommendations require complex changes in clinical practice, improved collaboration between disciplines or better organisation of care.[27] Failure often relates to a lack of realisation of the extent of commitment required and to the wide scope of activities needing change. Managing diabetic foot complications effectively requires seamless collaboration between the primary and secondary care teams responsible for the provision of care for this patient group, and one of the great barriers to change is the difficulty in ensuring that the right groups and individuals work together.[24]

The Implementation Team

Implementation ensuring the sustainability of the new practice guidelines is the main responsibility of the implementation team. This team sets key priorities and timelines for the change agenda. Because of its central role, the team requires dedicated members and ideally some form of representation by all the key groups and individuals affected by the upcoming implementation process. Resources are invariably limited and any implementation strategies that exhaust these limited resources are unlikely to be sustainable in the long term.[26] Membership is likely to require a substantial amount of work and impose greatly on the individual team member's workload and time; therefore, it is vital that all the members of the core team are committed to the project. Key people leading the change, as well as continuity of leadership, has been associated positively with receptivity to change.[21] Success also requires that the team members have the appropriate support and, equally important, the required knowledge and skills.[12]

Successful management of the implementation project may require a full-time lead person for a duration that depends on the size and complexity of the project. In all cases, a dedicated project champion committed to the project should head up the team.

Dedicated clinical leaders and champions are critical to a successful implementation process.[22] Therefore, it may be worthwhile to consider engaging opinion leaders and/or well-respected leaders committed to the required changes, as mentors and champions for support. A dedicated facilitator, or opinion leader, who works with individuals and teams in the practice context may help facilitate the adoption of new guidelines into practice; however, it is worth noting that this strategy can turn out to be resource intensive.[8]

Diagnostic Analysis and Adapting Guidelines

Any process to bring about change should begin by identifying and analysing factors likely to influence the proposed change.[12] This will facilitate a better understanding of the scope of required changes in practice and allow identification of and planning around barriers to implementation. Analysis of barriers to doctors' willingness to change their routines have shown that obstacles to change in practice can arise at different levels in the health care system.[27] To understand the extent of the change requirements, a thorough so-called diagnostic analysis, i.e. an analysis of how the current practice compares to the practice outlined in the CPGs, is recommended.[12]

An algorithm can be an important tool accompanying the CPGs to be implemented. Producing detailed algorithms for the key elements in the organisation as a whole, the health care team and the individual professionals, of both current practice and the practice to be implemented, may facilitate comparisons and the subsequent identification of key issues. It is important to examine these key elements, and when recording and considering the required changes in practice, it is important to identify the steps needed to address any particular barriers and to tailor strategies to overcome them.

It is very likely that the adaptation of national CPGs will require modifications of the guideline recommendations to suit the local circumstances. Analysing and modifying a CPG to ensure local relevance has been shown to be a positive factor influencing change.[8] Successful implementation is more likely if the intended adopters have sufficient opportunity, autonomy and support to adapt and refine or otherwise modify the innovation to suit their own needs and to improve its fitness for purpose.[23] Subsequently, it is important to review the adapted CPGs to gain a good understanding of facilitators and possible obstacles, and for developing required interventions.[30]

It is critical to ensure that the final CPGs and recommendations, in addition to being relevant to local practitioners and practice, are clear and specific. Unless guidelines are limited to the major decision points, they are likely to be too unwieldy to use in practice.[31] The preferred format of the guideline may vary between professional groups, and this may be influenced by whether the professional group considers the topic to be of relevance or priority to them.[32] Presenting the guideline at the implementation stage as an algorithm has been suggested to be an acceptable format for practitioners and may contribute to its successful implementation.[8]

Baseline Data Collection

For the purpose of evaluating project impact, baseline data should be secured. Naturally, this must take place before implementing any of the new recommendations. Without access to baseline data it is impossible to obtain an accurate view of the true impact of the new practice. It is expected that CPGs will reduce inappropriate variations in practice and promote delivery of high-quality, evidence-based health care.[33] Verifying expectations such as these and credibly evaluating the impact of the project, reporting progress and building a better case for the local relevance of the guidelines are clearly not possible without relevant baseline data. Furthermore, having credible data may be of crucial importance when seeking sustained support for the new practice in terms of resources and financing. It is worth ensuring that the current records and database support this activity; if not, further resources and financial support may be required in order to obtain the baseline data.

Draft Implementation Plan and Pre-testing

Guidelines that are simply distributed to the end users without a formal strategy for their implementation are likely to be ineffective.[20] In the implementation of any CPGs, the ultimate goal is to ensure that the practice recommendations in the guidelines become part of the routine practice. Thus, designing a draft implementation plan assigning responsibility for each of the key steps, preferably with a timeline, and testing the feasibility and acceptance with the target users is of value.[15] The implementation team may consider circulating such a plan to key stakeholders for review prior to possible pre-testing.

The primary objectives of pre-testing are to verify that all issues have been considered, to identify any unexpected barriers and to assess the estimated impact on the current system and the perceived needs for change in the practice.[34] This provides confidence that all issues have been considered at the outset and that the guidelines indeed are applicable to the local practice. Sometimes, a barrier to change is simply the perception of the new recommendations as complex. The practical experience gained by pre-testing may ultimately assist in bringing about positive change in these perceptions.[23] Importantly, pre-testing should include data collection. A concise report based on such preliminary outcomes data may be of particular benefit if further resources or budget changes are required.[22] This will ultimately facilitate the implementation process and make the benefits more visible to stakeholders.[23]

The Implementation Plan

A detailed, specific implementation plan should follow the stakeholder review of the draft plan and pre-testing. All feedback and lessons learned at this stage should be carefully considered. Goals should be carefully constructed and they should bridge the differences between the current practice and the desired practice. Each goal should be accompanied by the strategies or methods to reach the goal, again preferably assigning responsibility. Timelines are essential and should be attached to all goals and key steps, which will facilitate progress monitoring.

It is also useful to identify parties essential to success and outline the components that are each party's responsibility. In addition, key organisational issues need to be considered in an implementation plan and efforts made to tying in to existing structures, processes and goals.[8]

Lack of specificity has been identified as a possible barrier to change. Hence, it follows that for implementation to be successful it is necessary that the plan is clear and everyone understands the goals and strategies.

Ideally, a budget should be attached to an implementation plan. It may be worth planning for sustainability from the outset, as the change is likely to continue past the current fiscal year and the project can stall or stop if not adequately resourced.[22] Data to support start-up, implementation and ongoing evaluation must be credible and persuasive to those who influence budget decisions.[22] Finally, the plan should include a section on monitoring, maintenance and reinforcement of change.

The resulting implementation plan should be a living document and should be updated as and when its core elements, such as the strategies and goals, require.

Communication

For any project to gain support and succeed, feedback and communication is vital. Ideally, all stakeholders should endorse the implementation plan and be kept informed of the progress, as this is important to sustain the process. Communication should be brief, relevant, easily accessible and preferably in a form familiar to the target audience.[12] For stakeholder buy-in, the focus of information should be on improving quality of patient care and how the guideline will help achieve this.[25]

Effective communication has been shown to be best achieved using existing communication systems.[12] This could be in the form of a newsletter, email, a Web site or a hotline. Meetings should be kept to an absolute minimum, as they require finding time in an already overloaded timetable and could be seen as an addition to an already heavy workload.

Education

Education and training are essential when implementing national guidelines at a local level. Interactive, targeted education interventions can be effective in developing practitioners' knowledge, skills and attitudes in relation to guideline recommendations.[8] It is important to understand the gap between current and intended roles and practices before designing individual training schedules. The degree of training required is dependent on the level of change required. Ideally, education can be integrated in a meaningful and professionally supportive way. In addition to the health care professionals, education and training should include support staff, as a lack of involvement on all levels may lead to delays and uneven implementation of the new practice guidelines.[25]

Raising the awareness of the guidelines in new staff members through induction programs can be a useful way to promote good practice.[35] Successful adoption is more likely if the intended adopters have sufficient training and support on task issues (e.g. fitting the changes into the daily work schedule).[23]

Monitoring and Collection of Outcomes Data

Guidelines that are simply distributed to the end users without regular review are likely to be ineffective.[20] Monitoring is essential to review progress against the established goals. Thus, any systematic approach to implementation of new CPGs and therefore changing professional practice should include plans to monitor and evaluate as well as to maintain and reinforce any change.[12] Different processes exist to monitor progress and outcomes. Identification of what needs to be measured and the means of capturing relevant data should be considered at an early stage in the planning process.[12] Simple user and target group surveys could be used, or more formal clinical audits may be performed. Audit and feedback are useful to measure adherence to guideline recommendations and may also provide a mechanism by which health care professionals can be made accountable for clinical implementation. Importantly, the process of audit will detect if aspects of the guidelines prove impracticable in local practice, and appropriate modifications can subsequently be made.[20] This importance of an audit to enable modifications or create new support systems should be emphasised. Audit results may be used as positive reinforcement if they are fed back in a constructive manner to participants.[8]

CONCLUSION

Whilst a guideline may be developed by experts, using a comprehensive and rigorous evidence base, it may still lack the necessary tools and recommendations to facilitate implementation. The guidelines selection and implementation process is fractured, and there is clearly a need for much attention to be given to the appropriate implementation strategies to accompany a guideline. Shortcomings exist in the appraisal of available guidelines and most lack a pilot test period prior to issuance. This suggests that the guidelines are being developed without their developers having the specific circumstances and problems of their implementation in mind.

This lack of pre-testing of CPGs by their developers prior to the dissemination of the guidelines may be a major reason why to date only limited evidence is available in the literature concerning those factors that are instrumental in achieving successful implementation of CPGs. The failure to pre-test may not be surprising as the mindset, skills, expertise and experience of developers of CPGs are often different than those who would implement CPGs in an organisation.

A successful facilitator of CPGs implementation is logically someone who is a project management, or change management, specialist or at a minimum has project management or change management skills, expertise and experience as well as the ability to be the 'translator' of the guidelines into daily clinical practice. Such specialists are not common in the primary care setting. If it is desired that CPGs be successfully implemented into primary care, the sector needs to have access to such specialists. In addition, in an ideal world, the teams of developers of CPGs would also include individuals who have the above-mentioned project or change management experience.

In light of the distinct lack of robust evidence concerning the delivery of CPGs into the primary sector, this chapter should be viewed as a presentation of recommendations and suggestions rather than as a definitive checklist for realising best practice in CPG delivery and translation. Our presentation of the subject has been based on a combination of not only the information available in the literature but the authors' own project and change management experience. Finally, it is hoped that this chapter will at least to a small extent assist in the ultimate implementation of CPGs and prevent them from becoming 'lost in translation'.

ACKNOWLEDGEMENTS

The authors wish to express their appreciation to Professor Patricia Price, Director Wound Healing Research Unit (WHRU), Cardiff University, Wales, for her review of this chapter and valuable comments. The authors also thank Professor Patricia Price and Elizabeth Mudge, Research Fellow WHRU, for their participation in the guidelines appraisal using the AGREE instrument.

REFERENCES

1. Engelgau MM, Venkat Narayan KM, Saaddine J, Vinicor F. Addressing the burden of diabetes in the 21st century: better care and primary prevention. *J Am Soc Nephrol* 2003;14:S88–S91.
2. Boulton AJM, Connor H, Cavanagh PR. *The Foot in Diabetes.* Chichester: Wiley; 2000.
3. Kenny C. Primary diabetes care: yesterday, today and tomorrow. *Pract Diabetes Int* 2004;21:65–68.
4. Lohr KN, Field MJ. A provisional instrument for assessing clinical practice guidelines. In: Field MJ, Lohr KN, eds. *Guidelines for Clinical Practice. From Development to Use.* Washington, DC: National Academy Press; 1992.
5. Davis DA, Taylor-Vaisey A. Translating guidelines into practice: a systematic review of theoretic concepts, practical experience and research evidence in the adoption of clinical practice guidelines. *Can Med Assoc J* 1997;157:408–416.
6. Woolf SH. Evidence-based medicine and practice guidelines – an overview. *Cancer Control* 2000;7:362–367.
7. Bedregal P, Ferlie E. Evidence based primary care? A multi-tier, multiple stakeholder perspective from Chile. *Int J Health Plan Manag* 2001;16:47–60.
8. Richens Y, Anderson EG, Rycroft-Malone J, Morrell C. Getting guidelines into practice: a literature review. *Nurs Stand* 2004;18:33–40.
9. Davis D, Evans M, Jadad A, *et al.* The case for knowledge translation: shortening the journey from evidence to effect. *BMJ* 2003;327:33–35.
10. Grol R, Wensing M. What drives change? Barriers to and incentives for achieving evidence-based practice. *Med J Aust* 2004;180:S57–S60.

11. DiCenso A, Virani T, Bajnok I, *et al.* A toolkit to facilitate the implementation of clinical practice guidelines in healthcare settings. *Hosp Q* 2002;5:55–60.

12. *Effective Health Care. Getting Evidence into Practice.* York: University of York; 1999.

13. Graham DI, Harrison MB, Brouwers M. Evaluating and adapting practice guidelines for local use: a conceptual framework. In: Pickering S, Thompson J, eds. *Clinical Governance in Practice.* London: Harcourt; 2001.

14. Cabana MD, Rand CS, Powe NR, *et al.* Why don't physicians follow clinical practice guidelines? A framework for improvement. *JAMA* 1999;282:1458–1465.

15. The AGREE Collaboration. Appraisal of guidelines for research and evaluation (AGREE) instrument. Available at: www.agreecollaboration.org, 2001. Accessed May 23, 2005.

16. NICE National Collaborating Centre for Primary Care. *Type 2 Diabetes Prevention and Management of Foot Problems.* National Institute for Clinical Excellence; 2004.

17. Scottish Intercollegiate Guidelines Network (SIGN). *Management of Diabetes.* Scottish Intercollegiate Guidelines Network; 2001. (SIGN Publication No. 55)

18. Hutchinson AMA, Cox S. Towards efficient guidelines: how to monitor guideline use in primary care. *Health Technol Assess* 2003;7:1–97.

19. New Zealand Guidelines Group. *Management of Type 2 Diabetes.* Wellington: New Zealand Guidelines Group; 2003.

20. International Working Group on the Diabetic Foot. *International Consensus on the Diabetic Foot*, Maastricht; 1999.

21. Newton J, Graham J, McLoughlin K, Moore A. Receptivity to change in a general medical practice. *Br J Manage* 2003;14:143–153.

22. Bradley E, Webster T, Baker D, *et al. Translating Research into Practice: Speeding the Adoption of Innovative Health Care Programs.* The Commonwealth Fund; 2004.

23. Greenhalgh T, Robert G, MacFarlane F, Bate P, Kyriakidou O. Diffusion of innovations in service organizations: systematic review and recommendations. *Milbank Q* 2004; 82:581–629.

24. Firth-Cozens J. Health promotion: changing behaviour toward evidence-based health care. *Qual Health Care* 1997;6:205–211.

25. Nicholas W, Farley DO, Vaiana ME, Cretin S. *Putting Practice Guidelines to Work in the Department of Defense Medical System: A Guide for Action.* Santa Monica, CA: RAND; 2001.

26. Foy R, Eccles M, Grimshaw J. Why does primary care need more implementation research? *Fam Pract* 2001;18:353–355.

27. Grol R, Grimshaw J. From best evidence to best practice: effective implementation of change in patients' care. *Lancet* 2003;362:1225–1230.

28. Ferlie E, Shortell S. Improving the quality of health care in the United Kingdom and in the United States: a framework for change. *Milbank Q* 2001;79:281–315.

29. Von Korff M, Gruman J, Scahefer J, Curry SJ, Wagner EH. Collaborative management of chronic illness. *Ann Intern Med* 1997;127:1097–1102.

30. Grol R. Personal paper. Beliefs and evidence in changing clinical practice. *BMJ* 1997;315:418–421.

31. Jackson R. Guidelines for clinical guidelines. *BMJ* 1998;317:427–428.

32. DeOreo P, Esbach J. Implementation of the anemia guidelines. *Can Med Assoc J* 1999;157:408–416.

33. Thomas L. Clinical practice guidelines. *Evidence Based Nurs* 1999;2:38–39.

34. Grol R, Dalhuijsen J, Thomas S, in 't Veld Cees, Rutten G, Mokkink H. Attributes of clinical guidelines that influence use of guidelines in general practice: observational study. *BMJ* 1998;317:858–861.

35. Xakellis G, Frantz R, Lewis A, Harvey P. Translating pressure ulcer guidelines into practice: it's harder than it sounds. *Adv Wound Skin Care* 2001;14:249–258.

36. Royal College of General Practitioners Clinical Guidelines Working Group. *The Development and Implementation of Clinical Guidelines.* London: Royal College of General Practitioners; 1995.

38 Practical Aspects of Establishing a Multidisciplinary Diabetic Foot Clinic

M. Edmonds and A. Foster

INTRODUCTION

When the diabetic foot clinic at King's College Hospital was set up in 1981, it led to a 50% reduction in major amputations and was able to prevent almost all major amputations of neuropathic feet.[1] With the onset of modern techniques to revascularise the ischaemic leg and active management of early infection, it was able to achieve a further 50% reduction in major amputations of the ischaemic foot.[2] In this chapter, we discuss both the setting up of this diabetic foot clinic and the manner in which the clinic has grown, changed and gradually evolved over many years.

The main thrust of the clinic has been to provide rapid multidisciplinary treatment to patients with active foot problems and then to follow them up to attempt to prevent recurrence. It has acted as a first-aid centre for patients who can attend in an emergency without an appointment. This is a crucial part of its role, as diabetic foot problems progress extremely quickly. Delays of a few days, and sometimes a few hours, cannot be accepted. The diabetic foot can deteriorate with alarming rapidity, and any delays can lead to the loss of a leg that could have been saved, or to the need for many months of treatment for ulcers and infections, or to the death of the patient. The clinic has also acted as a focal point for regular follow-up treatment of diabetic patients, who identify the diabetic foot clinic as a specific forum committed to the care of the foot. While the situation we describe is not, of course, the only way of organising care for patients with diabetic foot problems, the multidisciplinary, hospital-based diabetic foot clinic has proved to be a very successful way of reducing amputations and improving outcomes for diabetic patients with foot problems.

WHAT ARE THE AIMS OF A DIABETIC FOOT CLINIC?

The aims of the King's College Hospital diabetic foot clinic have been twofold: first, to provide the best possible multidisciplinary care for patients with foot problems, and secondly, to

The Foot in Diabetes, 4th Edition. Editors Andrew J.M. Boulton, Peter R. Cavanagh and Gerry Rayman.
© 2006 John Wiley & Sons, Ltd.

investigate the pathogenesis of these problems and to research new treatments. The natural history of the diabetic foot is to progress from the at-risk foot to ulceration and then to infection and necrosis. The aim is to intervene early and to prevent further progression by close attention to the wound, and to the microbiological, mechanical, vascular, metabolic and educational aspects of treatment. The specific aims are

- to provide good wound care including sharp debridement, dressings and advanced wound healing products;

- to diagnose infection early and treat it aggressively;

- to provide an efficient offloading service by the provision of footwear education, footwear, orthotics, braces and casts;

- to diagnose ischaemia early and to manage it aggressively;

- to encourage patients to achieve optimal metabolic control of hyperglycaemia, hypertension, hyperlipidaemia and encourage patients to cease smoking;

- to educate patients, their families, their friends and other health care professionals in ways of preventing and treating diabetic foot problems.

An important role of the diabetic foot clinic is to research into the pathogenesis and treatment of diabetic foot problems. Foot clinics should investigate new treatments. In order to carry out useful research, it may be necessary to link up with other diabetic foot clinics so as to carry out multicentre studies that are sufficiently powered to give meaningful results.

WHERE TO SITE THE DIABETIC FOOT CLINIC

The authors strongly believe that optimal management of the foot with problems is in the hospital-based diabetic foot clinic. It needs to be able to manage emergencies by having the capability to perform urgent investigations, carry out debridements, start immediate antibiotics, including parenteral antibiotics, organise rapid vascular and orthopaedic opinions and arrange emergency admissions. The clinic ideally should be open 5 days a week and be sited on the ground floor with easy wheelchair access. Arrangements should be made for diabetic foot emergencies, which present in the evenings or weekends to be seen in the emergency department.

The physician who started our diabetic foot clinic worked within a hospital with support from podiatrists, orthotists, surgeons and nurses, and it was therefore decided that the foot clinic should be based at the hospital. This prevented the need for extra staff-travelling time, avoided the necessity of expensive duplication of services such as X-ray, microbiology and other investigative methodologies and made it much easier for the team members to make extra visits to the clinic at short notice. Specimens could be delivered and reported on without delays. Investigations could be undertaken without necessitating yet another journey to a different site for the patient. Rapid admissions and support for very sick patients were quickly available, and as the clinic grew over the years and the proportion of patients who were ischaemic increased, this aspect of work of the clinic became very important. An established diabetic foot clinic will succeed in salvaging many diabetic feet in patients who will continue to attend the foot clinic for the rest of their lives, and will eventually suffer from peripheral vascular disease together with most or all the complications of diabetes. The diabetic foot clinic is a magnet for the most frail and complicated of diabetic patients. These patients, if they develop a diabetic foot infection, can become destabilised and very sick with alarming rapidity. Timely access to support services is thus essential.

WHAT IS A MULTIDISCIPLINARY DIABETIC FOOT CLINIC?

Establishing a multidisciplinary diabetic foot clinic involves the setting up of a clinical area where different members of the multidisciplinary team will work together within the same space at the same time. A podiatrist working in a separate room within a diabetic clinic is not the ideal diabetic foot clinic. A diabetic foot clinic is a place where patients can regularly be seen by multidisciplinary team members who work together regularly, at specific times, within the same clinic and usually within the same clinical room, and where multidisciplinary case conferences can be conducted.

In 1981, our first diabetic foot clinic was based within the podiatry room at our hospital, where a joint clinic was held on Thursday mornings with a physician, a podiatrist, an orthotist and a surgeon. It was born out of a desire of these professionals to work together on a regular basis. Subsequently, there was an ever-increasing number of new referrals and this resulted in the clinic being held, eventually, throughout the week. Now the podiatry room is an open layout room with five podiatry chairs where podiatric treatment and casting and multidisciplinary consultations are carried out. The open plan layout of the room is to accommodate relatives, who take part in the care of the patient, and visitors to the clinic, including community and hospital staff and students from all disciplines. The benefits of privacy and separate treatment cubicles must be weighed against the advantages of a large open plan room where patients and staff can gain valuable lessons from observation, and where it is easier for the multidisciplinary team to work together. In the presence of neuropathy and ischaemia, there is lack of usual signs and symptoms, and diagnosis is difficult. Thus, joint consultation between the disciplines is helpful. If a large, open plan approach is chosen, then this area can double up as an education room. The need for good infection control procedures is of key importance within the diabetic foot clinic. We have held separate clinics for patients known to have methicillin-resistant *Staphylococcus aureus* (MRSA) infection or other infections with resistant organisms.

In 1983, an investigations room was added to the diabetic foot clinic, to facilitate neurological and vascular investigations. It is now equipped with a neurothesiometer, thermal discrimination equipment and Doppler stethoscopes to measure ankle–brachial pressure index, toe–brachial pressure index and also an apparatus to measure transcutaneous oxygen. The investigations room also contains a small inner room for confidential discussions with patients and/or relatives.

The work of the diabetic foot clinic should not be confined to management of diabetic foot outpatients: it should also take part in the management of patients who are admitted as inpatients, working closely with staff on the ward. Ward staff may include a 'diabetic foot practitioner'. This is a new role, which overlaps aspects of the roles within podiatry, nursing and medicine, and the diabetic foot practitioner works closely with the physician and surgeon on the wards.

CLINICAL STAFF AND THEIR ROLES WITHIN THE DIABETIC FOOT CLINIC

In our diabetic foot clinic, we have established the following clinical roles for staff members:

- The *podiatrists* man the clinic's emergency service throughout the week, and undertake specialist wound care of ulcers, including debridement, plaster casting for indolent ulcers and Charcot osteoarthropathy. The podiatrists play a part in diagnosing problems, call in other members of the team, as appropriate, and also educate patients, their families and friends and other health care professionals. They also provide routine preventive foot care.

- The *physician* plays a key role in the diagnosis of foot complications and is also crucial in the diagnosis and management of infection, working closely with the medical microbiologists. The physician also decides on the need for admission and facilitates this admission, liaises with all members of the foot team and is responsible for the medical care of patients, including the management of diabetes and its complications.

- The *nurses* are also involved in ensuring optimal care of diabetes and its complications and also play an important role in the investigation of the ischaemic patient, using Doppler sonography and transcutaneous oxygen, and also in the assessment and management of the patient with neuropathy including those with painful neuropathy. The health care assistant prepares the dressing trolleys and also assists in addressing the ulcers.

- The *orthotists* measure and take casts for the manufacture of insoles, shoes, orthotics and braces; they also deliver footwear education to patients and staff. The orthotists carry out joint consultations in the podiatry rooms and then measure and cast the patients in the orthotists' rooms, which are adjacent to the foot clinic.

- An important role of the *surgeon* is to take part in joint consultation when the foot is infected and to decide on the need for incision and drainage, surgical debridement and digital or ray amputations. Historically, in our multidisciplinary team, the orthopaedic surgeon works with the neuropathic patients, and an important role is to assess their suitability for surgical treatment of osteomyelitis. The vascular surgeon works in conjunction with the interventional radiologist to assess those patients suitable for revascularisation of the ischaemic foot.

- The *diabetic foot practitioner* works closely with the physician and ward staff to ensure that all inpatients receive rapid and optimal treatment, that the feet are inspected on a daily basis so that deterioration or failure to progress are detected quickly, there are no delays in organising investigations, results are acted upon promptly and patients are discharged home, with a good care plan, as quickly as possible, for follow-up in the outpatient diabetic foot clinic.

- Other members of the team include the microbiologist, the physiotherapist, the rehabilitation physician and the psychiatrist, whose roles are very important but who often do not work within the foot clinic.

Many of the above roles have changed and developed over time, and some aspects of each role will vary according to the skills and interests of the individual. There may be areas of overlap, and it is important that all members of the team understand the roles of their colleagues and support them where necessary, so that patients and their families receive uniform messages. There is no room for interdisciplinary rivalries within the close team of the diabetic foot clinic.

SUPPORT STAFF

Diabetic foot clinics benefit from the presence of the following support staff, who have the following roles:

- The *receptionist* greets patients on arrival at the clinic, makes appointments, fields telephone calls and extracts and files notes safely and securely. There is a direct telephone line into the clinic to allow patients to seek immediate advice, in the form of a helpline.

- The *secretary* provides a secretarial and clerical service for the clinical staff, writing and posting letters and reports, organising clinical meetings and courses and contacting other hospital and community staff as necessary.

- The *managers* support the work of the diabetic foot clinic, maintaining its complement of personnel, and support the development of novel procedures and new approaches to the management of the diabetic foot.

- The *cleaner* ensures that the entire department, including clinics, offices, corridors, windows and recreational areas are kept clean and tidy according to local infection-control policies.

THE FOOT CLINIC TIMETABLE

It is not possible for the entire team to be working together throughout the entire week, as most people have additional responsibilities and commitments outside the area of diabetic foot disease. However, it is useful if all members of the team are accessible in emergency, in addition to having a formal commitment to work within the diabetic foot clinic with other team members at certain times.

The podiatrists should be based within the diabetic foot clinic throughout the entire working week, if at all possible, to maintain an emergency diabetic foot service, where 'walk-in' patients can be seen immediately.

The consultant physician in our team carries a pager so that he is accessible to give advice at all times. We do not think it is demeaning for a senior physician to carry a pager, and regard it as an essential practice for the diabetic foot physician to be contactable at all times during the working day. The physician also works within the diabetic foot clinic for specific sessions during the week, conducts two ward rounds per week and takes part in the joint vascular ward round.

A nursing presence is ideal, as many patients are elderly and ischaemic with multiple co-morbidities. They are prone to hypoglycaemic episodes of which they are often unaware and which require early diagnosis and intervention. We often treat infection with intramuscular antibiotics, initially administered in the clinic by the nurses and then given once daily at home by the community nurses.

The orthotists should work within the diabetic foot clinics for a regular period each week and should be available in emergency. They should keep a supply of shoes and devices so that no patient with a diabetic foot ulcer ever has to leave the clinic wearing the very pair of shoes that caused the ulcer.

The surgeons – both vascular and orthopaedic – should attend joint clinics eve[r]
possible. We have developed a joint vascular clinic that enables the team to org[anize]
vascular assessments including duplex angiography. A decision is made as to the suitability of
angioplasty, and this is now often performed as a day case procedure in the radiology department. A vascular radiology meeting attended by the diabetic foot clinic staff together with the
interventional radiologist, and vascular laboratory scientists and vascular surgeons, is held every week, where angiograms are reviewed and joint decisions are made. Following angioplasty,
the patients are followed up closely in the joint vascular clinic. The joint orthopaedic clinic,
which is currently held monthly, reviews patients with indolent neuropathic ulcers and acute
Charcot osteoarthropathy and considers whether surgical intervention might be beneficial.

It is important that there is continuity of care for the patient who is admitted from the diabetic
foot clinic. Thus, the consultant physician who works in the foot clinic is also responsible for
the care of the patients when they are admitted to the hospital. The diabetic foot practitioner
looks after the feet from day to day and is aided by the nurses from the clinic, who carry out
vascular investigations including transcutaneous oxygen measurements. All diabetic feet on
the ward should also be checked every day by a member of the diabetic foot team.

CONCLUSION

The pathology of the diabetic foot can be overwhelming. However, it is not an incurable condition and the outcome of treating diabetic foot problems is related to the amount of care that is
given. With the appropriate diligence and attention to detail, most legs can be saved. The diabetic
ischaemic foot does respond to treatment but does so very slowly, and it is important to have a diabetic foot clinic in which to monitor and look after these patients on a long-term basis. Reports
from Sweden,[3] Denmark,[4] Italy[5] and the Netherlands[6] have also shown a reduction in major amputations, and all four reports stressed the importance of a multidisciplinary service. Successful
management of the diabetic foot needs the expertise of a multidisciplinary foot care service.

REFERENCES

1. Edmonds ME, Blundell MP, Morris ME, Thomas EM, Cotton LT, Watkins PJ. Improved survival of
   the diabetic foot: the role of a specialized foot clinic (related articles). *Q J Med* 1986;60:763–771.
2. Edmonds M, Foster AVM. Reduction of major amputations in the diabetic ischemic foot: a strategy
   to 'take control' with conservative care as well as revascularisation. *VASA* 2001;58:6–14.
3. Larsson J, Apelqvist J, Agardh CD, Stenstrom A. Decreasing incidence of major amputation in diabetic
   patients: a consequence of a multidisciplinary foot care team approach? *Diabet Med* 1995; 12:770–776.
4. Holstein P, Ellitsgaard N, Olsen BB, Ellitsgaard V. Decreasing incidence of major amputations in
   people with diabetes. *Diabetologia* 2000;43:844–847.
5. Faglia E, Favales F, Aldeghi A, *et al*. Change in major amputation rate in a center dedicated to diabetic
   foot care during the 1980s: prognostic determinants for major amputation. *J Diabetes Complications*
   1998;12:96–102.
6. Van Houtum WH, Rauwerda JA, Ruwaard D, Schaper NC, Bakker K. Reduction in diabetes-related
   lower-extremity amputations in The Netherlands: 1991–2000. *Diabetes Care* 2004;27:1042–
   1046.

39 Practical Issues in Diabetes Foot Care: Podiatry – Linking Primary and Secondary Care

Neil Baker

The key to a successful diabetic foot care service is providing a structured and integrated multidisciplinary team operating seamlessly between primary and secondary care boundaries. Good and frequent communication, cooperation and an appreciation of the working environment, skills, knowledge and expertise of all team members forge strong links between all involved. Links need regular maintenance, as once broken they are difficult to repair and lead to weakness of service. This can be achieved by working to a common goal, providing practical tools for communication, flexibility of practice, debate and continuing professional education, underpinned by support, encouragement and recognition.

INTRODUCTION

The establishment of specialist multidisciplinary diabetic foot clinics in the early 1980s has had a significant impact upon reducing lower extremity amputations due to diabetic foot complications.[1-5] The models established by King's College Hospital and Manchester Royal Infirmary[1,3] have been adopted throughout many hospitals within the United Kingdom, with modifications according to local resources, staffing and service infrastructures. The presence of a podiatrist is a major consistent feature of virtually all multidisciplinary foot clinics. The skills, knowledge and expertise of a podiatrist play a major role in[1,3,6] helping to reduce lower limb amputation by effective foot ulceration management and improved hospital inpatient care.[7] This has resulted in the majority of attention, focus, service developments and research regarding podiatric diabetic foot care being centred within secondary care settings.[1,3,8] Additionally, this has been furthered by reported publications and conference presentations from the high-profile specialist secondary care foot teams extolling the role of podiatric practice within these clinics. This has certainly been a very positive achievement for the podiatry profession, as it has raised general awareness of some of the scope of podiatric practice.

However, the focus upon the more 'glamorous' hospital multidisciplinary team may have cast a shadow over the equally important role of the diabetic foot team functioning within

The Foot in Diabetes, 4th Edition. Editors Andrew J.M. Boulton, Peter R. Cavanagh and Gerry Rayman.
© 2006 John Wiley & Sons, Ltd.

primary care settings. Furthermore, it may have possibly even inadvertently stunted the development of the equally important role of diabetic podiatry within primary care. It is possible that this may account for some of the discrepancies in the community/hospital patient care interface. Rectifying this is important and perhaps publishing the achievements of existing successful models may be the first step in raising the profile of primary diabetic foot care and how it links with specialist hospital foot teams. Successfully managing the increasing burden of diabetic foot disease requires the establishment of unhindered foot care protection programmes that are evidence based, fully integrated and resourced, crossing all working environments in each locality. This is even more important in light of the evidence provided by several sources that describe care as erratic and of poor standard of supervision in patients discharged to primary care.[9] Similarly, others have reported suboptimal supervision of elderly patients in hospital, residential care and general practice.[10–12]

BACKGROUND – POTENTIAL FOR DISASTER

At present, around 1.8 million people in the United Kingdom have diagnosed diabetes,[13] and it is widely believed that a further 1 million are thought to have diabetes but are as yet undiagnosed.[14,15] With improving health care and social conditions the elderly population continues to grow and, as the prevalence of diabetes increases with age,[16] we are likely to see a steady rise in newly diagnosed type 2 diabetes. It has been shown that up to 26% of people with type 2 diabetes may have neuropathy at diagnosis[17]; additionally, arterial diseases are common in this group of patients; thus, the potential for foot ulceration complicated by neuropathy and ischaemia is high. Consequently, developing effective diabetic foot care services with integrated care pathways and rapid referral mechanisms and utilising the skills of podiatrists within primary and secondary care settings is of paramount importance if the burden of diabetic foot disease is to be reduced or even contained. Although the roles of podiatrists within these settings may be different, neither is more or less important than the other, and a clear understanding and mutual respect of these is essential to facilitate good team working.

ROLES AND SETTINGS

Firstly, it is important to briefly outline the differing roles and scope of practice within the two health care settings. Screening for ulceration risk, preventing recurrence, education, ulcer healing and amputation prevention are objectives that are generic to all, irrespective of work location, but are only truly effective when used in a structured framework of care.[18] Although differences may be clearly apparent, this must not be seen as one setting or scope of practice being more or less important than the other. When this does happen elitism rears its ugly head, causing disunity, derision, team breakdown and ultimately poor patient care.

PRIMARY CARE

The role of diabetes specialist podiatrists in primary care settings is diverse, involving many skills. The principal emphasis within this setting is focused upon risk identification, education, routine foot care, wound care, biomechanical therapies and ulcer prevention. Boulton stated that primary foot care in diabetic patients involves adequate monitoring and the opportunity to reinforce messages of self-care.[19] The important concept of this message is to empower patients to self-care following appropriate education. However, many diabetic patients are unable to perform foot monitoring because of poor eyesight and reduced mobility, thus making foot inspection difficult.[20,21] Thus, Edmonds states that regular contact between professionals and patients is important,[22] but involving carers and other allied professionals in this process is equally vital. The skills needed here to motivate, empower and educate patients, carers and colleagues cannot be understated and require time, effort and perseverance.

Annual foot screening undertaken by podiatrists may soon increase significantly due to the shift of diabetes care from secondary to primary care and the rising incidence of diabetes. Therefore, having direct and unhindered referral methods and pathways for identified high-risk, ulcerated, infected or acute Charcot patients is essential, supported by defined methods of communication. It is equally important not only to originate referrals but also to have capacity to receive referrals and initiate care swiftly.

SECONDARY CARE

The podiatric role within specialist foot clinics includes diagnosis, education, debridement, wound care, counselling, offloading skills and research.[23,24] Close liaisons with all members of the multidisciplinary team, including ward staff for admitted foot patients, forms an integral part of many specialist podiatrists' role. Certainly, some treatments such as radical debridement and casting are best placed here, where support is readily available.

One striking difference is that certain resources are more readily available, such as diagnostic imaging, microbiology and surgical opinion; however, this does not mean that these should not be available to specialist clinics within the community in the future.

Despite these apparent differences, shared and integrated care is essential, and although one can exist without the other it cannot function as well without it. Many of the skills mentioned above are common to podiatrists working in both settings and differing only in their level of skill, understanding and application. As previously stated, clear, swift and open routes that are supported by good exchange of relevant information for timely referral are essential. A review in 1996 found that the exchange of information between specialists, general practitioners (GPs) and patients following discharge to general practice was delayed and inadequate in content.[25]

Developing Links for Shared Care

Shared care has been defined as 'the joint participation of hospital consultants and general practitioners in the planned delivery of care for patients with a chronic condition, informed by enhanced information exchange over and above routine discharge and referral notices'.[26] This definition is equally applicable to diabetic podiatry, where the passage of new, healed, recurrent or infected foot ulcers, etc., takes place between different care settings. Successful shared care requires a team of dedicated individuals working together to a common set of goals, supported by well-defined pathways of care and communication, with a clear understanding and respect for each member's role.

FOOT CARE PROTECTION PATHWAYS

Several areas within the United Kingdom have initiated foot care pathways with structured screening and education[27,28]; however, these are not commonplace. The National Institute for Clinical Excellence in conjunction with the Royal College of General Practitioners Effective Clinical Practice Programme have put forward an evidence-based model for diabetic foot care service pathways – Clinical Guideline 10.[29] This model suggests clear pathways, referral criteria to all levels of care and key priorities for its implementation. Adopting such a model, supplemented with regular team meetings and clearly defined methods of communication, should not only improve diabetic foot care but also provide a framework for effective team working and continuing professional education. Involving the community podiatry service manager is absolutely essential in developing and linking community and hospital services.

COMMUNICATION

Good communication pathways are pivotal in achieving successful and effective clinical outcomes.

With so many different individuals involved in the care of a patient with a foot ulcer, it is inevitable that misunderstandings, confusion and personal treatment preferences are likely to occur. A lack of clarity regarding treatment rationale can lead to conflicts between and within professions' will; furthermore, the patients may lose confidence in their care providers.

Making sure that everyone in patient care is kept up to date is the key to effective and harmonious team working; however, this is not always easy. Information relating to changes or developments in the day-to-day management of foot ulcers is perhaps best achieved by telephone calls to those directly involved. Significant changes in patient care such as identifying uncontrolled hypertension, changes in risk status, and infection need to be conveyed in writing.

REFERRALS

Providing adequate and relevant information facilitates appropriate appointment allocation and makes patient clerking easier. To this end, locally developed and agreed standardised referral forms to all levels of care can be very useful. All new or discharged patients should have a summary of findings or events, with outcome recommendations sent to the referral source and patients' GP.

TELEPHONE FOOT 'HOT' LINE

Providing a dedicated telephone 'hot' line and fax facility is a valuable method of assuring quick referrals for urgent foot problems, dealing with treatment queries and for advice to colleagues and patients alike. When unmanned, an answer phone that is checked frequently throughout the day solves the dilemma of staff resources.

SATELLITE SPECIALIST CLINICS

Establishing satellite foot clinics within community settings that act as gatekeepers for those at high ulcer risk or with healed ulcers and for shared care patients with specialist foot clinics is invaluable and help maintain a seamless care service. Rotating staff between the specialist clinic and satellite clinics facilitates good education, skill attainments and more importantly team working. These also provide a training placement for junior staff.

PATIENT-HELD RECORDS

Using a simple patient-held record book may help provide effective communication links between all team members. It has several benefits, which include the following:

1. A treatment plan can be clearly laid out.

2. It allows all involved practitioners to input their activity and treatment rationale/goals.

3. Any alterations in the patients' treatment or condition can be recorded.

4. Patients become more involved in their own care, taking responsibility for the record book.

5. Patients are able to read about the care and the status of their condition.

There are some common problems associated with the use of patient-held record books, including forgetting or losing the record book, unmade entries, duplication of record keeping, use of unfamiliar terminology and of course illegible handwriting.

We have found that since the introduction of this modality to our practice, it has improved communication interfaces and patient care significantly. Surprisingly, patients now feel their care is incomplete if the record book is not completed at each visit.

TRAINING NEEDS, MENTORSHIP

One very effective way of promoting and strengthening links between and within foot care teams is to hold regular meetings that provide a forum for training, debate, research, audit and service issues. The formulation of a local diabetic foot specialist group can be used to disseminate information and provide support and encouragement. The more contact the team members have with each other in this type of situation, the greater will be the chance of forming good working partnerships. Establishing a local mentorship scheme if approached sensitively as part of continued professional development is also very helpful for all concerned.

Ideally, community podiatrists involved in foot care protection pathway teams should have regular rotation placements into hospital specialist foot clinics, and equally, it is a good idea for those working in secondary care to spend time working alongside the primary care team. This has the advantage of not only breaking down perceived barriers but also clarifying pathways of care.

It is imperative that there are sufficient health care professionals involved in all aspects and levels of diabetic foot care, who have appropriate knowledge, understanding, skills and expertise or can obtain these via structured education.[30]

REFERENCES

1. Edmonds ME, Blundell MP, Morris ME, Cotton LT, Watkins PI. Improved survival of the diabetic foot: the role of the specialised foot clinic. *Q J Med* 1986;60:763–771.
2. Apelquist J, Agardh CD. The association between clinical risk factors and outcome of diabetic foot ulcers. *Diabetes Res Clin Pract* 1992;18:43–45.
3. Thomson FJ, Veves A, Ashe H, *et al.* A team approach to diabetic foot care – The Manchester experience. *Foot* 1991;1:75–82.
4. Macfarlane RM, JeffcoateWJ. Factors contributing to the presentation of diabetic foot ulcers. *Diabet Med* 1997;14:867–870.
5. McCabe CJ, Stevenson RC, Dolan AM. Evaluation of a diabetic foot screening and protection program. *Diabet Med* 1998;15:520–523.
6. Murray HJ, Young MJ, Hollis S, Boulton AJM. The association between callus formation, high pressures and neuropathy in diabetic foot ulceration. *Diabet Med* 1996;13:979–982.
7. Rayman G, Murali-Krishnan STM, Baker N, Wareham A, Rayman A. Are we underestimating diabetes lower extremity amputation rates? Results and benefits of the first prospective study. *Diabetes Care* 2004;27:1892–1896.
8. Spraul M, Chantelau E, Schmid M. Education of the patient. The diabetic foot clinic: a team approach. In: Bakker K, Niewenhuijzen Kruseman AC, eds. *The Diabetic Foot*. Amsterdam: Excerpta Medica; 1991:150–159.
9. Dunn NR, Bough P. Standards of care of diabetic patients in a typical English community. *Br J Gen Pract* 1996;46:401–405.
10. Fletcher AK, Dolben J. A hospital survey of the care of elderly patients with diabetes mellitus. *Age Ageing* 1996;25:349–352.
11. Benbow SJ, Walsh A, Gill GV. Diabetes in institutionalised elderly people: a forgotten population? *BMJ* 1997;314:1868–1869.
12. Dornan TL, Peck GM, Dow JD, Tattershall RB. A community survey of diabetes n the elderly. *Diabet Med* 1992;9:860–865.
13. Morris AD, Boyle DI, MacAlpine R, *et al.* The diabetes audit and research in Tayside Scotland (DARTS) study: electronic record linkage to create a diabetes register. DARTS/MEMO Collaboration. *BMJ* Aug 30, 1997;315:524–528.
14. Forrest RD, Jackson CA, Yudkin JS. Glucose tolerance and hypertension in North London; The Islington Diabetes Survey. *Diabet Med* 1986;3:338–342.
15. Simmons D, Williams DRR, Powell MJ. The Coventry Diabetes Study: prevalence of diabetes and impaired glucose tolerance in Europids and Asians. *Q J Med* (*New Series*) 1991;81:1021–1030.
16. Jean Ho P, Turtle JR. Establishing the diagnosis. In: Finucane P, Sinclair AJ, eds. *Diabetes in Old Age*. Chichester: Wiley; 1995:69–91.
17. Young MJ, Boulton AJM, MacLeod AF, Williams DRR, Sonksen PH. A multi-centre study of the prevalence of diabetic peripheral neuropathy in the United Kingdom hospital clinic population. *Diabetologia* 1993;36:150–154.
18. Gadsby R, McInnes A. The at-risk foot: the role of the primary care team in achieving St Vincent targets for reducing amputation. *Diabet Med* 1998;15:S61–S64.
19. Boulton AJM, Gries FA, Jervell JA. Guidelines for the diagnosis and outpatient management of diabetic peripheral neuropathy. *Diabet Med* 1998;15:508–514.
20. Thomson FJ, Masson EA. Can elderly diabetic patients co-operate in routine foot-care? *Age Ageing* 1992;21:333–337.

21. Masson EA, Angle S, Roseman I, *et al.* Diabetic foot ulcers: do patients know how to protect themselves? *Pract Diabetes* 1989;6:22–25.
22. Edmonds ME, Boulton AJM, Buckeman T, *et al.* Report of the diabetic foot and amputation group. *Diabet Med* 1996;13:S27–S42.
23. Foster AVM. The role of the chiropodist in diabetic foot care. In: Bakker K, Niewenhuijzen Kruseman AC, eds. *The Diabetic Foot.* Amsterdam: Excerpta Medica; 1991:137–149.
24. McInnes AD. The role of the chiropodist. In: Boulton AJM, Connor H, Cavanagh PR, eds. *The Foot in Diabetes.* 2nd edn. Chichester: Wiley; 1994:77–91.
25. Hampson JP, Roberts RI, Morgan DA. Shared care: a review of the literature. *Fam Pract* 1996;13:264–279.
26. Hickman M, Drummond N, Grimshaw J. A taxonomy of shared care for chronic disease. *J Public Health* 1994;16:447–454.
27. Abbott C, Carrington AL, Ashe H, *et al* The North-West Diabetes Foot Care Study: incidence of, and risk factors for, new diabetic foot ulceration in a community-based cohort. *Diabet Med* 2002;19:377–384.
28. Middleton A, Young RJ, Webb F, Brown C, Chadwick P. An integrated, district wide team approach to diabetic foot care (letter). *Diabet Foot* 2000;3:124.
29. NICE Clinical Guideline 10. Type 2 diabetes – prevention and management of foot problems. Available at: www.nice.org.uk/CGO10NICEguideline2004.
30. Rayman G, Baker NR, Barnett S. Diabetes specialist podiatrists: time for recognition. *Diabet Foot* 2000;3:38–40.

40 Algorithms for Assessing Risks for Ulcerations and Amputations

David G. Armstrong, Stephanie C. Wu and Ryan C. Crews

Foot ulceration is one of the commonest precursors to lower extremity amputations among persons with diabetes.[1,2] Ulceration allows an avenue for infection[3] and can cause progressive tissue necrosis and poor wound healing, particularly in the presence of critical ischaemia. Foot ulcers therefore play a pivotal role in the causal pathway to lower extremity amputation.[4]

Diabetic foot ulceration is commonly associated with the presence of peripheral neuropathy and repetitive trauma from normal walking activities to areas of the foot exposed to moderate or high pressure and increased shear forces.[5] Foot deformities, limited joint mobility, partial foot amputations and other structural deformities often predispose diabetics with peripheral neuropathy to abnormal weight bearing, areas of concentrated pressure and abnormal shear forces that may significantly increase their risk of ulceration.[6-8] Brand[9] theorised that when these types of forces were applied to a discrete area over an extended period, they would cause a local inflammatory response, focal tissue ischaemia, tissue destruction and ulceration. Since most ulcerations are entirely avoidable, the concept of prevention takes on an entirely new urgency. Clearly, identification of persons at risk for ulceration is of central importance in any plan for amputation prevention and diabetes care.

In this chapter, we will discuss the key, evidence-based risk factors for diabetic foot ulceration as well as those for assessing amputation risk.

ASSESSING THE RISK FOR ULCERATION

Preventing foot complications begins with identifying those at risk. When screening to identify patients at risk for diabetic foot ulcers, there are three key words that can help identify ulcer risk[10] – history, numbness and deformity.

The Foot in Diabetes, 4th Edition. Editors Andrew J.M. Boulton, Peter R. Cavanagh and Gerry Rayman.
© 2006 John Wiley & Sons, Ltd.

History

Does the patient have a previous history of foot amputation, ulceration or Charcot arthropathy?

Clinicians should inquire about factors known to be associated with foot ulcers, such as previous foot ulceration, prior lower extremity amputation or the presence of neuropathic fractures,[10–12] as these risk factors heighten the risk for further ulceration, infection and subsequent amputation.[4,10,13] Following ulceration, the skin at that site is often less resilient and less well fortified to accept repetitive stress and therefore more prone to subsequent breakdown. Partial foot amputation changes the architecture of the foot and may therefore affect its intrinsic stability. Thus, persons with a partial foot amputation often develop local foot deformities secondary to biomechanical imbalances that may cause further foci of increased pressure.[14–16] Patients with a high-level amputation such as below or above the knee tend to be much more reliant on their remaining limb for transfer or ambulation and may therefore increase the risk for tissue breakdown. In general, people with a history of ulceration or amputation have all the risk factors to re-ulcerate. This is evidenced by the fact that up to six in ten persons with a history of ulceration will develop another one within 1 year of wound healing.[17,18]

Numbness

Is there loss of protective sensation?

Neuropathy is the major component of nearly all diabetic ulcerations.[19] Diabetic persons who have lost the gift of pain will wear a hole in their foot similar to the way we may wear a hole in our sock. Without loss of protective sensation, patients generally will not ulcerate. This is defined as a level of sensory loss that allows patients to injure themselves without recognising the injury. The consequent vulnerability to physical and thermal trauma increases the risk of foot ulceration sevenfold.[20] The absence of protective sensation may be determined by a number of means described elsewhere in this book. These methods include, but are not limited to, a Semmes–Weinstein log 5.07 (10–g) nylon monofilament, a calibrated vibration perception threshold (VPT) meter (biothesiometer) or a comprehensive physical examination.[12]

Deformity

Is there deformity or limited joint mobility?

The second causative factor in foot ulceration is excessive plantar pressure from foot deformities. Neuropathy and foot deformity, in combination with repetitive or constant stress, will ultimately lead to failure of the protective integument and ulceration. Characteristically, ulceration occurs at the site of highest plantar pressure.[5,6,21–23] Foot deformity may be defined as any contracture or prominence that cannot be manually reduced. Diabetic peripheral neuropathy may also affect motor nerves, often causing atrophy of intrinsic musculature of the hand and foot. When this occurs, the extrinsic musculature functions unopposed, thus causing hammering of the toes, anterior displacement of the fat pad and retrograde buckling of the metatarsal heads. This results in bony prominences of the metatarsal heads on the plantar aspect of the foot, and of the dorsal surface of the proximal interphalangeal joints of the toes, predisposing these areas to neuropathic ulceration.[24–26]

In addition, foot deformity is often accompanied by limited joint mobility secondary to the non-enzymatic glycosylation of periarticular soft tissues. Limitation of motion reduces the foot's ability to accommodate for ambulatory ground reactive force and, therefore, increases plantar pressures.[8,27–30] We have previously defined limited joint mobility as simply less than 50° of non-weight-bearing passive dorsiflexion of the hallux.[10,31] Glycosylation may also deleteriously affect the resiliency of the Achilles tendon, thereby functionally pulling the foot into plantar flexion. This leads to increased forefoot pressure (increasing risk for plantar ulceration) and, in some patients, may be a component of midfoot collapse and Charcot arthropathy.

Clinicians should therefore also examine the feet for structural abnormalities including hammer or claw toes, flat feet, bunions and calluses and reduced joint mobility, to help identify pressure points that are susceptible to future ulceration.

CUMULATIVE RISK

When the above three questions have been answered, one may then begin to assess degree of risk for ulceration. Lavery *et al.* reported that a patient with neuropathy but no deformity or history of ulcer or amputation has a 1.7 times greater risk for ulceration, compared with a patient without neuropathy.[10] Neuropathy with concomitant deformity or limited joint mobility yields a 12.1 times greater risk. Lastly, a patient with a history of previous ulceration or amputation has a 36.4 times greater risk for presenting with another ulcer. The assessment of these three risk questions correlates well with those promoted by the International Working Group on the Diabetic Foot[32] as well as by other authors.[33]

CONTRIBUTORY FACTORS

Clinicians should also examine the patient for other contributing risk factors. Footwear should be inspected to ensure proper fit. Among 699 persons with a foot ulcer, 21% of the foot ulcers were attributed to rubbing from footwear.[34] Cutaneous manifestations associated with diabetes such as dry or fissured skin, calluses, tinea or onychomycosis should also be noted. Persons with diabetes have a higher rate of onychomycosis and digital interspace tinea infections that can lead to skin disruption.[35,36] When present, the callused tissue (as with all callused tissues) should generally be debrided and inspected for the possible presence of underlying neuropathic ulceration or abscess. Failure to do this could lead to exacerbation of the condition by both covering up a potential fluid collection and further increasing plantar pressure.[19,37–42]

ASSESSMENT FOR AMPUTATION RISK

The three key risk factors for lower extremity amputation are ischaemia, infection and wound depth.[43] However, of these key factors, ischaemia is the only one that can, in and of itself, precipitate a primary amputation. The other two factors listed rely on a host of concomitant or preceding factors to develop. For instance, most ulcers are preceded by neuropathy, deformity and repetitive stress. In turn, most diabetic foot infections are preceded by an ulcer.

Is the Wound Ischaemic?

In general, vascular disease is not the commonest cause of foot ulceration, being a component factor in only about a quarter of all cases.[44,45] It is, however, a powerful risk factor for the *non-healing* of an ulcer once present, and therefore a risk factor for amputation.

Certainly, macrovascular disease is more common in the diabetic population. It has been reported that patients with peripheral arterial disease (PAD) and diabetes experience worse lower extremity function than those with PAD alone.[46] Commensurately, PAD is twice as common in persons with diabetes as in persons without diabetes[47] and is also a major risk factor for lower extremity amputation especially in patients with diabetes.[46]

The American Diabetes Association (ADA) consensus statement, the most comprehensive document on this issue, recommends that the initial assessment of PAD in patients with diabetes begins with a thorough medical history and physical examination.[46] A thorough walking history is especially important, as it will help elicit classic claudication symptoms and variations thereof; furthermore, patients should be asked specifically about these types of symptoms, as they are often not volunteered by people with diabetes.[46]

Vascular assessment should include palpation of all lower extremity pulses, including femoral, popliteal, posterior tibial and dorsalis pedis pulses. In addition, clinical evidence of dependent rubor, pallor on elevation, absence of hair growth, dystrophic toenails and cool, dry, fissured skin should also be noted, as they may be concomitant signs of vascular insufficiency.[46] Ankle–brachial pressure index (ABPI) is an easily reproducible and reasonably accurate method of diagnosing vascular insufficiency in the lower limbs but, as described in Chapter 20, cannot be used to exclude PAD, as it may be falsely elevated in those with vascular calcification.[46] Peripheral circulation may also be assessed by transcutaneous oxygen tension measurement, a non-invasive measurement of limb perfusion.[48] Patients with occlusive disease have significantly reduced transcutaneous oxygen tension, and this has been used to determine the possibility of ulcer healing and optimal amputation healing.

As discussed above, identification of ischaemia is of utmost importance when evaluating a wound. Ischaemic wounds were found to have a longer duration of healing, compared with neuropathic wounds without deformities.[49] If pulses are not palpable, or if a wound is sluggish to heal even in the face of appropriate offloading and local wound care, non-invasive vascular studies are warranted, followed by a prompt vascular surgery consultation and possible intervention to improve perfusion and thereby effect healing.

Is the Wound Infected?

The definition of wound infection is not an easy one. Although cultures, laboratory values and subjective symptoms are often helpful, the diagnosis of an infection's genesis and resolution has and continues to be a clinical one. While criteria for infection may be something less than clear-cut, there is little question that presence of infection is a prime cause of lower extremity morbidity and frequently eventuates into wet gangrene and subsequent amputation. Therefore, in an effort to facilitate communication and effect consistent results, the foot care team should agree on the criteria for this very important risk factor.

Depth of the Wound

When examining the wound, it is important to determine depth of the ulceration as well as the involvement of underlying structures. There is a possible contribution of depth to ulcer-healing times.[49] We have known for some time that wounds that penetrate to bone are frequently osteomyelitic.[50] Additionally, we have observed that morbid outcomes are intimately associated with progressive wound depth. Depth of the wound and involvement of underlying structures may best be appreciated through the use of a sterile blunt metallic probe. The instrument is gently inserted into the wound and the dimensions of the wound may be explored. Additionally, bony involvement is typically readily appreciable through this method.

A flowchart for screening and treatment of the diabetic foot is depicted in Figure 40.1. This algorithm is adapted from the University of Texas diabetic foot risk classification and the International Working Group on the Diabetic Foot risk classification systems. It is designed to comprehensively assess for risk of diabetic foot ulceration and amputation. The clinician begins by asking questions assessing for the risk of amputation (ischaemia, infection and ulceration). Subsequently, the clinician may ask questions related to ulcer risk (neuropathy, deformity, history of previous ulcer or amputation). While the specific classification system utilised is not overtly important, what is critical is to ask the key questions (some described above) and subsequently utilise consistent operational definitions during every workup. This, more than anything else, will drive consistency of care and ultimately a reduction in lower extremity complications in persons with diabetes.

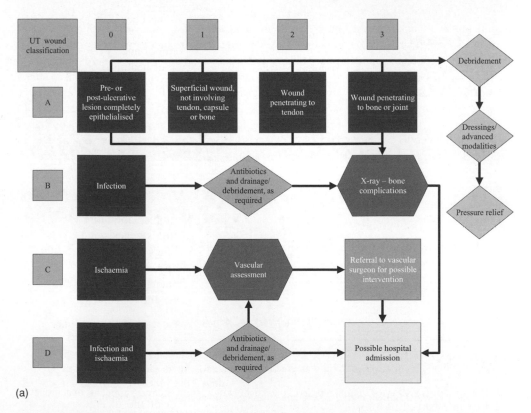

(a)

Figure 40.1 Sample algorithms for assessing (a) diabetic foot wounds and (b) generalised foot risk
Copyright © 2000, DG Armstrong. Modified for print by Andrew Findlow

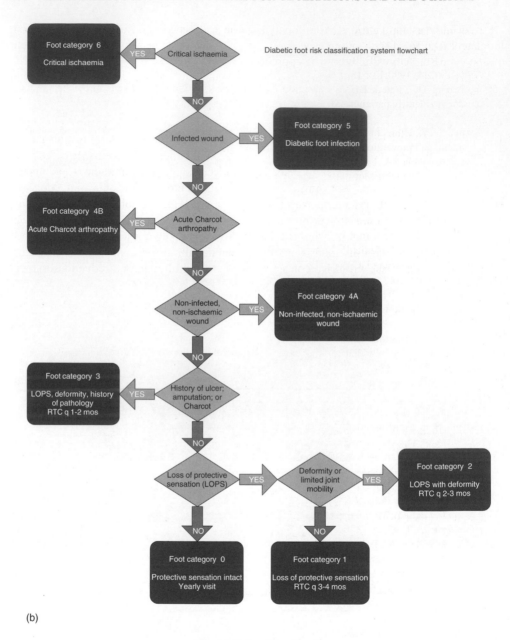

(b)

Figure 40.1 (*Continued*)

REFERENCES

1. Boulton AJM, Vileikyte L. Pathogenesis of diabetic foot ulceration and measurements of neuropathy. *Wounds* 2000;12:12B–18B.
2. Reiber GE, Smith DG, Carter J, *et al.* A comparison of diabetic foot ulcer patients managed in VHA and non-VHA settings. *J Rehabil Res Dev* May/Jun 2001;38:309–317.

3. Armstrong DG, Lipsky BA. Advances in the treatment of diabetic foot infections. *Diabetes Technol Ther* 2004;6:167–177.
4. Pecoraro RE, Reiber GE, Burgess EM. Pathways to diabetic limb amputation: basis for prevention. *Diabetes Care* 1990;13:513–521.
5. Armstrong DG, Peters EJ, Athanasiou KA, Lavery LA. Is there a critical level of plantar foot pressure to identify patients at risk for neuropathic foot ulceration? *J Foot Ankle Surg* 1998;37:303–307.
6. Cavanagh PR, Ulbrecht JS, Caputo GM. Biomechanical aspects of diabetic foot disease: aetiology, treatment, and prevention. *Diabet Med* 1996;13:S17–S22.
7. Lavery LA, Vela SA, Lavery DC, Quebedeaux TL. Reducing dynamic foot pressures in high-risk diabetic subjects with foot ulcerations. A comparison of treatments. *Diabetes Care* 1996;19:818–821.
8. Lavery LA, Lavery DC, Quebedeax-Farnham TL. Increased foot pressures after great toe amputation in diabetes. *Diabetes Care* 1995;18:1460–1462.
9. Brand PW. The diabetic foot. In: Ellenberg M, Rifkin H, eds. *Diabetes Mellitus, Theory and Practice.* 3rd edn. New York: Medical Examination Publishing; 1983:803–828.
10. Lavery LA, Armstrong DG, Vela SA, Quebedeaux TL, Fleischli JG. Practical criteria for screening patients at high risk for diabetic foot ulceration. *Arch Intern Med* 1998;158:158–162.
11. Boyko EJ, Ahroni JH, Stensel V, Forsberg RC, Davignon DR, Smith DG. A prospective study of risk factors for diabetic foot ulcer. The Seattle Diabetic Foot Study. *Diabetes Care* Jul 1999;22:1036–1042.
12. Abbott CA, Carrington AL, Ashe H, *et al.* The North-West Diabetes Foot Care Study: incidence of, and risk factors for, new diabetic foot ulceration in a community-based patient cohort. *Diabet Med* May 2002;19:377–384.
13. Goldner MG. The fate of the second leg in the diabetic amputee. *Diabetes* 1960;9:100–103.
14. Armstrong DG, Lavery LA, Vela SA, Quebedeaux TL, Fleischli JG. Choosing a practical screening instrument to identify patients at risk for diabetic foot ulceration. *Arch Intern Med* 1998;158:289–292.
15. Quebedeaux TL, Lavery LA, Lavery DC. The development of foot deformities and ulcers after great toe amputation in diabetes. *Diabetes Care* 1996;19:165–167.
16. Murdoch DP, Armstrong DG, Dacus JB, Laughlin TJ, Morgan CB, Lavery LA. The natural history of great toe amputations. *J Foot Ankle Surg* 1997;36:204–208.
17. Uccioli L, Faglia E, Monticone G, *et al.* Manufactured shoes in the prevention of diabetic foot ulcers. *Diabetes Care* 1995;18:1376–1378.
18. Helm PA, Walker SC, Pulliam GF. Recurrence of neuropathic ulcerations following healing in a total contact cast. *Arch Phys Med Rehabil* 1991;72:967–970.
19. Reiber GE, Vileikyte L, Boyko EJ, *et al.* Causal pathways for incident lower-extremity ulcers in patients with diabetes from two settings. *Diabetes Care* 1999;22:157–162.
20. Singh N, Armstrong DG, Lipsky BA. Preventing foot ulcers in persons with diabetes. *JAMA* (in press).
21. Boulton AJM. The importance of abnormal foot pressure and gait in causation of foot ulcers. In: Connor H, Boulton AJM, Ward JD, eds. *The Foot in Diabetes.* 1st edn. Chilchester: Wiley; 1987: 11–26.
22. Duckworth T, Betts RP, Franks CI, Burke J. The measurement of pressure under the foot. *Foot Ankle* 1982;3:130–141.
23. Birke JA, Novick A, Graham SL, Coleman WC, Brasseaux DM. Methods of treating plantar ulcers. *Phys Ther* Feb 1991;71:116–122.
24. Grant WP, Sullivan R, Sonenshine DE, *et al.* Electron microscopic investigation of the effects of diabetes mellitus on the Achilles tendon. *J Foot Ankle Surg* Jul/Aug 1997;36:272–278; discussion 330.

25. Rosenbloom AL, Silverstein JH, Lezotte DC, Riley WJ, Maclaren NK. Limited joint mobility in diabetes mellitus of childhood: natural history and relationship to growth impairment. *J Pediatr* Nov 1982;101:874–878.

26. Rosenbloom AL. Skeletal and joint manifestations of childhood diabetes. *Pediatr Clin North Am* 1984;31:569–589.

27. Birke JA, Franks D, Foto JG. First ray joint limitation, pressure, and ulceration of the first metatarsal head in diabetes mellitus. *Foot Ankle* 1995;16:277–284.

28. Frykberg RG, Lavery LA, Pham H, Harvey C, Harkless L, Veves A. Role of neuropathy and high foot pressures in diabetic foot ulceration (in process citation). *Diabetes Care* 1998;21:1714–1719.

29. Fernando DJS, Masson EA, Veves A, Boulton AJM. Relationship of limited joint mobility to abnormal foot pressures and diabetic foot ulceration. *Diabetes Care* 1991;14:8–11.

30. Armstrong DG, Stacpoole-Shea S, Nguyen HC, Harkless LB. Lengthening of the Achilles tendon in diabetic patients who are at high risk for ulceration of the foot. *J Bone Joint Surg Am* 1999;81A:535–538.

31. Birke J, Cornwall MA, Jackson M. Relationship between hallux limitus and ulceration of the great toe. *Sports Phys Ther J Orthop* 1988;10:172–176.

32. International Working Group on the Diabetic Foot. *International Consensus on the Diabetic Foot.* Maastricht: International Working Group on the Diabetic Foot; 1999.

33. Rith-Najarian S, Branchaud C, Beaulieu O, Gohdes D, Simonson G, Mazze R. Reducing lower-extremity amputations due to diabetes. Application of the staged diabetes management approach in a primary care setting. *J Fam Pract* Aug 1998;47:127–132.

34. Macfarlane RM, Jeffcoate WJ. Factors contributing to the presentation of diabetic foot ulcers. *Diabet Med* Oct 1997;14:867–870.

35. Altman MI, Altman KS. The podiatric assessment of the diabetic lower extremity: special considerations. *Wounds* 2000;12:64B–71B.

36. Boike AM, Hall JO. A practical guide for examining and treating the diabetic foot. *Cleve Clin J Med* Apr 2002;69:342–348.

37. Murray HJ, Young MJ, Hollis S, Boulton AJ. The association between callus formation, high pressures and neuropathy in diabetic foot ulceration. *Diabet Med* 1996;13:979–982.

38. Young MJ, Cavanagh PR, Thomas G, Johnson MM, Murray H, Boulton AJ. The effect of callus removal on dynamic plantar foot pressures in diabetic patients. *Diabet Med* 1992;9:55–57.

39. Pitei DL, Foster A, Edmonds M. The effect of regular callus removal on foot pressures. *J Foot Ankle Surg* 1999;38:251–255; discussion 306.

40. Collier JH, Brodbeck CA. Assessing the diabetic foot: plantar callus and pressure sensation. *Diabetes Educ* 1993;19:503–508.

41. Rosen RC, Davids MS, Bohanske LM, Lemont H. Hemorrhage into plantar callus and diabetes mellitus. *Cutis* 1985;35:339–341.

42. Ahroni JH, Boyko EJ, Forsberg RC. Clinical correlates of plantar pressure among diabetic veterans. *Diabetes Care* 1999;22:965–972.

43. Armstrong DG, Lavery LA, Harkless LB. Validation of a diabetic wound classification system. The contribution of depth, infection, and ischemia to risk of amputation (see comments). *Diabetes Care* 1998;21:855–859.

44. Edmonds ME. Experience in a multidisciplinary diabetic foot clinic. In: Connor H, Boulton AJM, Ward JD, eds. *The Foot in Diabetes.* Chichester: Wiley; 1987:121–131.

45. Thompson FJ, Veves A, Ashe H, *et al.* A team approach to diabetic foot care – the Manchester experience. *Foot* 1991;1:75–82.

46. American Diabetes Association. Peripheral arterial disease in people with diabetes. *Diabetes Care* Dec 2003;26:3333–3341.

47. Gregg EW, Sorlie P, Paulose-Ram R, *et al.* Prevalence of lower-extremity disease in the US adult population ≥40 years of age with and without diabetes: 1999–2000 national health and nutrition examination survey. *Diabetes Care* Jul 2004;277:1591–1597.
48. Franzeck UK, Talke P, Bernstein EF, Golbranson FL, Fronek A. Transcutaneous PO_2 measurements in health and peripheral arterial occlusive disease. *Surgery* 1982;91:156–163.
49. Armstrong DG, Peters EJ. Classification of wounds of the diabetic foot. 2001;1:233–238.
50. Grayson ML, Balaugh K, Levin E, Karchmer AW. Probing to bone in infected pedal ulcers. A clinical sign of underlying osteomyelitis in diabetic patients. *J Am Med Assoc* 1995;273:721–723.

Conclusions

Andrew J.M. Boulton, Peter R. Cavanagh and Gerry Rayman

This fourth edition of *The Foot in Diabetes* is almost twice as large as the previous one – a fact that is emblematic of the expansion of the field over the last 6 years. There has clearly been considerable progress in both research and practice since the third edition was published. The focus on foot complications during World Diabetes Day in 2005 and the simultaneous publication of a special edition of *The Lancet* devoted to the diabetic foot (Vol. 366, 12 November 2005) are landmark events that could hardly have been imagined as recently as the end of the twentieth century. The widespread publication, in many languages, of consensus documents by the International Working Group on the Diabetic Foot (http://www.diabetic-foot-consensus.com) has had an important impact on dissemination of the current knowledge base (Chapter 35 by Schaper and Bakker). But a close reading of the chapters written by our distinguished panel of authors indicates that there is still much to be learned before the field of diabetic foot complications can be said to have reached a high level of maturity.

There are beacons of progress (Chapter 8 by Robbins, Chapter 32 by Pedrosa, Boulton and Dias) that demonstrate that well-organised, multidisciplinary care (Chapter 9 by Donohoe, Powell and Tooke, Chapter 38 by Edmonds and Foster) can make a difference to outcomes and quality of life. But there is no evidence that the increased focus of attention on diabetic foot disease has made a consistent worldwide difference in improving such critical outcomes as faster ulcer-healing times or reduction in lower extremity amputations (Chapter 1 by LeMaster and Reiber, Chapter 2 by Chaturvedi). As with so many diseases, Third-World countries bear an excessive burden of diabetic foot complications (Chapter 33 by Viswanathan, Chapter 34 by Abbas and Archibald), and we are beginning to understand more about the role that ethnic and cultural factors can play in diabetic foot complications (Chapter 2 by Chaturvedi).

One of the most significant challenges is that re-ulceration occurs in about 60% of persons with prior ulcers (Chapter 1 by LeMaster and Reiber). Thus, although there are many new therapies to improve ulcer healing (Chapter 29 by Armstrong, Wu and Crews, Chapter 30 by van Schie and Ulbrecht, Chapter 31 by Armstrong and Boulton), new diagnostic modalities (Chapter 19 by Whitehouse) and much-improved surgical approaches (Chapter 21 by Simms, Chapter 23 by Salamon and Saltzman, Chapter 24 by Brodsky), the considerable economic and psychological burdens of diabetic foot pathology (Chapter 1 by LeMaster and Reiber, Chapter 11 by Vileikyte, Chapter 27 by van Ross and Carlsson) will continue to take their toll unless re-ulceration rates can be reduced. Therapeutic footwear must play a key role in this

The Foot in Diabetes, 4th Edition. Editors Andrew J.M. Boulton, Peter R. Cavanagh and Gerry Rayman.
© 2006 John Wiley & Sons, Ltd.

overall strategy (Chapter 28 by Cavanagh and Ulbrecht), but progress towards biomechanically sound, evidence-based footwear design and prescription has been glacially slow. Thanks to new techniques (Chapter 25 by Lavery and Murdoch), we now know more about the lack of patient adherence to recommendations designed to promote ulcer healing, and it appears likely that patients' poor understanding of the root cause of foot pathology may be a major factor in such behaviours (Chapter 11 by Vileikyte). Despite improved understanding, effective educational strategies to improve outcomes still remain elusive (Chapter 12 by Radford, Chipchase and Jeffcoate), and this area urgently demands further research.

In the United Kingdom, the much-anticipated Diabetes National Service Framework (http://www.nhs.uk/england/aboutTheNHS/nsf/diabetes.cmsx) seemed to all but ignore the *diabetic lower extremity and foot* (Chapter 10 by Gadsby), although the new general practitioner contract included a Quality and Outcomes Framework that systematically rewards foot examination. The NICE (National Institute of Health and Clinical Excellence; http://www.nice.org.uk/) guidelines go beyond examination for pulses and sensation and include the identification of foot *deformity* and examination of patients' footwear (Chapter 36 by Young). The guidelines also define an action plan based on the findings, but the provision of an infrastructure to enable implementation of the plan is still inadequate. Organisational change is as difficult in the health care field as it is in other areas (Chapter 37 by Heinrich and Clark), and the development of guidelines needs to be accompanied by a well-developed implementation plan and, always, a cheque!

There continue to be new challenges, such as the increased prevalence of methicillin-resistant *Staphylococcus aureus* (Chapter 13 by Lipsky and Berendt). Existing gaps in our knowledge, such as a need for clearer understanding of the aetiopathogenesis of Charcot neuroarthropathy (Chapter 22 by Jude), remain to be filled. Practice in some areas, such as wound debridement and dressings (Chapter 15 by Knowles), is still guided by past anecdotal experience rather than a strong evidence base.

This updated volume provides a broad sweep of current knowledge in the field of diabetic foot complications. It allows us to reflect on, and to celebrate, the successes that have occurred and to use the challenges that are identified herein to define a research agenda for the next several years. We are invigorated by the progress and energised by the challenges. It is our hope that you will find a reading of this volume similarly informative and rewarding, and we look forward to providing a fifth edition at some point in the future in which further evidence and progress can be reported.

Index